Radiology: A Practical Approach to Diagnostic Imaging

Radiology: A Practical Approach to Diagnostic Imaging

Edited by Coby Hawkins

hayle
medical

New York

Hayle Medical,
750 Third Avenue, 9th Floor,
New York, NY 10017, USA

Visit us on the World Wide Web at:
www.haylemedical.com

ISBN: 978-1-63241-584-4

Cataloging-in-Publication Data

Radiology : a practical approach to diagnostic imaging / edited by Coby Hawkins.
    p. cm.
Includes bibliographical references and index.
ISBN 978-1-63241-584-4
1. Diagnostic imaging. 2. Medical radiology. 3. Radiography, Medical.
4. Diagnosis, Radioscopic. I. Hawkins, Coby.
RC78.7.D53 R33 2019
616.075 4--dc23

Table of Contents

Permissions

List of Contributors

Index

Preface

Diagnostic imaging is the practice of creating visual representations of the interior of a body. It is done for assessing organ and tissue function and for designing medical interventions for the treatment of abnormalities and disorders. Some of the common imaging procedures include radiography, medical ultrasonography, magnetic resonance imaging (MRI) and X-ray computed tomography (CT). Such diagnostic techniques make use of X-rays, ultrasound, strong magnetic fields, radiopharmaceuticals, etc. Research in the application and interpretation of the medical images generated by diverse imaging techniques is covered under the field of radiology. The act of performing medical procedures with the guidance of imaging technologies is called interventional radiology. Most of the topics introduced in this book cover new techniques and applications of radiology. From theories to research to practical applications, case studies related to all contemporary topics of relevance to this field have been included in it. This book is appropriate for students seeking detailed information in this area as well as for experts and researchers.

This book is a comprehensive compilation of works of different researchers from varied parts of the world. It includes valuable experiences of the researchers with the sole objective of providing the readers (learners) with a proper knowledge of the concerned field. This book will be beneficial in evoking inspiration and enhancing the knowledge of the interested readers.

In the end, I would like to extend my heartiest thanks to the authors who worked with great determination on their chapters. I also appreciate the publisher's support in the course of the book. I would also like to deeply acknowledge my family who stood by me as a source of inspiration during the project.

Editor

Imaging the Facial Nerve: A Contemporary Review

Sachin Gupta,[1] Francine Mends,[2] Mari Hagiwara,[2]
Girish Fatterpekar,[2] and Pamela C. Roehm[1]

[1] Department of Otolaryngology, New York University School of Medicine, New York, NY 10016, USA
[2] Department of Radiology, New York University School of Medicine, New York, NY 10016, USA

Correspondence should be addressed to Pamela C. Roehm; pamela.roehm@nyumc.org

Academic Editor: Philippe Soyer

Imaging plays a critical role in the evaluation of a number of facial nerve disorders. The facial nerve has a complex anatomical course; thus, a thorough understanding of the course of the facial nerve is essential to localize the sites of pathology. Facial nerve dysfunction can occur from a variety of causes, which can often be identified on imaging. Computed tomography and magnetic resonance imaging are helpful for identifying bony facial canal and soft tissue abnormalities, respectively. Ultrasound of the facial nerve has been used to predict functional outcomes in patients with Bell's palsy. More recently, diffusion tensor tractography has appeared as a new modality which allows three-dimensional display of facial nerve fibers.

1. Introduction

Imaging plays an important role in the evaluation of facial nerve disorders. The facial nerve has a complex anatomical course, and dysfunction can be due to congenital, inflammatory, infectious, traumatic, and neoplastic etiologies. Computed tomography is useful for identifying bony abnormalities of the intratemporal facial nerve, which can occur with congenital malformations, trauma, and cholesteatoma. Magnetic resonance imaging (MRI) is useful for identifying soft tissue abnormalities around the facial nerve, as seen in inflammatory disorders, neoplasms, and hemifacial spasm. Facial nerve ultrasound has been used in a recent study to predict functional outcomes in Bell's palsy [1]. Diffusion tensor (DT) tractography, which uses MRI to make three-dimensional (3D) reconstructions of the facial nerve, has recently been developed. This technique has been shown to be potentially useful in the identification displacement of cranial nerve fibers by vestibular schwannomas [2]. In all cases, choice of the imaging modality utilized should be determined by specifics of the patient's symptoms and the differential diagnosis. In this paper we describe the development and anatomy of the facial nerve, then radiographic techniques used in facial nerve evaluation, and finally the pathologic entities that affect the facial nerve.

2. Development and Anatomy of the Facial Nerve

The facial nerve is composed of motor, sensory, and parasympathetic fibers. Complete separation of the facial and acoustic nerves and development of the nervus intermedius (or nerve of Wrisberg) occurs by 6 weeks of gestation. By the 16th week, the neural connections are completely developed. The bony facial canal develops until birth, enclosing the facial nerve in bone throughout its course except at the facial hiatus (the site of the geniculate ganglion) in the floor of the middle cranial fossa [3, 4]. The only difference between the anatomy of the facial nerve in infants compared with adults is in the region of the stylomastoid foramen. As the mastoid tip develops, the extratemporal facial nerve is positioned in a more inferior and medial position.

Facial motor fibers originate from cell bodies located in the precentral and postcentral gyri of the frontal motor cortex. These fibers travel in the posterior limb of the internal capsule inferiorly to the caudal pons. There, the motor fibers supplying the facial musculature beneath the brows cross the midline to reach the contralateral motor nucleus in the reticular formation of the lower pons (anterior to the fourth ventricle). The majority of motor fibers that supply the musculature of the forehead also cross the midline; however,

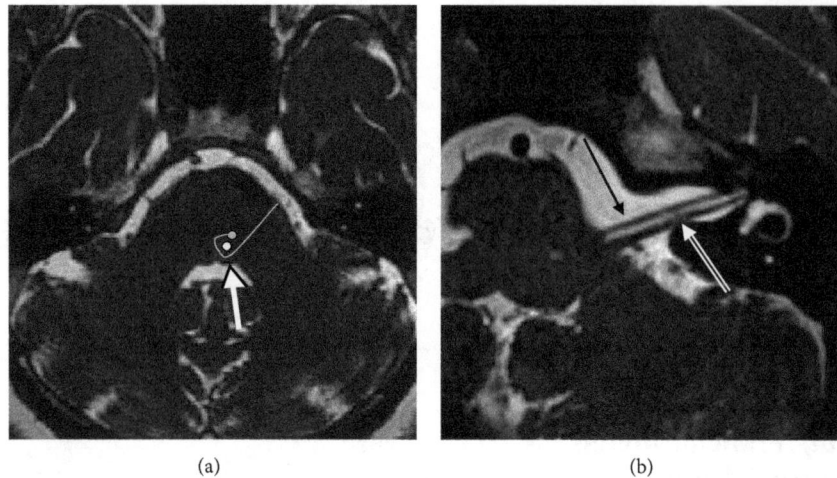

(a)   (b)

FIGURE 1: Normal facial nerve on MRI. (a) Axial CISS image at the level of the pons demonstrates the facial colliculus (arrow) seen as a small bump along the anterior wall of the fourth ventricle. This is formed by the motor tracts of the facial nerve (purple curved line) coursing around the abducens nucleus (yellow dot). (b) Axial CISS sequence of the left CPA and IAC demonstrates the normal cisternal and intracanalicular segments of the left CN VII (solid arrow), anterior to CN VIII (double lined arrow).

a few fibers do not, instead traveling in the ipsilateral motor nucleus. Thus, muscles of the forehead receive innervation from both sides of the motor cortex, and so forehead-sparing facial paralyses can be indicative of a central etiology. The motor fibers the pass dorsally, loop medial-to-lateral around the abducens nucleus, and create the facial colliculus, which bulges into the floor of the fourth ventricle (Figure 1). This loop of the facial nerve forms the internal genu of the facial nerve [5, 6].

The nervus intermedius contains sensory, special sensory and parasympathetic fibers. It provides sensation to the posterior concha and external auditory canal. The nervus intermedius' special sensory fibers supply taste sensation to the anterior two-thirds of the tongue. The afferent fibers synapse with cell bodies in the geniculate ganglion at the first genu of the facial nerve. These sensory afferents then join the parasympathetic fibers, passing via the nervus intermedius to the nucleus tractus solitarius in the medulla. The parasympathetic portion of the nervus intermedius originates in the superior salivatory nucleus in the dorsal pons and provides the secretomotor function of the ipsilateral lacrimal gland, submandibular glands, sublingual glands, and minor salivary glands.

Both the motor root of the facial nerve and the nervus intermedius leave the brainstem near the dorsal pons at the pontomedullary junction (the cisternal segment of the facial nerve). Within the cerebellopontine angle (CPA), the nerve travels anterolaterally into the porus acousticus of the internal auditory canal (IAC), anterior to the vestibulocochlear nerve (Figure 1(b)). This segment is 24 mm [7]. The nervus intermedius either joins the motor root as it emerges from the brainstem or near the meatus of the IAC [8]. The facial nerve runs in the anterior-superior quadrant of the IAC. At the lateral end of the IAC, a horizontal segment of bone (the transverse of falciform crest) separates the facial nerve from the cochlear nerve inferiorly. Within this area of the IAC,

a vertical segment of bone (Bill's bar) separates the facial nerve from the posteriorly located superior vestibular nerve.

The anterior inferior cerebellar artery (AICA) arises from the basilar artery near the junction of the pons and medulla. The AICA can have a variable course and territory. The AICA runs within the IAC and is frequently in proximity with the nerve within the IAC. In some cases, the AICA may run in the IAC between the facial and vestibulocochlear nerve [9]. The blood supply to this region of the facial nerve is the labyrinthine artery, a branch of AICA.

The bony facial nerve canal (or fallopian canal) begins as the facial nerve exits the IAC at the fundus. The major blood supply for the facial nerve proximally within the canal is the superficial petrosal artery, a branch of the middle meningeal artery. The stylomastoid artery supplies the fallopian canal distally [11]. The bony canal has three segments: labyrinthine, tympanic, and mastoid (Figures 2 and 3). The labyrinthine segment runs from the fundus of the IAC to the geniculate ganglion. It is both the narrowest (<0.7 mm diameter) and shortest (3–5 mm length) segment of the facial nerve. The labyrinthine segment travels anterior-laterally from the IAC and superior to the cochlea until it reaches the geniculate ganglion.

While the geniculate ganglion is typically covered by bone, in up to 18% of cases the ganglion is in direct contact with the dura of the middle cranial fossa [8]. The first branch of the facial nerve, the greater superficial petrosal nerve (GSPN), exits anteriorly from the geniculate ganglion. The GSPN carries preganglionic parasympathetic fibers from the superior salivatory nucleus, and runs along the anterior surface of the temporal bone into the pterygoid canal (Vidian canal). It synapses at the pterygopalatine ganglion in the pterygopalatine fossa. Postganglionic parasympathetic fibers then join the maxillary nerve to innervate the lacrimal gland and small salivary glands in the nose and palate. At the geniculate ganglion, the facial nerve makes a 75 degree turn

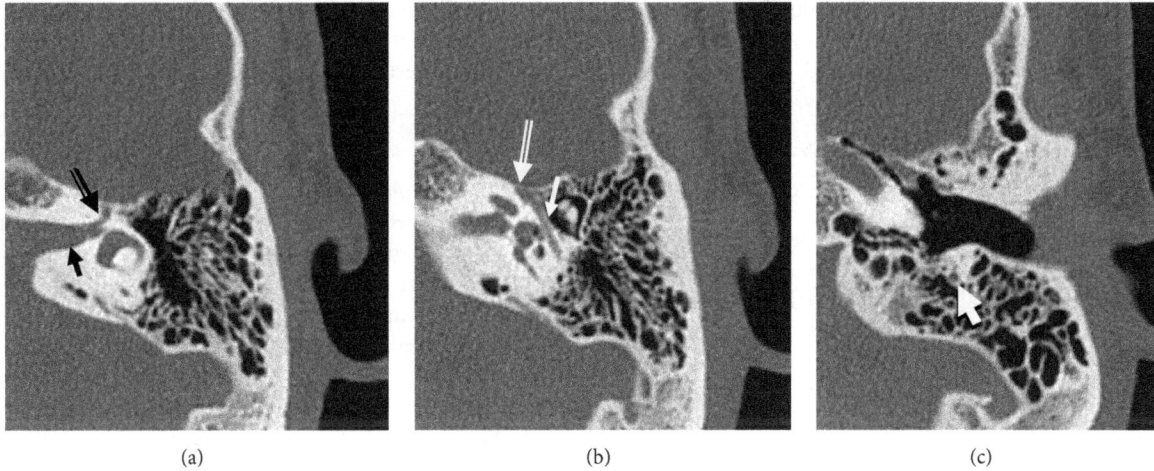

(a)　　　　　　　　　　(b)　　　　　　　　　　(c)

Figure 2: Normal facial nerve canal on CT. Axial temporal bone CT images demonstrate the intracanalicular (solid arrow in (a)), labyrinthine (double lined arrow in (a)), geniculate ganglion (double lined arrow in (b)), tympanic (solid arrow in (b)), and mastoid (arrow in (c)) segments of the facial nerve.

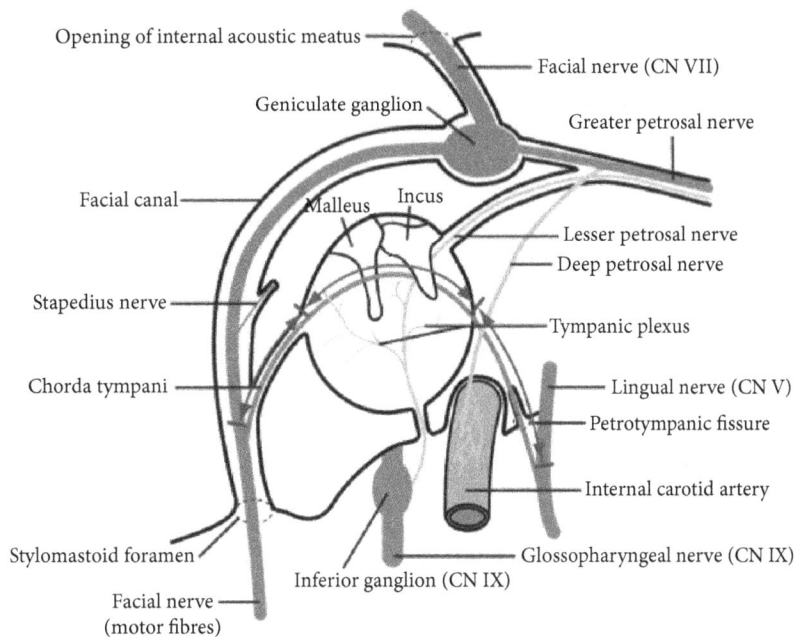

Figure 3: Diagram of the course of the intratemporal facial nerve from the fundus of the IAC to the stylomastoid foramen [10].

posteriorly to become the tympanic segment (the first or anterior genu).

The tympanic segment runs from the geniculate ganglion to the second (or posterior) genu [12]. Within the tympanic cavity, the facial nerve passes medial to the incus. It runs posterior-superior to the cochleariform process, superior and lateral to the oval window, and then inferior to the lateral semicircular canal. Bony dehiscence of the facial nerve canal is seen in 41–75% of people within this segment [4, 11, 12]. At the pyramidal process, the tympanic segment turns inferiorly at a 95°–125° angle (at the second genu) to become the mastoid or vertical segment [12].

The mastoid segment of the facial nerve runs postero-medially along the external auditory canal to its exit from the temporal bone at the stylomastoid foramen (13 mm in adults) [12]. Two branches arise from the mastoid segment: the nerve to the stapedius and the chorda tympani (Figure 3). The stylomastoid foramen arises between the styloid process anteriorly and the mastoid process posteriorly. The nerve exits the temporal bone at the stylomastoid foramen, entering the substance of the parotid gland.

Extratemporally, the facial nerve separates into two main branches at the pes anserinus: the temporofacial branch and the cervicofacial branch. Within the parotid gland, these branches further divide into five main branches that supply the facial musculature: temporal (or frontal), zygomatic, buccal, marginal mandibular, and cervical.

3. Imaging Techniques for the Evaluation of the Facial Nerve

Imaging of the facial nerve should be tailored to both the suspected pathology and clinical localization of the lesion along the nerve's course. Typically, if a facial palsy is localized to the cisternal or intracanalicular segments of the facial nerve or the pontine nuclei, contrast-enhanced MRI is indicated. If the lesion can be localized to the mastoid, tympanic, or labyrinthine segments of the facial nerve, high-resolution temporal bone CT is recommended to evaluate the fallopian canal. Contrast-enhanced MRI should be performed first in cases when the palsy cannot be definitively localized. Both MRI and temporal bone CT are typically performed for the evaluation of tumors involving the facial nerve.

3.1. CT. CT is preferable for imaging the lateral course of the facial nerve from the porus acusticus to the stylomastoid foramen. CT evaluation of the facial nerve lateral to the porus acusticus should include high-resolution temporal bone CT. Temporal bone CT is particularly useful in the evaluation of the caliber and the course of the IAC and bony facial nerve canal in the temporal bone. Erosion and destruction of the facial nerve canal are best depicted with high-resolution temporal bone CT. In addition, CT has the advantage of demonstrating the relationship of the facial nerve canal to normal anatomic landmarks such as the ossicles which are not seen on MR. These relationships are critical during surgical planning. At our institution, we acquire noncontrast 0.3 mm axial slices through the bilateral temporal bones for our raw data, with 0.6 mm thick axial, coronal, and Pöschl reformats through the individual temporal bones. Dose settings are typically 120 kVp, CTDI volume 55.5—62.6, and 140–220 mAs. Administration of intravenous contrast is not part of the standard protocol but may be included if there is a clinical suspicion of a neoplasm or vascular abnormality.

Temporal bone CT can detect deviations in the course and caliber of the intratemporal facial nerve, which can provide key information regarding facial nerve pathology and prove critical in surgical planning for otologic surgery. Bony dehiscences of the fallopian canal can be identified preoperatively, leading to a decreased rate of iatrogenic facial nerve trauma. In cases of aural atresia, the facial nerve can vary in its course, making it more susceptible to injury during atresiaplasty and limiting the diameter of the reconstructed external auditory canal [13]. High-resolution temporal bone CT can also identify temporal bone fractures that violate the facial nerve canal. Using 16- or 64-slice CT, helical mode acquisition, 0.6 mm slice thickness, and 0.3 mm reconstruction increments, Mu et al. [14] found a significant correlation between findings of increased transverse geniculate ganglion diameter on CT and intraoperative identification of fractures involving the geniculate ganglion ($P < 0.001$). All patients with an enlarged geniculate ganglion fossa (transverse diameter 1.9 ± 0.3 mm)

were found to have geniculate ganglion fossa fractures during surgical exploration. Two of these patients did not have visible temporal bone fractures on high-resolution temporal bone CT.

3.2. MRI. When using CT to evaluate the facial nerve, pathology often can only be inferred by visualization of erosion or destruction of the adjacent bony facial nerve canal. In contrast, MRI visualizes soft tissues well and so is better suited for evaluating soft tissue facial nerve abnormalities. MRI can be used to image the facial nerve from the brainstem to the fundus of the internal auditory canal and to determine the presence of perineural spread from parotid malignancies (Figure 9). At our institution, standard MRI imaging for evaluation of the facial nerve and inner ear pathology includes an IAC protocol with the following sequences: a noncontrast axial 5 mm whole brain T2-weighted sequence; an axial 3 mm, T1-weighted sequence of the IAC angled perpendicular to dorsal aspect of the brainstem; an axial constructive interference in the steady-state (CISS) sequence (heavily T2-weighted sequence, 0.6 mm) from the occipital bone to superior petrous ridge; axial 5 mm whole brain postcontrast FLAIR and T1-weighted sequences; a coronal 4 mm postcontrast T1-weighted sequence of the IAC; and an axial 3 mm T1-weighted fat-saturated sequence of the IAC.

In high-resolution T2-weighted images or CISS images, the normal facial nerve appears as a hypointense linear structure extending from the brainstem to the IAC, anterior to the vestibulocochlear nerve, surrounded by T2 hyperintense cerebrospinal fluid (Figure 1). The labyrinthine, tympanic, and mastoid segments of the facial nerve are not typically well visualized in noncontrast images. The proximal extracranial portion of the facial nerve in the parotid gland is best visualized with axial high-resolution T1-weighted images using a microscopic coil.

When gadolinium contrast is used, the normal facial nerve faintly enhances in the geniculate ganglion, tympanic, and mastoid segments (Figure 10) [7]. The cisternal, intracanalicular, labyrinthine, and parotid segments of the facial nerve do not normally enhance. Enhancement of the facial nerve in these regions raises suspicion of inflammatory or neoplastic processes. Asymmetric enhancement and/or thickening of the tympanic mastoid segments relative to the contralateral side should also be considered abnormal. For instance, in Bell's palsy, MRI with gadolinium contrast often demonstrates enhancement of the intracanalicular and labyrinthine segments of the facial nerve, as well as a greater degree of enhancement of the geniculate ganglion, tympanic, and mastoid segments (Figure 4) [7].

MRI can also reveal enlargement of the facial nerve, as may be seen in a neoplastic process. Particularly in the areas outside of the bony fallopian canal, this enlargement can be missed in high-resolution temporal bone CT. Facial nerve schwannomas may appear as fusiform masses in the labyrinthine and mastoid segments. In the cisternal, intracanalicular, and tympanic segments, schwannomas can appear lobulated (Figure 11). These lesions show strong enhancement with gadolinium on T1-weighted images. On

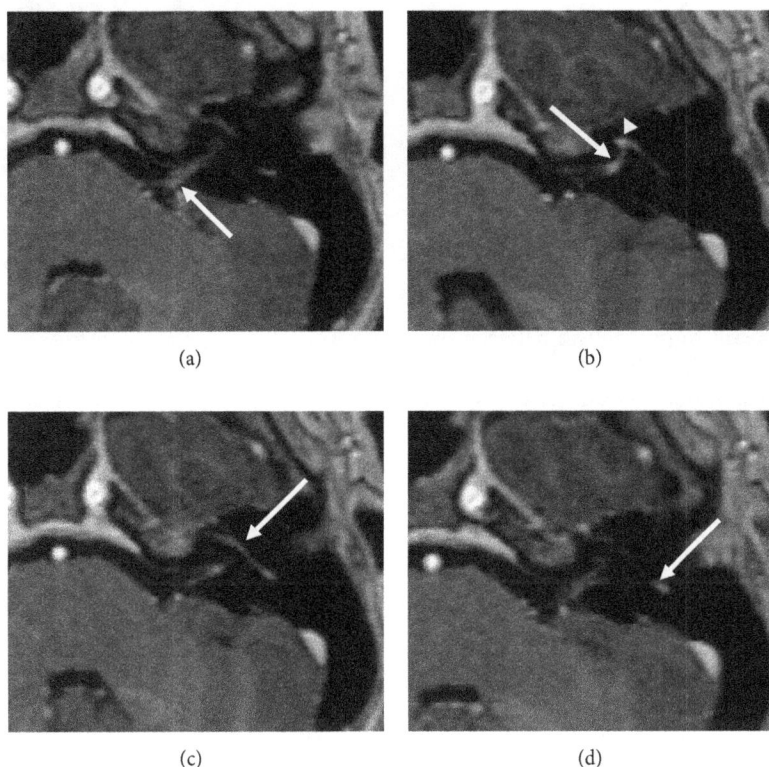

(a)

(b)

(c)

(d)

FIGURE 4: Bell's palsy. T1- weighted contrast-enhanced MR images demonstrate abnormal enhancement of the distal left cisternal (arrow, (a)), labyrinthine (arrow, (b)), first genu (arrowhead, (b)), and mastoid (arrow, (d)) segment of the facial nerve. Enhancement of the first genu, tympanic and mastoid segments was asymmetrically greater than the normal contralateral side (not shown).

CISS images, facial schwannomas will appear as nodular lesions along the nerve within the CPA or IAC. When large enough, they can fill the diameter of the internal auditory canal and may be difficult to differentiate from schwannomas of the vestibulocochlear nerve (Figure 11) [8].

MRI characteristics can be used to distinguish masses around the facial nerve that require surgical excision from those that should not be surgically removed until facial function has been affected. For instance, lipomas of the internal auditory canal and first genu will appear hyperintense on T1-weighted imaging without additional gadolinium and can be reliably identified with T1-weighted imaging with fat saturation (Figure 12). Hemangiomas of the facial nerve typically occur at the geniculate ganglion and show avid contrast enhancement. Surgical removal of lipomas or hemangiomas often results in facial paralysis and so is typically only performed when preoperative facial function is poor [15, 16]. In contrast, cholesteatomas in the petrous apex classically appear hypointense on T1, hyperintense on T2, and show no or little contrast enhancement. Further confirmation of presence of cholesteatoma can be made with diffusion-weighted imaging, which reveals significantly decreased diffusion within the lesion (Figure 13) [17]. Cholesteatomas should be surgically removed when identified to avoid future decrease in facial function as they increase in size [18].

Reconstructed sagittal oblique CISS images through the internal auditory canals obtained perpendicular to the course of the IAC enable the evaluation of the caliber of the facial nerve. In patients with Moebius syndrome, CISS imaging is particularly useful in confirming the absence or small caliber of the facial nerve within the CPA and IAC (Figure 14).

For patients with hemifacial spasm, a loop of the anterior inferior cerebellar artery, posterior inferior cerebellar artery, or vertebral artery compresses the ipsilateral facial nerve at the root exit zone, leading to involuntary contractions of the facial musculature. High-resolution T2-weighted or CISS images can directly visualize the vascular loop and compressed facial nerve (Figure 15).

3.3. Ultrasound. In a recent study, ultrasound has been utilized to predict facial nerve outcomes in Bell's palsy. In this prospective, controlled study, patients with Bell's palsy, ultrasound was performed 2–7 days after the onset of paralysis using a General Electric Logiq 7 Pro with a 5 to 10 MHz linear array transducer [1]. Facial nerve diameter was measured proximally at the stylomastoid foramen, distally just proximal to the pes anserinus, and midway between these two points. The average diameter of the facial nerve was calculated using these three measurements and then compared with blink reflex studies and nerve conduction studies. A normal ultrasound measurement on the affected side had a 100% positive predictive value for normal facial function recovery at 3 months, a value significantly higher than values for nerve conduction (72–80%) and blink reflex studies (90%). Abnormal facial nerve ultrasound had a negative predictive value of 77% of House-Brackmann Grade II or worse facial nerve function at 3 months. This was again higher than that of nerve conduction studies (25–35%) and blink reflex studies (33%).

3.4. Diffusion Tensor Tractography. In cases of large vestibular schwannomas, it can be difficult to distinguish between the facial nerve and the tumor on MRI. Both the facial nerve and the schwannoma have similar signal intensities, and larger tumors cause thinning of the facial nerve, making the nerve even more difficult to identify. Additionally, there is typically no intervening cerebrospinal fluid between the schwannoma and the facial nerve [2]. In these cases, diffusion tensor (DT) tractography may be useful for assessing facial nerve course and displacement. Taoka et al. [2] evaluated the accuracy of facial nerve DT tractography in 8 patients using a 1.5 Tesla scanner and a single-shot echo-planar sequence. Tracts of the facial nerve were determined from the pons to the internal auditory meatus using the DT images and compared with the facial nerve course visualized on high-resolution, heavily T2-weighted sequence of the brainstem. Tractography images were also compared with the facial nerve course observed intraoperatively. In 7 of 8 patients with tumors greater than 20 mm in size and whose facial nerves were indistinguishable from tumor on conventional imaging, DT tractography successfully visualized the facial nerve from the pons to the internal auditory meatus [2].

Chen et al. [19] used a 3 Tesla scanner to obtain 3-dimensional (3D) visualization of the facial nerve in patients with vestibular schwannoma. DT images were acquired with an echo-planar/spin-echo sequence, and T1 anatomic axial images were used to construct a 3D tumor model. Detailed anatomy of the fibers was better visualized in larger tumors, with small fibers seen coursing inferior to the tumor from the porus acusticus to the brainstem. For the smallest tumor, the VII/VIII complex was visualized at the porus, but the cisternal segment of the facial nerve could not be seen with as much detail. However, the authors' ability to distinguish between cranial nerves VII and VIII was limited due to their proximity and similar size.

Overall, DT tractography shows potential in evaluation of the course of the facial nerve, particularly in cases involving large vestibular schwannomas. Currently, this technique is computationally intensive and not automated, typically requiring intensive involvement of Ph.D. level personnel in the construction of these images. Further technological advancements in sensitivity and automation of the technique will likely lead to its greater clinical use.

4. Disorders of the Facial Nerve

The facial nerve can be affected by a number of different disorders resulting in weakness or paralysis of the facial

TABLE 1: Disorders of the facial nerve.

Infectious	Acute OM
	Chronic OM
	Cholesteatoma
	Herpes zoster oticus
	Lyme disease
Traumatic	Temporal bone fracture
	Iatrogenic injury
	Avulsion at brainstem
	Penetrating trauma
Neoplastic	Facial schwannoma
	Vestibular schwannoma
	Hemangioma
	Lipoma
	Glomus tumors
	Malignancy of skin/parotid
Congenital	Moebius syndrome
	Displacement (atresia)
	Aural atresia
	CHARGE syndrome
	Dehiscence of FC
Vascular	MCA infarct
	Pontine artery infarct
	Lacunar infarct
Idiopathic	Bell's palsy
	Multiple sclerosis
	Sarcoidosis
Inflammatory	Guillain-Barre

OM: otitis media; FC: fallopian canal; and MCA: middle cerebral artery.

musculature (Table 1). One of the critical steps in the clinical evaluation of facial paralysis is discerning whether a central nervous system process (cerebrovascular accident, brain tumor, and multiple sclerosis) or peripheral disease (Bell's palsy, middle ear infection/cholesteatoma, and facial nerve tumor) is the cause of the weakness. Due to the bilateral innervation of the forehead musculature, forehead-sparing facial paralyses suggest a central pathology. Many of the common causes of peripheral facial paralysis (Bell's palsy, chronic ear disease, cholesteatoma, and schwannomas) affect the distal branches of the ipsilateral facial nerve equally. In contrast, malignancies of the parotid and other structures lateral to the mastoid tip may cause paralysis of only one or a few of the distal branches of the facial nerve. Paralysis caused by tumors may be preceded by facial twitching. Timing of paralysis with respect to rapidity of onset, patient age at onset, and associated symptoms can also narrow the differential diagnosis. These clinical insights guide further evaluation, including the choice of imaging modality.

Facial dystonias and hyperkinetic states (hemifacial spasm, essential blepharospasm, and Meige's syndrome) can also occur. All of these pathologies are discussed in detail below.

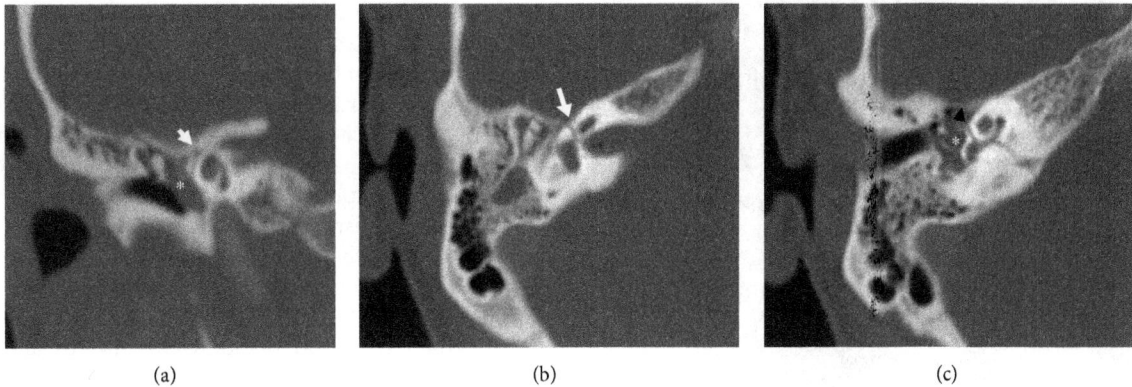

(a) (b) (c)

FIGURE 5: Transverse temporal bone fracture. Coronal (a) and axial (b) CT images demonstrate a transverse fracture through the labyrinthine segment of facial nerve canal (arrows). Axial CT image (c) shows the fracture involving the otic capsule and basal turn of the cochlea (arrowhead). Note blood products in the middle ear cavity (asterisks).

4.1. Idiopathic Facial Paralysis. The most common cause of facial paralysis, Bell's palsy, is characterized by the sudden onset of facial weakness. It has been associated with the reactivation of herpes simplex type 1 in the geniculate ganglion, leading to inflammatory edema of the facial nerve [20]. Imaging studies are not typically indicated in the early evaluation of this disorder. However, within the first month of onset of paralysis, MRI of the brain and brainstem with gadolinium contrast demonstrates abnormal enhancement of the intracanalicular, labyrinthine, tympanic and mastoid segments and asymmetric enhancement of the tympanic, and mastoid segments of the nerve (Figure 4). The presence of a parotid mass, antecedent facial twitching, or other neurologic signs in addition to a unilateral facial paralysis is an indication for earlier imaging of unilateral facial paralysis. MRI imaging is indicated later in the course of Bell's palsy if full recovery of facial function does not occur within 9 months of onset [21]. Recently, ultrasound has been utilized to predict outcomes in Bell's palsy, as discussed above [1].

Several other idiopathic and inflammatory processes can cause facial paralysis. These include sarcoidosis, Guillain-Barre syndrome, and multiple sclerosis. These paralyses may have a more indolent onset than Bell's Palsy, which is characterized by full onset of weakness within 72 hours. Typically these processes will involve other cranial nerves or parts of the brain in addition to the facial nerve. These pathologies are best evaluated utilizing MRI with gadolinium enhancement [3, 22].

4.2. Infectious Disorders of the Facial Nerve. A variety of infectious disorders can affect the facial nerve. For instance, dehiscences of the fallopian canal can lead to facial paralyses in the setting of chronic or acute otitis media. These are best evaluated with high-resolution CT of the temporal bones. In cases where extension of the infection into the central nervous system is suspected, both high-resolution temporal bone CT and MRI of the brain with gadolinium will be indicated. Lyme disease is increasingly common in the United States and is the most common cause of acquired bilateral facial paralysis. MRI of the brain with gadolinium may be

normal or may show bilateral enhancement of the facial nerves and, potentially, other nerves as well [23]. Ramsey-Hunt syndrome is the result of reactivation of the varicella zoster virus can lead to facial paralysis and vesicles in the ear, on the face, or on the palate. Accompanying symptoms include otalgia, hearing loss, and vertigo. Enhancement of the facial and trigeminal nerves and spinal trigeminal tract can be detected on MRI. However, MRI is not usually indicated in the evaluation of this disorder, as the diagnosis is typically clear from the clinical presentation.

4.3. Traumatic Injury to the Facial Nerve. Traumatic injury to the facial nerve can occur at a variety of levels, from the brainstem to the distal periphery. Blunt force trauma from high-speed motor vehicle accidents can fracture the temporal bone, leading to either direct involvement of the fallopian canal and nerve injury or indirect injury via post-concussive injury and edema. Delayed facial palsy results from reactivation of herpes simplex type I virus within the geniculate ganglion and occurs 3–14 days after a traumatic injury [24–26]. In the setting of a critically ill, initially comatose patient, distinguishing delayed facial palsy from a potentially reversible injury to the nerve can be impossible based on clinical information alone. In this setting, imaging can provide crucial information that can impact patient management.

Facial nerve injuries more commonly occur in transverse fractures (38–50% of cases), rather than longitudinal fractures (20% of cases) of the temporal bone [3]. However, since longitudinal temporal bone fractures are much more common, they ultimately result in the highest number of facial injuries. Transverse fractures often affect the labyrinthine segment, while longitudinal fractures more often affect the geniculate ganglion, greater superficial petrosal nerve, tympanic segment, and mastoid segment (Figure 5). Potential mechanisms of direct facial injury following temporal bone fracture include fractures crossing through the facial canal, bony spicules impinging on the facial canal, or hematomas compressing the facial nerve. These are best visualized on noncontrast high-resolution CT of the temporal bones.

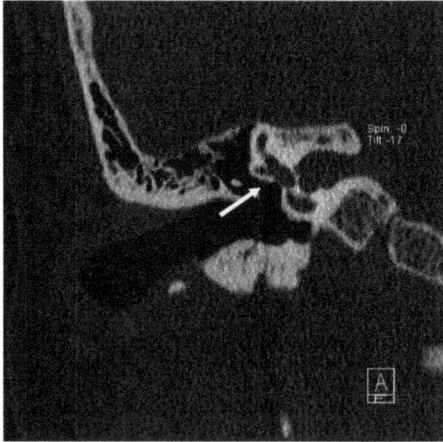

FIGURE 6: Facial nerve dehiscence. Coronal CT image of right temporal bone demonstrates dehiscence of right CN VII tympanic segment at the level of oval window (arrow).

4.4. Congenital Facial Nerve Malformations. Congenital malformations of the facial nerve can clinically be asymptomatic or present with facial weakness. Bony dehiscences of the facial nerve canal are the most common of these and typically occur in the tympanic segment superior to the oval window (Figure 6). These dehiscences predispose the facial nerve to damage from inflammatory processes such as cholesteatoma and otitis media and are important to recognize prior to otologic surgery. Typically, these dehiscences are best visualized on high-resolution CT of the temporal bones [3]. In patients with aural atresia, the second genu and mastoid segment may be displaced anteriorly and laterally (Figure 7). The stylomastoid foramen may also be displaced anteroraterally in atretic ears, making the facial nerve more susceptible to intraoperative injury. High-resolution temporal bone CT can detect clinically significant changes in the course of the facial nerve prior to aural atresia repair.

Congenital facial paralysis can occur as a result of facial nerve nucleus abnormalities in a variety of syndromes that include Moebius, DiGeorge, Goldenhar, CHARGE, trisomy 13, and trisomy 18. In Moebius syndrome, a constructive interference in steady-state (CISS) sequence can assist in early diagnosis by demonstrating the absence of the facial nerve [27]. Patients with CHARGE syndrome (colobomas, heart defects, choanal atresia, mental retardation, genitourinary anomalies, and ear anomalies) often have alterations in the course of the facial nerve. Posterior displacement of the labyrinthine segment is commonly seen [3]. Congenital hypoplasia or aplasia of the facial nerve can also occur as an isolated phenomenon and is best visualized by MRI.

4.5. Vascular and Other Central Processes Affecting the Facial Nerve. A variety of central pathologies can affect the intracranial portion of the facial nerve, including cerebrovascular accident (CVA), brain tumors (primary and metastatic), and multiple sclerosis. Presentation of the paresis or paralysis is determined by the site of the intracranial lesion. Central paralyses occur when the lesion disrupts the facial nerve

fibers prior to their decussation in the reticular formation of the caudal pons. Lesions affecting the facial nerve distal to the decussation can be mistaken for peripheral facial palsies; however, these are rare. Millard-Gubler syndrome is a mixed syndrome that is caused by lesions of the pons which lead to ipsilateral facial paresis, ipsilateral abducens paralysis, and contralateral hemiplegia. Millard-Gubler syndrome results from pathology disrupting the corticospinal tract prior to decussation plus the sixth and seventh nerve nuclei [28]. Eight-and-a-half syndrome results from involvement of the dorsal tegmen of the caudal pons involving the parapontine reticular formation or abducens nucleus and medial longitudinal fasciculus as well as the facial nerve nucleus. Symptoms of eight-and-a-half syndrome include intranuclear opthalmoplegia plus horizontal gaze palsy and ipsilateral facial paresis [29]. Regardless of the etiology of the lesion, these pathologies are best visualized on MRI.

Pontine infarcts comprise approximately 7% of all ischemic strokes. These infarcts are most frequently lacunar infarcts involving paramedian, short, and long circumferential perforators arising from the basilar artery [30, 31]. There are three main subtypes of pontine infarction: ventral, tegmental, and bilateral [31]. Ventral pontine infarcts are the most common type and are due to ischemia of the anteromedial and anterolateral pontine arteries, which supply the corticospinal tract, medial lemniscus, and cranial nerve nuclei. Clinically, patients present with severe ipsilateral paresis of the face, upper and lower extremities, dysarthria, and ipsilateral upper and lower extremity ataxia. Tegmental pontine infarcts result from ischemia of the short circumferential arteries which supply the tegmental area of the middle-upper pons. Patients present with eye movement disturbances, lemniscal and spinothalamic sensory deficits, and ipsilateral palsies of cranial nerves V, VI, and VII. Bilateral pontine infarcts are the least common and are associated with multiple brainstem infarcts. These patients present with pseudobulbar palsy and bilateral motor deficits of upper and lower extremities in addition to the signs seen in tegmental pontine infarction [31].

Central facial paralysis can also follow a CVA in the territory of the middle cerebral artery (MCA) or anterior cerebral artery (ACA) [32]. In the case of MCA stroke, patients can present with contralateral upper and lower extremity hemiparesis, contralateral hemianesthesia, and eye deviation towards the side of the infarct. When there is ischemia of the insula and operculum, forehead-sparing facial weakness also occurs [33]. For ACA strokes involving the dominant hemisphere, patients can present with contralateral-sided hemiparesis, contralateral hemianesthesia, dysarthria, aphasia, apraxia, and contralateral forehead-sparing facial paralysis.

MRI with multiple sequences can accurately detect ischemic changes in patients with acute neurologic deficits. The following sequences are typically included: diffusion weighted imaging (DWI), T2-weighted (T2W) and fluid-attenuated inversion recovery (FLAIR), MR angiography (MRA), perfusion-weighted imaging (PWI), and gradient-recalled echo (GRE). DWI sequence can detect acute

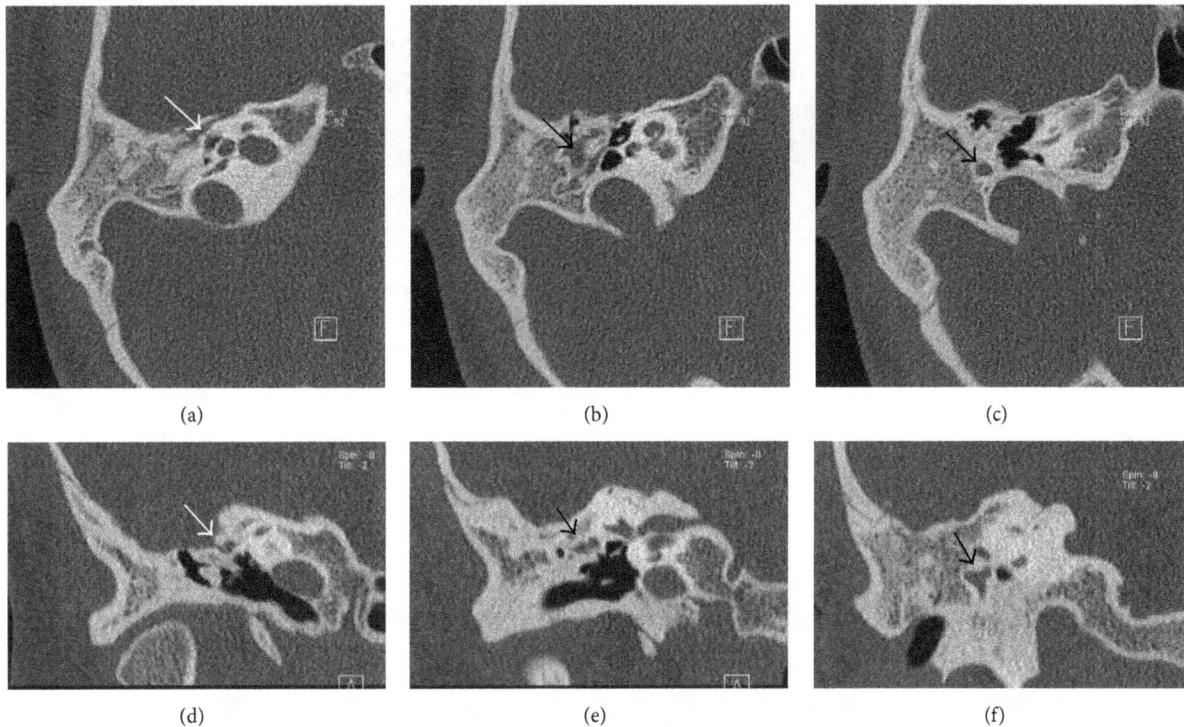

FIGURE 7: Aural atresia. Axial CT images (a)–(c) demonstrate abnormal facial nerve canal tympanic segment coursing posterolaterally to the middle ear cavity (arrows), instead of the normal posteromedial course. Coronal CT image (d) demonstrates the abnormal proximal tympanic segment of the facial nerve canal coursing superior to the middle ear cavity and ossicles (arrow), instead of its normal medial course. Coronal CT images (e)-(f) showing the abnormal distal tympanic segment and second genu of the facial nerve canal (arrows).

ischemia within minutes of onset as a focal area of hyperintensity [34], while T2W and FLAIR can detect acute ischemia within the first 3–8 hours after onset. Noncontrast time-of-flight MRA is used to evaluate the intracranial arterial system. PWI sequence with gadolinium contrast detects areas of the brain that have decreased cerebral blood flow but have not yet been severely injured. GRE sequences are tailored to be sensitive to the detection of iron products, thereby indicating the presence of prior hemorrhage [34].

4.6. Facial Dystonias.

Patients with hemifacial spasm suffer unilateral twitching or spasms of facial muscles. Tortuosity of the anterior inferior cerebellar artery, posterior inferior cerebellar artery, basilar artery, or vertebral artery can compress the facial nerve at the root exit zone, resulting in unilateral spasms. MRI can identify the artery compressing the facial nerve and, thus, serve as a guide for microvascular decompression. In essential blepharospasm, involuntary blinking occurs with increased frequency, particularly in response to stimuli such as wind, sunlight, noise, or stress [35]. The etiology is unknown, although it is hypothesized to result from disinhibition of blinking due to a disorder of the basal ganglia [36]. In clinically equivocal cases, MRI can assist in diagnosis by excluding vascular compression of the facial nerve in the posterior cranial fossa. Lastly, Meige's syndrome is a rare disorder characterized by blepharospasm

and involuntary contractions of the muscles in the jaw and tongue (oromandibular dystonia). MRI is used to exclude intracranial pathology in the evaluation of this idiopathic disorder.

4.7. Neoplastic Processes Affecting the Facial Nerve.

A variety of neoplastic processes can affect facial nerve function. Schwannomas can occur anywhere along the course of the facial nerve. Most commonly, they arise in the perigeniculate, tympanic, or mastoid segments. Lipomas can occur in the CPA or IAC, entrapping unmyelinated facial nerve fibers. Hemangiomas arise from the vascular plexus surrounding the facial nerve, most commonly in the perigeniculate region. Less commonly, these lesions are found in the IAC or mastoid segment [37]. Hemangiomas cause facial nerve dysfunction by direct neural compression or neural ischemia due to vascular steal [37]. Hemangiomas located in the geniculate ganglion can cause facial nerve weakness; tumors in the IAC may lead to progressive sensorineural hearing loss with poor speech discrimination [38]. Temporal bone CT can visualize mineralization of ossifying hemangiomas, distinguishing these tumors from facial nerve schwannomas (Figure 8). MRI is useful for proper identification of schwannomas, lipomas, and hemangiomas.

Paragangliomas are highly vascular tumors that originate in the paraganglionic tissue of the carotid bifurcation (carotid

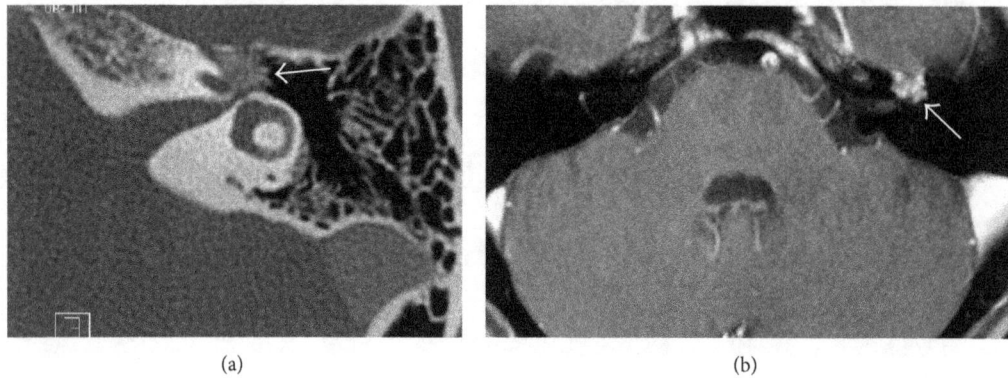

(a)   (b)

FIGURE 8: Facial nerve hemangioma. Axial CT (a) demonstrates a mass with trabecular bony matrix centered in the first genu of the facial nerve (arrow). Axial T1 postcontrast fat-saturated MRI (b) demonstrates the enhancing hemangioma (arrow).

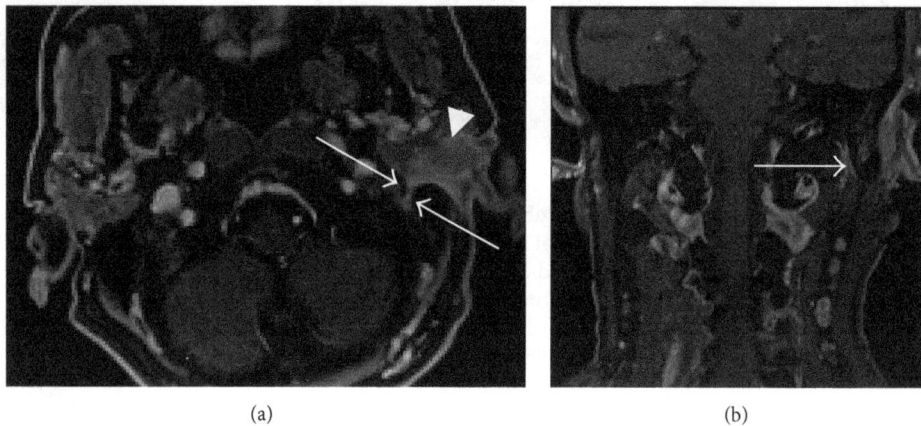

(a)   (b)

FIGURE 9: Perineural tumor spread along CN VII. Axial T1 (a) and coronal (b) postcontrast fat-saturated images demonstrate an enlarged, enhancing left facial nerve in the stylomastoid foramen and mastoid segment of the facial nerve canal (arrows), indicating perineural tumor spread from invasive squamous cell carcinoma (arrowhead) of the left external auditory canal.

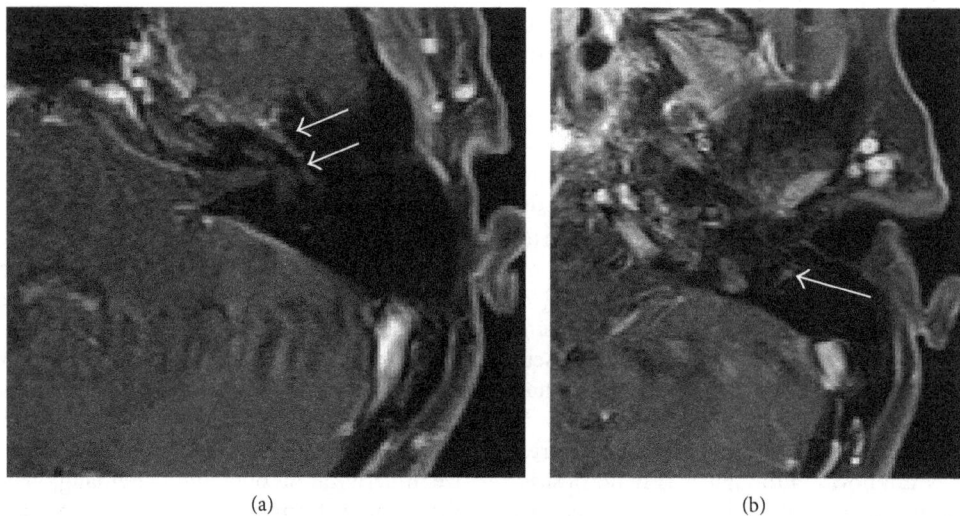

(a)   (b)

FIGURE 10: Normal facial nerve on MRI. Postcontrast fat-saturated T1-weighted MRI images of normal enhancing tympanic (a) and mastoid (b) CN VII segments.

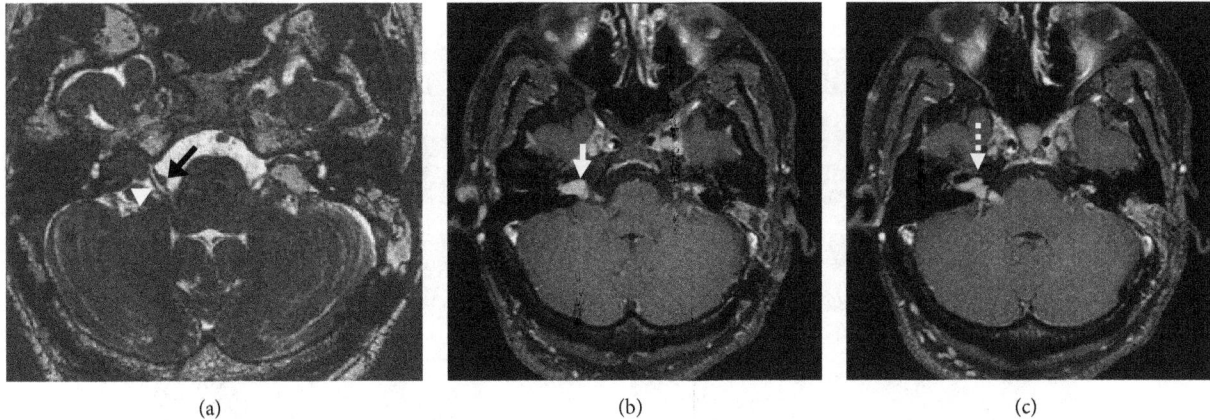

FIGURE 11: Right CN VII schwannoma in the cerebellopontine angle (CPA) in a patient with neurofibromatosis type II. Axial CISS sequence (a) demonstrates a small lesion along CNVII (black arrow), which courses anterior to CNVIII (white arrowhead) in the right CPA cistern. Axial T1 postcontrast fat-saturated images (b)-(c) demonstrate the enhancement of the right facial schwannoma (solid white arrow, (b)). Also note the vestibular schwannoma in the right IAC (dashed white arrow, (c)) and residual enhancement with postsurgical changes in the region of the left IAC.

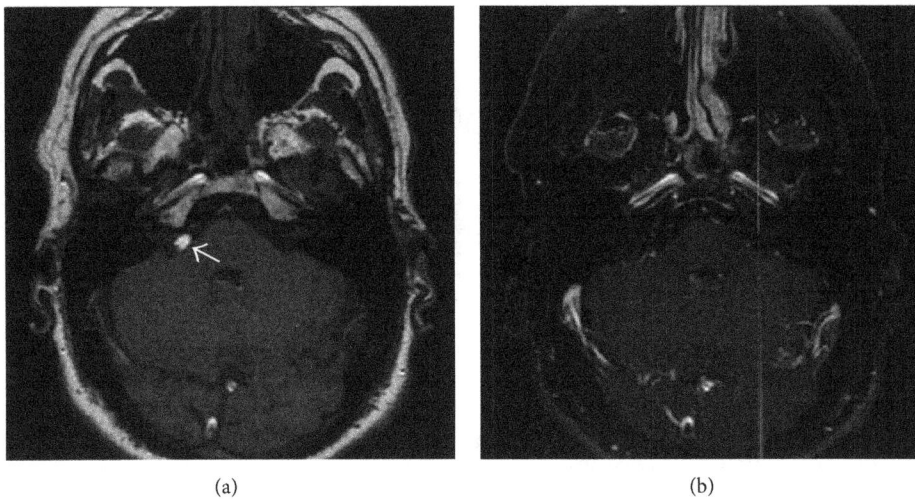

FIGURE 12: CPA Lipoma. Noncontrast T1-weighted image (a) demonstrates a globular hyperintense lesion in the right CPA (white arrow). (b) Postcontrast fat-saturated T1-weighted MR image shows signal dropout indicating that this lesion is composed of fat. There is no associated enhancement of this lesion.

body tumors), jugular foramen (glomus jugulare), vagus nerve (glomus vagale), and tympanic plexus on the promontory (glomus tympanicum). They can occur sporadically or in association with tumor syndromes such as multiple endocrine neoplasia type II (MEN II), von Hippel-Lindau syndrome, or neurofibromatosis type I. Rare cases of facial nerve paragangliomas occurring along the mastoid segment have also been reported [39]. CT and MRI are essential for defining the extent of these lesions and for surgical planning. On contrast-enhanced T1-weighted MRI, the lesions exhibit a "salt-and-pepper" appearance; they are hyperintense on T2. Unlike cholesteatomas, they enhance with contrast [39].

Neoplasms in the middle ear can infiltrate or compress the tympanic segment of the facial nerve. These lesions include adenomas, schwannomas, and paragangliomas. Adenomas arise from the glands of the middle ear mucosa and often present as a middle ear mass with conductive hearing loss. CT typically shows a middle ear mass without evidence of bony erosion.

Malignant tumors of the parotid can affect the extratemporal facial nerve. Primary malignant neoplasms include mucoepidermoid carcinoma, adenoid cystic carcinoma, adenocarcinoma, malignant mixed tumors, acinic cell carcinoma, lymphoma, and squamous cell carcinoma. In particular, adenoid cystic carcinoma frequently exhibits perineural invasion (70–75%) [40]. Head and neck primaries may metastasize to intraparotid lymph nodes, which provide lymphatic drainage to the scalp, face, external auditory canal,

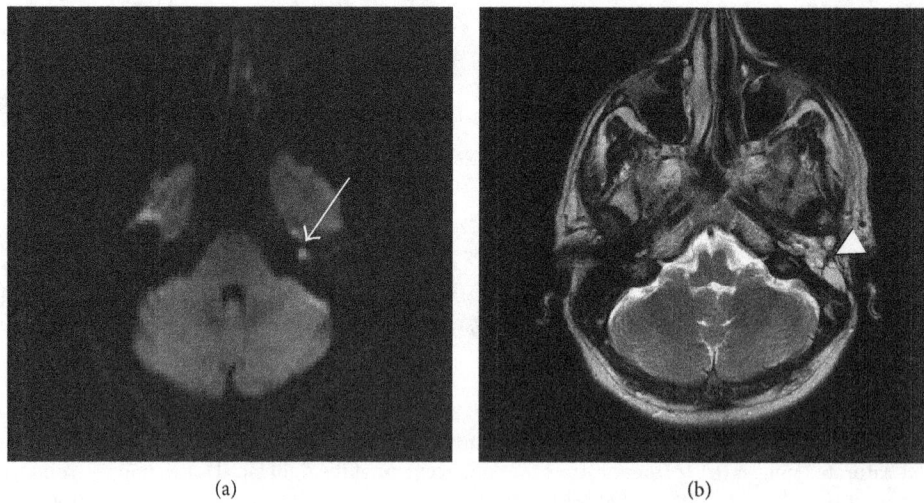

(a)   (b)

FIGURE 13: Recurrent cholesteatoma. Axial diffusion-weighted image (a) demonstrates abnormal hyperintense signal in the left temporal bone consistent with a focus on recurrent cholesteatoma (white arrow). Axial T2-weighted sequence (b) shows fat packing material in the left temporal bone (arrowhead) following mastoidectomy with blind sac closure.

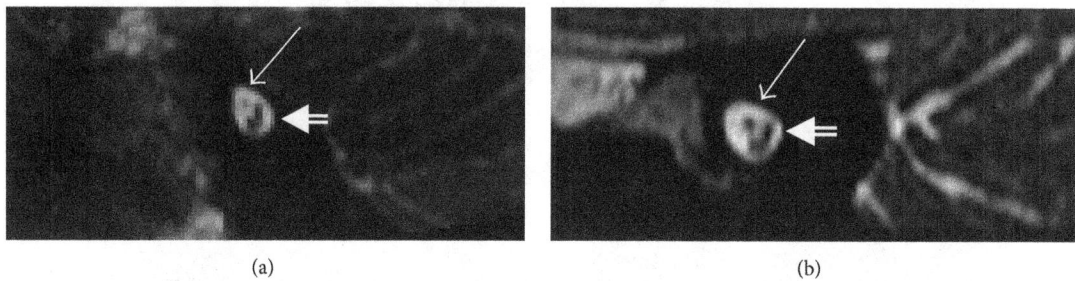

(a)   (b)

FIGURE 14: Moebius syndrome. Sagittal oblique CISS sequence of the internal auditory canal in a patient with Moebius syndrome (a) demonstrates the small caliber of the hypoplastic facial nerve in the anterior superior aspect of the canal (arrow). The normal vestibulocochlear nerve is seen posteriorly (double lined arrow). Sagittal oblique CISS image in a normal patient (b) demonstrates the normal caliber of the facial (solid arrow) and vestibulocochlear (double lined arrow) nerves for comparison.

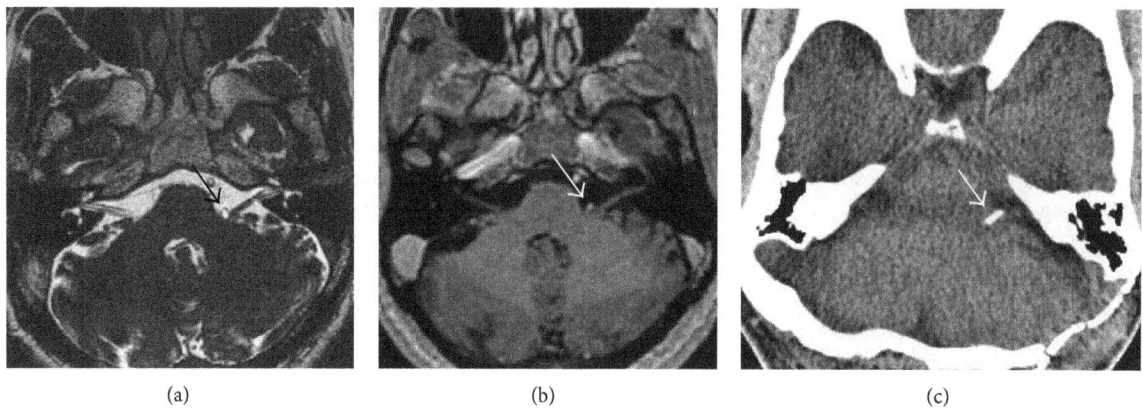

(a)   (b)   (c)

FIGURE 15: Neurovascular compression in a patient presenting with left hemifacial spasm. Axial CISS (a) and T1 postcontrast MRI (b) images demonstrate the left vertebral artery (arrow) abutting the left facial nerve at the root entry zone. Axial noncontrast CT scan (c) demonstrates the hyperdense postsurgical material from microvascular decompression surgery.

and tympanic membrane. Skin tumors such as squamous cell carcinoma and melanoma account for 80–90% of parotid metastases [41]. MRI with gadolinium is useful for detecting perineural spread from parotid and minor salivary gland malignancies along the facial nerve.

5. Conclusion

Imaging can provide critical information for diagnosis and treatment of facial nerve disorders. MRI of the brain and brainstem is most useful for central pathologies affecting the facial nerve as well as lesions of the facial nerve proximal to the porus acusticus. High-resolution CT of the temporal bone best visualizes the course of the nerve within the fallopian canal to the stylomastoid foramen. Soft tissue CT with contrast or MRI can be used to evaluate areas of the distal course of the facial nerve within the parotid and soft tissues of the face. Facial nerve ultrasound may be useful in predicting functional outcomes 3 months after the onset of paralysis in patients with Bell's palsy. DT tractography is a new modality that shows promise for 3D visualization of facial nerve fibers, potentially lowering the risk of facial nerve injury during treatment of vestibular schwannomas.

References

[1] Y. L. Lo, S. Fook-Chong, T. H. Leoh et al., "High-resolution ultrasound in the evaluation and prognosis of Bell's palsy," *European Journal of Neurology*, vol. 17, no. 6, pp. 885–889, 2010.

[2] T. Taoka, H. Hirabayashi, H. Nakagawa et al., "Displacement of the facial nerve course by vestibular schwannoma: preoperative visualization using diffusion tensor tractography," *Journal of Magnetic Resonance Imaging*, vol. 24, no. 5, pp. 1005–1010, 2006.

[3] P. Raghavan, S. Mukherjee, and C. D. Phillips, "Imaging of the facial nerve," *Neuroimaging Clinics of North America*, vol. 19, no. 3, pp. 407–425, 2009.

[4] A. Cisneros, J. R. W. Orozco, J. A. O. Nogues et al., "Development of the stapedius muscle canal and its possible clinical consequences," *International Journal of Pediatric Otorhinolaryngology*, vol. 75, no. 2, pp. 277–281, 2011.

[5] M. May and B. M. Schaitkin, *The Facial Nerve*, Thieme, New York, NY, USA, Second edition, 2000.

[6] H. D. Curtin, P. C. Sanelli, and P. M. Som, "Chapter 19 temporal bone: embryology and anatomy," in *Head and Neck Imaging*, P. M. Som and H. D. Curtin, Eds., vol. 2, Mosby, St. Louis, Mo, USA, 4th edition, 2003.

[7] K. Al-Noury and A. Lotfy, "Normal and pathological findings for the facial nerve on magnetic resonance imaging," *Clinical Radiology*, vol. 66, no. 8, pp. 701–707, 2011.

[8] L. Jäger and M. Reiser, "CT and MR imaging of the normal and pathologic conditions of the facial nerve," *European Journal of Radiology*, vol. 40, no. 2, pp. 133–146, 2001.

[9] F. Veillon, L. Ramos-Taboada, M. Abu-Eid, A. Charpiot, and S. Riehm, "Imaging of the facial nerve," *European Journal of Radiology*, vol. 74, no. 2, pp. 341–348, 2010.

[10] L. Liu, R. Arnold, and M. Robinson, "Dissection and exposure of the whole course of deep nerves in human head specimens after decalcification," *International Journal of Otolaryngology*, vol. 2012, Article ID 418650, 7 pages, 2012.

[11] S. C. Crawford, H. R. Harnsberger, and J. D. Swartz, "Chapter 7: the facial nerve (cranial nerve VII)," in *Imaging of the Temporal Bone*, J. D. Swartz and H. R. Harnsberger, Eds., Thieme, New York, NY, USA, 1998.

[12] G. T. Nager and B. Proctor, "Anatomic variations and anomalies involving the facial canal," *Otolaryngologic Clinics of North America*, vol. 24, no. 3, pp. 531–553, 1991.

[13] R. F. Yellon and B. F. Branstetter, "Prospective blinded study of computed tomography in congenital aural atresia," *International Journal of Pediatric Otorhinolaryngology*, vol. 74, no. 11, pp. 1286–1291, 2010.

[14] X. Mu, Y. Quan, J. Shao, J. Li, H. Wang, and R. Gong, "Enlarged geniculate ganglion fossa: CT sign of facial nerve canal fracture," *Academic Radiology*, vol. 19, no. 8, pp. 971–976, 2012.

[15] J. R. Brodsky, T. W. Smith, S. Litofsky, and D. J. Lee, "Lipoma of the cerebellopontine angle," *American Journal of Otolaryngology*, vol. 27, no. 4, pp. 271–274, 2006.

[16] B. Isaacson, S. A. Telian, P. E. McKeever, and H. A. Arts, "Hemangiomas of the geniculate ganglion," *Otology and Neurotology*, vol. 26, no. 4, pp. 796–802, 2005.

[17] B. De Foer, J. P. Vercruysse, M. Spaepen et al., "Diffusion-weighted magnetic resonance imaging of the temporal bone," *Neuroradiology*, vol. 52, no. 9, pp. 785–807, 2010.

[18] E. Yorgancilar, M. Yildirim, R. Gun et al., "Complications of chronic suppurative otitis media: a retrospective review," *European Archives of Oto-Rhino-Laryngology*, vol. 270, no. 1, pp. 69–76, 2013.

[19] D. Q. Chen, J. Quan, A. Guha, M. Tymianski, D. Mikulis, and M. Hodaie, "Three-dimensional in vivo modeling of vestibular schwannomas and surrounding cranial nerves with diffusion imaging tractography," *Neurosurgery*, vol. 68, no. 4, pp. 1077–1083, 2011.

[20] P. G. Kennedy, "Herpes simplex virus type 1 and Bell's palsy a current assessment of the controversy," *Journal of NeuroVirology*, vol. 16, no. 1, pp. 1–5, 2010.

[21] M. J. Lanser and R. K. Jackler, "Gadolinium magnetic resonance imaging in Bell's palsy," *Western Journal of Medicine*, vol. 154, no. 6, pp. 718–719, 1991.

[22] D. Pickuth and S. H. Heywang-Kobrunner, "Neurosarcoidosis: evaluation with MRI," *Journal of Neuroradiology*, vol. 27, no. 3, pp. 185–188, 2000.

[23] B. Vanzieleghem, M. Lemmerling, D. Carton et al., "Lyme disease in a child presenting with bilateral facial nerve palsy: MRI findings and review of the literature," *Neuroradiology*, vol. 40, no. 11, pp. 739–742, 1998.

[24] F. Salvinelli, M. Casale, L. Vitaliana, F. Greco, C. Dianzani, and L. D'Ascanio, "Delayed peripheral facial palsy in the stapes surgery: can it be prevented? " *American Journal of Otolaryngology*, vol. 25, no. 2, pp. 105–108, 2004.

[25] G. J. Gianoli, "Viral titers and delayed facial palsy after acoustic neuroma surgery," *Otolaryngology*, vol. 127, no. 5, pp. 427–431, 2002.

[26] D. E. Brackmann, L. M. Fisher, M. Hansen, A. Halim, and W. H. Slattery, "The effect of famciclovir on delayed facial paralysis after acoustic tumor resection," *Laryngoscope*, vol. 118, no. 9, pp. 1617–1620, 2008.

[27] H. T. F. M. Verzijl, J. Valk, R. De Vries, and G. W. Padberg, "Radiologic evidence for absence of the facial nerve in Möbius syndrome," *Neurology*, vol. 64, no. 5, pp. 849–855, 2005.

[28] I. E. Silverman, G. T. Liu, N. J. Volpe, and S. L. Galetta, "The crossed paralyses. The original brain-stem syndromes of Millard-Gubler, Foville, Weber, and Raymond-Cestan," *Archives of Neurology*, vol. 52, no. 6, pp. 635–638, 1995.

[29] E. Eggenberger, "Eight-and-a-half syndrome: one-and-a-half syndrome plus cranial nerve VII palsy," *Journal of Neuro-Ophthalmology*, vol. 18, no. 2, pp. 114–116, 1998.

[30] V. Saia and L. Pantoni, "Progressive stroke in pontine infarction," *Acta Neurologica Scandinavica*, vol. 120, no. 4, pp. 213–215, 2009.

[31] C. Bassetti, J. Bogousslavsky, A. Barth, and F. Regli, "Isolated infarcts of the pons," *Neurology*, vol. 46, no. 1, pp. 165–175, 1996.

[32] L. Cattaneo, E. Saccani, P. De Giampaulis, G. Crisi, and G. Pavesi, "Central facial palsy revisited: a clinical-radiological study," *Annals of Neurology*, vol. 68, no. 3, pp. 404–408, 2010.

[33] J. Y. S. Kim, "Facial nerve parlaysis," in *Medscape Reference*, D. Narayan, Ed., 2012.

[34] L. M. Nentwich and W. Veloz, "Neuroimaging in acute stroke," in *Emergency Medicine Clinics of North America*, vol. 30, pp. 659–680, 2012.

[35] B. R. Spencer Jr. and K. B. Digre, "Treatments for neuro-ophthalmologic conditions," *Neurologic Clinics*, vol. 28, no. 4, pp. 1005–1035, 2010.

[36] D. Boghen, V. Tozlovanu, A. Iancu, and R. Forget, "Botulinum toxin therapy for apraxia of lid opening," *Annals of the New York Academy of Sciences*, vol. 956, pp. 482–483, 2002.

[37] N. Ahmadi, K. Newkirk, and H. J. Kim, "Facial nerve hemangioma: a rare case involving the vertical segment," *Laryngoscope*, vol. 123, no. 2, pp. 499–502, 2013.

[38] O. Friedman, B. A. Neff, T. O. Willcox, L. C. Kenyon, and R. T. Sataloff, "Temporal bone hemangiomas involving the facial nerve," *Otology and Neurotology*, vol. 23, no. 5, pp. 760–766, 2002.

[39] J. Kunzel, J. Zenk, M. Koch, J. Hornung, and H. Iro, "Paraganglioma of the facial nerve, a rare differential diagnosis for facial nerve paralysis: case report and review of the literature," *European Archives of Oto-Rhino-Laryngology*, vol. 269, no. 2, pp. 693–698, 2012.

[40] A. S. Garden, R. S. Weber, W. H. Morrison, K. K. Ang, and L. J. Peters, "The influence of positive margins and nerve invasion in adenoid cystic carcinoma of the head and neck treated with surgery and radiation," *International Journal of Radiation Oncology Biology Physics*, vol. 32, no. 3, pp. 619–626, 1995.

[41] C. M. Malata, I. G. Camilleri, N. R. McLean et al., "Malignant tumours of the parotid gland: a 12-year review," *British Journal of Plastic Surgery*, vol. 50, no. 8, pp. 600–608, 1997.

2

Stereoscopic Visualization of Diffusion Tensor Imaging Data: A Comparative Survey of Visualization Techniques

Osama Raslan,[1] **James Matthew Debnam,**[1] **Leena Ketonen,**[1] **Ashok J. Kumar,**[1] **Dawid Schellingerhout,**[1] **and Jihong Wang**[2]

[1] *Department of Radiology, Section of Neuroradiology, MD Anderson Cancer Center, The University of Texas, 1400 Pressler Street, Unit 1482, Houston, TX 77030, USA*
[2] *Deparment of Imaging Physics, MD Anderson Cancer Center, The University of Texas, 1400 Pressler Street, Unit 1482, Houston, TX 77030, USA*

Correspondence should be addressed to James Matthew Debnam; matthew.debnam@mdanderson.org

Academic Editor: Weili Lin

Diffusion tensor imaging (DTI) data has traditionally been displayed as a grayscale functional anisotropy map (GSFM) or color coded orientation map (CCOM). These methods use black and white or color with intensity values to map the complex multidimensional DTI data to a two-dimensional image. Alternative visualization techniques, such as V_{max} maps utilize enhanced graphical representation of the principal eigenvector by means of a headless arrow on regular nonstereoscopic (VM) or stereoscopic display (VMS). A survey of clinical utility of patients with intracranial neoplasms was carried out by 8 neuroradiologists using traditional and nontraditional methods of DTI display. Pairwise comparison studies of 5 intracranial neoplasms were performed with a structured questionnaire comparing GSFM, CCOM, VM, and VMS. Six of 8 neuroradiologists favored V_{max} maps over traditional methods of display (GSFM and CCOM). When comparing the stereoscopic (VMS) and the non-stereoscopic (VM) modes, 4 favored VMS, 2 favored VM, and 2 had no preference. In conclusion, processing and visualizing DTI data stereoscopically is technically feasible. An initial survey of users indicated that V_{max} based display methodology with or without stereoscopic visualization seems to be preferred over traditional methods to display DTI data.

1. Introduction

Diffusion tensor imaging (DTI) is a magnetic resonance (MR) imaging technique that enables the quantitative measurement of molecular diffusion in biologic tissues *in vivo* [1–7]. Diffusion signal changes are caused by the anisotropy (or directionality) of WM fibers; the fibers restrict water molecule movement across the axons while leaving movement along the axons relatively unrestricted. This results in unequal (or anisotropic) diffusivities along the axons. The ability to measure these very specific tissue characteristics *in vivo* is unique to DTI and has many applications in clinical neuroimaging including the delineation of tumor infiltration, assessing the integrity of neuronal fibers and neurosurgical planning [8–19].

Many techniques and schemes have been proposed for visualizing DTI data [20–28] such as using ellipsoids with their principal axes corresponding to the eigenvectors and using volumetric rendering or shading to present these ellipsoids' directional information [23]. These are rigorous approaches but are still subject to the limiting problems of any technique that visualizes 3D information in two dimensions (2D). Often the 3D shading of diffusion tensor ellipsoids [23] or superquadric glyphs [24] at all voxels does not give a global view of tensor data in an imaging plane or in a volume at the zoomed-out view. To get a true 3D perspective, one must use computer animation tools to rotate the image plane or image volume thereby obtaining multiple views of the 3D tensor data [20]. Research into new and intuitive methods of analyzing and representing DTI data continues [29].

DTI data needs to be displayed in an interpretable manner in order to support clinical decision making. This is a challenging proposition, because unlike other volumetric grayscale images, in which the value at each voxel can be represented by a single number (scalar), DTI image display needs to communicate multiple values reflecting directional and magnitude information at every voxel. In fact, the value at each voxel is a tensor, which requires the use of multiple parameters for its representation. A tensor is typically represented by a 3×3 matrix with a total of nine elements, of which six are independent. The tensor matrix can be diagonalized, yielding three eigenvalues and their corresponding eigenvectors. A full representation of DTI information would include all three eigenvalues and eigenvectors for every voxel.

In order to simplify this tensor dataset for display on a 2D grayscale image, grayscale fractional anisotropy (GSFA) maps are often constructed (Figure 1(a)). GSFA maps are simply plots of the fractional anisotropy (FA) values at those voxels with a large difference between the principal and other eigenvalues as bright values and those with little differences as dark values:

$$FA = \sqrt{\frac{1}{2}} \frac{\sqrt{(\lambda_1 - \lambda_2)^2 + (\lambda_1 - \lambda_3)^2 + (\lambda_2 - \lambda_3)^2}}{\sqrt{(\lambda_1^2 + \lambda_2^2 + \lambda_3^2)}}, \quad (1)$$

where λ_1, λ_2, and λ_3 are three eigenvalues at each voxel.

Alternatively, color can be used to indicate direction and brightness to indicate the magnitude of the directional component, and color-coded orientation maps (CCOM) are displayed (Figure 1(b)).

Sometimes displaying all tensor information at every voxel at once may be cumbersome and even counterproductive for clinical diagnosis. Therefore, many have proposed and implemented visualization schemes that display only a portion of the tensor data [20–29]. For instance, in DTI-related publications, it is common to see fractional anisotropy (FA) maps, which are grayscale images of anisotropy indices that are composites of all three eigenvalues. As the principal eigenvector (V_{max}) represents the direction of fiber tracts, some DTI visualization schemes choose to present only the directional information of V_{max} and another parameter that indicates anisotropy. One popular DTI representation scheme uses three colors to represent the directional information of V_{max} in orthogonal planes [27].

Although color has been used extensively in medical imaging, sometimes as an indication of directional information, that is, color Doppler ultrasonography, many human observers are not sensitive to the subtle changes in color hue that represent directional information for DTI tensors. Therefore, the current, nontraditional technique of using colors to encode DTI eigenvector direction may not be intuitive, especially for eigenvectors with directions (CCOM) not parallel to any of the three orthogonal Cartesian coordinate axes, even with the use of a reference color circle [27].

Alternatively, stereoscopic vision can also be employed; this adds another dimension to 2D grayscale images. For DTI, a natural and true 3D view of V_{max}, (Figure 1(c)) as well as the WM fiber tracts can be easily achieved using stereoscopic vision principles. Creating a stereoscopic image pair (i.e., the left- and right-eye views) and presenting the images to the respective eyes enables a human viewer with normal stereo vision to get a 3D perception of the spatial and directional information of diffusion tensors' eigenvectors and WM fiber tracts by reconstructing the left- and right-eye retinal images in his visual system (Figure 2). In theory, stereoscopic perceptions (VMS) can be generated by calculating the projected left- and right-eye-view images of the V_{max} or WM fiber tracts and displaying these images with a stereoscopic image displaying device. Alternatively, we can put the pair of images side by side on paper (Figure 2) or on a computer monitor (Figure 3) and use a simple device (described below) that allows the left eye to see only the left-eye-view image and the right eye to see only the right-eye-view image.

The purpose of this study was to assess the clinical utility of V_{max} maps, both nonstereoscopic (VM) and stereoscopic (VMS), and to compare V_{max} maps to traditional DTI display method (GSFA and CCOM).

2. Materials and Methods

Eight neuroradiologists participated in the study and evaluated the DTI of 5 patients (5 females, ages 4–62 years, mean 43 years, and median 47 years) with the following intracranial pathology: metastatic breast carcinoma, brainstem glioma, glioblastoma, anaplastic astrocytoma, and lymphoma. The patients were imaged with MRI scanners (GE Healthcare, Milwaukee, WI) using single-shot EPI pulse sequences to obtain DTI data (b value = 1200, number of diffusion gradient directions = 27, FOV = 22 cm, slice thickness of 3.5 mm with no gap, and matrix size 128×128). The same DTI image data set was generated for each patient with all four of the visualization techniques to be compared.

2.1. Conventional/Traditional DTI Processing Tool. A commercial DTI data processing software package (AW version 4.4, GE Healthcare, Milwaukee, WI) was used in the generation of the grayscale functional anisotropy maps (GSFM) and coded orientation maps (CCOM) images on the selected patients (Figures 1(a) and 1(b)).

2.2. Stereoscopic DTI Processing. A DTI processing and stereoscopic visualization software was developed in-house with C++ (Microsoft Visual Studio, Microsoft Corp., Redmond, WA) using the OpenGL library for 3D rendering. From the diffusion weighted images, this software calculates the eigenvalues and eigenvectors as well as the ADC values first. Then it creates a headless arrow to represent the dominant eigenvector at each voxel, with the length of the arrow (as well as the color temperature) corresponding to the magnitude of the eigenvalue (VM). For stereoscopic view, the visualization program generates the two stereoscopic image pairs of these arrows at each voxel for all the image slices. Dominant principal eigenvector stereoscopic (VMS) images were generated by the stereoscopic visualization tool.

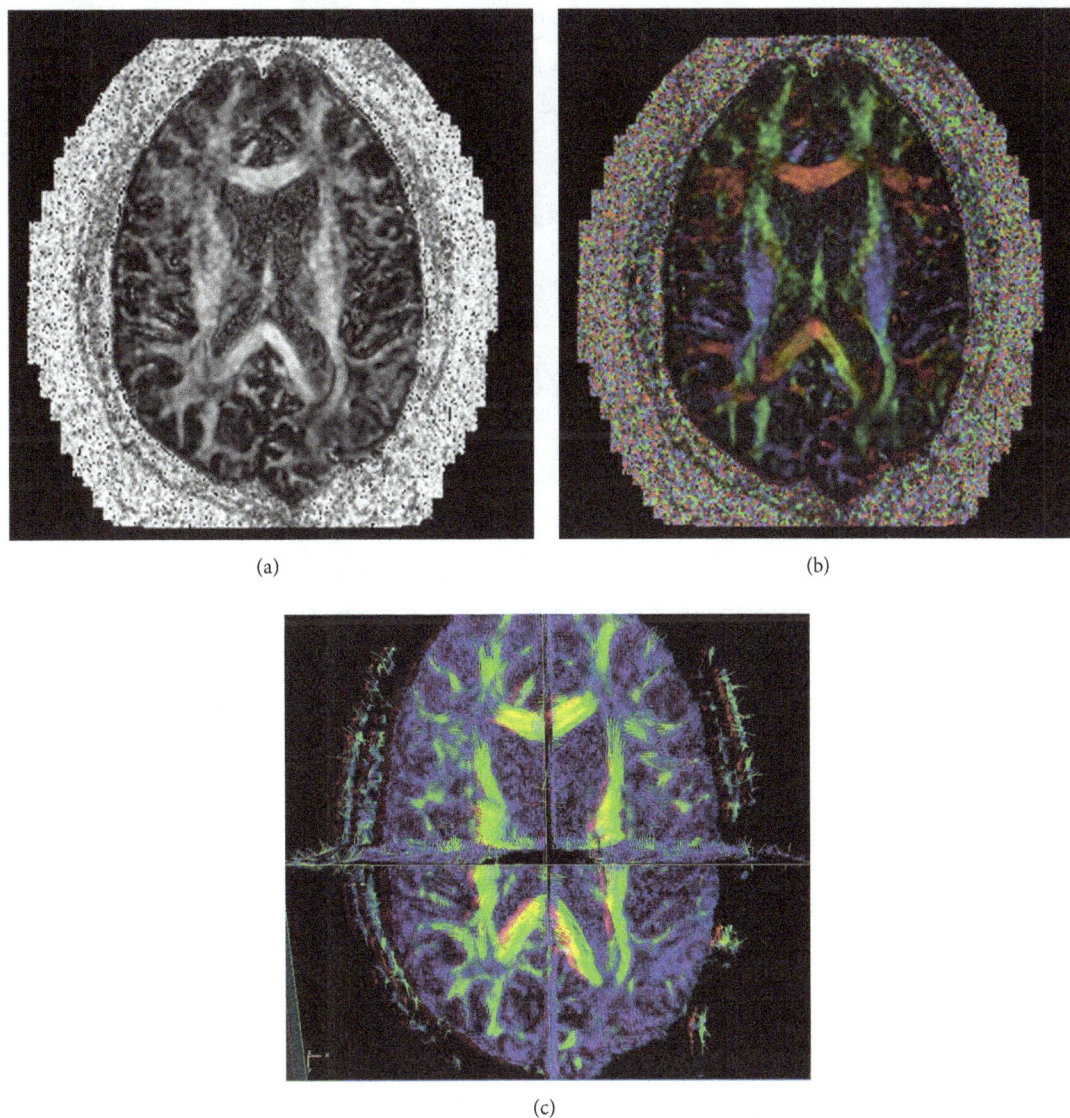

(a)

(b)

(c)

FIGURE 1: For comparison, the principal eigenvectors are presented in (grayscale (GSFA) map, color coded orientation view (CCOM), and headless arrow view (V_{max})). (a) GSFA. The intensity represents the FA value while no directional information is given. (b) CCOM. In the color coded orientation view, which is commonly seen in today's DTI literature, blue color represents the craniocaudal (in-out of paper) direction, red represents the left-right direction, and green represents the anterior-posterior (up-down) direction. The mixed colors represent directions somewhere in between. The intensity of color represents the FA value. (c) V_{max} map. In the stereoscopic view, eigenvectors' directional information is presented intuitively as headless arrows in 3D stereoscopically and colors represent the FA values.

2.3. Visualization Tool. All images were transferred to a stereoscopically enabled laptop computer (PC-AL3DU laptop, Sharp Electronics Corp., Mahwah, NJ) (Figure 3). This device enables stereoscopic vision by a specially designed monitor. More specifically, stereoscopic viewing was achieved using Sharp's StereoGL and its glasses-free stereoscopic LCD monitor. For this stereoscopic monitor, a stereoscopic view was created by having the left- and right-eye views interlaced as the even and odd vertical lines on the monitor. At a certain viewing distance, the right-eye view is visible only to the right eye and the left-eye view is visible only to the left eye. This generates a 3D perception for human observers with normal stereoscopic vision without the use of polarizing glasses,

and the visualization could be switched between stereoscopic (VMS) and nonstereoscopic (VM) mode with a control key button.

This software tool has two DTI data visualization functions: the eigenvector view function and the fiber-tracking (or tractography) function. In the eigenvector view function, the 3D vector fields of the principal eigenvectors (V_{max}) in the three orthogonal planes of the image volume are displayed stereoscopically. The eigenvectors are displayed as headless arrows and superimposed over the image of the FA values. The colors of the arrows correspond to the tensors' anisotropy indices (i.e., the FA values). Any of the three orthogonal planes can be turned on/off and looped through the image

(a)

(b)

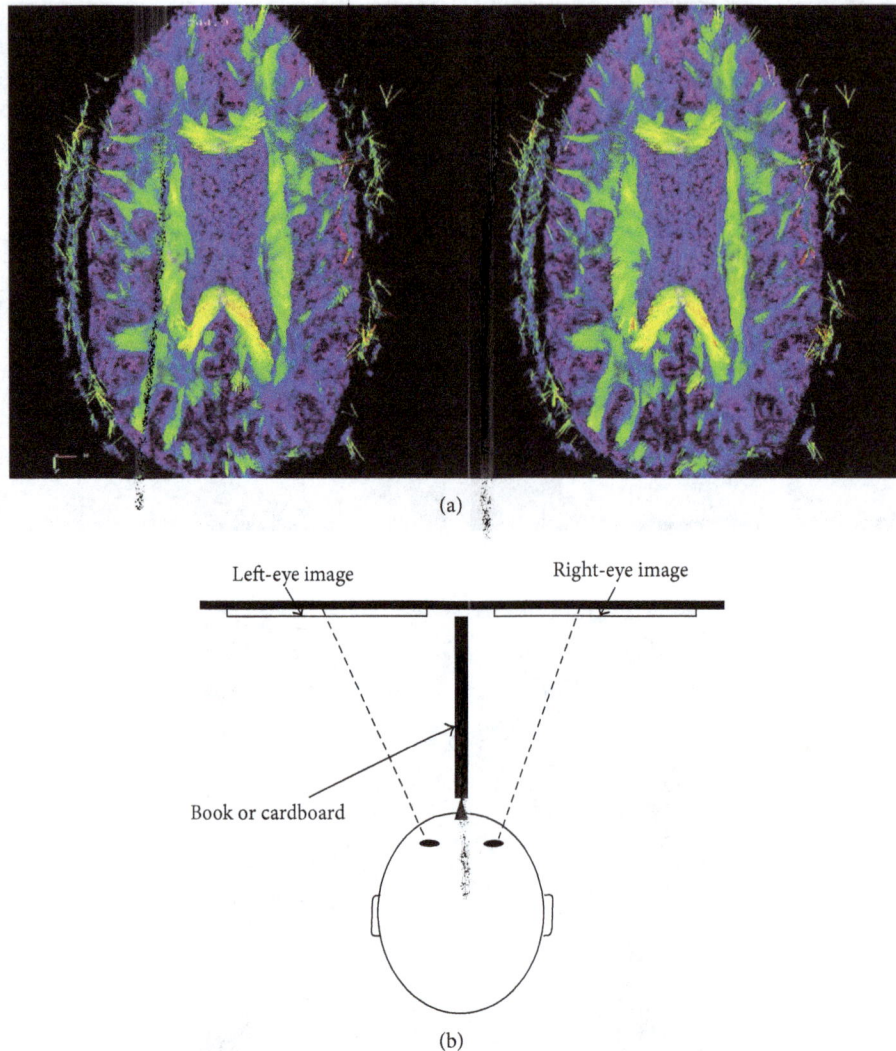

FIGURE 2: 3D visualization tool. Stereoscopic left- and right-eye-image generated by the visualization tool; one can achieve the stereo effect by focusing beyond the image plane or with the help of a stereoscope, or by using a piece of cardboard put between the two images (as shown schematically in (b) the top-down view) such that each eye is able to see only one of the two images. Once the stereo effect is achieved, one can clearly appreciate the 3D effect of the headless arrows pointing out of the paper plane at various angles.

volume along with the eigenvectors in those planes. The tool also allows the user to zoom in on any point within the image volume for a detailed view of the eigenvectors and to rotate the image volume to view it from any angle.

In the fiber-tracking function (Figure 4(a)), this tool performs WM fiber tracking using a simple line-propagation algorithm that follows the paths of V_{max} through the 3D tensor imaging volume. It assigns a color to each point along the fiber tracts corresponding to the local properties (e.g., FA value), using a typical rainbow color scale, and displays the tracts stereoscopically in 3D (Figure 4(b)).

2.4. Clinical Study. The data sets for all 5 patients were presented to the neuroradiologists on the same computer upon which the stereoscopic visualization tool resides. This minimized any potential differences of preference due to computer monitor characteristics such as brightness and monitor sizes, luminance. Pairwise comparison utilization studies were performed by utilizing a structured questionnaire to assess the following visualization techniques: (a) GSFM, (b) CCOM, and (c) V_{max} maps utilizing enhanced graphical representation of the principal eigenvector by means of a headless arrow without (VM) and with (VMS) stereoscopic display.

The 8 neuroradiologists were provided with a T1 post-gadolinium image showing each of the five lesions, as well as the patient's demographics, the pathologic diagnosis of the lesion, and the lesion location (see Table 1). Paired sets of different DTI images for the five lesions were also provided, and arranged for direct comparison as follows: (study group 1: GSFM versus CCOM; study group 2: VM versus CCOM; and study group 3: VM versus VMS.

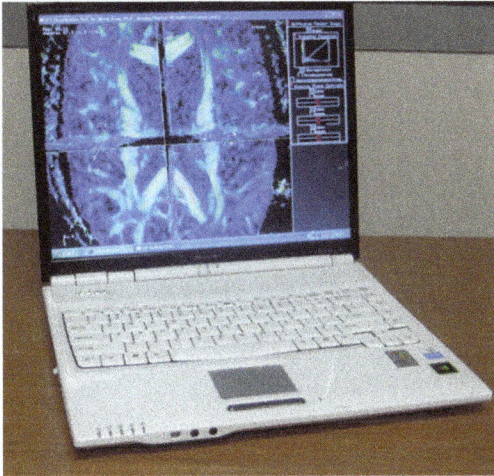

FIGURE 3: Photograph of the stereoscopic DTI processing and visualization tool. The laptop is equipped with a glasses-free LCD monitor. The laptop computer can operate in stereo or nonstereoscopic mode: the user can switch between modes by pushing a button. In stereoscopic mode, the LCD operates in 512×768 matrix size, and while in nonstereoscopic mode the LCD operates at 1024×768.

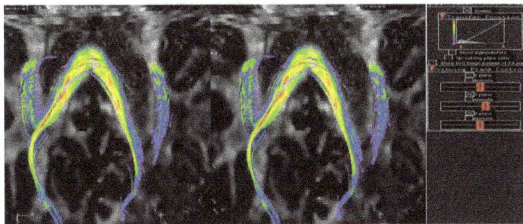

(a)

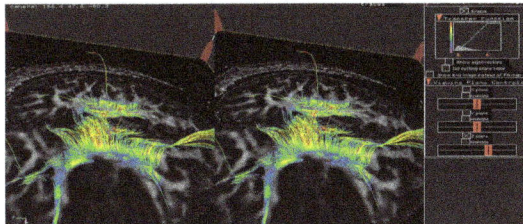

(b)

FIGURE 4: (a) DTI, fiber-tracking function. The fiber-tracking function of the DTI visualization tool is shown stereoscopically in the left-right eye stereo views. Notice the clear spatial separation of all the overlapping tracts once stereoscopic effect is achieved. (b) DTI, stereoscopic view. Color is used to depict other DTI parameters (such as the FA values in figures above) along the tracts.

2.5. Survey Questionnaire (Questions 1–3). For each of the three tests of comparison images (study groups 1–3), the reviewers were asked the following three questions.

Question 1: For the provided pair of images, which of the 2 is the most informative?

Question 2: Rate the strength of your preference. [Equivalent (0), weak (1), moderate (2), strong (3)].

Question 3: Explain the subjective reason for your choice.

TABLE 1: Patient demographics.

Patient no.	Age/sex	Lesion	Location
1	43/F	Breast cancer metastasis	Right frontal
2	4/F	Glioma	Brainstem
3	42/F	Glioblastoma	Left temporal lobe
4	60/F	Astrocytoma	Right frontoparietal
5	62/F	Lymphoma	Corpus callosum

2.6. Survey Questionnaire (Questions 4-5)

Question 4: The neuroradiologists were asked to determine if the adjacent white matter tracts in cases 1 and 3 or middle cerebellar peduncles in case 2 were either (a) involved by the lesion, (b) displaced by the lesion, (c) not affected by the lesion, or (d) if the reviewers were unsure about tract involvement. For the other two cases, (cases 4 and 5), the neuroradiologists were asked which part of the corpus callosal fibers remained intact?

Question 5: The reviewers were then asked about the confidence of their answer. [very unsure (1), unsure (2), undecided (3), confident (4), or very confident (5)].

The study questionnaire is summarized as follows.

Question 1: For the current pair of images which is the most informative?

(a) Image 1
(b) Image 2
(c) No difference.

Question 2: Mark the box that best describes the strength of your preference. [(Equivalent (0), weak (1), moderate (2), strong (3)].

Question 3: Can you explain why you made this choice?

Question 4: Are the corticospinal tracts (cases 1 and 3) or middle cerebellar peduncles (case 2)?

(a) Involved by the lesion
(b) Displaced by the lesion
(c) Not affected by the lesion
(d) Not sure of the answer.

Questions 4 (case 4): Which part of the Corpus Callosum fibers (CC) remains intact?

(a) Rostrum
(b) Genu
(c) Body
(d) Splenium
(e) None
(f) Not sure of the answer.

TABLE 2: Study results—questions 1 and 2.

Case	Study group 1 GSFA versus CCOM		Study group 2 CCOM versus VM		Study group 3 VM versus VMS	
	Prefer	Rank (0–3)	Prefer	Rank (0–3)	Prefer	Rank (0–3)
1	CCOM 8/8	2.38	VM 6/8	2.67	VMS 4/8	1.75
2	CCOM 5/8	2.8	VM 5/8	2.2	VMS 4/8	1.5
3	CCOM 5/8	2.6	VM 7/8	2.57	VMS 3/8	3
4	CCOM 7/8	2.29	VM 6/8	2.5	VMS 3/8	2
5	CCOM 3/8	2.33	VM 8/8	2.38	VMS 4/8	2.25

Questions 4 (case 5): Which part of the Corpus Callosum fibers (CC) is affected?

  (a) Rostrum
  (b) Genu
  (c) Body
  (d) Splenium
  (e) None
  (f) Not sure of the answer.

Questions 5: How confident are you of that answer? [(Very unsure (1), unsure (2), undecided (3), confident (4) very confident (5)].

3. Results

3.1. Questions 1-2

Study Group 1—GSFM versus CCOM. The CCOM was preferred in 70%, (28/40) (40 selections = 8 readers × 5 cases). The ranking for the strength of preference of CCOM (0–3) ranged between 2.3–2.8 (mean 2.5). The GFSA map and "no preference" between the two choices were selected in 15% of the cases each.

Study Group 2—VM versus CCOM. When comparing the VM nonstereoscopic to the CCOM maps, the VM nonstereoscopic was preferred in 80%, (32/40). The ranking for preference of VM nonstereoscopic (0–3) ranged between 2.2–2.7 (mean 2.5). The CCOM and "no preference" between the two choices were each selected in 10% of the cases.

Study Group 3—VM versus VMS. When comparing the VM nonstereoscopic to the VM stereoscopic maps, the VMS stereoscopic was preferred in 45% (18/40) and the VM nonstereoscopic in 35% (14/40). There was no preference in 20% (8/40). The ranking for preference of VM stereoscopic (0–3) ranged between 1.5 and 3.0 (mean 2.1). These results for questions 1 and 2 are further summarized in Table 2.

3.2. Question 3 (Study Groups 1-3).

Subjective reason for preference of CCOM, VM nonstereoscopic and VM stereoscopic, respectively, included more information provided, better delineation of white matter tracts, and easier to determine loss of anisotropy.

3.3. Questions 4-5.

In case 1 (Figure 5), when the neuroradiologists compared the GSFA maps to the CCOM, only 5 of 8 reviewers correctly identified that white matter tracts were invaded by the lesion. The number of reviewers who correctly identified involvement of the tracts rose to 7 of 8 with the CCOM maps and to 8 of 8 with the VM and VMS maps. In case 3 (Figure 6), 3 of 8 reviewers correctly identified that there was displacement of the white matter tracts when reviewing the GSFA maps. This increased to 4 of 8 with the CCOM, VM, and VMS maps.

In the other 3 test questions (cases 2, 4, and 5), there was no difference in detection of white matter tract involvement between the 4 sets of DTI display maps. The results for the test questions and confidence ranking of the reviewers are summarized in the accompanying Table 3.

4. Discussion

Despite the relatively small sample size, our preliminary results demonstrate that the traditional color-coded DTI display (CCOM) seems preferred over the grayscale display (GSFA), and that the nontraditional V_{max} maps (VM and VMS) seem preferred over the traditional color-coded display (CCOM). The subjective reasons for the preference of color-coded display and the V_{max} maps includes better delineation of white matter tracts and ease in determining loss of anisotropy. In 2 of 5 test cases (patients 1 and 3), the color-coded display and V_{max} maps provided better demonstration of white matter tract displacement or involvement. All the neuroradiologists who used this stereoscopic DTI visualization tool were able to achieve the stereoscopic effect with ease, and all stated that stereoscopic display of DTI eigenvectors was more intuitive than the color-encoded method (CCOM).

Traditionally, medical images ranging from X-ray films to computed tomography (CT) and MR images are presented in grayscale. Historically, the reason stemmed from the use of black and white film as the medium for X-ray images, but displaying medical images in grayscale was and still is an intuitive way to visualize scalar images (i.e., images in which each pixel can be represented by a single number) such as X-ray and later CT and MR images. Although there were past attempts to use color or pseudocolor in place of grayscale, they did not take hold in displays of scalar images. The intensity in X-ray and CT images often corresponds to some underlying physiological process, such as tissue density.

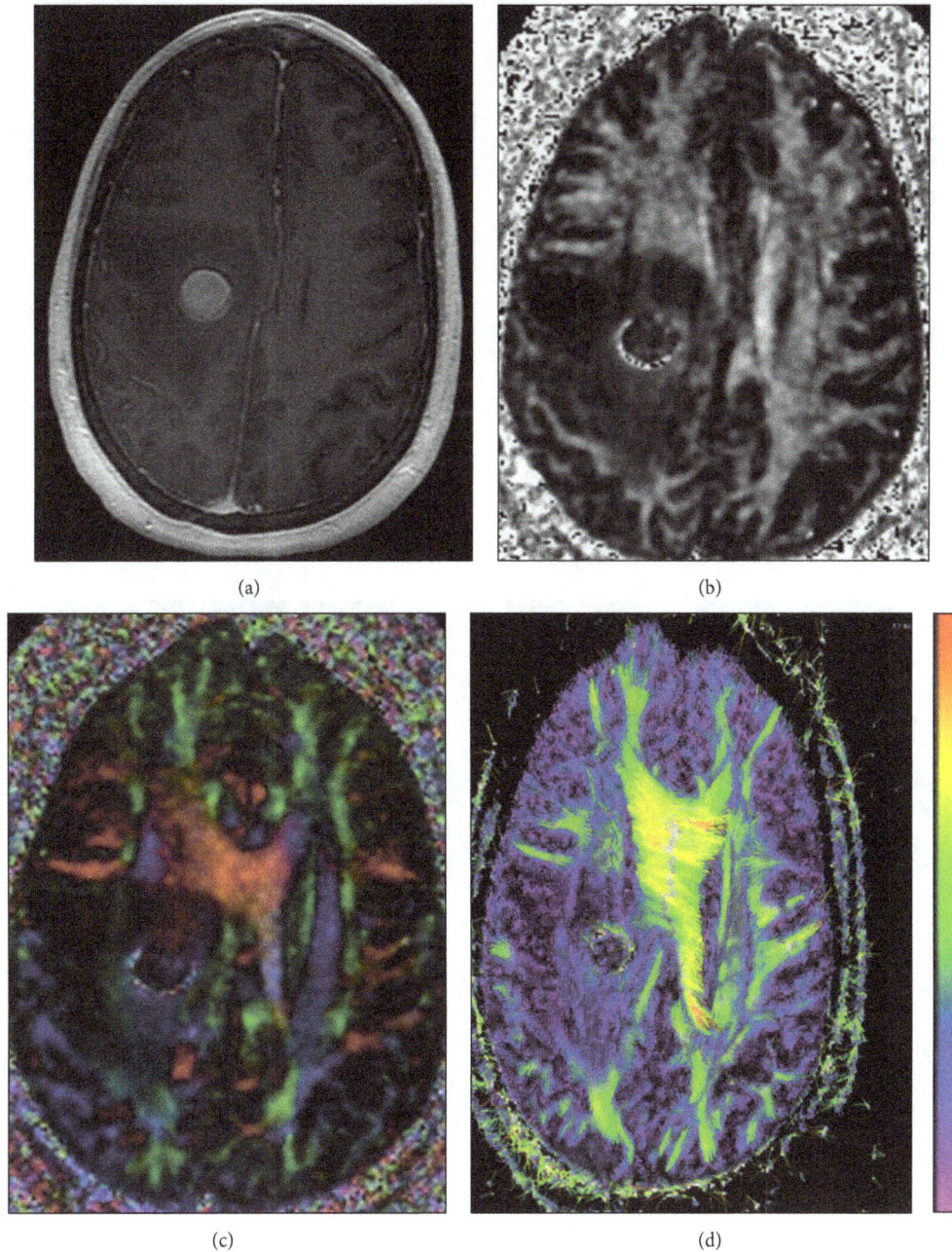

FIGURE 5: A 43-year-old female with breast cancer metastasis to the posterior right frontal lobe. (Case 1): (a) axial T1 postgadolinium; (b) grayscale FA (GSFA) map; (c) color coded orientation map (CCOM); and (d) stereoscopic view. There was an increase from 5 of 8 to 8 of 8 correct responses regarding white matter tract involvement between the GSFA map and VM nonstereoscopic and stereoscopic maps.

TABLE 3: Study results—questions 4 and 5.

Case	Test 1 Tract involvement Correct-Incorrect-Unsure	Test 1 Confidence (1–5)	Test 2 Tract involvement Correct-Incorrect-Unsure	Test 2 Confidence (1–5)	Test 3 Tract involvement Correct-Incorrect-Unsure	Test 3 Confidence (1–5)
1	5-1-2	4	7-1-0	3.57	8-0-0	3.38
2	7-1-0	3.43	7-1-0	3.29	7-1-0	3.57
3	3-5-0	3.67	4-4-0	3	4-4-0	3.25
4	8-0-0	3.75	8-0-0	3.13	8-0-0	3.25
5	7-0-1	3.71	7-0-1	3.57	7-1-0	3.43

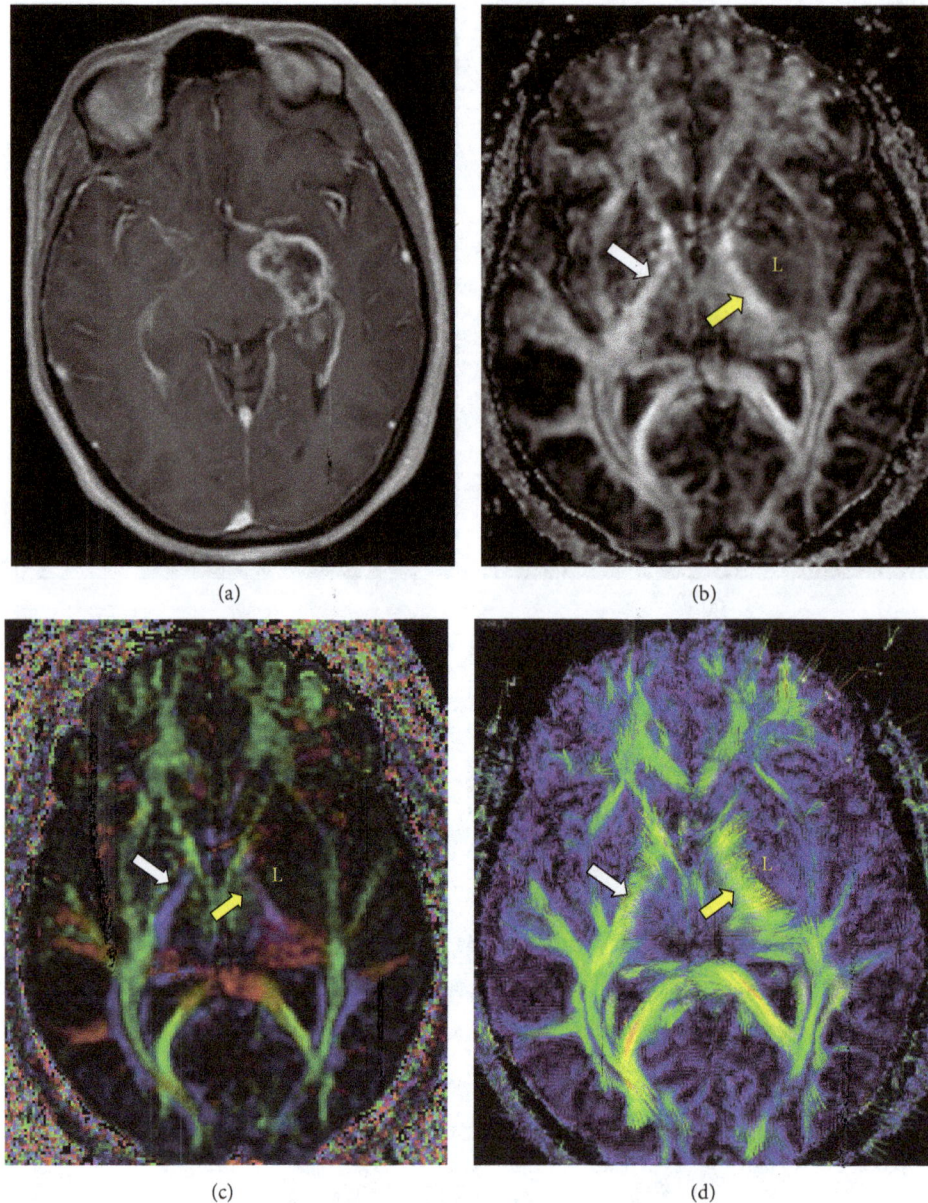

FIGURE 6: A 47-year-old female with left temporal glioblastoma multiform (L). (Case 3): (a) axial T1 postgadolinium; (b) grayscale FA (GSFA) map; (c) color coded orientation map (CCOM); and (d) nonstereoscopic V_{max} view. The question is the left corticospinal tract (CST) (yellow arrow) affected by the lesion or not? The CCOM suggested that the CST was affected by the lesion evidenced by change in its blue color (i.e., fibers have changed their direction), as well as the intensity of the blue color (i.e., fibers have changed their FA value); so conclusion was the CST is infiltrated by the lesion. The V_{max} images suggest that the ipsilateral CST is almost normal, apart from being slightly displaced, and having a higher FA values compared to opposite side (more yellow areas); so the conclusion was that the fibers are only displaced. The higher FA value could reflect the fibers becoming more compact as a result of the mass effect. To resolve this discrepancy, we resorted to the GSFA images as well as the clinical data. The GSFA showed that both CST have almost the same intensity (i.e., FA values) (white arrow = normal CST), so our conclusion was that the fibers are most likely not infiltrated. A through clinical exam revealed that there is no motor affection.

When intensity is considered with spatial distribution (the morphology), the underlying disease process can often be diagnosed.

With the addition of functional and dynamic imaging in recent decades, imaging data became multidimensional and alternative ways to visualize these data had to be implemented. Color, and sometimes the intensity of color, has been successfully employed in the visualization of some multidimensional data, such as in color Doppler ultrasonography. In color Doppler images, a binary color visualization scheme (red and blue) is employed to represent the direction of blood flow in arteries and veins, and the intensity represents the flow speed. Color adds a degree of freedom (or a dimension) in the data representation. Similarly, stereovision can potentially add a degree of freedom in the representation of multidimensional image data.

The current popular visualization tool CCOM uses one dimension, which is the color to represent two variable indices, the direction and the FA value of the axons. Although this might seem to be a more intuitive way to interpret the DTI, great caution must be taken when analyzing the data using this tool that is, when you have a change in the color, should we interpret this as change in the direction of the fibers, in the FA value of the fiber or both? Should we interpret this as infiltration of the fibers by the lesions, or just mere displacement? Further study may provide answers to these questions. Other topics for future investigation may include determining if this technique is applicable in the operating room during the neurosurgical procedures, and if any benefit is added by reviewing diffusion tensor glyphs to the headless arrow.

An obvious advantage of utilizing a stereoscopic view in DTI is that even with a single pair of static images (Figure 3) users can perceive the orientation of the eigenvectors plus the relative spatio-directional information of the WM tracts in the tractography mode. This enables an intuitive visual assessment of FA values along the WM tracts. Since FA values are believed to correlate with some physiological properties of WM tracts, one may use this tool to assess the integrity of WM tracts near or inside a tumor, leading to potential applications in treatment planning and assessment of treatment efficacy in patients with brain tumors. We believe that with the colors of the WM tracts indicating FA values and the stereoscopic views providing spatial information about the tumor volume and the tracts, a user will get a more intuitive visual assessment of the changes (or lack of changes) in the FA values along the WM tracts as they pass near or through a tumor.

5. Conclusion

Processing and visualizing DTI data stereoscopically is feasible, and an initial survey of users indicated that stereoscopic DTI visualization is more intuitive than the color coded orientation maps to humans with normal stereoscopic vision. The tool enables the use of color to indicate the FA values along WM fiber tracts, providing an intuitive technique to visually assess the integrity of the tracts.

Acknowledgments

This work was funded by an institutional grant from the M. D. Anderson Technical Review Committee. The authors thank Dr. Roderick McColl from University of Texas Southwestern Medical Center, Drs. Jason Stafford, Srikanth Mahankali, and Edward Jackson, and Ashok J. Kumar for their valuable feedback in the development of the DTI visualization tool. Osama Raslan and James Matthew Debnam are considered the co-first authors. Dawid Schellingerhout and Jihong Wang are considered the co-senior authors.

References

[1] P. J. Basser, J. Mattiello, and D. Lebihan, "Estimation of the effective self-diffusion tensor from the NMR spin echo," *Journal of Magnetic Resonance B*, vol. 103, no. 3, pp. 247–254, 1994.

[2] P. J. Basser, "Inferring microstructural features and the physiological state of tissues from diffusion-weighted images," *NMR in Biomedicine*, vol. 8, no. 7-8, pp. 333–344, 1995.

[3] P. J. Basser, "New histological and physiological stains derived from diffusion-tenser MR images," *Annals of the New York Academy of Sciences*, vol. 820, pp. 123–138, 1997.

[4] D. Le Bihan, J.-F. Mangin, C. Poupon et al., "Diffusion tensor imaging: concepts and applications," *Journal of Magnetic Resonance Imaging*, vol. 13, no. 4, pp. 534–546, 2001.

[5] E. R. Melhem, S. Mori, G. Mukundan, M. A. Kraut, M. G. Pomper, and P. C. M. Van Zijl, "Diffusion tensor MR imaging of the brain and white matter tractography," *American Journal of Roentgenology*, vol. 178, no. 1, pp. 3–16, 2002.

[6] P. J. Basser and D. K. Jones, "Diffusion-tensor MRI: theory, experimental design and data analysis—a technical review," *NMR in Biomedicine*, vol. 15, no. 7-8, pp. 456–467, 2002.

[7] D. Le Bihan, J.-F. Mangin, C. Poupon et al., "Diffusion tensor imaging: concepts and applications," *Journal of Magnetic Resonance Imaging*, vol. 13, no. 4, pp. 534–546, 2001.

[8] M. R. Wiegell, H. B. W. Larsson, and V. J. Wedeen, "Fiber crossing in human brain depicted with diffusion tensor MR imaging," *Radiology*, vol. 217, no. 3, pp. 897–903, 2000.

[9] C. Nimsky, O. Ganslandt, P. Hastreiter et al., "Preoperative and intraoperative diffusion tensor imaging-based fiber tracking in glioma surgery," *Neurosurgery*, vol. 56, no. 1, pp. 130–137, 2005.

[10] L. Concha, D. W. Gross, B. M. Wheatley, and C. Beaulieu, "Diffusion tensor imaging of time-dependent axonal and myelin degradation after corpus callosotomy in epilepsy patients," *NeuroImage*, vol. 32, no. 3, pp. 1090–1099, 2006.

[11] T. Schonberg, P. Pianka, T. Hendler, O. Pasternak, and Y. Assaf, "Characterization of displaced white matter by brain tumors using combined DTI and fMRI," *NeuroImage*, vol. 30, no. 4, pp. 1100–1111, 2006.

[12] S. J. Price, A. Pena, N.G. Burner et al., "Tissue signature characterization of diffusion tensor abnormalities in cerebral gliomas," *European Radiology*, vol. 14, no. 10, pp. 1909–1917, 2004.

[13] K. Kamada, Y. Sawamura, F. Takeuchi et al., "Functional identification of the primary motor area by corticospinal tractography," *Neurosurgery*, vol. 56, no. 1, pp. 98–108, 2005.

[14] A. S. Field, A. L. Alexander, Y.-C. Wu, K. M. Hasan, B. Witwer, and B. Badie, "Diffusion tensor eigenvector directional color imaging patterns in the evaluation of cerebral white matter tracts altered by tumor," *Journal of Magnetic Resonance Imaging*, vol. 20, no. 4, pp. 555–562, 2004.

[15] S. C. Partridge, P. Mukherjee, R. G. Henry et al., "Diffusion tensor imaging: serial quantitation of white matter tract maturity in premature newborns," *NeuroImage*, vol. 22, no. 3, pp. 1302–1314, 2004.

[16] Z. Ding, J. C. Gore, and A. W. Anderson, "Classification and quantification of neuronal fiber pathways using diffusion tensor

MRI," *Magnetic Resonance in Medicine*, vol. 49, no. 4, pp. 716–721, 2003.

[17] M. R. Wiegell, H. B. W. Larsson, and V. J. Wedeen, "Fiber crossing in human brain depicted with diffusion tensor MR imaging," *Radiology*, vol. 217, no. 3, pp. 897–903, 2000.

[18] Y. Jiang, K. Pandya, O. Smithies, and E. W. Hsu, "Three-dimensional diffusion tensor microscopy of fixed mouse hearts," *Magnetic Resonance in Medicine*, vol. 52, no. 3, pp. 453–460, 2004.

[19] T. G. Reese, R. M. Weisskoff, R. N. Smith, B. R. Rosen, R. E. Dinsmore, and V. J. Wedeen, "Imaging myocardial fiber architecture *in vivo* with magnetic resonance," *Magnetic Resonance in Medicine*, vol. 34, no. 6, pp. 786–791, 1995.

[20] H. Jiang, P. C. M. Van Zijl, J. Kim, G. D. Pearlson, and S. Mori, "DtiStudio: resource program for diffusion tensor computation and fiber bundle tracking," *Computer Methods and Programs in Biomedicine*, vol. 81, no. 2, pp. 106–116, 2006.

[21] G. J. M. Parker, "Analysis of MR diffusion weighted images," *British Journal of Radiology*, vol. 77, no. 2, pp. S176–S185, 2004.

[22] S. Zhang, M. E. Bastin, D. H. Laidlaw, S. Sinha, P. A. Armitage, and T. S. Deisboeck, "Visualization and analysis of white matter structural asymmetry in diffusion tensor MRI data," *Magnetic Resonance in Medicine*, vol. 51, no. 1, pp. 140–147, 2004.

[23] G. Kindlmann, D. Weinstein, and D. Hart, "Strategies for direct volume rendering of diffusion tensor fields," *IEEE Transactions on Visualization and Computer Graphics*, vol. 6, no. 2, pp. 124–138, 2000.

[24] D. B. Ennis, G. Kindlman, I. Rodriguez, P. A. Helm, and E. R. McVeigh, "Visualization of tensor fields using superquadric glyphs," *Magnetic Resonance in Medicine*, vol. 53, no. 1, pp. 169–176, 2005.

[25] C.-F. Westin, S. E. Maier, H. Mamata, A. Nabavi, F. A. Jolesz, and R. Kikinis, "Processing and visualization for diffusion tensor MRI," *Medical Image Analysis*, vol. 6, no. 2, pp. 93–108, 2002.

[26] T. E. Conturo, R. C. McKinstry, E. Akbudak, and B. H. Robinson, "Encoding of anisotropic diffusion with tetrahedral gradients: a general mathematical diffusion formalism and experimental results," *Magnetic Resonance in Medicine*, vol. 35, no. 3, pp. 399–412, 1996.

[27] S. Pajevic and C. Pierpaoli, "Color schemes to represent the orientation of anisotropic tissues from diffusion tensor data: application to white matter fiber tract mapping in the human brain," *Magnetic Resonance in Medicine*, vol. 42, no. 3, pp. 526–540, 1999.

[28] S. Peled, H. Gudbjartsson, C.-F. Westin, R. Kikinis, and F. A. Jolesz, "Magnetic resonance imaging shows orientation and asymmetry of white matter fiber tracts," *Brain Research*, vol. 780, no. 1, pp. 27–33, 1998.

[29] D. B. Ennis and G. Kindlmann, "Orthogonal tensor invariants and the analysis of diffusion tensor magnetic resonance images," *Magnetic Resonance in Medicine*, vol. 55, no. 1, pp. 136–146, 2006.

3

Whole Body Microwave Irradiation for Improved Dacarbazine Therapeutical Action in Cutaneous Melanoma Mouse Model

Monica Neagu,[1] Carolina Constantin,[1] Diana Martin,[2]
Lucian Albulescu,[3] Nicusor Iacob,[2] and Daniel Ighigeanu[2]

[1] *Immunology Department, Immunobiology Laboratory, "Victor Babes" National Institute of Pathology,*
99-101 Splaiul Independentei, sector 5, Bucharest 050096, Romania
[2] *National Institute for Laser, Plasma and Radiation Physics, 409 Atomistilor Street, Magurele 077125, Romania*
[3] *Department of Infectious Diseases and Immunology, Virology Division, Faculty of Veterinary Medicine,*
Utrecht University, Yalelaan 1, 3584 CL Utrecht, The Netherlands

Correspondence should be addressed to Monica Neagu; neagu.monica@gmail.com

Academic Editor: David Maintz

A cutaneous melanoma mouse model was used to test the efficacy of a new therapeutical approach that uses low doses of cytostatics in conjunction with mild whole body microwave exposure of 2.45 GHz in order to enhance cytostatics antitumoral effect. *Materials and Methods.* A microwave exposure system for C57BL/6 mouse whole body microwave irradiation was designed; groups of 40 mice (males and females) bearing experimental tumours were subjected to a combined therapy comprising low doses of dacarbazine in combination with mild whole body irradiation. Clinical parameters and serum cytokine testing using xMAP technology were performed. *Results.* The group that was subjected to combined therapy, microwave and cytostatic, had the best clinical evolution in terms of overall survival, tumour volume, and metastatic potential. At day 14 the untreated group had 100% mortality, while in the combined therapy group 40% of mice were surviving. Quantifying serum IL-1β, IL-6, IL-10, IL-12 (p70), IFN-γ, GM-CSF, TNF-α, MIP-1α, MCP-1, and KC during tumorigenesis and therapy found that the combined experimental therapy decreases all the inflammatory cytokines, except chemokine MCP-1 that was found increased, suggesting an increase of the anti-tumoral immune response triggered by the combined therapy. The overall metastatic process is decreased in the combined therapy group.

1. Introduction

Malignant melanoma (MM) is one of the most aggressive human cancers, since a few mm thick tumors have full potential to kill the host in more than 80% of the cases [1]. Besides the surgical elimination of the primary tumor, there is no other effective cure for MM [1, 2]. MM is resistant to ionizing radiations (radiotherapies) as well as to conventional chemotherapies. The combination of ionizing radiation as well as nonionizing radiation (such as microwaves) with other therapies is reported as a promising strategy in cancer therapy [2].

Microwaves (MW) are presently used or under study for therapeutic applications in areas such as cardiology, urology, general surgery, ophthalmology, and oncology. MW is used as well for organ imaging in the clinical diagnostic of cancer [3].

In the last years there is a revival of therapeutical possibilities to use MW in oncology, in both animal *in vivo* models studies and in clinical trials. Low-intensity microwave radiation used in animal model inoculated with sarcoma 45 cell line has shown that in 50% of animals' tumor growth and partial regression was obtained. The treatment was efficient due to the actual destruction of tumors and accumulation of antitumoral immune cells [4].

Recent technical study revealed that MW can generate *in vivo* a larger ablation zone compared with multipolar radio-frequency (RA) [5]. When used in actual patients presenting hepatocellular carcinoma as liver metastases, MW has the potential to decrease local recurrence when compared to RF-based therapy [6].

A study comprising results gathered for 10 years regarding microwave therapy in scapular tumors has shown that *in situ* microwave therapy for malignant tumors in the scapula can lead to reliable clinical effects and patient acceptability [7]. Treatment of bile duct carcinoma with thin coaxial antenna was recently showing the relation between tissue coagulation size and radiation power shown [8].

Thoroughly reviewed in 2010 [9] the hyperthermia-based therapy, used individually or as additional therapy, can adjoin the surgery for inoperable tumors, can treat relapsed patients without increasing toxicity, and so on. In this seminal review results of phase III randomized trials were shown. The conclusion of this study is that a microwave generator can induce a superficial hyperthermia or a radiofrequency applicator can enter more deeply into the tissues. MW appears to be the fourth treatment pillar beside surgery, radiotherapy, and chemotherapy [10].

MW, as nonionizing radiation, interacts with matter by different physical action, interaction, that is related to their physical parameters: frequency, polarization, modulation, power density, field uniformity, and temperature. The interaction is dependent on the properties of biological materials, expressed in terms of the complex relative permittivity $\varepsilon = \varepsilon' - j\varepsilon''$ with loss tangent $\tan\delta = \varepsilon''/\varepsilon$, biological sample parameters (nature, size and geometry of samples, and sample orientation relative to polarization), and environmental factors (temperature, humidity) [11, 12]. Since the quantum energy of the MW is not sufficient to cause atom ionization [13], its biological effects on tissues may be explained by thermal and nonthermal mechanisms [14]. From this complex array of possible effects, only one biological effect of MW is well known, namely, heating. The effect of MW is explained especially by their heating property on the polar or polarizable molecules of biological systems considered as water dominated dielectrics richly endowed with electrolytes and intricately packaged polar and nonpolar molecules [3, 11, 12, 15]. Some MW biological effects occur over a limited range ("windows") of frequencies or modulations and other biological effects have been reported to occur in multiple dose or intensity ranges, referred to as intensity windows, instead of showing classical ionizing radiation dose-response relationships [11, 14, 16–20]. These effects include, altered cell proliferation, cell membrane receptor-mediated events, alterations of the membrane channels, and many more cellular events.

In cancer treatment, one of the major side effects of chemotherapy is that it can suppress natural killer (NK) cell activity and enhance tumor evolution and metastasis. It was shown that the millimeter-waves (MMWs) irradiation (42.2 GHz) can inhibit tumor metastasis enhanced by cyclophosphamide (CPA), a known anticancer drug [21]. CPA was reported to induce a fivefold enhancement of the tumor process, which was significantly reduced when CPA-treated animals were irradiated with MMWs. MMWs also increased NK cell activity suppressed by CPA, suggesting that the observed reduction of tumor metastasis is mediated through activation of NK cells [21].

Whole body hyperthermia, a procedure in which the body temperature is elevated by MW exposure to 41–43°C, has been investigated as a treatment for cancer, most commonly as an adjunct to radiotherapy (thermoradiotherapy) or chemotherapy (thermochemotherapy) [22–24]. In 2011, it was reported that when combining microwave-based whole body hyperthermia with cytostatics cis-diaminedichloroplatinum (CDDP) and dacarbazine (DTIC) a good antitumoral response was obtained, namely, inhibition of melanoma tumor cell proliferation, reduced neovascularization, and an increase in the specific immune responses [25].

The transient permeable state of the cell membrane obtained by applying short, intense electric pulses, designated as "cell electroporation," was intensively studied both *in vitro* and *vivo*, technique that aimed to introduce nonpermeable molecules into living cells. European clinical experience gathered in the last years regarding this therapy showed good therapeutical results in skin and soft tissue tumours [26–30]. The reported data analysis have showed that proper whole body irradiation with MW enhances the tumoricidal effects of chemotherapy, overcomes acquired drug resistance, and stimulates certain components of the immune system involved in the antitumoral action. Our *in vitro* experiments, on melanoma cell lines [31], have suggested that similarly to the cell membrane electroporation effect, the MW exposure could be able to increase the drug delivery into melanoma cells only at high enough Specific Absorption Rate (SAR) values, that is, at high electric field strength values of the MW electric field component and appropriate Specific Absorption (SA) that overcome the temperature rise over 37-38°C.

DTIC, the only FDA-approved cytostatic for metastatic melanoma [32] is an imidazole carboxamide derivative with several proposed mechanisms of action [33]. Besides the secondary effects, there are several down-falls in DTIC treatment, one being the fact that high dose of DTIC can select a more aggressive form of melanoma phenotype [34]. Overall the main draw back in cutaneous melanoma therapy is its high resistance to cytostatics. Taking into account the DTIC toxicity the main goal of this work was to investigate the effects of small doses chemotherapy in conjunction with total body MW irradiation. Thus, we aimed to enhance tumour sensitivity to cytostatic and enlarged the panel of efficacious therapies using a mouse experimental model. We used low doses of cytostatics combined with MW irradiation in order to enhance drug sensitivity of skin tumours. In terms of DTIC concentration prior published studies in mice models have shown DITC doses as high as 80 mg/kg, with a 5-day administration [35] or 60 mg/kg administration [36]. Thus, we have used a low dose of DTIC, namely, 5 mg/kg/mice. The survival rate of mice, tumour volume, and soluble cytokine monitorization were followed during therapy. Using concomitant detection through multiplexing techniques we have tested cytokines/chemokines highly involved in immune processes triggered by tumour development. The serum pattern of cytokine production was used as efficacy markers for the skin melanoma experimental therapy.

In the last 15 years very few papers were published regarding cutaneous melanoma animal models for experimental therapy with MW. In our model using this combined therapy we decreased the concentration of therapeutical doses of DTIC increasing its clinical efficacy.

2. Material and Methods

2.1. Murine Experimental Model. We have used an established animal model for developing cutaneous melanoma [37], namely, the *in vivo* model of subcutaneous growth of B16 melanoma. Female and male C57BL/6J mice purchased from Jackson Laboratory (Bar Harbor, ME) were maintained in standard conditions in "Victor Babes" National Institute of Pathology Animal Husbandry. Recognized principles of laboratory animal care were followed [38] in the framework of *EU Directive 2010/63/EU for animal experiments.* All animal protocols were approved by "Victor Babes" National Institute of Pathology Animal Care and Use Committee.

All mice 6 weeks old having a mean weight of 20 ± 2 g entered the experimental procedures in groups consisting of 20 males and 20 females. The groups that were supposed to develop the skin melanoma were subcutaneously inoculated with 1×10^5 B16F10 (ECACC 92101204) melanoma cell lines/mouse. In the 7th day after inoculation mice were treated intramuscularly with low doses of DTIC (5 mg/kg/mouse) for 5 days at intervals of 24 h between treatments and subjected to whole body irradiation with MW (SAR = 1.63 W/mouse/day and SA = 74.98 J/mouse/day) in the below described original apparatus. Mice were retroorbitally bled at day 0, day 7 from B16 inoculation, and after treatment. Blood was subjected to serum harvesting and afterwards stored at $-70°$C until testing.

The following groups were tested.

(i) Control mice, tumor free animals, divided in the following groups: untreated (control), subjected to MW irradiation, subjected to combined therapy (MW and DTIC), and subjected only to DTIC.

(ii) Mice bearing B16F10 melanoma tumor untreated.

(iii) Mice bearing B16F10 melanoma tumor divided in the following groups: subjected to MW irradiation, subjected to combined therapy MW, and DTIC and subjected only to DTIC.

MW irradiation was applied concurrently with, prior to, or following DTIC administration. The presented results displayed the best clinical outcome and irradiation followed DTIC inoculation.

2.2. Experimental Procedure: Total Body Irradiation. The MW exposure system (MWES) used for C57BL/6 mouse in a whole body irradiation procedure with microwaves of 2.45 GHz is an innovative and flexible experimental installation (special designed for separate, successive and combined irradiation with MW, and accelerated electron beam) that was previously described and reported in [31]. For better understanding of experiments performed in the frame of this work, we decided to render several features of MWES. It consists mainly of a radiation exposure chamber (REC) and a microwave source of 2.45 GHz with adjustable output power (0–50 W), generated as 10 ms pulses at 50 Hz repetition rate, as REC the multimode rectangular cavity of a proper mechanical and electrical modified MW oven (MEM-MWO) is used. In this installations the conventional operation of

2.45 GHz oven magnetron supplied by an L.C. single-phase-half-wave doublers (L.C. HWD) was modified in order to permit the use of a manually or PC-controlled electronic regulator for the MW power adjustment and remote control [39]. The magnetron main power units consisting of a high voltage diode, a high voltage capacitor, and a high voltage anode transformer (HVAT) are similar to the units used for the conventional magnetron supplying system. Modification consisted in the use of a separate transformer for the filament supply and of a triad controlled regulator added to the HVAT primary circuit. Also, several electronic units are added for MW exposure time presetting as well as for magnetron peak and average current measurement. Another feature added to the MWES operation was obtained by modifying the geometry and rotation velocity of the sample rotary system, as shown in Figures 1(a), 1(b), and 2.

By this procedure the sample rotation velocity can be modified from one rotation per second to one rotation per 30 seconds depending on the desired dose at certain MW power levels. For the experiments with MWES, the C57BL/6 mouse is placed into a special designed cylindrical cage. Figure 2 shows the photograph of this cage containing inside a C57BL/6 mouse. The C57BL/6 mouse cage is made up from a marked cylinder of 250 mL, PMP 2574 type cut at 112 mm from its sole. Two Teflon pistons with aeration apertures assure the mouse immobilization during radiation exposure. During the radiation exposure time the mouse cage can perform two rotation motion types: in the horizontal plane and around its axis (Figure 2).

During one horizontal rotation the mouse cage accomplishes two axial rotations. Horizontal motion transmission to the mouse cage is performed by a Teflon arm fitted to the upper end with an aperture in which a Teflon axle is rotating. On the one Teflon axle end a mouse cage is mounted and on the other end a Teflon friction wheel that is in permanent contact with a fixed platform that generates the cage axial rotation. The desired radiation exposure homogeneity and reproducibility of the C57BL/6 mouse in the cage is obtained by presetting the exposure time so that each mouse is to perform only complete rotations (one, two, or more) inside MEM-MWO multimode cavity during irradiation process. The mouse cage motion starts and interrupts simultaneously with MW switch on and switch off, respectively.

For an approximate evaluation of the MW power amount absorbed by a mouse of certain mass, we determined the dependence of the absorbed MW power by different distilled water and culture medium samples placed in the same geometrical configuration as the mouse's cage. The experimental arrangement (EA) is shown in Figure 3. Because we selected for experiments mice with an initial mass of 20 ± 2 g, it was assumed that during treatment the mouse mass may increase up to 30 g; the sample volumes used in the experiments performed with the installation shown in Figure 3 were 20, 25, and 30 mL.

The proper correlation between magnetron average current and MW power as well as between MW power and SAR characterizing MW exposure is a very difficult procedure because the SAR depends strongly on geometry and electromagnetic properties of exposed material as well as on

(a)

(b)

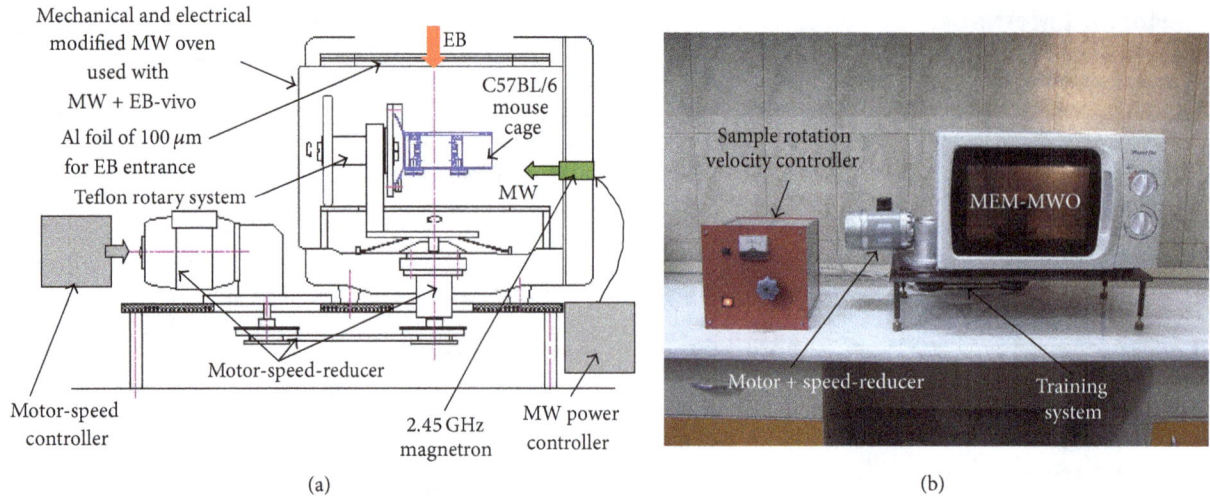

FIGURE 1: (a) Schematic drawing of the MEM-MWO; (b) photograph of the MEM-MWO.

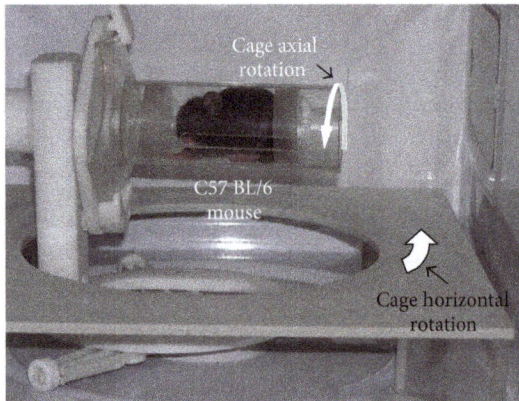

FIGURE 2: Photograph of MEM-MWO internal configuration used with MWES.

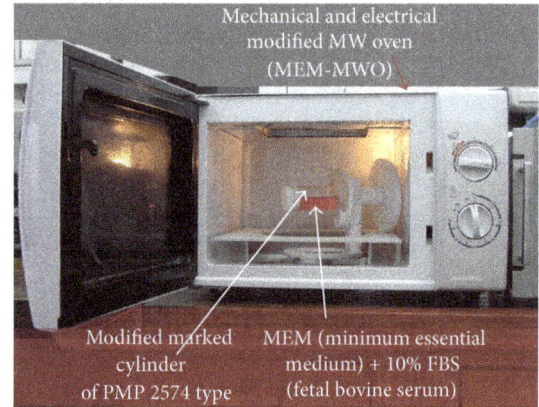

FIGURE 3: Photograph of the MEM-MWO used for an approximate evaluation of the MW power amount absorbed by a mouse.

environmental factors that are variable and cannot be well controlled during treatment especially in *in vivo* conditions. Also, only a small amount of offered MW energy is absorbed by small sample volumes [40]. Different sample volumes absorb different MW energies from the same offered MW energy in the exposure applicator. In our opinion SAR and SA could be given by W per mass of sample mass and J per mass of sample, respectively, pointing out each time the sample nature, geometry, applicator type, and exposure geometry.

The dependence of MW absorbed power (P_A), SAR, and SA versus magnetron average current for distilled water samples is presented in Figure 4(a).

As seen in Figure 4, the MW absorbed power, SAR, and SA depend strongly on water volume of samples (20, 25, and 30 mL) at the same value of magnetron average current. The usage of homogenous animal mass at the procedure start was essential due to SAR and SA parameters that can fluctuate in regard to each mouse mass. During treatment over many days, this need is very difficult to be kept as well as in the case of mice bearing cutaneous melanoma. In these

circumstances, the SAR and SA will increase or decrease depending on the evolution of each mouse mass and tumor volume. As a consequence, the SAR and SA cannot be well controlled during microwave irradiation. The only parameters that can be controlled during microwave irradiation are magnetron average current and MW exposure duration that is correlated with the number of complete rotations of the mouse cage in the horizontal plane and around its axis. Finally we set out to use in our experiments a magnetron average current of 5 mA and a MW irradiation time of 46 s (i.e., two complete horizontal and four complete axial rotations of the cage with C57BL/6J mouse into radiation exposure chamber). The corresponding values for SAR and SA for mice of 20 ± 2 g initial mass are SAR = 1.63 W/mouse (0.0815 W/g) and SA = 74.98 J/mouse (3.749 J/g). These values were established to satisfy our demands that the estimated SAR is as high as possible, while the variation of mouse skin surface temperature during MW exposure is kept in the range of 2–5°C. For these experimental conditions the obtained results were presented in Figure 4(b) and Table 1. As seen

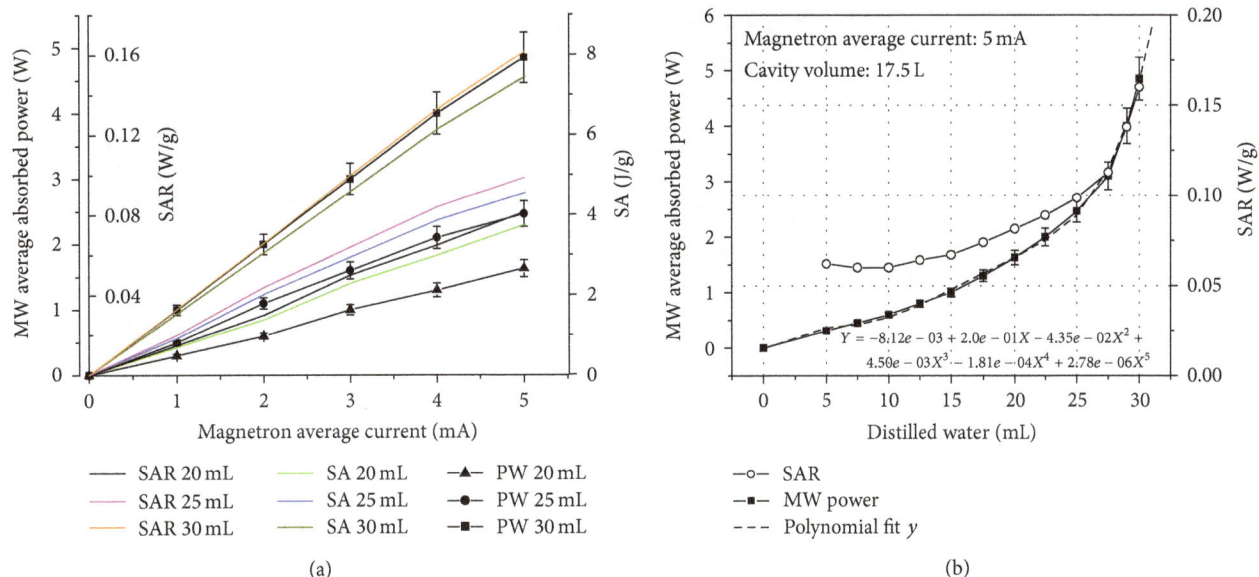

FIGURE 4: (a) P_A, SAR and SA versus magnetron average current for distilled water samples; (b) P_A versus distilled water volume.

TABLE 1: The effect of average mass (AM) of different MW exposed groups on MW absorbed power (P_A) and SAR.

Group	AM (SD) g			P_A (SD) W			SAR (SD) W/g		
	F	M	F + M	F	M	F + M	F	M	F + M
G1	21.7075 (1.0248)	24.81 (2.69293)	23.25875 (2.5116)	1.842 (0.131)	2.485 (0.515)	2.164 (0.494)	0.085 (0.002)	0.099 (0.012)	0.092 (0.011)
G2	21.5875 (1.6229)	24.775 (2.6753)	23.18125 (2.6643)	1.835 (0.200)	2.473 (0.538)	2.160 (0.519)	0.088 (0.006)	0.104 (0.017)	0.096 (0.015)
G3	22.1125 (1.1019)	23.873 (1.3832)	22.9925 (1.4918)	1.901 (0.160)	2.212 (0.592)	2.056 (0.458)	0.086 (0.003)	0.094 (0.011)	0.090 (0.009)
G4	21.6125 (1.4389)	25.15 (1.3143)	23.38125 (2.281)	1.840 (0.205)	2.627 (0.669)	2.234 (0.631)	0.085 (0.003)	0.101 (0.016)	0.094 (0.015)
Mean value	21.755 g	24.6519 g	23.2034 g	1.855 W	2.449 W	2154 W	0.086 W/g	0.100 W/g	0.093 W/g
SD of mean value	0.2439 g	0.5464 g	0.1630 g	0.0311 W	0.1729 W	0.0733 W	0.0014 W/g	0.0042 W/g	0.0026 W/g

Legend: AM: average mass over all treatment days (g); P_A: microwave absorbed power (W); SAR = P_A/AM; F: female; M: male; SD: standard deviation; G1: tumor-free irradiated group; G2: tumor-free irradiated + cytostatic group; G3: tumor bearing irradiated group; G4: tumor bearing irradiated + cytostatic group.

in Figure 4(b) the SAR variation versus sample volume has a lower growth rate than P_A experimental determined versus water volume increasing up to 30 mL. This demonstrates that SAR increasing due to the increasing P_A is partially compensated because its variation is inversely proportional to sample volume. Also, this suggests that although the MW absorbed power could increase or decrease during MW exposure due to the mouse mass variation, assessed SAR expressed as P_A per mouse mass (W/g) will have a lower variation rate than P_A as is shown in Table 1.

As seen in Table 1, the AM (measured average mass of all mice, female and male, over all treatment days with MW) is 23.2034 ± 0.1630 g, corresponding P_A (determined from polynomial fit "y" plotted in Figure 4(b)) is 2.0471 ± 0.02257 W and estimated SAR is 0.0882 ± 0.0005 W/g. This example demonstrates that although AM and P_A are different

values compared with initial values (20 g and 1.63 W) from first treatment day with MW, the SAR value of 0.0882 W/g, averaged over all treatment days, is close to its initial value of 0.0815 W/g.

Figure 5 shows final temperature (T_f) versus number of complete horizontal rotation of mouse cage during MW irradiation with 5 mA magnetron average current for culture medium sample of 20 mL.

The mouse skin surface temperature was measured before and after MW exposure with a non-contact-type infrared thermometer. The mouse surface temperature increased in the range of 3–5°C for healthy mice group and 1.5–3°C for tumor-bearing mice group. The MW irradiation in conjunction with DTIC administration in melanoma bearing mice increased by about 2°C.

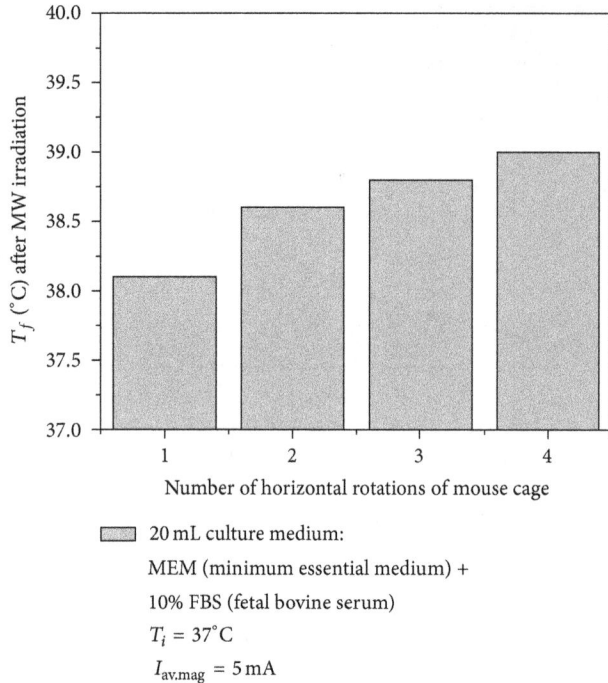

FIGURE 5: Final temperature (T_f) versus number of complete horizontal rotation of mouse cage during MW irradiation with 5 mA magnetron average current ($I_{av.mag}$).

2.3. Clinical Parameters. Tumor volume was measured and expressed in mm^3 according to Egorov [41] after the following formula:

$$V = \frac{\pi}{6} \times (\text{Length}) \times (\text{Width}) \times (\text{Height}). \quad (1)$$

Results are presented as mean ± SD mm^3.

Postmortem necropsies were performed for confirming the presence and extent of neoplastic growth. The sampled tissues were subjected to histological analyses. Survival of mice was monitored until the animals' quality of life was not drastically affected and they were euthanized when required.

2.4. Serum Cytokine Testing Using xMAP Technology. Using Mouse Cytokine/Chemokine Lincoplex Kit (Cat. number MCYTO-70K) and Luminex 200 concomitant serum cytokine were quantified: IL-1β, IL-6, IL-10, IL-12 (p70), IFN-γ, GM-CSF, TNF-α, monocyte chemoattractant protein (MCP-1), macrophage inflammatory protein (MIP-1), and keratinocyte-derived chemokine (KC) after producer's recommendations.

The calibration curves were obtained using the provided standards and the method accuracy was analyzed using the registered high and low controls provided by the producer and laid within the recommended ranges. Results are presented as indexes of the actual pg/mL serum concentrations compared to each proper control (mean ± SD).

For statistical analysis the unpaired Student's t-test was used.

3. Results

3.1. Clinical Parameters in Combined Therapy: Cytostatics and Whole Body Irradiation. Measuring the tumor volume, we have observed that immediately after starting the therapy the groups just "split" in terms of tumor volume (Figure 6(a)). Therefore, as expected, the untreated group has had the highest increase in tumour volume and the increase had the highest rate, while the groups treated with irradiation or only cytostatics have had a similar development. Immediately from the beginning of the experiment, the group subjected to both therapeutical approaches has had a lower volume and a decreased rate of tumour development. At day 14, all mice from the untreated groups have died (Figure 6(b)) and the *postmortem* necropsies and pathology tests have shown, as expected, massive melanoma metastases in all organs, with an increased burden on the brain, lung, pleural membrane, liver, kidney, adrenal glands, lymph nodes, and muscles. The tumor volume of animals treated with cytostatic or irradiated increased at the same rate and, at day 18, all the animals from these groups have died. The tumour of animals subjected to both treatments also had an increased volume, but they were still surviving at day 20 and were euthanized. No significant differences were registered in terms of tumour volume or survival rates between males and females.

Survival rate matches in a good manner the tumour volume increase especially in the untreated group. At day 14 when the untreated group had 100% mortality, in the combined therapy, 40% of mice were surviving. At day 18, whether treated only with the cytostatic or only irradiated, all mice were dead while 25% of the combined therapy group was surviving. This group although bearing tumours as large as 1/3 of their body volume had low extent metastasis. Overall metastasis in combined treated therapy group had lower organ extent compared to controls and/or singular therapy groups.

3.2. Serum Cytokines in Mice Subjected to Combined Therapy. In order to find serum cytokines that can be in the future used as disease or therapy monitoring indicators we have quantified them during clinical evolution. The concentration ranges of serum cytokines varies from 0 to 10,000 pg/mL; thus, we have presented the indexes calculated to each subsequent control.

After 7 days of B16F10 melanoma cell line postinoculation, animals displayed higher serum concentrations of the tested proinflammatory cytokines. This result was to be expected (Figure 7), and overall we have a 7-fold increase for serum IL-1β and for KC, while MIP-1α and IL-6 displayed a 4-fold and 2-fold increase, respectively. It seems that in tumor bearing animals, soluble KC is a parameter that is steadily increasing in the serum. One probable explanation is that melanoma cells can intensively secrete KC [42]; therefore, an on-going tumoral process can be associated with an increase in serum KC.

In the combined therapy groups (Figure 8), after 11 days of therapy, we obtained a clear decrease of inflammatory cytokines. Only the chemotactic molecule, MCP increases statistically significant, while the other cytokines remained

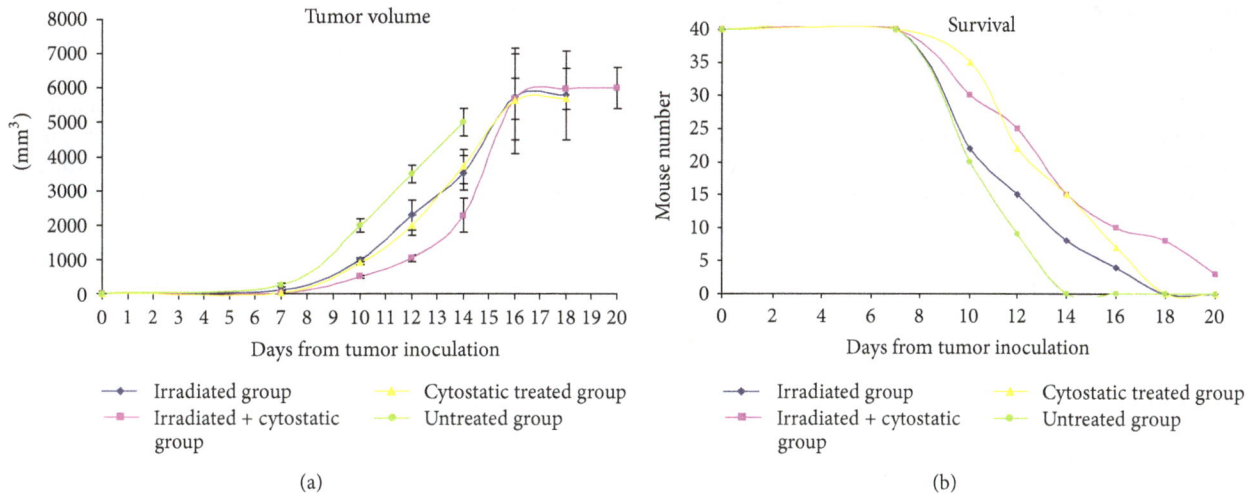

FIGURE 6: Tumor volume (a) and survival rate (b) in mice experimental model.

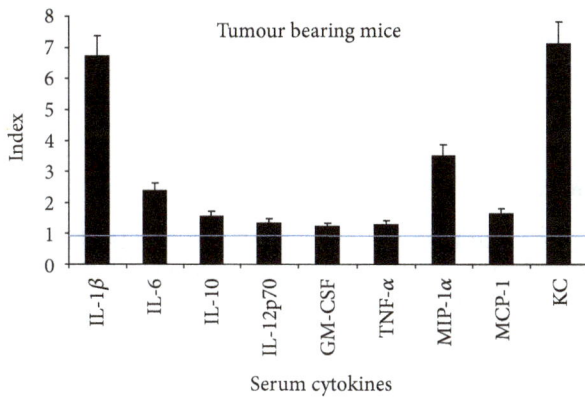

FIGURE 7: Serum cytokines in tumour bearing animals—index calculated in comparison to control group (mean ± SD); straight line depicts control value.

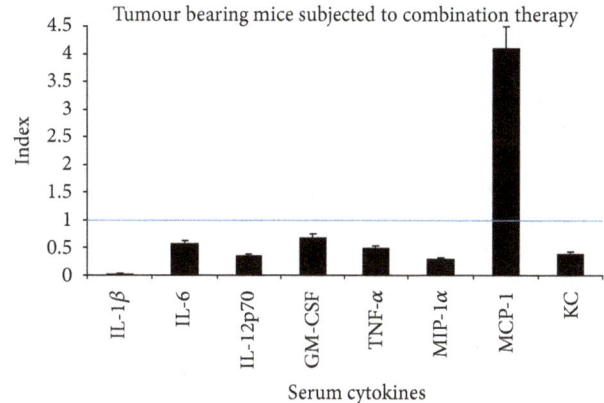

FIGURE 8: Serum cytokines concentrations in tumour bearing animals subjected to combined therapy—index calculated in comparison to untreated group (mean ± SD); straight line depicting cytokines values in untreated tumour bearing animals.

under the ranges detected in nontreated group. MCP is a chemokine involved in attracting and activating both innate and adaptive immune cells and finding it increased is a beneficial sign for the combined therapy antitumor action [43].

4. Discussion

In a previous study that used MW combined with another cytostatic, cyclophosphamide (CPA) [44], it was shown that MW can restore cytokine production that is suppressed by the drug. The study showed that when used with CPA, MW did not present significant clinical improvement. While CPA acts by adding an alkyl group to the guanine base of DNA, for DTIC several mechanisms of action were proposed. As it has a structure similar to a purine it can inhibit DNA synthesis by acting as a purine analog. Moreover, it can act as CPA, namely, acting as an alkylating agent or it can interact with SH groups. We cannot rule out that all these mechanisms could be involved *in vivo*.

The cytokines that we have tested have different functions and in tumour development they intervene at different stages. It was reported that MCP-1 favors tumor angiogenesis and early tumor growth by inducing TNFα, IL-1α, and VEGF by TAMs [45]. Only one recent publication reports the quantification of serum MCP in melanoma bearing mice [46]. In melanoma bearing mice the serum levels of MCP-1, MIP-1β, MCP-3, and inducible protein-10 (IP-10) was found significantly increased compared to controls. A report published few years ago demonstrated that melanoma cells cultured in presence of IFN-γ or TNF-α secreted KC [42]. This finding is more interesting when we add that in tumor bearing animals this chemokine was found significantly increased and after the combined therapy the level of KC decreases considerably.

Investigating the levels of circulating cytokines, IL-1β, 6, 12 p70, GM-CSF, TNF-α, MIP-1α, and KC decreased statistically significantly after combined therapy, while IL-10 was insensitive. MCP-1 proved to have a different behaviour compared to the other circulating tested molecules out of all the tested one, only MCP-1 increased in relation to combined therapy. The possibility of monitoring by means of cytokine serum level the evolution of melanoma was recently published by us in longitudinal melanoma patients followed up for several years [47], thus opening the possibility to enlarge the panel of biomarkers predictors in melanoma therapy.

Another noninvasive new therapy, high intensity focussed ultrasound (HIFU), has gained a large amount of interest due the fact that it provides adequate heating to the full tumor volume, in particular for deep seated tumors, and allows noninvasive tissue heating with high spatial accuracy (~mm). Also, the HIFU combination with classical cancer therapies such as chemo- or radiation therapy, as well as immunotherapy, is attracting growing clinical interest [48]. However, in our opinion, "laser-initiated hyperthermia by heat shock using nanoparticles (NPs)" (such gold NPs) will have a higher potential use in nanomedicine for cancer therapy. These nanoparticles can absorb laser light strongly and then rapidly convert this energy into heat, allowing for the selective destruction of cancer cells at laser energies not sufficient to harm surrounding healthy cells. When such NPs are conjugated to cancer antibodies or other cancer targeting molecules, the cancer cells selectively labeled with those nanoparticles can be easily detected under a simple microscope, due to their strongly enhanced light scattering properties [49]. HIFU therapy has been used in Japan [50], but in other countries this therapy has been reported with contradictory results, sometimes failing [51] and sometimes showing improved results in secondary hyperparathyroidism treatment in patients with chronic kidney disease [52]. More radical negative results were published this year when all the prostate cancer patients treated with HIFU relapsed after approximately 6 years after HIFU treatment [53]. The conclusion of the results published until now using HIFU is the need to accumulate more clinical experience in this type of treatment.

The major problem in cutaneous melanoma is the highly metastatic potential of the tumour and the fact that after surgery cytostatics have low efficacy. In the animal model results herein presented, using whole body mild irradiation, the antitumoral effect of the cytostastics is favoured, lowering its unwanted side effects, such as hindering the immune-based antitumoral action. Moreover, it is known that the metastatic process has a stage where tumour cells are circulating in blood/lymph, so by this therapy these cells can be better triggered with a whole body irradiation than an off-target localized one.

5. Conclusions

We aimed in this study to use microwave therapy to increase the efficacy of DTIC cytostatic and monitor soluble cyto/chemokine production as possible markers for disease evolution in cutaneous melanoma animal model. Whole body irradiation with microwave was performed in an original equipment. The mice group that were subjected to combined therapy had the best clinical evolution and these findings encourage us to state that the used microwave therapy can increase the therapeutical effect of dacarbazine. We have purposely used low dacarbazine dose in order to demonstrate that in conjunction with mild total body microwave irradiation, it could contribute with positive effects to the cancer therapies. The mild total body MW irradiation and drug exposure could be a novel cutaneous melanoma therapy if MW and drug application sequences and doses are optimized and carefully controlled.

Authors' Contribution

Authors Monica Neagu, Carolina Constantin, Diana Martin, Nicusor Iacob, and Daniel Ighigeanu had equally contributed in designing, performing the experiments, and preparing the paper. The authors are thankful to Dr. Gheorghe Savi and Dr. Ileana Savi from "Victor Babes" National Institute of Pathology Animal Husbandry for their help in developing the mice model and the authors regret the too early departure of our colleague Dr. Gheorghe Savi.

Acknowledgment

The presented work was financially supported by the NATO Project Science for Peace Program 982838/2007, PCE-IDE-0318/2011 (Grant no. 113/2011), PN-II-RU-TE-2011-3-2049, PN 01.01/2008, National Research Grants PNII 61-009/2007, and PNII 62-074/2008.

References

[1] J. Tímár, L. Mészáros, A. Ladányi, L. G. Puskás, and E. Rásó, "Melanoma genomics reveals signatures of sensitivity to bio- and targeted therapies," *Cellular Immunology*, vol. 244, no. 2, pp. 154–157, 2006.

[2] J. Yang, G. Jin, X. Liu, and S. Liu, "Therapeutic effect of pEgr-IL18-B7.2 gene radiotherapy in B16 melanoma-bearing mice," *Human Gene Therapy*, vol. 18, no. 4, pp. 323–332, 2007.

[3] A. Rosen, M. A. Stuchly, and A. Vander Vorst, "Applications of RF/microwaves in medicine," *IEEE Transactions on Microwave Theory and Techniques*, vol. 50, no. 3, pp. 963–974, 2002.

[4] T. N. Gudzkova, G. V. Zhukova, L. H. Garkavi, M. I. Sukhanova, O. F. Evstratova, and T. A. Barteneva, "Morphofuctional aspects of antitumor activity of low-intensity microwave resonance radiation in experiment," *Bulletin of Experimental Biology and Medicine*, vol. 150, no. 5, pp. 659–663, 2011.

[5] W. Fan, X. Li, L. Zhang, H. Jiang, and J. Zhang, "Comparison of microwave ablation and multipolar radiofrequency ablation in vivo using two internally cooled probes," *American Journal of Roentgenology*, vol. 198, no. 1, pp. W46–W50, 2012.

[6] Y. Liu, S. Li, X. Wan et al., "Efficacy and safety of thermal ablation in patients with liver metastases," *European Journal of Gastroenterology & Hepatology*, vol. 25, no. 4, pp. 442–446, 2013.

[7] Y.-C. Hu, J.-T. Ji, and D.-X. Lun, "Intraoperative microwave inactivation in-situ of malignant tumors in the scapula," *Orthopaedic Surgery*, vol. 3, no. 4, pp. 229–235, 2011.

[8] K. Saito, K. Tsubouchi, M. Takahashi, and K. Ito, "Practical evaluations on heating characteristics of thin microwave antenna for intracavitary thermal therapy," *Proceedings of the Annual International Conference of the IEEE Engineering in Medicine and Biology Society*, pp. 2755–2758, 2010.

[9] M. Palazzi, S. Maluta, S. Dall'Oglio, and M. Romano, "The role of hyperthermia in the battle against cancer," *Tumori*, vol. 96, no. 6, pp. 902–910, 2010.

[10] R. C. Ward, T. T. Healey, and D. E. Dupuy, "Microwave ablation devices for interventional oncology," *Expert Review of Medical Devices*, vol. 10, no. 2, pp. 225–238, 2013.

[11] S. M. Michaelson and E. C. Elson, "Interaction of nonmodulated and pulse modulated radiofrequency fields with living matter: experimental result," in *Handbook of Biological Effects of Electromagnetic Fields*, CRC Press, 1996.

[12] W. R. Adey, "Biological effects of radiofrequency electromagnetic radiation," in *Interaction of Electromagnetic Waves With Biological Systems*, J. C. Lin, Ed., Plenum Press, New York, NY, USA, 1998.

[13] U. Kaatze, "Fundamentals of microwaves," *Radiation Physics and Chemistry*, vol. 45, no. 4, pp. 539–548, 1995.

[14] M. A. Emekaya, N. Seyhan, and S. Ömeroğlu, "Pulse modulated 900 MHz radiation induces hypothyroidism and apoptosis in thyroid cells: a light, electron microscopy and immunohistochemical study," *International Journal of Radiation Biology*, vol. 86, no. 12, pp. 1106–1116, 2010.

[15] "CSIRO Report, Biological Effects and Safety of EMR," June 1994, http://electricwords.emfacts.com/csiro.

[16] M.-C. Parker, T. Besson, S. Lamare, and M.-D. Legoy, "Microwave radiation can increase the rate of enzyme-catalysed reactions in organic media," *Tetrahedron Letters*, vol. 37, no. 46, pp. 8383–8386, 1996.

[17] H. Bohr and J. Bohr, "Microwave-enhanced folding and denaturation of globular proteins," *Physical Review E*, vol. 61, no. 4B, pp. 4310–4314, 2000.

[18] I. Trosic, I. Busljeta, V. Kasuba, and R. Rozgaj, "Micronucleus induction after whole-body microwave irradiation of rats," *Mutation Research*, vol. 521, no. 1-2, pp. 73–79, 2002.

[19] I. Trosic, I. Busljeta, and B. Modlic, "Investigation of the genotoxic effect of microwave irradiation in rat bone marrow cells: in vivo exposure," *Mutagenesis*, vol. 19, no. 5, pp. 361–364, 2004.

[20] K. K. Kesari and J. Behari, "Effects of microwave at 2.45 GHz radiations on reproductive system of male rats," *Toxicological & Environmental Chemistry*, vol. 92, no. 6, pp. 1135–1147, 2010.

[21] M. K. Logani, I. Szabo, V. Makar, A. Bhanushali, S. Alekseev, and M. C. Ziskin, "Effect of millimeter wave irradiation on tumor metastasis," *Bioelectromagnetics*, vol. 27, no. 4, pp. 258–264, 2006.

[22] I. Green, *Hyperthermia in Conjunction with Cancer Chemotherapy*, Health Technology Assessment 2 Rockville, U.S. Department of Health and Human Services, 1991, http://www.ahcpr.gov/clinic/hypther2.htm.

[23] D. M. Katschinski, G. J. Wiedemann, W. Longo, F. R. d'Oleire, D. Spriggs, and H. I. Robins, "Whole body hyperthermia cytokine

[24] B. Hildebrandt, P. Wust, O. Ahlers et al., "The cellular and molecular basis of hyperthermia," *Critical Reviews in Oncology/Hematology*, vol. 43, no. 1, pp. 33–56, 2002.

[25] D. Jia, W. Rao, C. Wang et al., "Inhibition of B16 murine melanoma metastasis and enhancement of immunity by fever-range whole body hyperthermia," *International Journal of Hyperthermia*, vol. 27, no. 3, pp. 275–285, 2011.

[26] L. M. Mir, "Therapeutic perspectives of in vivo cell electropermeabilization," *Bioelectrochemistry*, vol. 53, no. 1, pp. 1–10, 2001.

[27] T. Kotnik, A. Maček-Lebar, D. Miklavčič, and L. M. Mir, "Evaluation of cell membrane electropermeabilization by means of a nonpermeant cytotoxic agent," *BioTechniques*, vol. 28, no. 5, pp. 921–926, 2000.

[28] S. Satkauskas, M. F. Bureau, M. Puc et al., "Mechanisms of in vivo DNA electrotransfer: respective contribution of cell electropermeabilization and DNA electrophoresis," *Molecular Therapy*, vol. 5, no. 2, pp. 133–140, 2002.

[29] A. Gothelf, L. M. Mir, and J. Gehl, "Electrochemotherapy: results of cancer treatment using enhanced delivery of bleomycin by electroporation," *Cancer Treatment Reviews*, vol. 29, no. 5, pp. 371–387, 2003.

[30] V. Muñoz Madero and G. Ortega Pérez, "Electrochemotherapy for treatment of skin and soft tissue tumours. Update and definition of its role in multimodal therapy," *Clinical and Translational Oncology*, vol. 13, no. 1, pp. 18–24, 2011.

[31] D. Martin, S. Cinca, I. Margaritescu et al., "Combined microwave and electron beam exposure facilities for medical studies and applications," *Journal of Microwave Power & Electromagnetic Energy*, vol. 43, no. 3, pp. 12–20, 2009.

[32] T. DiChiara, "Cancer Chemotherapy for Melanoma: Dacarbazine a Patient's Guide to Cancer Chemotherapy with Dacarbazine," 2009, http://skincancer.about.com/od/treatmentoptions/a/melanoma_chemo.htm.

[33] A. Y. Bedikian, M. Millward, H. Pehamberger et al., "Bcl-2 antisense (oblimersen sodium) plus dacarbazine in patients with advanced melanoma: the oblimersen melanoma study group," *Journal of Clinical Oncology*, vol. 24, no. 29, pp. 4738–4745, 2006.

[34] D. C. Lev, A. Onn, V. O. Melinkova et al., "Exposure of melanoma cells to dacarbazine results in enhanced tumor growth and metastasis in vivo," *Journal of Clinical Oncology*, vol. 22, no. 11, pp. 2092–2100, 2004.

[35] X. H. Zhang, E. Q. Qiao, Z. Gao et al., "Efficacy of combined axitinib with dacarbazine in a B16F1 melanoma xenograft model," *Oncology Letters*, vol. 6, no. 1, pp. 69–74, 2013.

[36] Z. Wang, J. Chen, J. Wang et al., "Novel tubulin polymerization inhibitors overcome multidrug resistance and reduce melanoma lung metastasis," *Pharmaceutical Research*, vol. 29, no. 11, pp. 3040–3052, 2012.

[37] W. W. Overwijk and N. P. Restifo, "B16 as a mouse model for human melanoma," *Current Protocols in Immunology*, vol. 39, pp. 20.1.1–20.1.29, 2001.

[38] *Guide for the Care and Use of Laboratory Animals*, Committee for the Update of the Guide for the Care and Use of Laboratory Animals, National Research Council, 8th edition, 2010.

[39] D. Martin, A. Jianu, and D. Ighigeanu, "A method for the 2.45-GHz magnetron output power control," *IEEE Transactions on Microwave Theory and Techniques*, vol. 49, no. 3, pp. 542–545, 2001.

[40] C. Persch and H. Schubert, "Characterization of household microwave ovens by their efficiency and quality parameter," in *Proceedings of the 5th International Conference on Microwave and High Frequency Heating*, pp. S31.1–S31.4, Cambridge, UK, 1995.

[41] I. K. Egorov, "Mouse models of efficient and inefficient anti-tumor immunity, with emphasis on minimal residual disease and tumor escape," *Cancer Immunology, Immunotherapy*, vol. 55, no. 1, pp. 1–22, 2006.

[42] H. Winter, N. K. van den Engel, D. Rüttinger et al., "Therapeutic T cells induce tumor-directed chemotaxis of innate immune cells through tumor-specific secretion of chemokines and stimulation of B16BL6 melanoma to secrete chemokines," *Journal of Translational Medicine*, vol. 5, article no. 56, 2007.

[43] K. Wetzel, S. Struyf, J. Van Damme et al., "MCP-3 (CCL7) delivered by parvovirus MVMp reduces tumorigenicity of mouse melanoma cells through activation of T lymphocytes and NK cells," *International Journal of Cancer*, vol. 120, no. 6, pp. 1364–1371, 2007.

[44] M. K. Logani, A. Bhanushali, A. Anga, A. Majmundar, I. Szabo, and M. C. Ziskin, "Combined millimeter wave and cyclophosphamide therapy of an experimental murine melanoma," *Bioelectromagnetics*, vol. 25, no. 7, pp. 516–523, 2004.

[45] M. Koga, H. Kai, K. Egami et al., "Mutant MCP-1 therapy inhibits tumor angiogenesis and growth of malignant melanoma in mice," *Biochemical and Biophysical Research Communications*, vol. 365, no. 2, pp. 279–284, 2008.

[46] C. E. Redona, J. S. Dickeya, A. J. Nakamuraa et al., "Tumors induce complex DNA damage in distant proliferative tissues in vivo," *Proceedings of the National Academy of Sciences of the United States of America*, vol. 107, no. 42, pp. 17992–17997, 2013.

[47] M. Neagu, C. Constantin, and S. Zurac, "Immune parameters in the prognosis and therapy monitoring of cutaneous melanoma patients: experience, role, and limitations," *BioMed Research International*, vol. 2013, Article ID 107940, 13 pages, 2013.

[48] G. Pietro and C. Roca, "Results of hyperthermia alone or with radiation therapy and/or chemotherapy," in *Hyperthermia in Cancer Treatment: A Primer, Medical Intelligence Unit*, pp. 119–127, 2006.

[49] P. K. Jain, I. H. ElSayed, and M. A. El-Sayed, "Au nanoparticles target cancer," *Nano Today*, vol. 2, no. 1, pp. 18–29, 2007.

[50] M. Fukugawa, M. Kitaoka, Y. Tominaga et al., "Guidelines for percutaneous ethanol injection therapy of the parathyroid glands in chronic dialysis patients," *Nephrology Dialysis Transplantation*, vol. 18, no. 3, pp. iii31–iii33, 2003.

[51] J. E. de Barros Gueiros, M. C. Chammas, R. Gerhard et al., "Percutaneous ethanol (PEIT) and calcitrol (PCIT) injection therapy are ineffective in treating severe secondary hyperparathyroidism," *Nephrology Dialysis Transplantation*, vol. 19, no. 3, pp. 657–663, 2004.

[52] R. D. Kovatcheva, J. D. Vlahov, J. I. Stoinov et al., "High-intensity focussed ultrasound (HIFU) treatment in uraemic secondary hyperparathyroidism," *Nephrology Dialysis Transplantation*, vol. 27, no. 1, pp. 76–80, 2012.

[53] F. Alongi, R. L. Liardo, C. Iftode et al., "11C choline PET guided salvage radiotherapy with volumetric modulation arc therapy and hypofractionation for recurrent prostate cancer after HIFU failure: preliminary results of tolerability and acute toxicity," *Technology in Cancer Research and Treatment*, 2013.

4

Low Dose X-Ray Sources and High Quantum Efficiency Sensors: The Next Challenge in Dental Digital Imaging?

Arnav R. Mistry,[1] Daniel Uzbelger Feldman,[1] Jie Yang,[2] and Eric Ryterski[3]

[1]*Department of Endodontology, Temple University Kornberg School of Dentistry, 3223 North Broad Street, Philadelphia, PA 19140, USA*

[2]*Oral and Maxillofacial Radiology Department, Temple University Kornberg School of Dentistry, 3223 North Broad Street, Philadelphia, PA 19140, USA*

[3]*E3 Medical, Inc., 941 Garfield Avenue, Louisville, CO 80027, USA*

Correspondence should be addressed to Daniel Uzbelger Feldman; duzbelger@gmail.com

Academic Editor: Sotirios Bisdas

Objective(s). The major challenge encountered to decrease the milliamperes (mA) level in X-ray imaging systems is the quantum noise phenomena. This investigation evaluated dose exposure and image resolution of a low dose X-ray imaging (LDXI) prototype comprising a low mA X-ray source and a novel microlens-based sensor relative to current imaging technologies. *Study Design.* A LDXI in static (group 1) and dynamic (group 2) modes was compared to medical fluoroscopy (group 3), digital intraoral radiography (group 4), and CBCT scan (group 5) using a dental phantom. *Results.* The Mann-Whitney test showed no statistical significance ($\alpha = 0.01$) in dose exposure between groups 1 and 3 and 1 and 4 and timing exposure (seconds) between groups 1 and 5 and 2 and 3. Image resolution test showed group 1 > group 4 > group 2 > group 3 > group 5. *Conclusions.* The LDXI proved the concept for obtaining a high definition image resolution for static and dynamic radiography at lower or similar dose exposure and smaller pixel size, respectively, when compared to current imaging technologies. Lower mA at the X-ray source and high QE at the detector level principles with microlens could be applied to current imaging technologies to considerably reduce dose exposure without compromising image resolution in the near future.

1. Introduction

With all other technical factors (e.g., kilovolts, distance, time, etc.) held constant, patient radiation dose is directly proportional to the milliamperes (mA). A 50% reduction in mA would result in a decrease in radiation dose by 50% [1]. Previously, the mA range has not been taken into consideration in any attempt to reduce radiation dose to which dental patients are being exposed [2–6]. The sensitivity of a digital sensor is measured at a constant wavelength in nanometers (nm) on the basis of the detective quantum efficiency (DQE). This value is used primarily to describe imaging detectors in optical imaging and medical radiography [7]. The quantum efficiency (QE) is the ratio of impinging photons on a pixel to the number of collected electrons. The QE of the pixel is equal to the QE of the complementary metal oxide semiconductor (CMOS) photodiode multiplied for the fill factor of the pixel

[8]. Fluoroscopy is a dynamic X-ray or X-ray movie showing images of video frame rates produced by a low mA X-ray source and image intensification at the detector level [9]. An image intensifier unit is capable of multiplying 1,000 to 20,000 times, electron-by-electron, of the produced image, therefore increasing the system QE while allowing dose reduction [10, 11]. Unfortunately, image intensifier units and direct radiography large flat panel detectors have heretofore been too bulky to be used inside the mouth as well as being expensive for a dental setting [12–14]. Another disadvantage of intensifiers is image distortion [15]. With regard to visualization of a stent created from 50 microns (μm) diameter wires in flat panel X-ray fluoroscopy, for the idealized direct detector, the 100 μm pixel size resulted in maximum measured contrast sensitivity. For an idealized indirect detector, with a scintillating layer, the maximal measured contrast sensitivity was obtained at 200 μm pixel size [16].

The major challenge encountered to decrease the mA level in X-ray imaging systems is the quantum noise phenomena. In electronic imaging systems such as fluoroscopy or intraoral radiography digital sensors, we find three principal sources of noise. The first and most relevant arises from quantum statistics, in which the discrete nature of the radiographic signal (which often is photon-starved) introduces uncertainty into the image. The second is electronic noise which is generated in the detector or detector electronics. The third is quantization error that occurs in digital electronic imaging systems when the signal is digitized. For a quantum statistics noise limited system, if the number of photons used is quadrupled, the noise in the resultant image should be halved [17–20]. Not only X-ray systems but also digital cameras are noise limited and quantum limited. Randomly spaced speckles, called noise, can appear in digital images. Noise is similar to grain that appears in photos taken with traditional cameras using high International Organization of Standardization (ISO) films. Noise increases in photos taken with a digital camera using a high ISO number. The higher ISO number leads to more noise. When noise is present, image detail and clarity are reduced, sometimes significantly. The ISO level indicates the film and digital camera's sensitivity to light. According to the ANSI/ISO classification, a dental film with raw speed of ISO 29–56 would be classified as E speed, while one with speed of ISO 57–112 would be classified as F speed [21]. Photographic film typically has a QE of much less than 10% [22]. Current digital cameras have improved their ISO settings which can achieve up to ISO 204,800 [23–25]. To improve the sensitivity or QE of front illuminated charged couple device (CCD) and CMOS image sensors without increasing their pixel size, digital cameras manufacturers apply a thin (0.5–1.0 mm thickness) and inexpensive microlens array to the sensors to reach high ISO levels [26]. The microlens principle was invented in the 17th century where Hooke and Van Leeuwenhoek developed techniques to make small glass lenses for use with their microscopes [27]. The microlens collects and focuses light that would have otherwise fallen onto the nonsensitive areas of the sensor chip, improving the QE significantly (Figure 1) [28].

Attempts for improving digital sensors QE without compromising the system's noise have been made through the introduction of back illuminated and electron multiplied CCD and CMOS image sensors. Their major drawbacks are complicated manufacturing processes and elevated cost [29, 30]. As a result, the most common used image sensor in dentistry is the front illuminated type [31].

Consequently, a lower milliamperes (mA) setting at the X-ray source and the use of front illuminated sensors with microlens or back illuminated sensors at the detector level for an increased QE that reduces the required radiation dose and sensor pixel size without impacting image quality should have a dramatic positive impact on dental radiology and oral diagnosis. The purpose of this investigation was to prove the concept of radiation exposure reduction and dynamic fluoroscopy feasibility in dentistry without compromising image quality by testing a low-dose X-ray imaging (LDXI) prototype comprising a low-dose X-ray source and a high QE front illuminated sensor with microlens and comparing it to standard of care in terms of dose exposure in milligrays (mGy) and image resolution in lines per millimeters (lp/mm) [6].

2. Materials and Methods

The Temple University Environmental Health and Radiation Safety Institutional Department approved this study. A LDXI prototype (Real Time Imaging Technologies, LLC, Cleveland, OH) was used. The LDXI was comprised of a 35–80 kilovolt peak (kVp), 0.1–0.5 mA X-ray source (9.95′ L × 5.27′ W × 5.35′ H) (SourceRay, Bohemia, NY), and a 8′ rectangular collimator (Margraf Dental, Jenkintown, PA) and an X-ray detector utilizing a CMOS front illuminated sensor (EOS 5D Mark III, Canon, Japan) having 36 × 24 mm effective area, 6.25 × 6.25 um pixel size, 22.3 megapixels resolution, and 49% [32] QE with microlens and capable of performing up to 30 frames per second (fps) for the dynamic video mode. The CMOS sensor modular transfer function (MTF) was >30% at the 18 lp/mm range. Upon low-pass filter and sensor removal, the scintillator/fiber optic plate (AppliedScintech, UK) was coupled at the sensor [33, 34] on top of the microlens [35] with optic glue (BEW Engineering, Ketsch, Germany). The scintillator/fiber optic plate measured 20.8×20.8 mm and was comprised of a 6 um columnar cesium iodide with thallium (CsI : Tl) coating with a MTF curve showing and ultimate resolution >18 lp/mm at 60 kVp with 98% attenuation at 70 kVp. Camera software (EOS Utility Ink, Japan) and a kid's watch (Disney Store, Orlando, FL) were used in order to establish and calibrate sensor's ISO settings. Images obtained were raw positive still shots and video. Raw images (A) were converted to negative radiographic images (B) through a software and then cropped (Microsoft Digital Suite 2006 Editor, Microsoft, Redmond, WA) (Figure 2).

Ionization chambers Radcal 9010 (Radcal Corp., Monrovia, CA) and RaySafe Xi (RaySafe, Hopkinton, MA) were used to measure the dose exposure in mGy (obtained through rad formula conversion) received by a patient phantom (DXTTR, RINN, Elgin, IL) in all groups and sixteen dosimeters (Landauer, Inc., Glenwood, IL) were utilized for obtaining the dose equivalent in millisievert (mSv) (obtained through rem formula conversion) received by the operator simulated distance at 30 cm for LDXI and fluoroscopy (Figure 3).

ISO settings were established at ISO 5,000 for group 1 and ISO 12,800 for group 2 and image acquisition was made at 1/30 shutter (0.03 seconds). Group 1 was exposed to the LDXI prototype (Real Time Imaging Technologies, LLC, Cleveland, OH) at 0.2 mA and 80 kVp in static mode during 10 intervals from 0 to 27 continuous seconds with a 6.25 × 6.25 um pixel size sensor and 49% QE. Group 2 was exposed to the LDXI prototype at 0.2 mA and 80 kVp in the dynamic video mode during 31 intervals from 0 to 300 seconds with a 6.25 × 6.25 um pixel size sensor and 49% QE. Group 3 was exposed to medical fluoroscopy (GE C-arm OEC 9800, Cleveland, OH) at 0.038 mA and 55 kVp in 31 intervals from 0 to 300 seconds with a 12.8 × 12.8 um pixel size sensor and a 9′ image

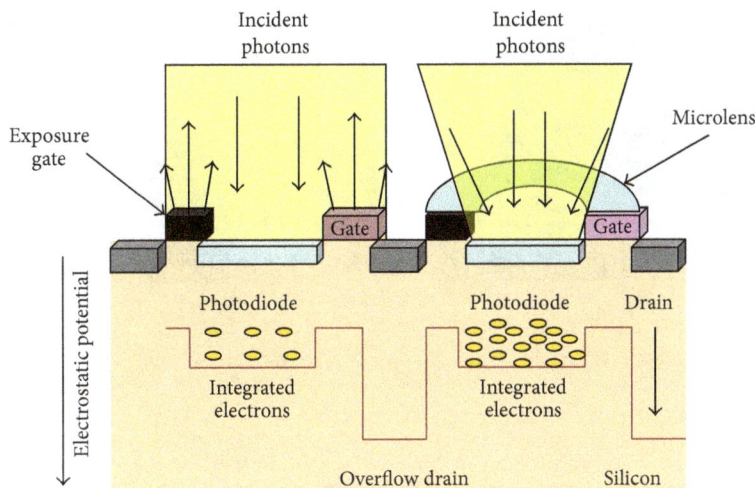

FIGURE 1: CMOS sensor and microlens (right side) architecture scheme.

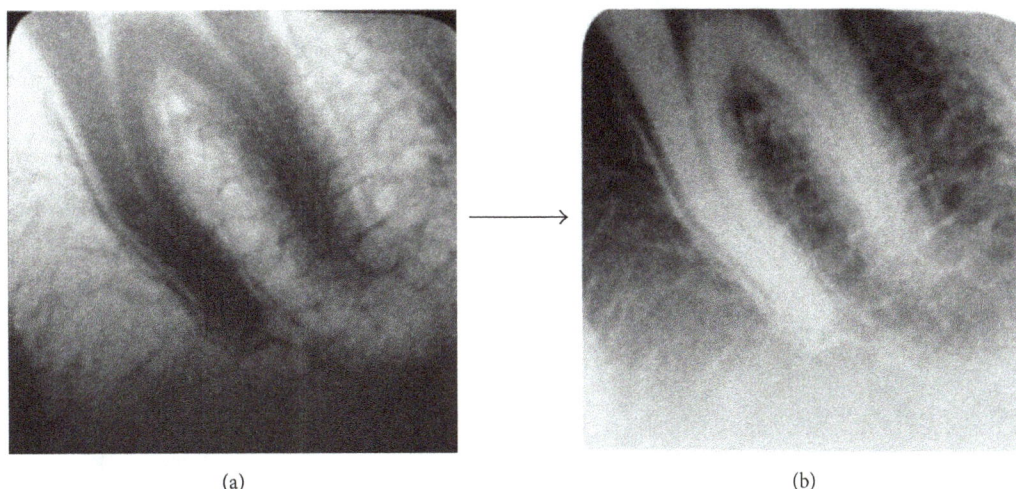

(a)   (b)

FIGURE 2: (a) Molar tooth raw positive image obtained at 0.2 mA and 1/30 camera shutter (0.03 seconds) with collimation and (b) negative image.

intensifier with 65% QE at 550 nm [36]. Group 4 was exposed to digital intraoral radiography (Gendex GX-770, Hatfield, PA/Planmeca Dixi 2 v3, Roselle, IL) at 7 mA and 70 kVp in 29 intervals from 0 to 1.65 seconds with a 19 × 19 um pixel size sensor. Group 5 was exposed to CBCT Scan (iCat Imaging Sciences International Inc., Hatfield, PA) at 5 mA and 120 kVp from 0 to 26.9 seconds in 28 intervals and several modalities with a 125 um voxel size sensor. Six thermoluminescent Luxel and ten optical stimulated luminescence technology Nanodots dosimeters (Landauer, Inc., Glenwood, IL) were used at the patient phantom, area monitor, and positive and negative controls for the LDXI. After research completion, all the dosimeters were mailed back to Landauer for analysis purposes. Image resolution for the LDXI was measured with a resolution test pattern (Fluke Corp., Cleveland, OH) in lp/mm. An endodontic file size 10 (Dentsply, Maillefer, York, PA) was placed within phantom's tooth number 27 at the radiographic apex for intraoral imaging subjective resolution assessment purposes in which two endodontists and one oral and maxillofacial radiologist from the institution were asked to confirm tooth's working length [6]. Dose exposure measurements and image resolution were calculated for all groups and dosimeters were analyzed.

3. Results

The Mann-Whitney test showed no statistical significance ($\alpha = 0.01$) in dose exposure (mGy) between groups 1 and 3 and 1 and 4 and timing exposure (seconds) between groups 1 and 5 and 2 and 3 (Figure 4).

Dosimeters for the LDXI operator simulated distance and controls did not register significant dose equivalent (mSv).

Image resolution test showed LDXI 1 > digital intraoral radiography > LDXI 2 > medical fluoroscopy > CBCT scan (Table 1).

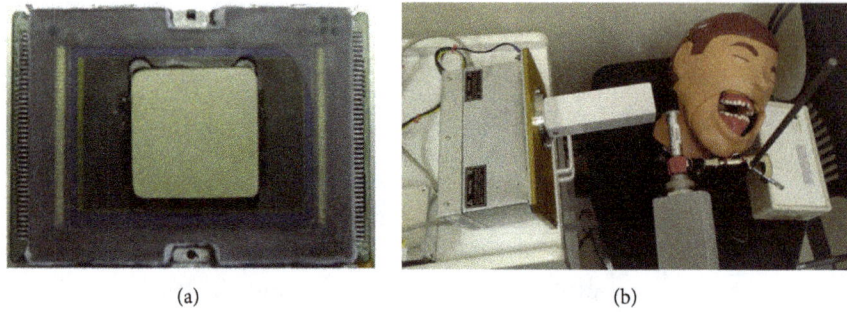

(a)   (b)

FIGURE 3: (a) Dental size sensor with microlens coupled with scintillator/FOP (front view) and (b) LDXI prototype testing on the DXTTR phantom at 0.2 mA and 80 kVp.

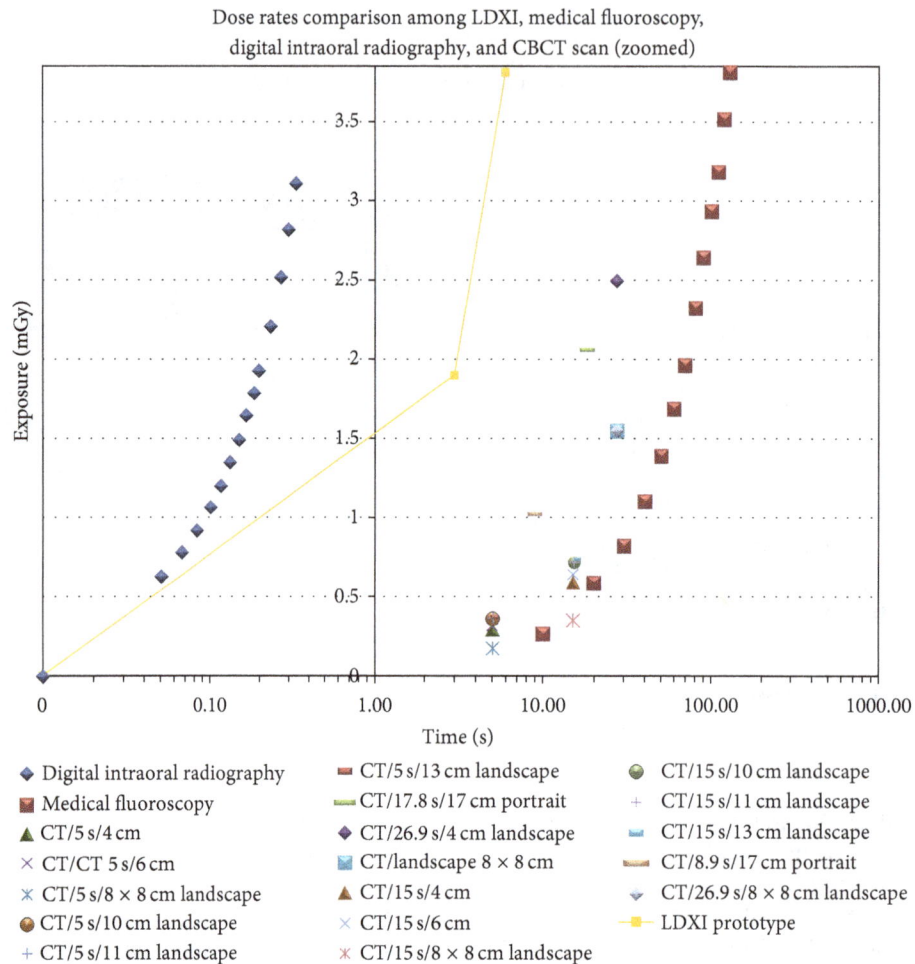

FIGURE 4: Radiation and timing exposures comparison amongst all groups.

File size 10 was observed at the working length as confirmed by two endodontists and one oral and maxillofacial radiologist (Figure 5).

4. Discussion

Technical advances enable cameras to better capture the drama of low-light photography/video. As a rule, bigger is indeed better when it comes to the overall dimensions of a sensor because a bigger sensor provides not only more pixels, but also bigger pixels, which more efficiently gather light. However, of all the improvements in the imaging field, perhaps the most notable are not the increases in sensor size but the innovations in increasing a sensor's ability to gather light in low-light situations and to record a wider range of light. Much improved sensors with microlens now allow one to

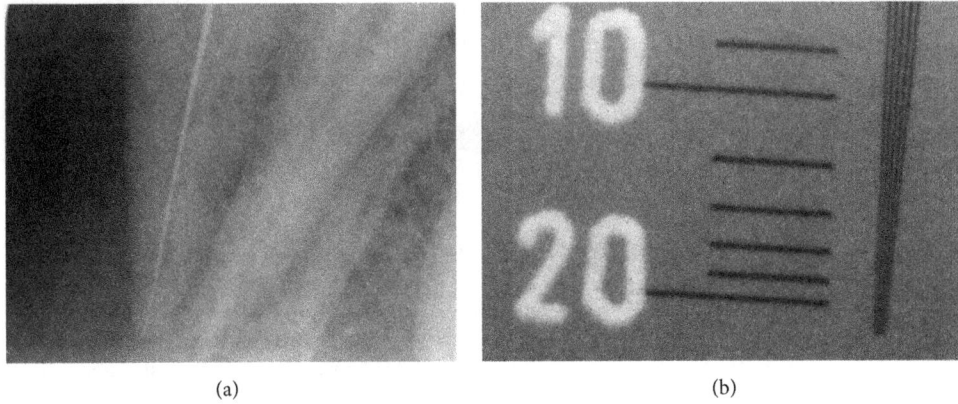

(a)   (b)

FIGURE 5: Group 1 LDXI static: (a) endodontic file number 10 at working length and (b) 18 lp/mm.

TABLE 1: mA, kVp, pixel size settings, and resolution outcome comparison of different devices.

Device type	mA	kVp	Pixel/voxel size (um)	Resolution (lp/mm)
LDXI 1 (static)	0.2	80	6.25 × 6.25	18
LDXI 2 (dynamic)	0.2	80	6.25 × 6.25	10
Medical fluoroscopy (image intensified)	0.038	55	12.8 × 12.8	1.75
Digital intraoral radiography	7	70	19 × 19	16
CBCT scan	5	120	125	1.6

obtain detailed low-light images by allowing shots at high ISO levels that previously generated unflattering digital "noise" or graininess in an image at smaller pixel sizes. From an image resolution dental perspective, studies have demonstrated that spatial resolution affects bone loss and caries diagnosis in dentistry. A research undertaken to determine the effect of X-ray beam alignment and spatial resolution on quantification of alveolar bone using radiometric techniques concluded that 50 um pixel spatial resolution is apparently superior to 200 um pixel images if radiometric data is to be evaluated [37]. Another study determined that spatial resolution affected radiometric analyses aimed at detecting progressive enamel loss. Cumulative percent histograms shifts associated with the smaller 59 um pixels accounted for 68% of the variation in weights caused by enamel reduction, whereas the shifts associated with the larger 200 um pixels accounted for 50%. The results indicated that pixel size does affect radiometric determinations of enamel reduction [38, 39]. In summary, the smaller the pixel size and the more pixels are arranged in a sensor, the better the quality of the image that is captured. In this study, microlens also allows decreasing the sensor's pixel size (6.25 × 6.25 um), therefore increasing image spatial resolution as compared to the larger pixel size of current sensors used in digital intraoral radiography (19 × 19 um), CBCT scans (125 um voxel), and medical fluoroscopy

(12.5 × 12.5 um for image intensifiers and 100 × 100 um for flat panel detectors). As compared to similar front illuminated intraoral sensors used in dentistry (DQE 3% CCD and DQE 18% CMOS) [40, 41] the LDXI prototype has used a large size (35 mm), full frame, and front illuminated CMOS sensor with a thin microlens array for improved DQE (49%) directly coupled to the scintillator/fiber optic plate, capable of acquiring low mA images at ISO 5,000 and ISO 12,800 as well as in dynamic video frame rates. From a radiation exposure perspective, we found that 3.05 and 3.95 seconds of LDXI are comparable to one single shot of 0.2 seconds of digital intraoral radiography and 26.9 seconds 4 cm landscape single area CBCT scan, respectively. As a result, the LDXI used for 0.2 seconds would reduce 93.4% dose exposure as compared to digital intraoral radiography used for 0.2 seconds. For a conventional root canal requiring a pre-op, working length, master cone, partial condensation, and final X-ray, the LDXI prototype could be used during 15 seconds without producing more dose exposure due to the addition of microlens for increased QE as compared to digital intraoral radiography. As a result, lower mA settings (up to 0.2 mA) as compared to digital intraoral radiography (7 mA) could be captured at 18 lp/mm and 10 lp/mm image resolution for the static and dynamic modalities, respectively [6]. In addition, an endodontic file size 10 was observed at the working length at the phantom as confirmed by two endodontists and one oral and maxillofacial radiologist from the institution (Figure 5). In addition to root canals, other clinical applications for low dose X-ray sources and high QE image sensors in the static mode would be full mouth X-rays, pre- and postradiographs, bitewings, and panoramic, cephalometric, and CBCT scans for oral diagnosis while the dynamic mode would allow the introduction of fluoroscopy in dentistry for dental implant placement, temporomandibular joint analysis, maxillofacial surgeries, and postplacement. Since the scintillator/fiber optic plate was coupled in the central area of the sensor, the effect of X-rays on the surrounding, residual, and uncovered area caused significant noise causing black spots at the image. In addition, despite the fact that sensor's housing was internally masked against light, light pollution was observed on one corner (Figure 6).

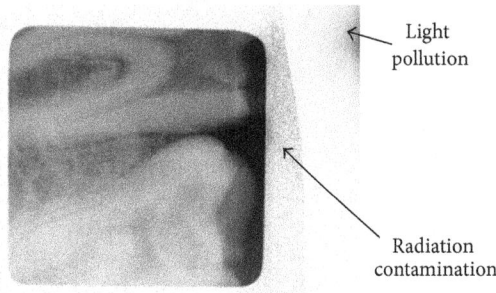

FIGURE 6: Preventable artifacts obtained in images.

These artifacts should be avoided in future studies by providing complete sensor shielding and a 100% light proof housing. In addition to further evaluations with higher QE (>65% at 550 nm) new generation front illuminated sensors with microlens, the authors recommend testing a back illuminated sensor due to its increased QE as compared to the front illuminated sensor used in this study [14, 35]. Finally, we propose testing the next generation LDXI using head and neck anthropomorphic phantoms following Sections C and D of the FDA guidance for Solid State X-Ray Imaging Devices (MTF, detective quantum efficiency, and signal-to-noise ratio) and compare it to digital intraoral radiography, medical fluoroscopy, and CBCT scan imaging devices.

5. Conclusions

The LDXI proved the concept for obtaining a high definition image resolution for static and dynamic radiography at lower or similar dose exposure and smaller pixel size, respectively, when compared to traditional imaging devices. Lower mA at the X-ray source and high QE at the detector level principles with microlens could be applied not only to digital intraoral radiography and dental fluoroscopy but also to panoramic, cephalometric, and CBCT scans devices to considerably reduce X-ray source dose exposure as well as sensor pixel size and more research is recommended to demonstrate this further.

Diclosure

The paper, or any part of it, has not been submitted or published and will not be submitted elsewhere for publication while being considered by the journal. The research has been shown as a poster presentation at Temple University Kornberg School of Dentistry Research Day and has been presented at the 64th AAOMR Annual Session as an abstract and as part of the 2013 William H. Rollins Award Lecture.

Acknowledgments

This study has been possible thanks to the funds received by Real Time Imaging Technologies, LLC (Cleveland, OH), from the Great Lakes Innovation & Development Enterprise Grant ($25,000) and the Indus Entrepreneurs (TiE) Ohio Business Plan Competition Award ($2,500) as well as by the research team from Temple University Kornberg School of Dentistry Student Research Grant ($2,000).

References

[1] Q. B. Carroll, *Fuchs's Radiographic Exposure and Quality Control*, Charles C Thomas Publisher, 7th edition, 2003.

[2] D. Uzbelger, "Comparison between medical fluoroscopy, digital dental imaging and intraoral radiography," *Journal of Dental Research*, vol. 97, p. 701, 2005.

[3] D. Uzbelger-Feldman, C. Susin, and J. Yang, "The use of fluoroscopy in dentistry: a systematic review," *Oral Surgery, Oral Medicine, Oral Pathology, Oral Radiology, and Endodontology*, vol. 105, article e61, 2008.

[4] D. Uzbelger Feldman, J. Yang, and C. Susin, "A systematic review of the uses of fluoroscopy in dentistry," *The Chinese Journal of Dental Research*, vol. 13, no. 1, pp. 23–29, 2010.

[5] D. Uzbelger Feldman, P. M. Panchal, and J. Yang, "Resolution and dose rates comparison among fluoroscopy, digital/film-based intraoral radiography and CBCT scan," in *Proceedings of the 61th Annual Meeting of the American Academy of Oral & Maxillofacial Radiology*, San Diego, Calif, USA, 2010.

[6] D. Uzbelger Feldman, A. Mistry, and J. Yang, "Radiation exposure and image resolution testing of a low-dose X-ray imaging," in *Proceedings of the 64th Annual Meeting of American Academy of Oral & Maxillofacial Radiology*, Beverly Hills, Calif, USA, October 2013.

[7] A. R. Cowen, A. G. Davies, and M. U. Sivananthan, "The design and imaging characteristics of dynamic, solid-state, flat-panel x-ray image detectors for digital fluoroscopy and fluorography," *Clinical Radiology*, vol. 63, no. 10, pp. 1073–1085, 2008.

[8] G. C. Holst and T. S. Lomheim, *CMOS/CCD Sensors and Camera Systems*, SPIE Press Book, Bellingham, Wash, USA, 2nd edition, 2011.

[9] B. D. Giordano, S. Ryder, J. F. Baumhauer, and B. F. DiGiovanni, "Exposure to direct and scatter radiation with use of mini-c-arm fluoroscopy," *Journal of Bone and Joint Surgery—Series A*, vol. 89, no. 5, pp. 948–952, 2007.

[10] J. T. Thirlwall, "The detective quantum efficiency of medical x-ray image intensifiers," *Review of Scientific Instruments*, vol. 69, no. 11, pp. 3953–3957, 1998.

[11] S. Hasham, F. D. Burke, S. J. Evans, M. K. Arundell, and D. N. Quinton, "An audit of the safe use of the mini c-arm image intensifier in the out-patient setting," *Journal of Hand Surgery*, vol. 32, no. 5, pp. 563–568, 2007.

[12] J. A. Seibert, "Flat-panel detectors: how much better are they?" *Pediatric Radiology*, vol. 36, no. 14, pp. 173–181, 2006.

[13] D. Uzbelger Feldman, "Real Time Imaging Technologies, LLC, Assignee. Apparatus for Diagnosis and/or Treatment in the Field of Dentistry using Fluoroscopic and Conventional Radiography," US Patent 6543936, 2003.

[14] D. Uzbelger Feldman, "Real Time Imaging Technologies, LLC, assignee. Dental Fluoroscopic Imaging System," US patent 8,430,563, April 2013.

[15] D. P. Chakraborty, "Image intensifier distortion correction," *Medical Physics*, vol. 14, no. 2, pp. 249–252, 1987.

[16] Y. Jiang and D. L. Wilson, "Optimization of detector pixel size for stent visualization in x-ray fluoroscopy," in *Medical Imaging 2004: Image Perception, Observer Performance, and Technology Assessment*, vol. 5372 of *Proceedings of SPIE*, p. 311, May 2004.

[17] B. A. Arnold and P. O. Scheibe, "Noise analysis of a digital radiography system," *American Journal of Roentgenology*, vol. 142, no. 3, pp. 609–613, 1984.

[18] D. W. Mah, J. A. Rowlands, and J. A. Rawlinson, "Measurement of quantum noise in fluoroscopic systems for portal imaging," *Medical Physics*, vol. 23, no. 2, pp. 231–238, 1996.

[19] M. Hensel, T. Pralow, and R. R. Grigat, "Modeling and real-time estimation of signal-dependent noise in quantum-limited imaging," in *Proceedings of the 6th WSEAS International Conference on Signal Processing, Robotics and Automation (ISPRA '07)*, World Scientific and Engineering Academy and Society, Corfu Island, Greece, February 2007.

[20] S. Suh, S. Itoh, S. Aoyama, and S. Kawahito, "Column-parallel correlated multiple sampling circuits for CMOS image sensors and their noise reduction effects," *Sensors*, vol. 10, no. 10, pp. 9139–9154, 2010.

[21] American National Standards Institute, *Photography—Direct-Exposing Medical and Dental Radiographic Film/Process Systems—Determination of ISO Speed and ISO Average Gradien*, American National Standards Institute ISO, New York, NY, USA, 1991.

[22] F. Träger, *Handbook of Lasers and Optics*, Springer, Berlin, Germany, 2012.

[23] M. K. Khoury, I. Parker, and D. W. Aswad, "Acquisition of chemiluminescent signals from immunoblots with a digital single-lens reflex camera," *Analytical Biochemistry*, vol. 397, no. 1, pp. 129–131, 2010.

[24] T. Ang, *Digital Photography: An Introduction*, DK Publishing, New York, NY, USA, 4th edition, 2012.

[25] The British Journal of Photography Report. The 50 Best Photography Products of 2012. The British Journal of Photography, Apptitude Media Ltd., London, UK, 2012.

[26] R. F. Stevens and N. Davies, "Lens arrays and photography," *The Journal of Photographic Science*, vol. 39, pp. 199–208, 1991.

[27] R. Hooke, *Micrographia: or some Physiological Descriptions of Minute Bodies made by Magnifying Glasses*, The Royal Society of London, London, UK, 1st edition, 1665.

[28] P. H. Nussbaum, R. Völkel, H. P. Herzig, M. Eisner, and S. Haselbeck, "Design, fabrication and testing of microlens arrays for sensors and microsystems," *Pure and Applied Optics*, vol. 6, no. 6, pp. 617–636, 1997.

[29] R. A. Stern, L. Shing, N. Waltham, H. Mapson-Menard, A. Harris, and P. Pool, "EUV and soft X-ray quantum efficiency measurements of a thinned back-illuminated CMOS active pixel sensor," *IEEE Electron Device Letters*, vol. 32, no. 3, pp. 354–356, 2011.

[30] S. N. Vasan, P. Sharma, C. N. Ionita et al., "Image acquisition, geometric correction and display of images from a 2x2 x-ray detector array based on electron multiplying charge coupled device (EMCCD) technology," in *Medical Imaging 2013: Physics of Medical Imaging*, vol. 8668 of *Proceedings of SPIE*, Lake Buena Vista, Fla, USA, 2013.

[31] A. G. Farman and T. T. Farman, "A comparison of 18 different x-ray detectors currently used in dentistry," *Oral Surgery, Oral Medicine, Oral Pathology, Oral Radiology and Endodontics*, vol. 99, no. 4, pp. 485–489, 2005.

[32] http://www.sensorgen.info/CanonEOS_5D_MkIII.html.

[33] R. G. van Silfhout and A. S. Kachatkou, "Fibre-optic coupling to high-resolution CCD and CMOS image sensors," *Nuclear Instruments and Methods in Physics Research Section A: Accelerators, Spectrometers, Detectors and Associated Equipment*, vol. 597, no. 2-3, pp. 266–269, 2008.

[34] H. Fan, H. L. Durko, S. K. Moore et al., "DR with a DSLR: digital radiography with a digital single-lens reflex camera," *Proceedings of the Society of Photo-Optical Instrumentation Engineers*, vol. 15, p. 7622, 2010.

[35] D. Uzbelger Feldman, "Real time imaging technologies, LLC, assignee. Imaging apparatus and methods," International patent application PCT/US13/49504, July 2013.

[36] W. K. Chu, C. Smith, R. Bunting, P. Knoll P, R. Wobig, and R. Thacker, "Application of the CCD camera in medical imaging," in *Sensors, Cameras, and Systems for Scientific/Industrial Applications, 121*, vol. 3649 of *Proceedings of SPIE*, San Jose, Calif, USA, January 1999.

[37] M. K. Shrout, J. Weaver, B. J. Potter, and C. F. Hildebolt, "Spatial resolution and angular alignment tolerance in radiometric analysis of alveolar bone change," *Journal of Periodontology*, vol. 67, no. 1, pp. 41–45, 1996.

[38] M. K. Shrout, C. M. Russell, and B. J. Potter, "Spatial resolution in radiometric analysis of enamel loss A pilot study," *Oral Surgery, Oral Medicine, Oral Pathology, Oral Radiology, and Endodontics*, vol. 81, no. 2, pp. 245–250, 1996.

[39] A. Wenzel, F. Haiter-Neto, and E. Gotfredsen, "Influence of spatial resolution and bit depth on detection of small caries lesions with digital receptors," *Oral Surgery, Oral Medicine, Oral Pathology, Oral Radiology and Endodontology*, vol. 103, no. 3, pp. 418–422, 2007.

[40] A. C. Mörner-Svalling, *Digital intraoral radiography: determination of technical properties and application evaluations [Dissertation]*, Department of Oral Radiology and Oral and Maxillofacial Surgery, Institute of Odontology, Karolinska Institute, Stockholm, Sweden, 2002.

[41] H. S. Cho, S. G. Choi, B. S. Lee, and S. Kim, "Image quality evaluation of a highly-integrated digital X-ray imaging sensor for dental intraoral-lmaging applications," *Journal of the Korean Physical Society*, vol. 51, no. 1, pp. 30–34, 2007.

5

Image Guidance in Radiation Therapy: Techniques and Applications

Shikha Goyal and Tejinder Kataria

Division of Radiation Oncology, Medanta Cancer Institute, Medanta-The Medicity, Gurgaon, Haryana 122001, India

Correspondence should be addressed to Shikha Goyal; drshikhagoyal@gmail.com

Academic Editor: Paul Sijens

In modern day radiotherapy, the emphasis on reduction on volume exposed to high radiotherapy doses, improving treatment precision as well as reducing radiation-related normal tissue toxicity has increased, and thus there is greater importance given to accurate position verification and correction before delivering radiotherapy. At present, several techniques that accomplish these goals impeccably have been developed, though all of them have their limitations. There is no single method available that eliminates treatment-related uncertainties without considerably adding to the cost. However, delivering "high precision radiotherapy" without periodic image guidance would do more harm than treating large volumes to compensate for setup errors. In the present review, we discuss the concept of image guidance in radiotherapy, the current techniques available, and their expected benefits and pitfalls.

1. Introduction

Radiotherapy has always required inputs from imaging for treatment planning as well as execution, when the treatment target is not located on the surface and inspection and visual confirmation are not feasible. Traditional radiotherapy practices incorporate use of anatomic surface landmarks as well as radiologic correlation with two-dimensional imaging in the form of port films or fluoroscopic imaging.

Broadly, imaging has two major roles in radiotherapy:

(a) Sophisticated imaging techniques such as contrast enhanced computed tomography (CECT) scans, magnetic resonance imaging (MRI), positron emission tomography (PET) scans, and angiography obtain three-dimensional (3D) structural and biologic information which is used to precisely define the target and thus enable precise and accurate treatment planning with shaped beams in isocentric or non-isocentric geometry.

(b) "In-room" imaging methods (planar, volumetric, video, or ultrasound-based) obtain periodic information on target position and movement (within the same session or between consecutive sessions),

compare it with reference imaging, and give feedback to correct the patient setup and optimize target localization. They also have the potential to provide feedback that may help to adapt subsequent treatment sessions according to tumor response.

More specifically, modern day radiotherapy regards the latter application with "in-room" imaging as "image guided radiation therapy" (IGRT).

Modern external beam radiotherapy techniques such as intensity modulated radiation therapy (IMRT), volumetric modulated arc therapy (VMAT), stereotactic radiosurgery (SRS), or stereotactic radiotherapy (SRT) have helped reduce the safety margin around the target volumes thus allowing for lower normal tissue doses without compromising delivery of tumoricidal doses. However, there is a great deal of uncertainty in accurately defining of the position of targets during the delivery of fractionated radiotherapy, both during a given fraction and between successive fractions. Targets that may move during treatment due to respiratory or peristaltic movements or with cardiac pulsations create an even bigger challenge. Hence, there is need to develop and implement strategies to measure, monitor, and correct these uncertainties. This has led to evolution of various in-room imaging technologies which enable evaluation and correction of setup errors, anatomic changes related to weight loss or deformation, or internal organ motion related to respiration, peristalsis, or rectal/bladder filling.

Brachytherapy treatment planning also incorporates orthogonal X-ray imaging and fluoroscopy for guiding brachytherapy catheter/applicator placement, volumetric imaging with CT or MRI for applicator identification and reconstruction, and plan optimization in three dimensions based on imaging. Isodose distribution is reviewed and optimized on visualizing dose distribution to the target as well as critical structures. This adds to treatment efficacy and safety.

2. The Concept of IGRT

Though technically complex, surgical procedures enable the operating surgeons to directly visualize and handle their targets, thus eliminating the ambiguity in identification and appropriate management. Radiotherapy, despite being a local therapy that aims to achieve similar goals, inherently carries the disadvantage of making a significant number of assumptions when using traditional treatment techniques. The 3D image dataset acquired at simulation is a snapshot of the tumor, its relation to normal structures, and the patient's shape and position at a single time point, and it is this model that is used for plan development and dose calculation. During the planning stage, a lot of assumptions based on prior experience and literature are used with regard to clinical target volume (CTV) margins to define the microscopic spread around the tumor and planning target volume (PTV) margins to incorporate the expected range of internal organ motion and setup errors. The treatment is then carried out with the belief that all those assumptions would hold true for any given patient during daily treatment sessions, the foremost being that the patient and tumor anatomy and their positions with respect to the positioning devices have remained unchanged since the time of simulation. However, the assumption that the dose calculated on the CT dataset on the planning system matches the dose delivered through each fraction or through the entire radiation therapy course is grossly in error. Additionally, the internal organs and targets move with respiration and peristalsis and planning radiotherapy on a static image dataset is unable to account for errors due to this motion. To ensure that all of these assumptions do not compromise the dose delivery to the CTV, wider PTV margins are taken. This causes a large volume of normal tissues to be included in the irradiated volume. IGRT gives a method to capture this information regularly during the treatment course in the form of serial "snapshots" and is a means of verifying accurate and precise radiation delivery. In simple terms, the IGRT process ensures that the delivered treatment matches the intended treatment in accurately targeting the tumor while minimizing "collateral damage." Changes to the composite delivered dose and their impact on disease control as well as toxicity may be minimized by use of appropriate localization devices and PTV margins. Occasionally, replanning may be required if gross deviations beyond predetermined tolerances are observed [1–3].

IGRT allows assessment of geometric accuracy of the "patient model" during treatment delivery. It provides a method whereby deviations of anatomy from initial plan are determined and this information is used to update dosimetric assumptions. Correction strategies may include daily repositioning to register patient position in accordance with the base plan or recalculation of treatment delivery in real time to reflect the patient's presentation during a given fraction. This philosophy of reevaluating treatment and accounting for the differences between actual patient anatomy on a given day and the snapshot of planned treatment is known as adaptive radiotherapy [4]. The eventual goal is to reevaluate and in certain situations redefine daily positioning for treatment to keep it on the same track as the intended treatment. Future applications may include dose titration for maximizing effect or mitigating side effects.

3. Errors and Margins

An error in radiotherapy delivery is defined as any deviation from intended or planned treatment. A great degree of uncertainty is inherent to radiotherapy practices and may be in the form of mechanical uncertainties related to treatment unit parameters such as couch and gantry motion, patient uncertainties related to ability to lie comfortably in a certain position and cooperate during the treatment time, geometric uncertainties related to position and motion of target, and dosimetric uncertainties. IGRT deals with the geometric uncertainties, which may be either intrafractional or interfractional [5, 6].

Both inter- and intrafractional uncertainties may be a result of a combination of systematic and random errors. A systematic error is essentially a treatment preparation error and is introduced into the chain during the process of positioning, simulation, or target delineation. This error, if uncorrected, would affect all treatment fractions uniformly. A random error, on the other hand, is a treatment execution error, is unpredictable, and varies with each fraction. Systematic errors shift the entire dose distribution away from the CTV, while random errors blur this distribution around the CTV. Of the two, systematic error is more ominous since it would have a much larger impact on treatment accuracy and hence the therapeutic ratio.

Margins are added to the CTV to take these errors into account. These margins are geometric expansions around the CTV and may be non-uniform in all dimensions depending on the expected errors. These margins ensure that dosimetric planning goals are met despite the variations during and between fractions. ICRU 62 defines the expansion of PTV around the CTV as a composite of two factors—internal target motion (internal margin) and setup variations (setup margin) [7]. Depending on observed systematic and random errors in a given setup for a particular treatment site, a variety of recipes for calculating PTV margins exist in literature [8, 9]. To enhance the therapeutic ratio, a host of correction strategies may be applied to reduce these margins and may include online or offline correction of interfraction errors or real time correction of intrafraction motion. Tracking and correcting organ motion helps reduce internal margin while improved accuracy of positioning reduces setup margins, thus reducing the required PTV margin.

4. Offline versus Online Corrections

Offline and online IGRT correction strategies refer to whether the patient is on the treatment couch while the verification is being done and whether the correction would be applied to the same or subsequent sessions.

In the offline strategy, images are acquired before treatment and matched to the reference image at a later time point. This strategy aims to determine the individual systematic setup error and thus reduce it. When combined with setup data of other patients treated under the same protocol, it helps define the population standard error for that treatment in that institution. Widely used offline correction protocols include Shrinking action level and No action level protocols [10, 11]. PTV margins in an institution depend on these determinations of individual and population systematic errors.

An online strategy, on the other hand, employs acquisition of images and their verification and correction prior to the day's treatment. It aims to reduce both random and systematic errors. The treatment site and the expected magnitude of error may determine the frequency of online imaging. Sites where large daily shifts are anticipated (abdomen, pelvis, and thorax) or where even slight shifts will alter the dose distribution within adjacent critical structures (paraspinal tumors, intracranial tumors in close proximity to optic structures) are best managed with daily imaging. Our experience with online corrections showed the maximum errors in thorax followed closely by abdomen and pelvis. The minimum errors were observed in head and neck region [12]. Additionally, treatments such as VMAT and SBRT carry the potential to translate minor shifts into major alterations in dose distribution and hence require daily online verification. For daily online correction, systematic and random errors may be calculated from the matched data. Post-treatment imaging is required to quantify both intrafraction motion and residual errors. If evaluated for a patient population, these data may help check the PTV margin for that treatment protocol. In fact, the use of daily online imaging with corrections in conjunction with use of automatic couch with 6 degrees of freedom has obviated the need for invasive frames for SRS treatments [13].

5. IGRT Technology Solutions

Depending on the imaging methods used, the IGRT systems may broadly be divided into radiation based and nonradiation based systems [14, 15].

5.1. Nonradiation Based Systems [16–22]. These may employ ultrasound, camera-based systems, electromagnetic tracking, and MRI systems integrated into the treatment room.

5.1.1. Ultrasound-Based Systems. These systems (e.g., BAT, SonArray, Clarity) acquire 3D images that help align targets to correct for interfractional errors. Geometric accuracy is 3–5 mm and the greatest advantage is lack of any ionizing radiation. Sites of common application include prostate, lung, and breast radiotherapy.

5.1.2. Camera-Based (Infrared) or Optical Tracking Systems. These systems identify the patient reference setup point positions in comparison to their location in the planning CT coordinate system, which aids in computing the treatment couch translation to align the treatment isocenter with plan isocenter. Optical tracking may also be used for intrafraction position monitoring for either gating (treatment delivery only at a certain position of target) or repositioning for correction. Tools such as AlignRT image the patient directly and track the skin surface to give real time feedback for necessary corrections. These systems have found application in treatment of prostate and breast cancer and for respiratory gating using external surrogates. Geometric accuracy is 1-2 mm, but application is limited only to situations where external surface may act as a reliable surrogate for internal position or motion.

5.1.3. Electromagnetic Tracking Systems. These systems (e.g., Calypso) make use of electromagnetic transponders (beacons) embedded within the tumor, and motion of these beacons may be tracked in real time using a detector array system. Beacons need to be placed through a minimally invasive procedure, their presence may introduce artifacts in MR images, and there are limitations to the patient size. Calypso has a geometric accuracy of <2 mm, but its use at present is limited to prostate radiotherapy.

5.1.4. MRI-Guided IGRT. These systems (e.g., ViewRay) help real time assessment of internal soft tissue anatomy and motion using continual soft tissue imaging and allow for intrafractional corrections. Geometric accuracy of the system is 1-2 mm. However, MRI has certain drawbacks such as motion artifacts, distortion with non-uniform magnetic fields, and cannot be performed for patients with pacemakers or metallic implants. All these limitations of diagnostic MRI apply to this IGRT system as well. A wide application potential exists in treatment of prostate, liver, and brain, as well as for brachytherapy.

5.2. Radiation Based Systems. These include static as well as real time tracking, using either kilovoltage (KV), megavoltage (MV), or hybrid methods.

5.2.1. Electronic Portal Imaging Devices (EPID). EPID was developed as a replacement of film dosimetry for treatment field verification and is based on indirect detection active matrix flat panel imagers (AMFPIs). They are offered as standard equipment by nearly all linear accelerator (LINAC) vendors as both field verification and quality assurance (QA) tools. Image acquisition is 2D, with a geometric accuracy of 2 mm. Bony landmarks on planar images are used as

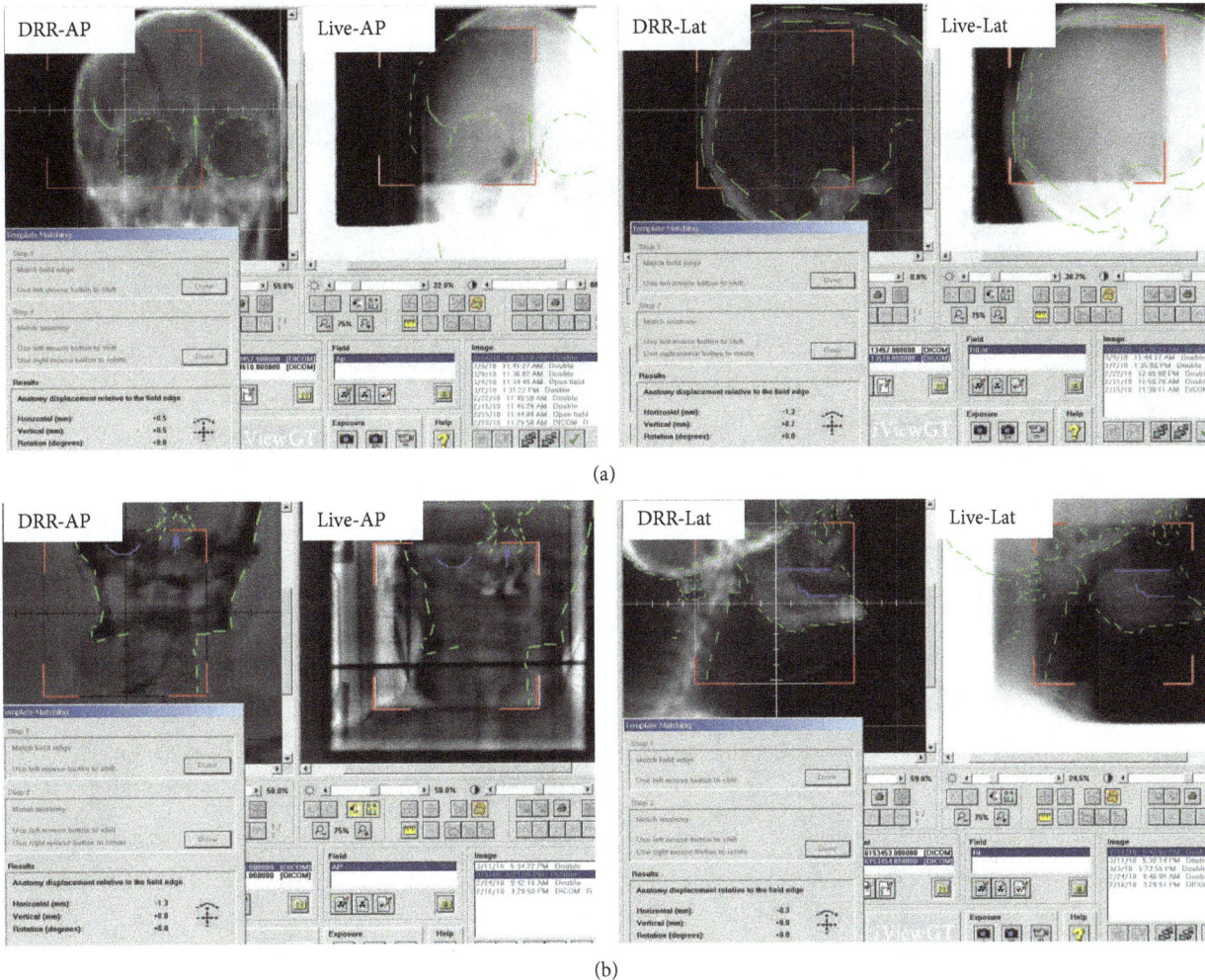

FIGURE 1: Use of MV EPID for online correction using orthogonal 2D images (anteroposterior and lateral). Both the field and the bony anatomy are matched sequentially to give an estimate of error. The comparison of live image with reference DRR helps assess and correct translational shifts but does not estimate rotational errors. (a) Right parietal glioma. (b) Head and neck cancer. MV: Megavoltage; EPID: Electronic portal imaging device; 2D: two-dimensional; DRR: Digital reconstructed radiograph.

surrogates for defining positional variations respective to the digital reconstructed radiographs (DRRs) developed from the planning CT dataset (Figure 1). Different systems may use either KV or MV X-rays for imaging, with the image contrast being superior with KV images while there is lesser distortion from metallic implants (dental, hip prostheses) in MV images. EPID systems are unable to detect or quantify rotations. Average dose per image is 1–3 mGy for KV systems while it is as high as 30–70 mGy for MV systems [23–25].

5.2.2. Cone Beam CT (CBCT), KV or MV. These systems consist of retractable X-ray tube and amorphous silicon detectors mounted either orthogonal to (Elekta Synergy, Varian OBI) or along the treatment beam axis (Siemens Artiste). These have capability of 2D, fluoroscopic and CBCT imaging. Another system (Vero, BrainLAB) consists of a gimbaled X-ray treatment head mounted on an O-ring with two KV X-ray tubes, two flat panel detectors, and an EPID.

The O-ring can be rotated 360 degrees around the isocenter and can be skewed 60 degrees around its vertical axis. Geometric accuracy is 1 mm or lesser with possibility of 2D and 3D matching with DRRs or X-ray volumetric images generated from planning CT data sets. Scanning is done through a continuous partial or complete gantry rotation around the couch, acquiring the "average" position of organs with respiratory motion. Both interfraction setup changes and anatomical changes related to weight changes or organ filling (bladder, rectum) may be monitored (Figure 2). Repeat scans at the end of treatment may give an estimate of intrafractional changes. For tumors discernible separately from surrounding normal tissue, treatment response may also be monitored and these scans may be used for dose recalculation or treatment plan adaptation after necessary image processing. KV CT gives better contrast resolution compared to MV CT but may be limited by artifacts from prostheses and scatter from bulky patient anatomy. Average dose per image is 30–50 mGy [26–29].

(a)

(b)

(c)

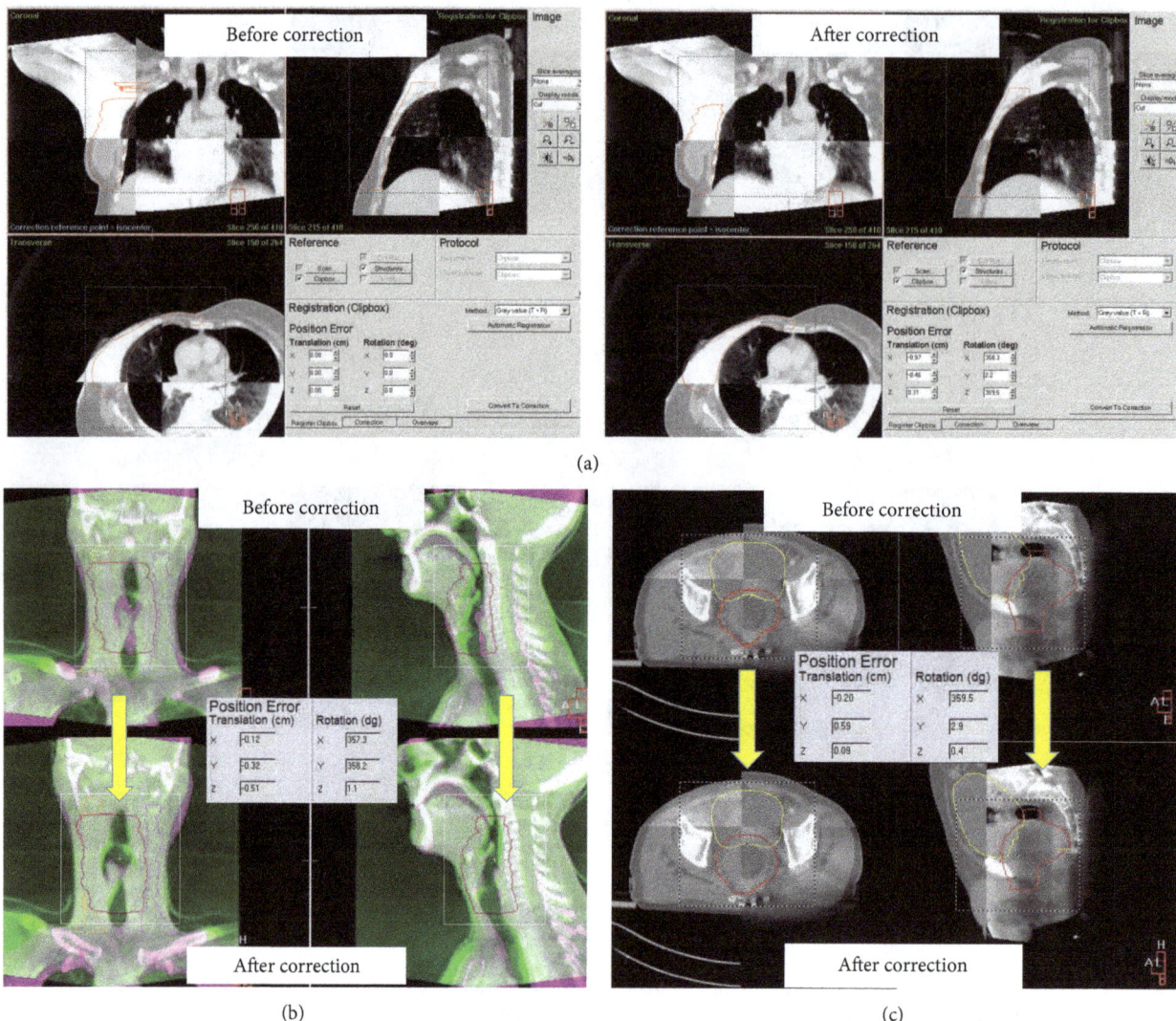

FIGURE 2: KV CBCT volumetric imaging. Both translational and rotational errors may be estimated. Translational errors are easily corrected whereas few systems have provisions for correcting rotational errors with couch rotations. (a) CBCT compared with reference scan before and after correction of setup error in a case of Carcinoma right breast, post-mastectomy. (b) CBCT correction in a case of Carcinoma larynx. (c) CBCT in a case of Carcinoma prostate not only corrects for setup errors, but also provides an estimate of reproducibility of prostate position with respect to bladder filling. In this particular case, the live image shows negligible bladder filling and treatment was delayed to allow for optimum bladder position for obtaining a reproducible position of prostate as well as moving the bowel out of treatment field. KV: kilovoltage; CBCT: cone beam computed tomography.

5.2.3. Fan Beam KV CT (CT-on-Rails). This system has an in-room CT scanner and gantry that moves across the treatment couch/patient, which can be rotated towards either the scanner or the gantry for imaging and treatment, respectively. 3D images are taken with the patient immobilized on the couch, the difference from a diagnostic CT being a larger bore size (>80 cm diameter) to accommodate bulky immobilization devices, and a multislice detector. Accuracy and applications are similar to CBCT with average dose of 10–50 mGy per image [30].

5.2.4. Fan Beam MV CT (TomoTherapy Hi ART II). This includes an on-board imaging system to obtain MV CT images of the patient in treatment position. The same LINAC

is used to generate both the treatment (6 MV) and imaging beam (3.5 MV). A xenon detector located on the gantry opposite the LINAC collects exit data for generation of MV CT images. Patient dose from imaging varies with pitch setting and is typically 10–30 mGy per scan [31].

5.2.5. Hybrid Systems for Real Time 4D Tracking

2D KV Stereoscopic Imaging (CyberKnife). The Accuray CyberKnife robotic radiosurgery system consists of a compact LINAC mounted on an industrial robotic manipulator arm which directs the radiation beams to the desired target based on inputs from two orthogonal X-ray imaging systems mounted on the room ceiling with flat panel floor detectors

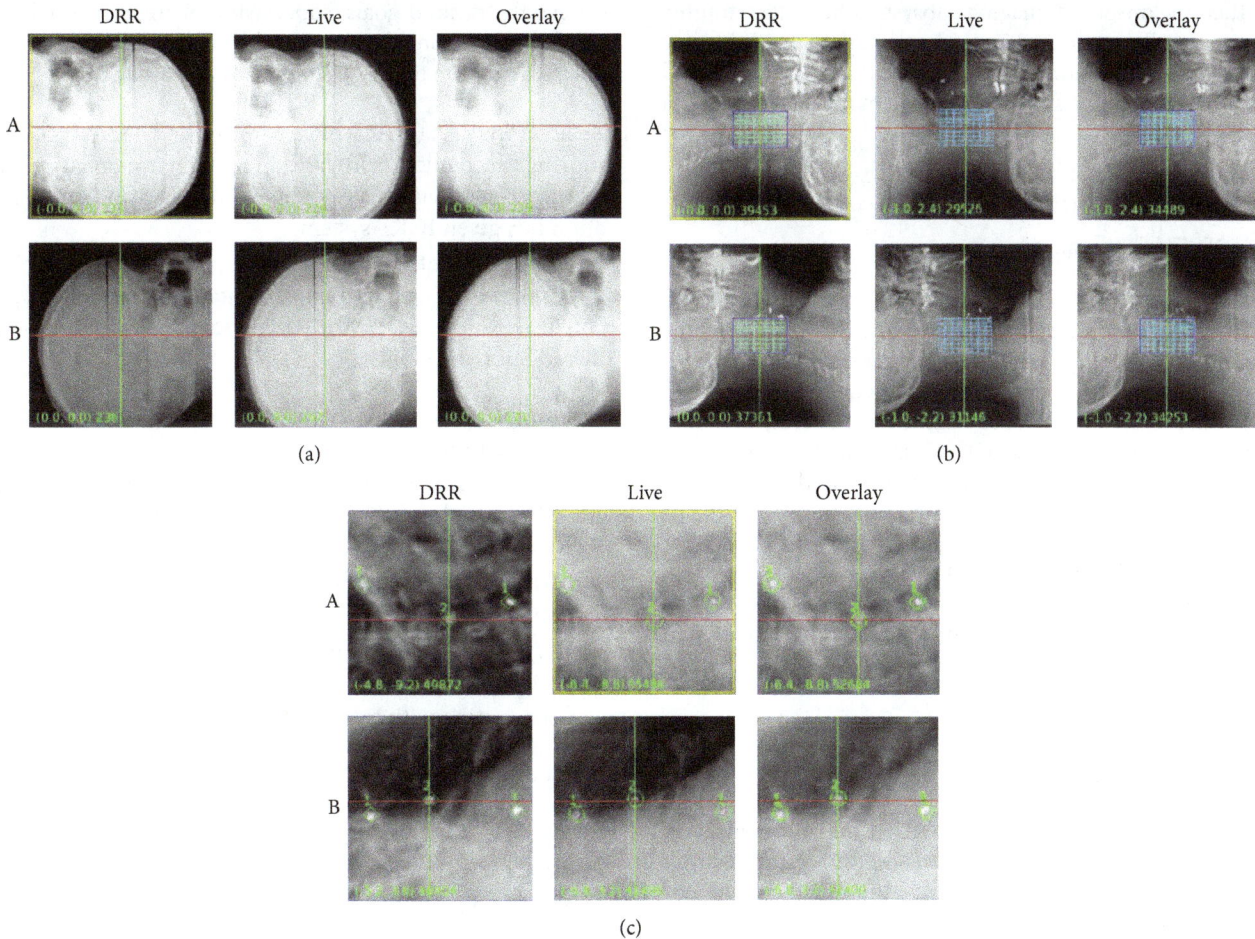

FIGURE 3: CyberKnife console showing the tumor tracking options in a case of head and neck malignancy. (a) 6D skull for skull base lesions. (b) Spine tracking for paravertebral tumors. (c) Fiducial tracking for all other lesions whose motion is independent of skull or spine position, such as base of tongue or neck nodes.

on either side of couch, integrated to provide image guidance for the treatment process. Images are acquired throughout the treatment duration at periodic intervals ranging from 5 to 90 seconds, and the couch and robotic head movements are guided through an automatic process. Several tracking methods may be used depending upon the treatment site (Figure 3). Skull, skull base, or brain tumors may be treated using 6D skull tracking, paravertebral tumors whose movement parallels that of spine may be treated with X-Sight spine tracking, and lung tumors that are surrounded by normal lung parenchyma may be tracked with X-Sight lung tracking. Lung tracking may employ automatic generation of internal target volume depending upon visibility of tumor through both, one or none of the X-ray imaging systems in the treatment position. For all other tumors (e.g., prostate, liver, neck nodes, abdominal masses, etc.), internal surrogates or fiducial markers may need to be placed within or in direct contact with the tumor and the tumor motion is tracked and corrected for through monitoring the fiducial position including translations, rotations, and deformation. Respiratory motion is also monitored and accounted for when correcting for target position and motion through

a synchrony model generated in real time. The system also has a couch that has 6 degrees of freedom to correct for positional variations. Treatment may be limited by patient position and size, and posterior treatment beams cannot be used. A semi-invasive procedure may be required if fiducial markers are needed for tracking. This system can be employed for both cranial (frameless) and extracranial radiosurgery or SRT [32, 33].

Real Time Tumor-Tracking (RTRT) System. This system is designed for real time tracking of tumors by imaging implanted fiducials and using this information for gating. It consists of four X-ray camera systems mounted on the floor, a ceiling-mounted image intensifier, and a high-voltage X-ray generator. The LINAC is gated to irradiate the tumor only when the marker is within a given tolerance from its planned coordinates relative to the isocenter [34, 35].

VERO. This system has two X-ray tubes and corresponding flat panel detectors and uses a combination of initial couch motion and a pair of radiographs for patient alignment. The couch is capable of 3D alignment for initial coarse setup and then the on-board imaging subsystem helps fine-tuning. A pair of radiographs is acquired and registered with prior DRRs using bony landmarks to evaluate the translational and rotational shifts. The system can also compensate for organ motion [36].

5.2.6. Combination Alignment Systems: Optical Imaging and 2D KV Orthogonal Imaging

ExacTrac X-Ray 6-D Stereotactic IGRT System. It uses a combination of optical positioning and KV radiographic imaging for online positioning corrections. There are two main subsystems: an infrared-based system for initial patient setup and precise control of couch movement using a robotic couch and a radiographic KV X-ray imaging system for position verification and readjustment based on internal anatomy or implanted markers. Infrared system may also be used for respiratory monitoring and signaling to LINAC for beam tracking and gating. Novalis Tx combines this system with an additional on-board imaging system (MV, KV X-rays, and KV CBCT) on a multiphoton/electron beam LINAC [37, 38].

6. Guidelines for Medical Personnel and Implementation

American College of Radiology (ACR) and the American Society for Radiation Oncology (ASTRO) jointly developed guidelines for IGRT that define the qualifications and responsibilities of personnel including radiation oncologists, medical physicists, dosimetrists and radiation therapists, QA standards, clinical implementation, and suggested documentation. Similar guidelines have also been proposed by European agencies [39–41]. A summary of the key points is given below.

6.1. Qualifications and Responsibilities

Qualifications. Respective personnel should obtain appropriate certification with specific training in IGRT before performing any stereotactic procedures.

Responsibilities

Radiation Oncologist. (i) Conduct of disease-specific treatment, staging, evaluation of comorbid conditions and prior treatments, exploration of all available treatments including discussion of pros and cons of IGRT, treatment, and subsequent follow-up.

(ii) Determination of the most appropriate patient positioning method, recommendation of the appropriate approach to manage organ motion, supervision of simulation paying particular attention to positioning, immobilization and appropriate motion management, determination and delineation of target volumes and relevant normal critical structures using available imaging techniques, communication of expected goals and constraints and collaboration with the physicist in the iterative process of plan development to achieve the desired goals, supervision of treatment delivery and determination of acceptable day-to-day setup variations, and participation in the QA process and subsequent approval.

Medical Physicist. (i) Acceptance testing and commissioning, assuring mechanical, software, and geometric precision and accuracy, as well as image quality verification and documentation in a given IGRT system.

(ii) Implementation and management of a QA program.

(iii) Development and implementation of standard operating procedures (SOPs) for IGRT use, in collaboration with the radiation oncologist.

Dosimetrist. (i) Normal structure delineation under the guidance of radiation oncologist.

(ii) Management of volumetric patient image data (CT and other fused data sets) on radiation treatment planning (RTP) system.

(iii) Generation of a treatment plan under oncologist's and physicist's guidance.

(iv) Generation of all technical documentation for IGRT plan implementation.

(v) Assisting with treatment verification.

Radiation Therapist. (i) Understanding and appropriate use of immobilization/repositioning systems.

(ii) Performance of simulation and generation of imaging data for planning, implementation of treatment plan, acquisition of periodic verification images under supervision and periodic evaluation of stability and reproducibility of the immobilization/repositioning system, and reporting inconsistencies immediately.

6.2. IGRT Implementation

Fiducial Markers. These serve as surrogates to soft tissue targets when they are difficult to visualize and their alignment cannot be related to bony anatomy. These may be tracked in real time to obtain 3D coordinates of the target for subsequent corrections.

Moving Targets and Delineation. Intrafraction target motion or interfraction displacement, deformation, or alteration of targets and other tissues should be accounted for during determination of PTVs. Appropriate motion management methods should be chosen depending on available expertise and degree and type of motion. This process starts at the time of simulation and continues throughout till the end of therapy.

Patient Positioning. It is imperative to ensure the accuracy of patient position and its reproducibility for fractionated treatments relative to the chosen IGRT device as well as treatment unit.

Image Acquisition. The IGRT system should be calibrated to ensure high imaging quality with attention to slice thickness uniformity, image contrast, spatial resolution, isocenter alignment between imaging and treatment planning and delivery systems, accuracy of software used for identification, and correction of couch misalignments. Relevant QA procedures should ensure reliability and reproducibility of the entire process.

Treatment Verification. Image review by radiation oncologist at the first fraction and then periodically is necessary to ensure treatment accuracy and reproducibility. Each department should determine its own threshold of couch positioning changes that would necessitate setup review or change before treatment delivery.

Quality Assurance and Documentation. A documentation of all the necessary QA procedures throughout the course of simulation, treatment, and periodic verification should be maintained. These would help determine departmental thresholds for action as well as serve as guides for modification of the processes involved following review of findings.

7. IGRT: Clinical Benefits

Use of the IGRT process has improved our awareness and understanding of daily inter- and intrafractional setup variations and motion. Real time tracking has helped quantify interpatient and intrapatient variations in lung and liver tumor motion related to breathing and complexities of such motion have become clearer. We now understand that even when breath-holds are repeated, the relative position of soft tissue and skeletal structures may vary, rendering use of bony landmarks useless for such endeavors. Changes in prostate position (translation, rotation, and shape) have been quantified and we can better correct for these errors as well as tailor PTV margins to these findings, thus allowing more accurate targeting. Understanding of the various IGRT techniques, their applicability, limitations, and additional radiation hazards helps the radiation oncologist take an educated decision on the method best suited to a particular clinical situation for maximizing benefit from radiation therapy. Changes in parotid position relative to the tumor in head and neck cases, change in body contour due to weight loss, seroma, or body fluid collections, change in prostate position relative to bladder or rectal filling and effect of bowel gas, reduction of tumor size during treatment, and changes in spinal position during spinal or head and neck radiotherapy are situations which were never even considered of significance in the pre-IGRT era and their respective roles and solutions are being developed as we are understanding their role during treatment. With better geometric precision, volume of irradiated healthy normal tissue can be significantly reduced with reduction in toxicity risks. Adaptation to reduction in tumor volume may lead to additional gains in normal tissue toxicity reduction.

Results from ongoing and future trials will hopefully demonstrate the net gain in therapeutic ratio from application of IGRT technologies and the onus lies on the radiation oncology community to take up the challenge of demonstrating the benefit of these potentially expensive approaches.

IGRT is most likely to benefit clinical situations where the tumor is in close proximity to sensitive healthy tissues, when doses required for disease control exceed the tolerance levels of adjacent normal tissues or when large organ motion and setup errors may result in severe consequences of positional errors. All patients treated with conformal radiotherapy, IMRT, and SBRT should, in theory, benefit from IGRT. Thoracic and upper abdominal targets with significant respiratory motion, obese patients, head and neck cancers, paraspinal and retroperitoneal sarcomas, and prostate cancer are situations that are expected to derive maximum benefit with some clinical experience forthcoming. Clinical situations where even low dose irradiation produces excellent local control, palliative radiotherapy delivered using large fields, and superficial tumors that are amenable to direct visual inspection are likely to derive least benefit from IGRT.

8. Concerns with IGRT

Limited availability of experienced trained staff is a major hurdle in wide application of the technique despite its demonstrable benefits, even with the simplest approaches. Other factors that need consideration include quality control, algorithms that define the decisions whether to change a plan or continue with original plan, and need for commercial development of software as well as hardware to match clinical needs and demands. Another major concern regarding frequent on-treatment imaging is the radiation dose to normal tissues. Although the doses from IGRT appear insignificant, only long term follow-up will define any potential risk of second malignancies from low dose exposure. Thus, there is an ongoing debate on the necessary frequency of verification imaging especially when using ionizing radiation. Recent developments in MR-LINACs have tried to address these concerns while allowing daily imaging for treatment verification. Another concern is that of treatment safety since the technologies available in the clinic require integration of hardware and software from different vendors. Clinical use of any system should be preceded by proper acceptance testing, commissioning, and routine QA used to assure accurate regular functionality. Education of all users (oncologists, physicists, and technologists) on safe use and clinical utility is mandatory, along with knowledge of additional dose and possible risks associated with use. No single technology is ideal in every scenario and no single institution can manage to integrate all or most technologies in one place. Only time will tell which of these methods gain wider popularity and acceptance, based on clinical relevance and ease of use.

9. Clinical Applications: Current and Future

Use of IGRT systems is essential to treatment of any site where setup deviations and organ motion are anticipated. Additional gains are monitoring of treatment response, weight changes, and organ filling on day-to-day basis. With improved precision of planning systems, use of SRS or SRT, and high dose hypofractionated regimens, the chances of small deviations leading to significant errors in treatment delivery are much higher, and the use of IGRT is far more critical in these situations. Integration of LINACs with MR-based soft tissue imaging and PET-based biological imaging may help even further improve targeting accuracy in the future [42, 43]. However, it is mandatory to ensure proper training of staff and QA at all steps for optimum use of such technology and its integration into routine use.

References

[1] L. A. Dawson and D. A. Jaffray, "Advances in image-guided radiation therapy," *Journal of Clinical Oncology*, vol. 25, no. 8, pp. 938–946, 2007.

[2] A. W. Beavis, "Image-guided radiation therapy: what is our Utopia?" *British Journal of Radiology*, vol. 83, no. 987, pp. 191–193, 2010.

[3] D. A. Jaffray, "Image-guided radiation therapy: from concept to practice," *Seminars in Radiation Oncology*, vol. 17, no. 4, pp. 243–244, 2007.

[4] Q. J. Wu, T. Li, and F.-F. Yin, "Adaptive radiation therapy: technical components and clinical applications," *Cancer Journal*, vol. 17, no. 3, pp. 182–189, 2011.

[5] M. van Herk, "Errors and margins in radiotherapy," *Seminars in Radiation Oncology*, vol. 14, no. 1, pp. 52–64, 2004.

[6] C. Rasch, R. Steenbakkers, and M. van Herk, "Target definition in prostate, head, and neck," *Seminars in Radiation Oncology*, vol. 15, no. 3, pp. 136–145, 2005.

[7] J. C. Stroom and B. J. M. Heijmen, "Geometrical uncertainties, radiotherapy planning margins, and the ICRU-62 report," *Radiotherapy and Oncology*, vol. 64, no. 1, pp. 75–83, 2002.

[8] M. van Herk, P. Remeijer, C. Rasch, and J. V. Lebesque, "The probability of correct target dosage: dose-population histograms for deriving treatment margins in radiotherapy," *International Journal of Radiation Oncology, Biology, Physics*, vol. 47, no. 4, pp. 1121–1135, 2000.

[9] J. C. Stroom, H. C. J. de Boer, H. Huizenga, and A. G. Visser, "Inclusion of geometrical uncertainties in radiotherapy treatment planning by means of coverage probability," *International Journal of Radiation Oncology Biology Physics*, vol. 43, no. 4, pp. 905–919, 1999.

[10] A. Bel, M. van Herk, H. Bartelink, and J. V. Lebesque, "A verification procedure to improve patient set-up accuracy using portal images," *Radiotherapy and Oncology*, vol. 29, no. 2, pp. 253–260, 1993.

[11] H. C. J. de Boer, M. J. H. van Os, P. P. Jansen, and B. J. M. Heijmen, "Application of the No Action Level (NAL) protocol to correct for prostate motion based on electronic portal imaging of implanted markers," *International Journal of Radiation Oncology Biology Physics*, vol. 61, no. 4, pp. 969–983, 2005.

[12] T. Kataria, A. Abhishek, P. Chadha, and J. Nandigam, "Set-up uncertainties: online correction with X-ray volume imaging," *Journal of Cancer Research and Therapeutics*, vol. 7, no. 1, pp. 40–46, 2011.

[13] T. Kataria, D. Gupta, K. Karrthick et al., "Frame-based radio-surgery: is it relevant in the era of IGRT?" *Neurology India*, vol. 61, no. 3, pp. 277–281, 2013.

[14] J. M. Balter and Y. Cao, "Advanced technologies in image-guided radiation therapy," *Seminars in Radiation Oncology*, vol. 17, no. 4, pp. 293–297, 2007.

[15] J. de los Santos, R. Popple, N. Agazaryan et al., "Image guided radiation therapy (IGRT) technologies for radiation therapy localization and delivery," *International Journal of Radiation Oncology Biology Physics*, vol. 87, no. 1, pp. 33–45, 2013.

[16] M. Fuss, B. J. Salter, S. X. Cavanaugh et al., "Daily ultrasound-based image-guided targeting for radiotherapy of upper abdominal malignancies," *International Journal of Radiation Oncology Biology Physics*, vol. 59, no. 4, pp. 1245–1256, 2004.

[17] C. Bert, K. G. Metheany, K. P. Doppke, A. G. Taghian, S. N. Powell, and G. T. Y. Chen, "Clinical experience with a 3D surface patient setup system for alignment of partial-breast irradiation patients," *International Journal of Radiation Oncology, Biology, Physics*, vol. 64, no. 4, pp. 1265–1274, 2006.

[18] A. Brahme, P. Nyman, and B. Skatt, "4D laser camera for accurate patient positioning, collision avoidance, image fusion and adaptive approaches during diagnostic and therapeutic procedures," *Medical Physics*, vol. 35, no. 5, pp. 1670–1681, 2008.

[19] D. W. Litzenberg, T. R. Willoughby, J. M. Balter et al., "Positional stability of electromagnetic transponders used for prostate localization and continuous, real-time tracking," *International Journal of Radiation Oncology Biology Physics*, vol. 68, no. 4, pp. 1199–1206, 2007.

[20] T. R. Willoughby, P. A. Kupelian, J. Pouliot et al., "Target localization and real-time tracking using the Calypso 4D localization system in patients with localized prostate cancer," *International Journal of Radiation Oncology Biology Physics*, vol. 65, no. 2, pp. 528–534, 2006.

[21] J. Dempsey, B. Dionne, J. Fitzsimmons, A. Haghigat, and J. Li, "A real-time MRI guided external beam radiotherapy delivery system," *Medical Physics*, vol. 33, article 2254, 2006.

[22] B. G. Fallone, B. Murray, S. Rathee et al., "First MR images obtained during megavoltage photon irradiation from a prototype integrated linac-MR system," *Medical Physics*, vol. 36, no. 6, pp. 2084–2088, 2009.

[23] M. G. Herman, "Clinical use of electronic portal imaging," *Seminars in Radiation Oncology*, vol. 15, no. 3, pp. 157–167, 2005.

[24] C. W. Hurkmans, P. Remeijer, J. V. Lebesque, and B. J. Mijnheer, "Set-up verification using portal imaging; review of current clinical practice," *Radiotherapy and Oncology*, vol. 58, no. 2, pp. 105–120, 2001.

[25] C. Walter, J. Boda-Heggemann, H. Wertz et al., "Phantom and in-vivo measurements of dose exposure by image-guided radiotherapy (IGRT): MV portal images vs. kV portal images vs. cone-beam CT," *Radiotherapy and Oncology*, vol. 85, no. 3, pp. 418–423, 2007.

[26] D. A. Jaffray, "Kilovoltage volumetric imaging in the treatment room," *Frontiers of Radiation Therapy and Oncology*, vol. 40, pp. 116–131, 2007.

[27] C. A. McBain, A. M. Henry, J. Sykes et al., "X-ray volumetric imaging in image-guided radiotherapy: the new standard in on-treatment imaging," *International Journal of Radiation Oncology, Biology, Physics*, vol. 64, no. 2, pp. 625–634, 2006.

[28] O. Morin, A. Gillis, J. Chen et al., "Megavoltage cone-beam CT: system description and clinical applications," *Medical Dosimetry*, vol. 31, no. 1, pp. 51–61, 2006.

[29] J. Pouliot, A. Bani-Hashemi, M. Svatos et al., "Low-dose mega-voltage cone-beam CT for radiation therapy," *International Journal of Radiation Oncology Biology Physics*, vol. 61, no. 2, pp. 552–560, 2005.

[30] R. de Crevoisier, D. Kuban, and D. Lefkopoulos, "Image-guided radiotherapy by in-room CT-linear accelerator combination," *Cancer/Radiotherapie*, vol. 10, no. 5, pp. 245–251, 2006.

[31] K. J. Ruchala, G. H. Olivera, E. A. Schloesser, and T. R. Mackie, "Megavoltage CT on a tomotherapy system," *Physics in Medicine and Biology*, vol. 44, no. 10, pp. 2597–2621, 1999.

[32] J. R. Adler Jr., S. D. Chang, M. J. Murphy, J. Doty, P. Geis, and S. L. Hancock, "The Cyberknife: a frameless robotic system for radiosurgery," *Stereotactic and Functional Neurosurgery*, vol. 69, no. 1–4, pp. 124–128, 1997.

[33] C. Antypas and E. Pantelis, "Performance evaluation of a CyberKnife G4 image-guided robotic stereotactic radiosurgery system," *Physics in Medicine and Biology*, vol. 53, no. 17, pp. 4697–4718, 2008.

[34] H. Shirato, S. Shimizu, K. Kitamura et al., "Four-dimensional treatment planning and fluoroscopic real-time tumor tracking radiotherapy for moving tumor," *International Journal of Radiation Oncology, Biology, Physics*, vol. 48, no. 2, pp. 435–442, 2000.

[35] H. Shirato, S. Shimizu, T. Kunieda et al., "Physical aspects of a real-time tumor-tracking system for gated radiotherapy," *International Journal of Radiation Oncology Biology Physics*, vol. 48, no. 4, pp. 1187–1195, 2000.

[36] Y. Kamino, K. Takayama, M. Kokubo et al., "Development of a four-dimensional image-guided radiotherapy system with a gimbaled X-ray head," *International Journal of Radiation Oncology, Biology, Physics*, vol. 66, no. 1, pp. 271–278, 2006.

[37] Z. Chang, Z. Wang, Q. J. Wu et al., "Dosimetric characteristics of Novalis Tx system with high definition multileaf collimator," *Medical Physics*, vol. 35, no. 10, pp. 4460–4463, 2008.

[38] J.-Y. Jin, F.-F. Yin, S. E. Tenn, P. M. Medin, and T. D. Solberg, "Use of the BrainLAB ExacTrac X-Ray 6D System in Image-Guided Radiotherapy," *Medical Dosimetry*, vol. 33, no. 2, pp. 124–134, 2008.

[39] L. Potters, L. E. Gaspar, B. Kavanagh et al., "American Society for Therapeutic Radiology and Oncology (ASTRO) and American College of Radiology (ACR) practice guidelines for image-guided radiation therapy (IGRT)," *International Journal of Radiation Oncology, Biology, Physics*, vol. 76, no. 2, pp. 319–325, 2010.

[40] S. Korreman, C. Rasch, H. McNair et al., "The European Society of Therapeutic Radiology and Oncology-European Institute of Radiotherapy (ESTRO-EIR) report on 3D CT-based in-room image guidance systems: a practical and technical review and guide," *Radiotherapy and Oncology*, vol. 94, no. 2, pp. 129–144, 2010.

[41] E. White and G. Kane, "Radiation medicine practice in the image-guided radiation therapy era: new roles and new opportunities," *Seminars in Radiation Oncology*, vol. 17, no. 4, pp. 298–305, 2007.

[42] E. Rusten, J. Rodal, Ø. S. Bruland, and E. Malinen, "Biologic targets identified from dynamic ^{18}FDG-PET and implications for image-guided therapy," *Acta Oncologica*, vol. 52, no. 7, pp. 1378–1383, 2013.

[43] X. Geets, "4D PET-CT guided radiation therapy," *JBR-BTR*, vol. 96, no. 3, pp. 155–159, 2013.

6

Ultrasound Findings in Hand Joints Involvement in Patients with Psoriatic Arthritis and Its Correlation with Clinical DAS28 Score

Priyanka Naranje,[1] Mahesh Prakash,[1] Aman Sharma,[2] Sunil Dogra,[3] and Niranjan Khandelwal[1]

[1]*Department of Radiodiagnosis, Postgraduate Institute of Medical Education and Research (PGIMER), Chandigarh 160012, India*
[2]*Department of Internal Medicine, Postgraduate Institute of Medical Education and Research (PGIMER), Chandigarh 160012, India*
[3]*Department of Dermatology, Venereology and Leprology, Postgraduate Institute of Medical Education and Research (PGIMER), Chandigarh 160012, India*

Correspondence should be addressed to Priyanka Naranje; priyanka11sh@gmail.com and Mahesh Prakash; image73@gmail.com

Academic Editor: Ali Guermazi

Objective. To determine the frequency of the various ultrasound findings in hand joints in patients with psoriatic arthritis and correlate grayscale and Power Doppler ultrasonography findings with Disease Activity Score 28. *Methods.* This prospective study was performed in 30 patients. Ultrasound evaluation of 28 joints of both hands was undertaken and various findings were recorded including synovial hypertrophy, Power Doppler abnormality, soft tissue thickening, tendonitis, joint effusion, periosteal reaction, and erosions. Composite ultrasound scores and Disease Activity Score 28 were calculated and compared. Spearman correlation was used to see relationship between the ultrasound and DAS28 scores. *Results.* Ultrasound detected more abnormalities in the hand joints than did clinical examination. The frequency of various ultrasound abnormalities was as follows: Synovial hypertrophy was seen in 100%, Power Doppler abnormality suggesting hypervascularity was seen in 36.7%, soft tissue thickening was seen in 66.7%, periosteal reaction was seen in 33.3%, erosions were seen in 30% (mostly in DIP and PIP joints), and flexor tendonitis was seen in 6.7% of patients. Significant correlation was found between Disease Activity Score 28 and grayscale joint score (GSJS) (Spearman's ρ: 0.499; P: 0.005), grayscale joint count (GSJC) (ρ: 0.398; P: 0.029), and Power Doppler joint score (PDJS) (ρ: 0.367; P: 0.046). There was a statistically significant difference between remission and low disease activity group and moderate disease activity group in terms of GSJC, GSJS, PDJC, and PDJS ($P < 0.05$). These ultrasound measures were higher in moderate disease activity zone patients. *Conclusion.* Ultrasound is a useful modality for the objective assessment of psoriatic arthritis. Ultrasound including Power Doppler can be used as a modality for assessment of severity of psoriatic arthritis as it correlates with the clinical scoring.

1. Introduction

Psoriatic arthritis (PsA) is commonly described as chronic, seronegative, inflammatory spondyloarthropathy seen in association with psoriasis. It has been shown that psoriatic arthritis patients may develop progressive joint damage, deformity, and disability [1]. Progression of the psoriatic arthritis adds to increase in morbidity. PsA occurs in a variable, albeit considerable, percentage of psoriatic patients that range from 10 to 30% depending on the studied population [2]. In India, prevalence of PsA in patients with psoriasis has been around 7 to 8% [3]. The arthropathy generally begins several years after the commencement of the disease [4, 5]. Serological investigations for RA are negative in most of these patients [6].

Among various imaging modalities, ultrasound (US) is routinely accessible, inexpensive, and noninvasive diagnostic imaging modality. It is a rapidly evolving technique that is gaining an increasing success in the assessment of PsA. It provides measures of synovial morphology and vascularity.

Grayscale (GS) ultrasound visualizes the structures of the joint and can discriminate amongst synovial hypertrophy and various other sources of perceptible swelling of the joint such as tenosynovitis or edema in subcutaneous plane [7]. Power Doppler (PD) sonography shows increased soft tissue vascularity with superior sensitivity and hence differentiates inflamed from noninflamed synovial swelling. Various scoring systems have been elicited to clinically assess the disease activity and severity in psoriatic arthritis, out of which Disease Activity Score 28 (DAS28) has shown to be of better accuracy and DAS28 is more suitable to assess PsA forms with joint involvement [8]. On an individual joint basis there has been a poor correlation between joint tenderness and swelling which are the clinical presentations of synovitis and grayscale as well as Power Doppler ultrasound measures of synovial pathology [9]. Previous studies done in patients with rheumatoid arthritis (RA) have revealed that US identifies more synovial changes than is clinically noticed and PD depicts that it is not essential for all the swollen joints to show hypervascularity and that yet a clinically normal joint may show synovial hypervascularity [9, 10]. It has been tried to overcome these differences between clinical and US findings in a particular joint in patients with RA by using composite counts or scores from many joints. Such scores would overall become indicative of entire disease activity in a patient [11]. The association between Power Doppler ultrasonography and clinical scores has not been evaluated in PsA. Therefore this study was done to assess the relation between DAS28 score and its components with compound GS and PD Ultrasound counts and scores of the metacarpophalangeal (MCP), proximal interphalangeal (PIP), and distal interphalangeal (DIP) joints in psoriatic arthritis.

2. Material and Methods

The Ethical Committee of Postgraduate Institute of Medical Education and Research (PGIMER), Chandigarh, approved this study. Written informed consent was taken from all controls and patients. The prospective study was carried out on the patients presenting to the rheumatology outpatient department (OPD) of PGIMER, Chandigarh. A total of 30 consecutive patients diagnosed to have psoriatic arthritis and presenting with symptoms of pain/swelling of the small joints of hands were included. The study was conducted in the Department of Radiodiagnosis and Imaging, in collaboration with Department of Internal Medicine, and Department of Dermatology, PGIMER, Chandigarh.

2.1. Inclusion Criteria. Patients diagnosed to have psoriatic arthritis according to ClASsification criteria for Psoriatic ARthritis (CASPAR) and presenting with pain and/or swelling of the small joints of hands were incorporated in the study.

2.2. Exclusion Criteria. Exclusion criteria included patients with symptoms of arthritis before the onset of skin disease and patients with rheumatoid factor positivity and coexistent infection of the digits and amputation/injury/plaster of any digit.

Detailed history was taken and complete clinical examination was done at the time of enrolment. For each participant, diagnosis of psoriatic arthritis was established by a rheumatologist in the rheumatology clinic by patient interview including history of pain and/or swelling of hand joints. Clinical examination was performed to assess for the swollen joints and tender joints. Erythrocyte sedimentation rate was determined by using Wintrobe's method on the same day of the clinical examination and Visual Analog Scale (VAS) was used for the patient's assessment of general health (GH).

DAS28 score was calculated to assess the disease activity of PsA.

2.3. Calculation of DAS28 Score. Examination of swollen and tender joints of patient was performed and each affected joint was noted. Sum of all swollen and tender joints was done and totals were recorded. Patient's erythrocyte sedimentation rate (ESR) was recorded in mm/h. Visual Analog Scale (VAS) of 100 mm was used to record the general health of the patient. DAS28 value was calculated using the following formula. A DAS28 calculator v1.1-beta was used to compute this value:

$$DAS28 = 0.56 * \sqrt{(\text{tender joints})} + 0.28$$
$$* \sqrt{(\text{swollen joints})} + 0.70 * Ln\left(\frac{ESR}{CRP}\right) \quad (1)$$
$$+ 0.014 * VAS.$$

On the same day of clinical evaluation, ultrasound was performed in bilateral metacarpophalangeal, proximal interphalangeal, and distal interphalangeal joints using Philips HD 11 system or Philips iU22 system, equipped with a 3 to 12 MHZ linear transducer. For Power Doppler studies, "low flow" settings with a medium to low wall filter (to minimize flash artifact) were used and a pulse repetition frequency of 500 to 700 Hz was set. The color gain was accustomed to just below the noise level. Each joint was scanned in both transverse and longitudinal planes for grayscale and Power Doppler study.

In every patient, scanning of 28 hand joints (10 MCP, 8 PIP, and 10 DIP joints) was done and the presence of abnormal synovial thickening, soft tissue thickening, tendonitis, periosteal reaction, joint effusion, erosions, and Power Doppler abnormality was noted. In addition, these joints were scored according to Table 1. Interphalangeal joint of first digit was considered as DIP joint. The severity grade of GS score was determined according to the following grading of synovial thickness (Figure 1) [12]:

Grade 0: no/minimal synovial thickening (considered normal).

Grade 1: synovial thickening bulging over the line joining the tops of the bones forming the joint without extension along the bone diaphyses.

Grade 2: synovial thickening extending to one of the metadiaphyses.

Grade 3: extension to both metadiaphyses.

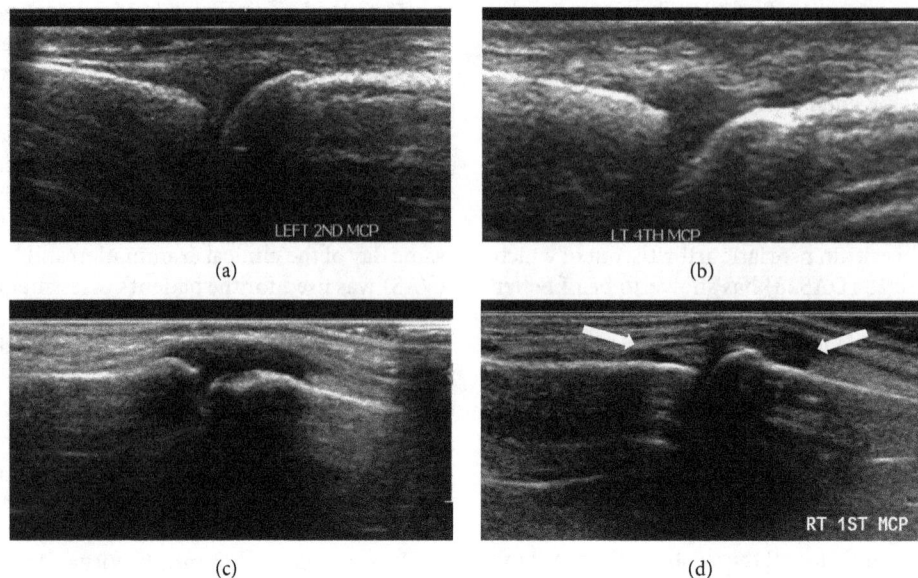

FIGURE 1: (a–d) Grading of synovial thickening is depicted; (a) Grade 0, (b) Grade 1, (c) Grade 2, and (d) Grade 3. Arrows indicate extension of synovial thickening to both metadiaphyses.

TABLE 1: Subjective GS and PD scoring system for US images of MCP, PIP, and DIP joints.

GS synovial score	PD score
0: absence of synovial hypertrophy	Absence of PD signal
1: small degree of synovial hypertrophy	Single vessel dots
2: moderate synovial hypertrophy	Confluent vessel dots over less than half the area of synovium
3: marked synovial hypertrophy	Confluent vessel dots over greater than half the area of synovium

Separate grayscale and Power Doppler subjective score were documented for each joint which ranged from 0 to 3. Scores of 1, 2, and 3 were considered abnormal, and 0 was considered as normal. These scores were used to derive the composite US measures of synovial pathology as follows: (i) grayscale joint count (GSJC): number of joints scoring either 1, 2, or 3, out of a total of 28; (ii) grayscale joint score (GSJS): sum of the GS scores in all 28 joints, out of a total of 84; (iii) Power Doppler joint count (PDJC): number of joints scoring either 1, 2, or 3, out of a total of 28; and (iv) Power Doppler joint score (PDJS): the sum of the PD scores in all 28 joints, out of a total of 84.

Accordingly, the GSJC and PDJC represented number of normal or abnormal joints, similar to TJC and SJC system employed in the DAS28, whereas the GSJS and PDJS suggested an assessment of severity. The correlation between US measures and clinical measures of the disease was determined amongst the following variables: the US measures and the DAS28 score and the DAS28 components, including SJC, TJC, ESR, and VAS.

The statistical analysis was performed using Statistical Package for Social Sciences (SPSS Inc., Chicago, IL, version 17.0 for Windows). Spearman correlation was used to see relationship between different continuous variables. Qualitative or categorical variables were described as frequencies and proportions (percentages). All statistical tests were two-sided and performed at a significance level of $\alpha = 0.05$.

3. Results: Psoriatic Arthritis Patients

3.1. Demographic Data of the Patients (Table 2). Thirty patients (16 males and 14 females) were enrolled in the study. The mean age was 38.97 ± 12.187 years (range 18–62 years). None of the patients had a family history of psoriasis. On examination, 8/30 patients (26.7%) had nail involvement due to psoriasis. 25/30 (83.3%) patients were on medical treatment in the form of methotrexate, steroids, or nonsteroidal anti-inflammatory drugs (NSAIDs).

3.2. Range of US Measures and Clinical Measures of Synovial Disease. Wide range of scores was seen in both clinical and US measures of synovial pathology (Table 3) in 30 recruited patients, indicating a wide spectrum of disease activity in them.

Most of the patients (19) were having DAS28 score within the moderate disease activity range, nine (9) patients were in remission and low disease activity, and only two (2) patients were in high disease activity zone, as shown in Figure 2.

In the 30 patients, a total of 840 MCP, PIP, and DIP joints were evaluated clinically and sonologically. Out of this total, clinically 50 were swollen joints and 113 were tender joints.

With GS, abnormal synovial thickening was observed in the joints of all the 30 patients (100%). Out of the scanned joints of the hand, it was seen in 182/840 joints (21.6%) and PD signal abnormality (suggested by scores or 1, 2, or 3) was seen in 25/840 joints and in 11/30 (36.7%) patients (Figures 3 and 4).

TABLE 2: Demographic data of the patients.

Total number of patients	Male	Female	Mean age	Age range	Family history of psoriasis	Nail involvement	Number and percentage of patients on medical treatment			
							None 5 (16.7%)	Methotrexate (MTX) 15 (50%)	MTX and Steroids 4 (13.3%)	NSAIDS 6 (20%)
30	16	14	38.97 ± 12.18 years	18–62 years	0	8 (26.7%)				

TABLE 3: Range of clinical and ultrasound measures of synovial disease.

Disease activity measures	Minimum	Maximum	Median	Mean	SD (±)
TJC	1	10	3.00	3.77	2.487
SJC	0	9	1.00	1.67	2.249
ESR	11	68	29.00	31.40	14.407
VAS	8	80	20.00	26.67	17.980
DAS28	2.52	6.36	3.68	3.8267	0.86204
GSJC	1	14	5.00	6.07	3.483
GSJS	1	21	7.5	8.27	5.558
PDJC	0	7	0.00	0.83	1.533
PDJS	0	11	0.00	1.37	2.619

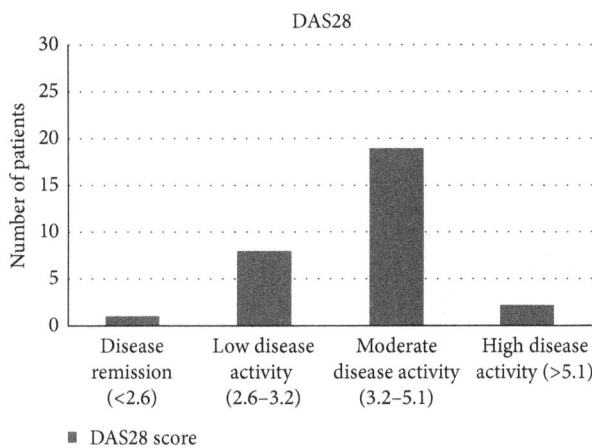

FIGURE 2: Distribution of patients in DAS28 subcategories.

Out of 182 joints with abnormal synovial hypertrophy, 71 (39.01%) were MCP, 69 (37.91%) were PIP, and 42 (23.07%) were DIP joints. Thus, more synovial hypertrophy was detected by US than by clinical examination; however PD signal abnormality was noted in fewer number of joints than were clinically tender or swollen.

Soft tissue thickening was observed in 20/30 (66.7%) patients. None of the scanned joints revealed joint effusion. In only 2/30 (6.7%) patients, flexor tendonitis was observed. Periosteal reaction was observed in 10/30 (33.3%) patients. Erosions were observed in 9/30 (30%) patients, mostly in the DIP and PIP joints. There were no PD signs inside or near the erosions.

3.3. *Correlation between Clinical and US Measures of Synovial Disease.* There was a significant positive correlation between the DAS28 score and the composite US scores. The strongest relation was noted with the GSJS (Spearman's ρ: 0.499; *P*: 0.005) (Figure 5) and the GSJC (ρ: 0.398; *P*: 0.029) (Figure 6), and also significant relation was noted with the PDJS (ρ: 0.367; *P*: 0.046) (Figure 7) but only weaker relation was noted with the PDJC (ρ: 0.348; *P*: 0.060, NS).

Correlation between the components of the DAS28 score [TJC, SJC, ESR, and VAS] and US measures was as follows: TJC is correlated positively with GSJC (ρ: 0.474; *P*: 0.008) (Figure 8), GSJS (ρ: 0.484; *P*: 0.007) (Figure 9), PDJC (ρ: 0.461; *P*: 0.010), and PDJS (ρ: 0.481; *P*: 0.007). There was no significant relation between the SJC and any of the GS or PD measures. ESR correlated with the GSJC (ρ: 0.478; *P*: 0.008) (Figure 10) and GSJS (ρ: 0.434; *P*: 0.017) and not with PDJC or PDJS. The VAS showed significant relation with GSJS (ρ: 0.541; *P*: 0.002), with GSJC (ρ: 0.423; *P*: 0.020), and with PDJC (ρ: 0.365; *P*: 0.047) and weaker relation with PDJS (ρ: 0.360; *P*: 0.051, NS).

On applying Mann-Whitney *U* test for comparison of US measures (GSJC, GSJS, PDJC, and PDJS), the difference between remission and low disease activity group and moderate disease activity group was statistically significant in terms of GSJC (*P*: 0.039), GSJS (*P*: 0.021), PDJC (*P*: 0.029), and PDJS (*P*: 0.027). Moderate disease activity zone patients demonstrated higher US measures as compared to the values within the remission and low disease activity zone patients.

However, no statistically significant difference was found between remission and low disease activity group and high disease activity group or between moderate disease activity group and high disease activity groups regarding the US measures. This was because of less number of patients (only 2) within the high disease activity zone, and hence the actual comparison between these groups could not be well evaluated.

4. Discussion

In our study we found various abnormalities on US evaluation of the joints which included abnormal synovial thickening, soft tissue thickening, tendonitis, periosteal reaction, erosions, and hypervascularity within the abnormal synovial thickening on Power Doppler. Out of four US measures, GSJC, GSJS, and PDJS demonstrated considerably significant correlation with DAS28 score.

MSUS with PD is routinely available, noninvasive, relatively inexpensive, patient friendly imaging method. It is a rapidly evolving technique in assessment of psoriatic

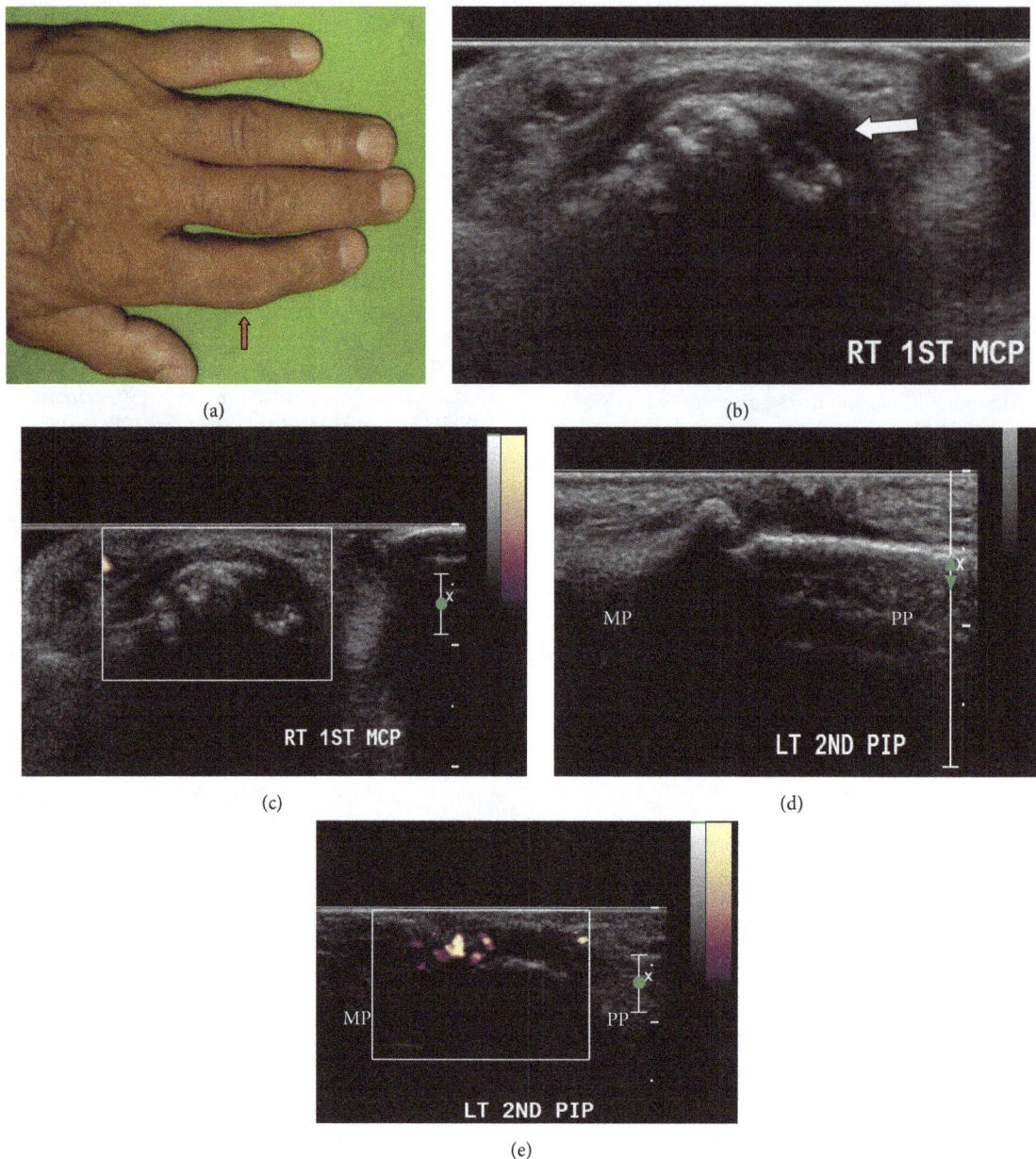

(a)

(b)

(c)

(d)

(e)

FIGURE 3: A 52-year-old male patient with PsA presented with pain in multiple joints of the hands in addition to other joints with swelling in left second PIP joint (a, arrow). DAS28 score was 4.78 (suggestive of moderate disease activity) at the time of presentation. US revealed extensive disease in multiple joints of the hands. The GS and PD scores were as follows: GSJC-12, GSJS-18, PDJC-4, and PDJS-8. Grade 2 GS synovial score with Grade 0 PD score in right first MCP joint (b and c). Grade 2 GS score with Grade 2 PD in left second PIP joint (d and e). Longitudinal view (d and e). Transverse view (b and c).

arthritis. It assesses synovial tissue, joint effusions, and erosions. Power Doppler sonography depicts increased soft tissue vascularity and synovial inflammation. It allows for the characterization of early inflammatory changes in arthritis [13].

Several studies have recognized the efficiency of ultrasound in detecting inflammation in the joints of patients with PsA, in addition to the degree of structural damage [14].

US synovial hypertrophy was identified according to the OMERACT definitions and published descriptions of US pathology. Synovial hypertrophy is defined as abnormal hypoechoic (relative to subdermal fat but sometimes may be isoechoic or hyperechoic) intraarticular tissue that is nondisplaceable and poorly compressible and which may exhibit Doppler signal [15, 16].

Our study demonstrated that abnormal synovial thickening was observed in the joints of all the 30 patients (100%). Other studies have shown a variable and high percentage (up to 52% to 60%) of synovial abnormality in PsA [17–19].

It was seen in our study that synovial hypertrophy was more often detected by US than by the clinical examination which seems to be in line with previous studies [12, 20].

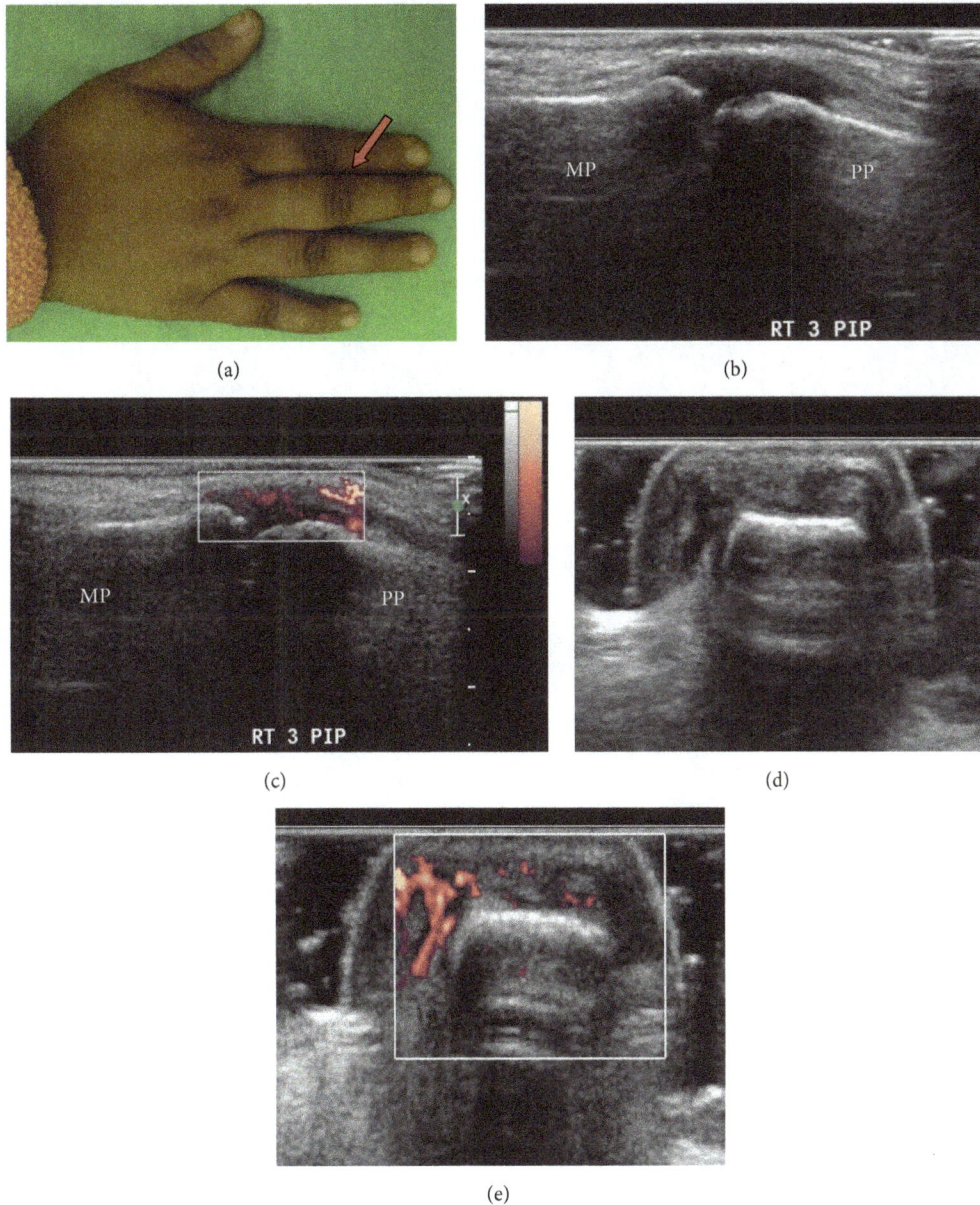

FIGURE 4: A 30-year-old female patient diagnosed as PsA presented with history of pain and swelling of right third PIP (arrow) (a). DAS28 score was 4.48 (suggestive of moderate disease activity). Ultrasound examination revealed Grade 2 synovial hypertrophy in right third PIP joint (b and d). PD evaluation showed increased signal (Grade 3) within the hypertrophied synovium in the joint (c and e). US scores derived were as follows: GSJC-11, GSJS-18, PDJC-3, and PDJS-7. Longitudinal view (b and c). Transverse view (d and e).

Another study has validated US in identifying the abnormalities involving the synovial tissue in the fingers and toes of patients with suspected PsA [21]. In a study by Wakefield et al., in 64% (51/80) of cases, US detected synovial inflammation in more number of joints than clinical examination [10].

Increased PD signal was seen in 25/840 joints corresponding to 11/30 (36.7%) patients. Out of 182 joints showing abnormal synovial hypertrophy, 25 (13.73%) joints showed PD signal abnormality.

Previous studies have revealed that the prevalence of PDUS synovitis was significantly higher in psoriatic patients than in controls [19].

A study by Caldarola et al. in 2011 found that most of the patients who had abnormalities on US also depicted vascular spots, suggesting active inflammation, in intra-articular and/or peritendinous spaces on PDUS, thereby providing additional information on disease activity. Twenty-nine of thirty-six patients who had grayscale US abnormalities suggestive of PsA also showed increased vascularity on PDUS in the abnormal synovial tissue [21].

The lower incidence of PD abnormality in the examined joints in our study can be attributed to the patient characteristics. Most of the patients were on treatment prior to assessment of the joints by PDUS which might have reduced

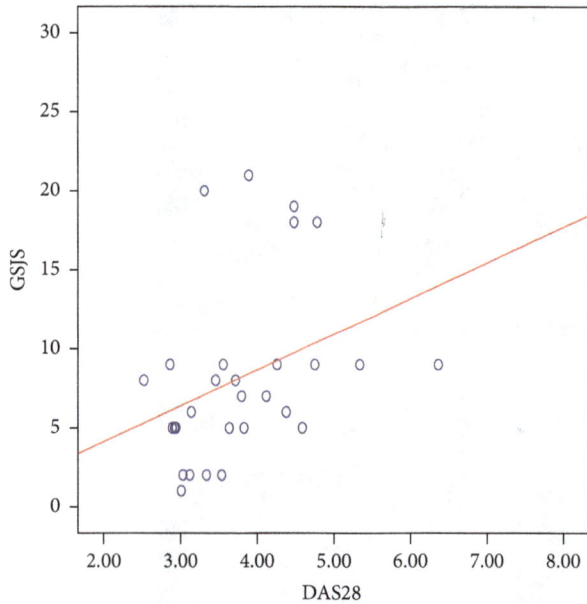

FIGURE 5: Relation between GSJS (taken from 28 MCP, PIP, and DIP joints) and DAS28 score in 30 patients with PsA. Spearman's ρ: 0.499; P: 0.005 suggesting a significant correlation.

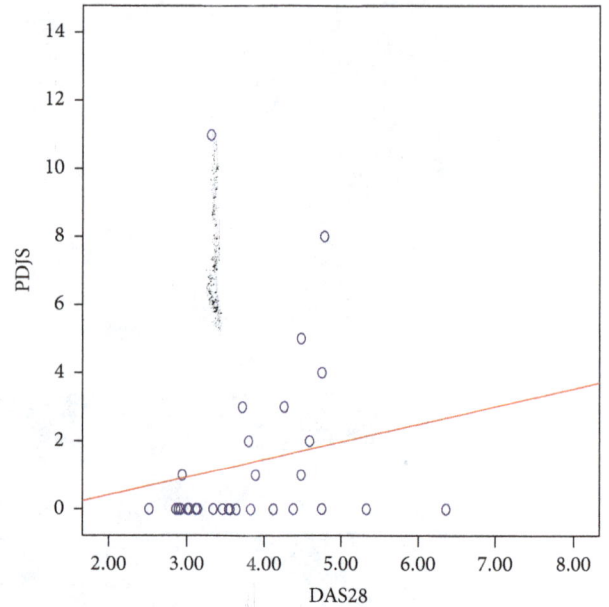

FIGURE 7: Relation between PDJS (taken from 28 MCP, PIP, and DIP joints) and DAS28 score in 30 patients with PsA. Spearman's ρ: 0.367; P: 0.046 suggesting a significant correlation.

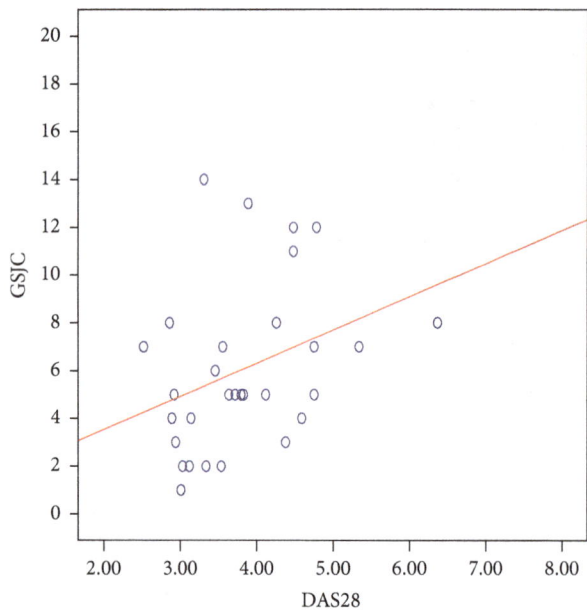

FIGURE 6: Relation between GSJC (taken from 28 MCP, PIP, and DIP joints) and DAS28 score in 30 patients with PsA. Spearman's ρ: 0.398; P: 0.029 suggesting a significant correlation.

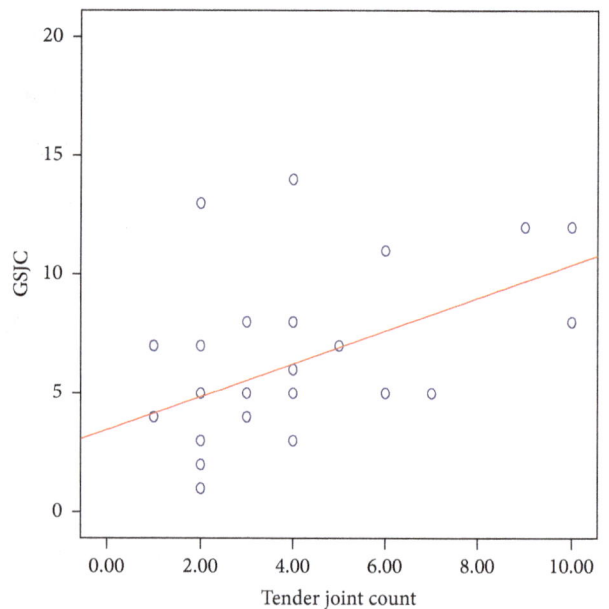

FIGURE 8: Relation between GSJC (taken from 28 MCP, PIP, and DIP joints) and TJC in 30 patients with PsA. Spearman's ρ: 0.474; P: 0.008 suggesting a significant correlation.

the inflammation within the joints which generates the PD signal. Such an effect of treatment has been demonstrated in RA as well as PsA patients in a study by Backhaus et al. 2009, wherein the PD scores significantly decreased after 6 months of therapy [22].

A study by Weiner et al. 2008 has shown that US had a sensitivity of 40% and 57% for erosions when compared to radiography and MRI [23]. In addition studies by Backhaus

et al. [22] and Weiner et al. [23] suggested that erosions are more frequently seen in PIP and DIP joints by US and radiography. This is in accordance with our data. PIP and DIP joints are also involved in primary OA and erosions might not be a specific finding. There were no PD signals inside or near the erosions. However, there was hypertrophied synovium identified in the region of erosion.

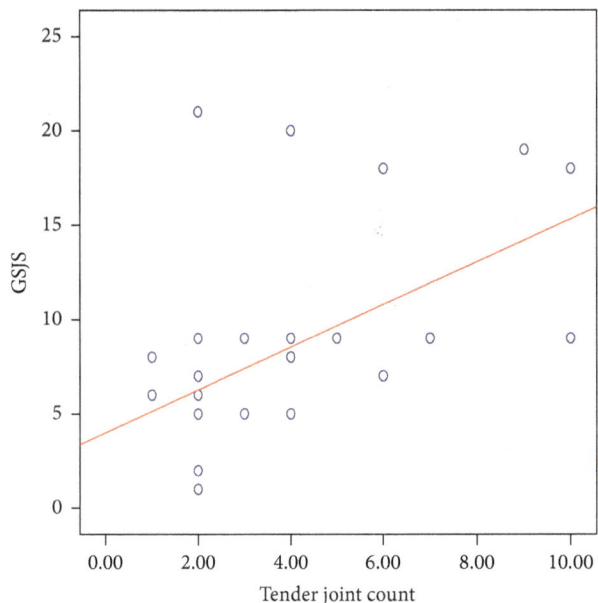

FIGURE 9: Relation between GSJS (taken from 28 MCP, PIP, and DIP joints) and TJC in 30 patients with PsA. Spearman's ρ: 0.484; P: 0.007 suggesting a significant correlation.

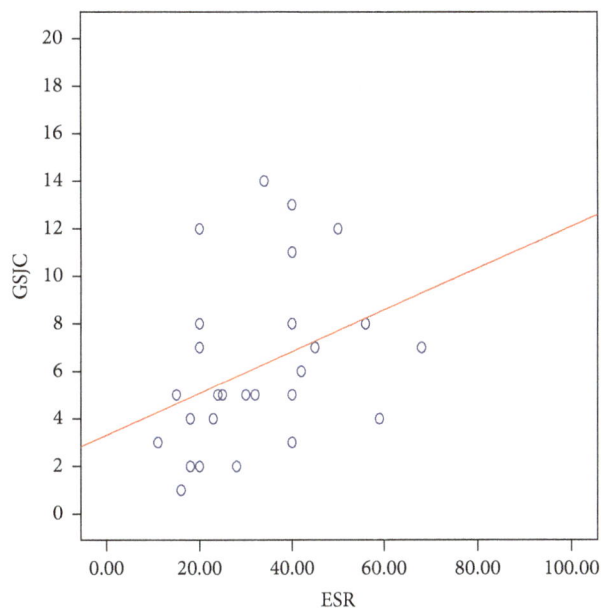

FIGURE 10: Relation between GSJC (taken from 28 MCP, PIP, and DIP joints) and ESR in 30 patients with PsA. Spearman's ρ: 0.478; P: 0.008 suggesting a significant correlation.

Prevalence of periosteal reaction in patients with PsA is up to 25%. In a previous study by Weiner et al., 10 out of 21 joints showing osteoproliferations on radiography also depicted them on US. On the contrary, US suggested osteoproliferative changes without corresponding changes in radiography in six joints. The reported sensitivity of US in comparison to the radiography in the detection of osteoproliferative changes was 10/21 (0.48) and the specificity was 163/169 (0.96) [23].

In our study, the presence of synovial thickening was scored on grayscale and Power Doppler into the Grades 0–3 as shown in Table 2. This semiquantitative scoring system introduced by Szkudlarek in 2003 has been widely used in other studies [24, 25]. Such a grading system has been used in previous studies by Backhaus et al. in which they have evaluated a novel 7-joint ultrasound score in daily rheumatologic practice. They did the study on 120 patients with RA (91%) and PsA (9%). They used the similar grading system for assessment of GS and PD findings [22].

Studies done in patients with RA have shown that GS and PD ultrasound measures have better reliability than the commonly used clinical indices in the evaluation of synovitis and that PD scores may be applied with greater accuracy than clinical scores of synovitis for treatment decisions [26]. The relationship between Power Doppler ultrasonography and clinical scores has not been extensively evaluated in psoriatic arthritis.

Using these scores, composite scores were derived as GSJC, GSJS, PDJC, and PDJS as has already been described. Such a composite scoring system has been used previously in evaluation of disease activity compared to clinical measures in patients with RA [11].

In our study, out of four US measures, GSJC, GSJS, and PDJS demonstrated considerably significant correlation with DAS28 score. Although GS measures showed stronger association than the PD measures, the PD score did correlate significantly and hence demonstrates its utility for the assessment of severity and hence an ongoing inflammation.

The GSJC, GSJS, PDJC, and PDJS were higher in the patients with moderate disease activity as compared to patients with remission and low disease activity. This implies that as the clinical severity score increases, the US scores also show increment.

In the US examination, we included the 28 joints of hands, rather than all those 28 joints that compose the DAS28 score, because PsA often involves DIP joints in addition to PIP and MCP joints. This may affect the analysis of the correlations between clinical data and US data in those cases that have synovitis involving the omitted joints that are knees, wrists, elbows, and shoulders. However, in the cohort studied, only those patients with complaints specific to hands were included and involvement of other joints which contribute to DAS28 was observed to be minimal.

The limitation of our study includes the use of two US machines, so different sensitivity of detecting changes by the US system would have affected the prevalence of various US findings in the hand joints. Lack of reference standard over an ultrasound examination is another limitation since ultrasound detects more abnormality than clinical exam but that may be due to ultrasound overdiagnosing abnormalities that are not clinically relevant.

5. Conclusion

Ultrasound is a useful modality for the objective assessment of PsA, which can detect joint inflammation to a larger extent than clinically expected. Ultrasound findings correlate well with clinical disease activity in patients with psoriatic arthritis. Hence, it may be said that ultrasound including PD can be used as a modality for assessment of severity of psoriatic arthritis in relation to the clinical scoring. Ultrasound including PD may provide useful information regarding the joint disease in the situations where the clinical assessments of severity as DAS28 or ESR are discordant.

Authors' Contribution

Priyanka Naranje and Mahesh Prakash contributed equally to this paper.

References

[1] J. C. T. Alonso, A. R. Perez, J. M. A. Castrillo, J. B. Garcia, J. L. R. Noriega, and C. L. Larrea, "Psoriatic arthritis (PA): a clinical, immunological and radiological study of 180 patients," *British Journal of Rheumatology*, vol. 30, no. 4, pp. 245–250, 1991.

[2] G. Ibrahim, R. Waxman, and P. S. Helliwell, "The prevalence of psoriatic arthritis in people with psoriasis," *Arthritis Care & Research*, vol. 61, no. 10, pp. 1373–1378, 2009.

[3] P. V. S. Prasad, B. Bikku, P. K. Kaviarasan, and A. Senthilnathan, "A clinical study of psoriatic arthropathy," *Indian Journal of Dermatology, Venereology and Leprology*, vol. 73, no. 3, pp. 166–170, 2007.

[4] H. Valdimarsson, A. Karason, and J. E. Gudjonsson, "Psoriasis: a complex clinical and genetic disorder," *Current Rheumatology Reports*, vol. 6, no. 4, pp. 314–316, 2004.

[5] D. D. Gladman, C. Antoni, P. Mease, D. O. Clegg, and O. Nash, "Psoriatic arthritis: epidemiology, clinical features, course, and outcome," *Annals of the Rheumatic Diseases*, vol. 64, supplement 2, pp. ii14–ii17, 2005.

[6] B. Frediani, P. Falsetti, L. Storri et al., "Ultrasound and clinical evaluation of quadricipital tendon enthesitis in patients with psoriatic arthritis and rheumatoid arthritis," *Clinical Rheumatology*, vol. 21, no. 4, pp. 294–298, 2002.

[7] P. Balint and R. D. Sturrock, "Musculoskeletal ultrasound imaging: a new diagnostic tool for the rheumatologist?" *British Journal of Rheumatology*, vol. 36, no. 11, pp. 1141–1142, 1997.

[8] P. J. Mease, C. E. Antoni, D. D. Gladman, and W. J. Taylor, "Psoriatic arthritis assessment tools in clinical trials," *Annals of the Rheumatic Diseases*, vol. 64, no. 2, pp. ii49–ii54, 2005.

[9] J. D. Rees, J. Pilcher, C. Heron, and P. D. W. Kiely, "A comparison of clinical vs ultrasound determined synovitis in rheumatoid arthritis utilizing gray-scale, power Doppler and the intravenous microbubble contrast agent 'Sono-Vue'," *Rheumatology*, vol. 46, no. 3, pp. 454–459, 2007.

[10] R. J. Wakefield, M. J. Green, H. Marzo-Ortega et al., "Should oligoarthritis be reclassified? Ultrasound reveals a high prevalence of subclinical disease," *Annals of the Rheumatic Diseases*, vol. 63, no. 4, pp. 382–385, 2004.

[11] B. Hameed, J. Pilcher, C. Heron, and P. D. W. Kiely, "The relation between composite ultrasound measures and the DAS28 score, its components and acute phase markers in adult RA," *Rheumatology*, vol. 47, no. 4, pp. 476–480, 2008.

[12] E. G. McNally, "Ultrasound of the small joints of the hands and feet: current status," *Skeletal Radiology*, vol. 37, no. 2, pp. 99–113, 2008.

[13] A. Evangelisto, R. Wakefield, and P. Emery, "Imaging in early arthritis," *Best Practice and Research: Clinical Rheumatology*, vol. 18, no. 6, pp. 927–943, 2004.

[14] R. D. Sturrock, "Clinical utility of ultrasonography in spondyloarthropathies," *Current Rheumatology Reports*, vol. 11, no. 5, pp. 317–320, 2009.

[15] R. J. Wakefield, P. V. Balint, M. Szkudlarek et al., "Musculoskeletal ultrasound including definitions for ultrasonographic pathology," *The Journal of Rheumatology*, vol. 32, no. 12, pp. 2485–2487, 2005.

[16] R. J. Wakefield and M.-A. D'Agostino, *Essential Applications of Musculoskeletal Ultrasound in Rheumatology*, Saunders, Philadelphia, Pa, USA, 2010.

[17] D. Kane, T. Greaney, B. Bresnihan, R. Gibney, and O. Fitzgerald, "Ultrasonography in the diagnosis and management of psoriatic dactylitis," *The Journal of Rheumatology*, vol. 26, no. 8, pp. 1746–1751, 1999.

[18] B. Fournié, N. Margarit-Coll, T. L. Champetier de Ribes et al., "Extrasynovial ultrasound abnormalities in the psoriatic finger. Prospective comparative power-doppler study versus rheumatoid arthritis," *Joint Bone Spine*, vol. 73, no. 5, pp. 527–531, 2006.

[19] E. Naredo, I. Möller, E. de Miguel et al., "High prevalence of ultrasonographic synovitis and enthesopathy in patients with psoriasis without psoriatic arthritis: a prospective case-control study," *Rheumatology*, vol. 50, no. 10, pp. 1838–1848, 2011.

[20] J. Milosavljevic, U. Lindqvist, and A. Elvin, "Ultrasound and power Doppler evaluation of the hand and wrist in patients with psoriatic arthritis," *Acta Radiologica*, vol. 46, no. 4, pp. 374–385, 2005.

[21] G. Caldarola, C. De Simone, M. D'Agostino et al., "Usefulness of ultrasound imaging in detecting psoriatic arthritis of fingers and toes in patients with psoriasis," *Clinical and Developmental Immunology*, vol. 2011, Article ID 390726, 5 pages, 2011.

[22] M. Backhaus, S. Ohrndorf, H. Kellner et al., "Evaluation of a novel 7-joint ultrasound score in daily rheumatologic practice: a pilot project," *Arthritis Care and Research*, vol. 61, no. 9, pp. 1194–1201, 2009.

[23] S. M. Weiner, S. Jurenz, M. Uhl et al., "Ultrasonography in the assessment of peripheral joint involvement in psoriatic arthritis," *Clinical Rheumatology*, vol. 27, no. 8, pp. 983–989, 2008.

[24] M. Szkudlarek, E. Narvestad, M. Klarlund, M. Court-Payen, H. S. Thomsen, and M. Østergaard, "Ultrasonography of the metatarsophalangeal joints in rheumatoid arthritis: comparison with magnetic resonance imaging, conventional radiography, and clinical examination," *Arthritis & Rheumatism*, vol. 50, no. 7, pp. 2103–2112, 2004.

[25] M. Szkudlarek, M. Court-Payen, S. Jacobsen, M. Klarlund, H. S. Thomsen, and M. Østergaard, "Interobserver agreement in ultrasonography of the finger and toe joints in rheumatoid arthritis," *Arthritis and Rheumatism*, vol. 48, no. 4, pp. 955–962, 2003.

[26] P. Mandl, P. V. Balint, Y. Brault et al., "Metrologic properties of ultrasound versus clinical evaluation of synovitis in rheumatoid arthritis: results of a multicenter, randomized study," *Arthritis and Rheumatism*, vol. 64, no. 4, pp. 1272–1282, 2012.

7

In Vivo MR Microneurography of the Tibial and Common Peroneal Nerves

Paolo F. Felisaz,[1] **Eric Y. Chang,**[2] **Irene Carne,**[3] **Stefano Montagna,**[4]
Francesco Balducci,[1] **Giulia Maugeri,**[1] **Anna Pichiecchio,**[5] **Fabrizio Calliada,**[1,6]
Maurizia Baldi,[4] **and Stefano Bastianello**[5,7]

[1]*Radiology Department, University of Pavia, 27100 Pavia, Italy*
[2]*Radiology Service, VA San Diego Healthcare System, San Diego, CA 92161, USA*
[3]*Medical Physics Department, IRCCS Salvatore Maugeri Foundation, Scientific Institute of Pavia, 27100 Pavia, Italy*
[4]*Radiology Department, IRCCS Salvatore Maugeri Foundation, Scientific Institute of Pavia, 27100 Pavia, Italy*
[5]*Neuroradiology Department, C. Mondino National Neurological Institute, 27100 Pavia, Italy*
[6]*Institute of Radiology, IRCCS Policlinico S. Matteo Foundation, 27100 Pavia, Italy*
[7]*Department of Brain and Behavioral Sciences, University of Pavia, 27100 Pavia, Italy*

Correspondence should be addressed to Paolo F. Felisaz; paulfel@hotmail.it

Academic Editor: Andreas H. Mahnken

MR microneurography is a noninvasive technique that provides visualization of the microanatomy of peripheral nerves, otherwise available only with histopathology. The objective of this study was to present a protocol to visualize the microstructure of peripheral nerves in vivo, using a 3T MRI scanner with a clinical set of coils and sequences. The tibial and the common peroneal nerves of healthy volunteers were imaged above the medial malleolus and at the level of the fibular head, respectively. The acquired images provided details about the internal structure of peripheral nerves, with visualization of the fascicles, the interfascicular fat, the epineurium, and the perineurium. MR microneurography can be performed in a clinical setting with acceptable imaging times and can be a potentially powerful tool that complements standard MR neurography.

1. Introduction

Magnetic resonance imaging (MRI) of peripheral nerves, also known as MR neurography, provides visualization of the main peripheral nerve trunks and allows detection of pathologic changes such as edema, loss of fascicular pattern, osteofibrous tunnel narrowing, and tumors [1]. Functional evaluation with diffusion weighted imaging (DWI) and diffusion tensor imaging (DTI) techniques have also been described [2]. One main issue with standard MR neurography is spatial resolution, in fact, the nerve fibers, the fascicles and the connective tissues within the peripheral nerves are not easily accessible with conventional imaging protocols.

However, the visualization of the microanatomy of peripheral nerves is a matter of clinical relevance. According to the commonly utilized Seddon and Sunderland classifications for peripheral nerve injuries [3, 4], the integrity of the connective tissues such as the epineurium and perineurium is related to clinical outcome [5]. Current standard of care utilizes a combination of clinical findings and electrophysiology for diagnosis. However, a technique that can visualize and evaluate earlier the integrity of the epineurium and the perineurium may potentially improve diagnosis.

MR microneurography is a noninvasive technique that provides visualization of anatomic details otherwise available only with histopathology. Since early ex vivo experiments that were performed with high field scanners, there has been little development in this field [5–7]. The objective of this study was to present a protocol of MR microneurography using a 3T scanner and a clinical set of coils and sequences,

TABLE 1

	Type	TR/TE (ms)	Flip α	FOV (cm)	Acq matrix	N of slices	Slice thick (mm)	Gap (mm)	ETL	NEX	BW (kHz)	Fat sup.	Time (min)
Localizer	3D SPGR	18/8	10	14	224×192	140	1	0	/	1	35	Yes	2–4
Fluid sensitive HR	3D SPGR	16/6	10	5	512×420	10	2	0	/	5	25	Yes	10–12
T1 weighted HR	2D FSE	625/12	90	5	512×420	10	2	0.5	5	6	31	No	8–10

which could potentially visualize the microarchitecture of peripheral nerves in vivo.

2. Materials and Methods

Imaging was performed on a Discovery MR750 3T scanner (GE Healthcare, Milwaukee) utilizing a 6-channel carotid array coil. Each antenna set articulates, rotates, and locks facilitating the setup in the ankle and knee regions.

After acquisition of written, informed consent, imaging was performed on five volunteers (24 to 30 years of age), all referred in good health without clinical complaints. Experiments were repeated several times with different standard coils and sequences with the aim of finding the optimal setup. Only a few published protocols are available in the literature [5–10] and, to the best of our knowledge, there are no published standard protocols for use on clinical scanners. The 6-channel carotid coil was utilized because it provided high signal-to-noise-ratio (SNR) for relatively superficial nerves. This coil allowed comfortable positioning on the lower limb for the study of the ankle and the knee regions. The tibial nerve was imaged several centimeters along its course, from above the tibiotalar joint into the tarsal tunnel. The common peroneal nerve (CPN) was imaged several centimeters along its course, from above the fibular head to the region of the fibular neck.

3D spoiled gradient echo technique (SPGR—GE, FLASH —Siemens, T1 FFE—Philips) was chosen because it has the advantages of 3D acquisition, with preservation of SNR and lower SAR compared with 3D fast-spin-echo (FSE) techniques such as SPACE (Siemens), CUBE (GE), or VISTA (Philips). Additionally, this particular class of sequences is available on nearly all 1.5T and 3T scanners, which is not the case with the 3D FSE sequences. The detailed parameters of the sequences used are reported in Table 1.

Low-resolution images were first acquired using 3D SPGR sequence with FOV of 10–14 cm. This was useful to localize the neurovascular bundle and visualize the nerve course, facilitating the selection of an exactly perpendicular plane to the nerve, a crucial point to counteract partial volume effects (see Section 4.2).

Thereafter, high-resolution images were acquired with smaller FOVs, ranging from 3 to 6 cm, 512×480 matrix, with scan time approximately 10–12 minutes per sequence. All sequences were acquired without contrast agent injection. Fluid sensitive images were obtained using 3D SPGR

sequences with a small flip angle (10°), adding a standard fat saturation preparation pulse. T1 weighted images were obtained using 2D fast spin echo sequences.

3. Results

Typical microneurograms of the tibial nerve at the ankle and the CPN at the fibular head-neck, using the above MRI protocols, are shown in Figures 1–4. Images of these two nerves were obtained from all the volunteers, but best results were possible when the acquisition plane was precisely orthogonal to the long axis of the nerve, thereby minimizing partial volume effects. Anatomical nerve course variations within the acquisition coverage (2 cm) such as curving, bending, or divisions were a limit to spatial resolution. The localizer protocol (3D SPGR, low resolution with large coverage) was critical to select straight nerve tracts. The tibial nerve was easier to study since its diameter is approximately twice of the CPN, and it exhibited usually a straight course above the tibial malleolus. The CPN instead travels in a curved tract before the fibular head and it divides into its two deep and superficial branches in the peroneal tunnel; therefore imaging of the CPN was more difficult.

On the images in Figures 1 and 2, sequential axial sections of the tibial nerve and the CPN demonstrate the typical fascicular pattern. Details on the neurovascular bundle at the ankle and the main branches of these two nerves are pointed out in the figures. Figure 3 shows the constituents of the neurovascular bundle at the ankle, composed of the tibial nerve, posterior tibial artery, and two veins, surrounded by a fatty, supporting tissue and enclosed within a thicker connective fascia. The tibial nerve is seen with approximately 100 μm in-plane resolution. On 3D SPGR fat suppressed images, the fascicles are hyperintense and highlighted against a hypointense background, mainly due to the suppressed epineurial fat and the epineurial fibrous tissue. This becomes clear in the T1 weighted image (Figure 4), where the epineurial fat is hyperintense and the fascicles are hypointense. The fibrous part of the epineurium is hypointense and surrounds the fascicles, which is the reason why it is not clearly visible. The perineurium is hyperintense in the 3D SPGR fat suppressed images and is best demonstrated when the imaging plane is precisely orthogonal to the long axis of the nerve, as shown in Figures 3 and 4. Finally the paraneural fascia, the outermost connective layer that surrounds the whole fascicles within the epineurium, is hyperintense in the 3D SPGR fat

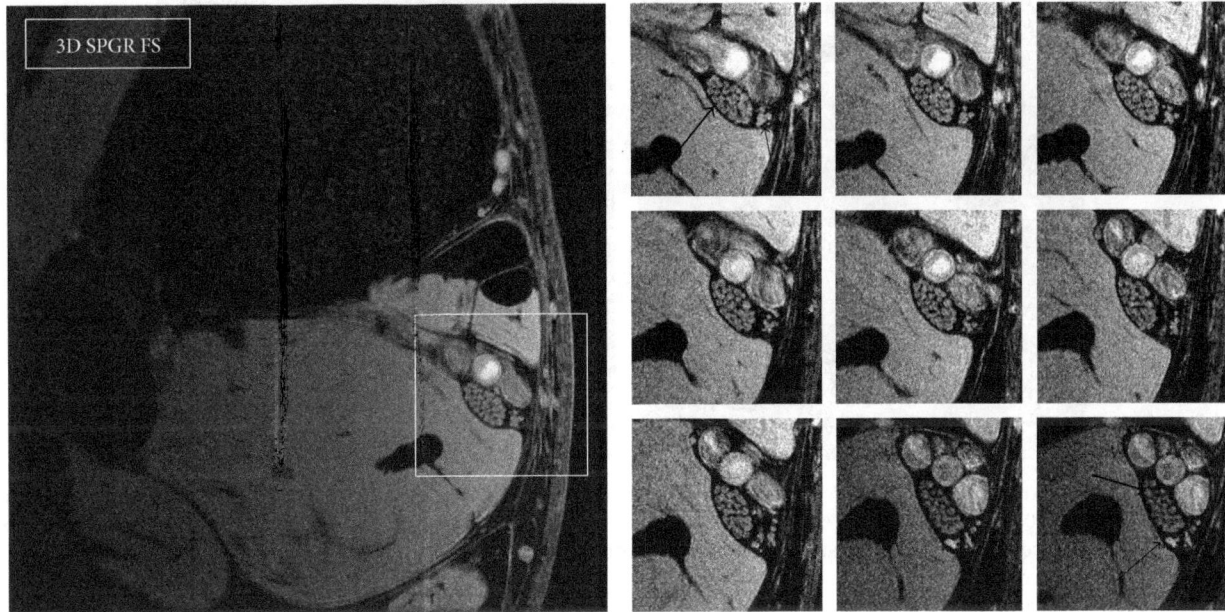

FIGURE 1: 3D SPGR FS, FOV 5 cm. Axial sections at the posteromedial aspect of the tibia, above the medial malleolus. The tibial nerve is visualized (large arrow) with the typical fascicular pattern. The neurovascular bundle is seen at the posteromedial aspect of the tibia. Sequential images at high resolution demonstrate the medial calcaneal nerve dividing into anterior and posterior branches, providing sensory innervation to the plantar aspect of the heel (small arrows).

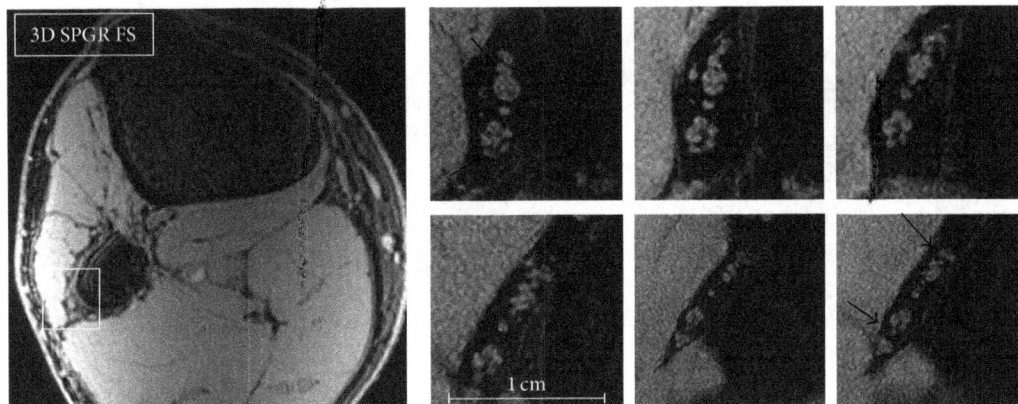

FIGURE 2: 3D SPGR FS, FOV 5 cm. Axial sections of the common peroneal nerve (CPN) at the level of the fibular neck. The CPN is approximately half the diameter of the tibial nerve and therefore contains fewer fascicles. It travels along the lateral aspect of the fibular neck and divides into two main branches, the deep and superficial peroneal nerves (arrows).

suppressed images and hypointense in the TSE T1 weighted images.

4. Discussion

4.1. Anatomy and MR Appearance of the Peripheral Nerves. Peripheral nerves are composed of organized bundles of nerve fibers. Nerve fibers are made by the axons, long protrusions of nerve cell bodies located in the anterior horn of the spinal cord (motor neuron) or in the dorsal root ganglia (sensory neuron). Most axons are surrounded by myelin sheaths, made of Schwann cells. Myelinated and unmyelinated nerve fibers are grouped together in bundles called fascicles, dispersed in a loose connective tissue called endoneurium, and then enclosed in a membrane of flattened cells called perineurium. Nerve fascicles may have different sizes and their number may change along the course of the nerve [11]. They are held together in a fibrous connective tissue called epineurium, which gradually becomes thicker extending to the periphery. Within the epineurium, fat is present in variable amounts depending on the location (typically in higher amount where the nerve slides over bones or within osteofibrous tunnels) or between different nerves (e.g., the sciatic nerve contains more fat than the nerves of the upper limbs [12]).

The MR appearance of the perineurium and the epineurium was first described nearly two decades ago in early studies using MR microneurography [5–7]. The perineurium is

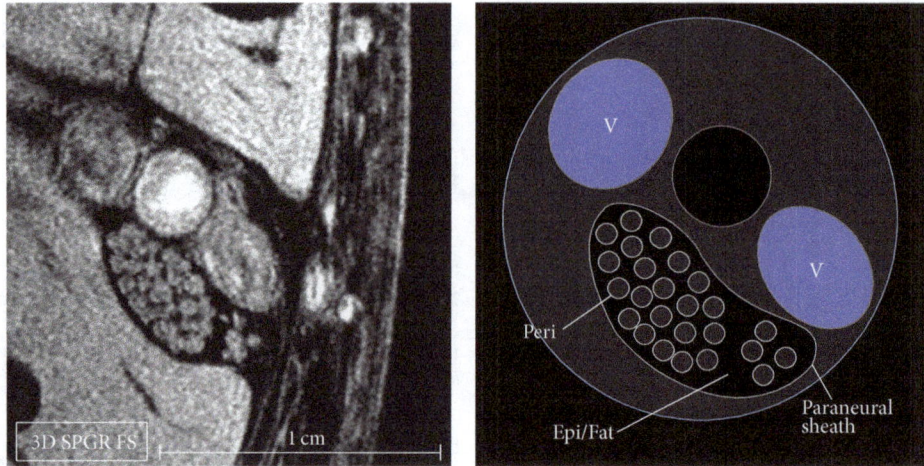

FIGURE 3: 3D SPGR FS. Axial section of the neurovascular bundle at the ankle with the tibial nerve and the corresponding schematic diagram. In-plane resolution is ~100 μm. The paraneural sheath is hyperintense. The epineurium and the epineurial fat (Epi/Fat) appear hypointense because the fat is suppressed and the epineurium has a fibrous structure with low signal. The perineurium (Peri) is hyperintense. The artery (A) demonstrates a thicker wall compared with the paired veins (V). The neurovascular bundle is surrounded by a fatty, supporting tissue and enclosed within a thicker connective fascia.

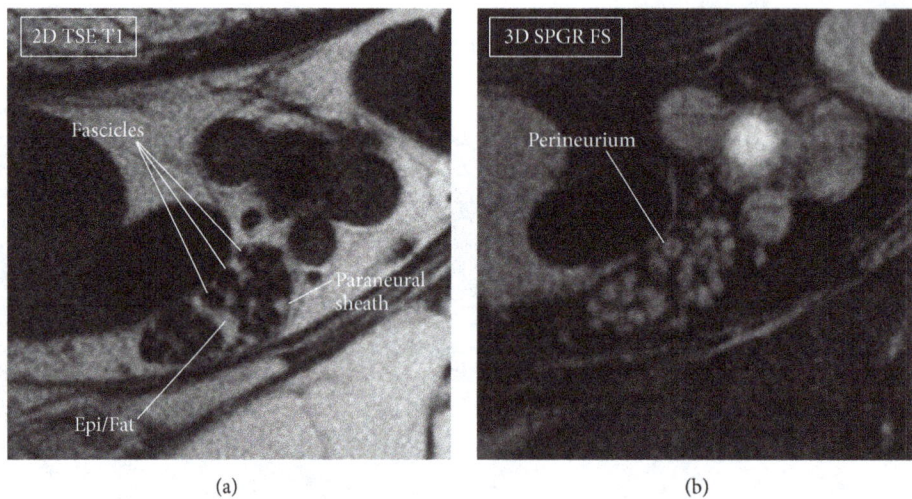

FIGURE 4: Tibial nerve, axial sections. In 2D TSE T1 weighted image (a) the fascicles are hypointense surrounded by a hyperintense tissue, mainly the epineurial fat (Epi/Fat), while the fibrous part of the epineurium has low signal and surrounds the fascicles; it is not clearly seen. The paraneural sheath is also detected. In SPGR fat suppressed image (b), the fascicles are covered by a bright thin layer, the perineurium, best seen when the acquisition plane is exactly perpendicular to the nerve orientation, therefore minimizing the partial volume effects.

the longest T2 component and appears bright in T2 weighted images. The tissue within the fascicles shows intermediate signal, while the internal epineurium is the shortest T2 component with low signal in any sequence with conventional TEs (10 ms or more). The high signal within the fascicles seen in T1 weighted images is mainly fat. This MR appearance may be related to the tissue properties. The epineurium is a dense matrix of thicker, longitudinally oriented collagen bundles that provides mechanical support. Because of this fibrous nature, the epineurium is a short T2 component and can be highlighted using ultrashort TE (UTE) pulse sequences [10]. The perineurium is a layered membrane made of interspaced flattened perineurial cells, basal

laminas rich of proteoglycans, and thinner collagen bundles [13]; the higher amount of free water within the perineurium may contribute to the longer T2 seen in these studies [9].

4.2. Technical Aspects. The definition of MR microscopy (MRM) is relatively vague, and some definitions include use of spatial resolution on the order of 100 μm or smaller [14]. The goal of MRM is to achieve a combination of high spatial resolution and adequate SNR with an acceptable acquisition time. In practice this is challenging, since smaller voxel size results in a decrease of SNR and a longer acquisition time. High field magnets (3T or more) and dedicated small surface coils are typically required to obtain high resolution while maintaining adequate SNR [15].

SNR increases approximately linearly with the field strength. However there are some drawbacks using high field strength such as changes in relaxation times (T1 increases, T2* decreases) and increase of susceptibility effects.

Small surface coils typically have a good SNR close to the coil and allow smaller FOVs; however the sensitivity to the signal drops as the distance increases. Solenoid coils with dimensions smaller than 1 mm allow for resolutions down to the cellular scale; however this can only be used with small ex vivo samples [16]. In the clinical setting, use of the carotid 6-channel coil may limit spatial resolution, but allows for imaging of larger body regions. Furthermore, the multiple channels allow for the possibility of parallel imaging with a further reduction in scan time.

Peripheral nerves demonstrate anatomical features that are advantageous for imaging with MR microscopy. They are anisotropic in shape and they are made of fascicles oriented along one predominant direction. This feature allows for larger slice thickness to be used (e.g. 2 mm), with corresponding increases in SNR, while minimizing the detrimental effects of partial volume averaging. An important technical point is that the acquisition plane should be precisely orthogonal to the long axis of the fibers. Moreover, many clinically relevant nerves of the upper and lower limbs (including tibial, common peroneal, median, and ulnar nerves) are close to the skin surface and accessible with small surface coils.

With regard to scanning technique, early imaging parameters of peripheral nerves typically utilized fat suppression based on chemical selective saturation pulses or the STIR method [17] and fast T2 weighting techniques such as fast spin echo [18]. T2 weighted fat saturated images are useful to demonstrate the presence of edema or hyperemia. Moreover, fat saturation eliminates chemical shift artifact from the epineurial fat along the frequency encoding direction which may obscure the visualization of the perineurium [6]. However additive lengthy spatial-spectral pulses or fat-saturation pulses are required in standard fat saturation techniques, with detriment in SNR and increase in scan time. The sequence 3D IDEAL (Iterative Decomposition of water and fat with Echo Asymmetry and Least-squares estimation—GE Healthcare, USA) do not use additive fat-saturation pulses but provides a three-point water-fat separation method to achieve the maximum possible SNR performance. IDEAL method can be combined with the SPGR sequences providing in a single scan only-fat and only-water images [19]. We did not attempt to use the IDEAL technique although this is feasible and available by other vendors (DIXON—Siemens, Germany; Mdixon—Philips, The Netherlands).

5. Conclusion

MR microneurography provides visualization of the ultra-structure of peripheral nerves. Nearly two decades have passed since its original introduction in the literature; however a simple and repeatable protocol for in vivo use on a clinical MR scanner has not yet been published until now. In this study, we demonstrate that the constituents of peripheral nerve such as the epineurium and perineurium can be readily visualized. Although these structures are typically ignored in conventional radiological practice, they are of great importance in the clinical arena and for the determination of patient outcomes. Future studies should be performed to explore the contribution of this technique to clinical practice. Potential applications include evaluation of the nerves in compressive syndromes, stretch injuries, metabolic diseases, and tumors. Alterations of signal on T2 weighted images, usually described as generalized edema or inflammation of the entire nerve, may be referred to the appropriate compartment such as perineurium, epineurium, or fascicles. Clear visualization of chronic changes such as fascicle involution and fat and fibrous substitution may help to discern a chronic condition from early, reversible damage. Microscopic evaluation of peripheral nerves in vivo may lead to a deeper understanding of the pathogenesis of neuropathies.

Future directions such as parallel imaging with a large array of narrow coils [20, 21] may allow for the characterization of longer nerve tracts with high resolution. Evaluation of function at the microscopic scale is already a part of the standard of care for the study of the central nervous system (including DWI and DTI techniques), and the translation of these MR microscopic techniques to peripheral nerve imaging will certainly lead to better diagnosis of peripheral neuropathies.

References

[1] A. Chhabra, "Magnetic resonance neurography-simple guide to performance and interpretation," *Seminars in Roentgenology*, vol. 48, no. 2, pp. 111–125, 2013.

[2] S. Jambawalikar, J. Baum, T. Button, H. Li, V. Geronimo, and E. S. Gould, "Diffusion tensor imaging of peripheral nerves," *Skeletal Radiology*, vol. 39, no. 11, pp. 1073–1079, 2010.

[3] H. J. Seddon, P. B. Medawar, and H. Smith, "Rate of regeneration of peripheral nerves in man," *The Journal of Physiology*, vol. 102, no. 2, pp. 191–215, 1943.

[4] S. Sunderland, "A classification of peripheral nerve injuries producing loss of function," *Brain*, vol. 74, no. 4, pp. 491–516, 1951.

[5] A. Heddings, M. Bilgen, R. Nudo, B. Toby, T. McIff, and W. Brooks, "High-resolution magnetic resonance imaging of the human median nerve," *Neurorehabilitation & Neural Repair*, vol. 18, no. 2, pp. 80–87, 2004.

[6] M. Bilgen, A. Heddings, B. Al-Hafez et al., "Microneurography of human median nerve," *Journal of Magnetic Resonance Imaging*, vol. 21, no. 6, pp. 826–830, 2005.

[7] K. Ikeda, V. M. Haughton, K.-C. Ho, and B. H. Nowicki, "Correlative MR-anatomic study of the median nerve," *The American Journal of Roentgenology*, vol. 167, no. 5, pp. 1233–1236, 1996.

[8] S. Farooki, C. J. Ashman, J. S. Yu, A. Abduljalil, and D. Chakeres, "In vivo high-resolution MR imaging of the carpal tunnel at 8.0 tesla," *Skeletal Radiology*, vol. 31, no. 8, pp. 445–450, 2002.

[9] G. M. Bydder, R. M. Znamirowski, M. Carl, and N. M. Szeverenyi, "MR imaging of peripheral nerves with short and ultrashort echo pulse sequences," in *Proceedings of the 21st Annual Scientific Meeting of International Society of Magnetic Resonance in Medicine*, Salt Lake City, Utah, USA, April 2013.

[10] P. F. Felisaz, S. Statum, J. Du et al., "Demonstration of the collagenous components of peripheral nerve with short and ultrashort (UTE) pulse sequences," in *Proceedings of the Joint Annual Meeting of ISMRM-ESMRMB*, Milan, Italy, May 2014.

[11] S. Sunderland, "The intraneural topography of the radial, median and ulnar nerves," *Brain*, vol. 68, no. 4, pp. 243–298, 1945.

[12] S. Sunderland, *Nerves and Nerve Injuries*, Churchill Livingstone, Edinburgh, UK, Longman, New York, NY, USA, 2nd edition, 1978.

[13] T. Ushiki and C. Ide, "Three-dimensional organization of the collagen fibrils in the rat sciatic nerve as revealed by transmission- and scanning electron microscopy," *Cell and Tissue Research*, vol. 260, no. 1, pp. 175–184, 1990.

[14] J. M. Tyszka, S. E. Fraser, and R. E. Jacobs, "Magnetic resonance microscopy: recent advances and applications," *Current Opinion in Biotechnology*, vol. 16, no. 1, pp. 93–99, 2005.

[15] M. V. Kulkarni, J. A. Patton, and R. R. Price, "Technical considerations for the use of surface coils in MRI," *American Journal of Roentgenology*, vol. 147, no. 2, pp. 373–378, 1986.

[16] P. Glover and S. P. Mansfield, "Limits to magnetic resonance microscopy," *Reports on Progress in Physics*, vol. 65, no. 10, pp. 1489–1511, 2002.

[17] G. M. Bydder and I. R. Young, "MR imaging: clinical use of the inversion recovery sequence," *Journal of Computer Assisted Tomography*, vol. 9, no. 4, pp. 659–675, 1985.

[18] A. G. Filler, F. A. Howe, C. E. Hayes et al., "Magnetic resonance neurography," *The Lancet*, vol. 341, no. 8846, pp. 659–661, 1993.

[19] C. M. Gerdes, R. Kijowski, and S. B. Reeder, "IDEAL imaging of the musculoskeletal system: robust water fat separation for uniform fat suppression, marrow evaluation, and cartilage imaging," *The American Journal of Roentgenology*, vol. 189, no. 5, pp. W284–W291, 2007.

[20] M. P. McDougall and S. M. Wright, "A parallel imaging approach to wide-field MR microscopy," *Magnetic Resonance in Medicine*, vol. 68, no. 3, pp. 850–856, 2012.

[21] S. Raghuraman, M. F. Mueller, Š. Zbýň et al., "12-channel receive array with a volume transmit coil for hand/wrist imaging at 7 T," *Journal of Magnetic Resonance Imaging*, vol. 38, no. 1, pp. 238–244, 2013.

8

Rapid Automated Target Segmentation and Tracking on 4D Data without Initial Contours

Venkata V. Chebrolu,[1,2,3] **Daniel Saenz,**[2,4] **Dinesh Tewatia,**[2]
William A. Sethares,[5] **George Cannon,**[6] **and Bhudatt R. Paliwal**[2,4]

[1] *Department of Biomedical Engineering, University of Wisconsin-Madison, Madison, WI 53706, USA*
[2] *Department of Human Oncology, University of Wisconsin-Madison, Madison, WI 53792, USA*
[3] *Wisconsin Institute of Medical Research, 1111 Highland Avenue, Madison, WI 53705, USA*
[4] *Department of Medical Physics, University of Wisconsin-Madison, Madison, WI 53792, USA*
[5] *Department of Electrical & Computer Engineering, University of Wisconsin-Madison, Madison, WI 53706, USA*
[6] *Department of Radiation Oncology, Intermountain Healthcare, Salt Lake City, UT 84107, USA*

Correspondence should be addressed to Venkata V. Chebrolu; venkata.v.chebrolu@gmail.com

Academic Editor: Sotirios Bisdas

Purpose. To achieve rapid automated delineation of gross target volume (GTV) and to quantify changes in volume/position of the target for radiotherapy planning using four-dimensional (4D) CT. *Methods and Materials.* Novel morphological processing and successive localization (MPSL) algorithms were designed and implemented for achieving autosegmentation. Contours automatically generated using MPSL method were compared with contours generated using state-of-the-art deformable registration methods (using Elastix© and MIMVista software). Metrics such as the Dice similarity coefficient, sensitivity, and positive predictive value (PPV) were analyzed. The target motion tracked using the centroid of the GTV estimated using MPSL method was compared with motion tracked using deformable registration methods. *Results.* MPSL algorithm segmented the GTV in 4DCT images in 27.0 ± 11.1 seconds per phase (512×512 resolution) as compared to 142.3 ± 11.3 seconds per phase for deformable registration based methods in 9 cases. Dice coefficients between MPSL generated GTV contours and manual contours (considered as ground-truth) were 0.865 ± 0.037. In comparison, the Dice coefficients between ground-truth and contours generated using deformable registration based methods were 0.909 ± 0.051. *Conclusions.* The MPSL method achieved similar segmentation accuracy as compared to state-of-the-art deformable registration based segmentation methods, but with significant reduction in time required for GTV segmentation.

1. Introduction

In the practice of radiation therapy better local control and survival are often associated with increased delivered dose [1]. The greatest limitation to increasing treatment dose is induced by normal lung toxicity. Due to nonperiodic breathing pattern in patients, the planned dose is very often not delivered as intended. Interfractional target motion considerably deteriorates the geometric accuracy of the delivery process. In the recent past, systems and methodologies such as TomoTherapy [2, 3] and cone-beam computer tomography (CBCT) [4, 5] were developed and used in clinical practice

to improve treatment planning and delivery. A quick and accurate method of contouring structures would be useful to improve the efficacy of these systems. Manual segmentation is too time-consuming, making rapid imaging and automated target delineation very attractive for motion management in radiation therapy.

A typical four-dimensional (4D) data for radiation treatment planning in lung cancer includes 10 phases (separated by 10% difference from 0 to 100% of the breathing cycle) and approximately 100 images per phase. To estimate target volume and motion, contours for the gross target volume (GTV) are required on all the phases of the 4D data.

Manual contouring often used for contouring GTV suffers from being very time consuming and subject to intra- and interobserver variability [6]. Reproducibility of the results with manual contouring is challenging due to variations in the experience and training of radiation oncologists. The problem of segmentation is accentuated by the complexity of tumor geometry and by the relatively similar intensity of the tumors as compared to the surrounding tissues or organs. Importantly, manual segmentation is prone to bias and error and is not suitable for rapid, adaptive treatment planning. The use of autocontouring algorithms is very attractive for introducing dynamic assessment of target shape, volume, and position. This work focuses on the design and implementation of computationally efficient automated image segmentation algorithms for rapid assessment of the shape, volume, and position of the target for radiotherapy planning using 4DCT.

Accurate delineation of the GTV is crucial in treatment planning because the construction of both the clinical target volume (CTV) and the planning target tumor volume (PTV) is based on the GTV. During the radiotherapy process, tumor regression often occurs, and when the change is beyond some threshold, the contours should be adapted to the new GTV. Similarly, accurate delineation of the tumor volume during the different phases of breathing cycle is crucial to reduce margins added around the clinical tumor volume. Further reduction in margin would be anticipated to decrease integral radiation dose, mitigating potential acute and late side effects to organs at risk (OAR), and allowing further dose escalation as indicated. The specific tumor trajectory and position often changes from day to day and during the delivery of radiation therapy treatment. When small margins are used, such variability may be detrimental when the treatment target is in motion. Intrafraction tumor motion due to the respiratory cycle and cardiac motion and interfraction differences in the patient's position, anatomy, tumor size, and shape during the course of treatment often result in suboptimal delivery of the planned radiation dose. Often in practice, an extended volume envelope is used to address the problem of uncertainties due to motion. Unfortunately, this increase in treatment volume limits the patient tolerance dose. Rapid and automatic delineation can therefore improve clinical workflow and efficiency, which can eventually improve the therapeutic ratio.

The state of the art for obtaining CT contours particularly in a 4DCT is deformable registration [7–9] based segmentation. These algorithms use manually created contours on one phase of 4D data to automatically segment the target volume(s) in the other phases of 4D data [10]. Deformable image registration delineates motion of any internal structure as well as deformation from the reference phase to each phase. This registration procedure outputs deformation maps, that is, voxel-to-voxel displacement between the reference image and each phase image. One limitation of deformable registration approach for application in adaptive treatment planning is that, before the deformable registration method can be used to determine target motion profiles, there is a need to manually segment one phase of the 4DCT data. Another limitation of deformable registration is that it is generally

computationally complex. In this work we design and implement novel computationally efficient automated segmentation algorithms that do not require manual contouring on one phase of 4DCT data. We apply these autocontouring algorithms to quantify changes in volume/position of the target during free breathing.

2. Methods and Materials

Nine lung cancer patients were imaged using 4DCT protocol under free-breathing condition with a GE Discovery Light-Speed CT Scanner (GE Healthcare Waukesha, WI) under the request of a physician interested in target motion. An appropriate institutional review board (IRB) approved the study. The imaging parameters include slice thickness of 2.5 mm, an energy of 120 kVp, and a tube current of 100 mA. Varian Real-time Position Management (RPM) system was used for acquiring the respiratory waveform for retrospective binning. The raw data was retrospectively binned using Advantage 4D software to divide the data into ten breathing phases.

2.1. Automated Image Segmentation Using Morphological Processing and Successive Localization. Novel and computationally efficient morphological processing and successive localization (MPSL) algorithms were developed for achieving automated segmentation of the body, lung, and the tumors [11, 12]. Morphological operations such as dilation and erosion are computationally efficient. If A and B are two subsets in a N-dimensional space, then the morphological operation such as dilation and erosion on subset A with a structuring element B is mathematically represented as

$$\text{Dilation}: A \oplus B$$

$$= \left\{ c \in Z^N \mid c = a + b \text{ for some } a \in A, b \in B \right\},$$

$$\text{Erosion}: A \ominus B = \left\{ x \in Z^N \mid x + b \in A \text{ for every } b \in B \right\}.$$

$$(1)$$

The following sections describe the utilization of these operations to achieve automated segmentation.

2.1.1. Segmenting the Tumors. Initially, the intensity range for the tumors and the surrounding regions were defined. In general, this a priori information required for automated segmentation can be obtained using the images from a prior CT scan. If there were no overlaps between the intensity range for the tumors and the surrounding regions, then a threshold on the maximum/minimum intensity would segment the tumors. However, in general there will be an overlap between the two intensity ranges. Therefore, a binary mask that includes the regions with intensity values within either of the two intensity ranges was generated.

The binary mask generated above was then eroded to produce disjoint regions. The amount of erosion was determined empirically by performing the erosion operation in a population of individuals. Each of the separate regions in the disjoint region data was then labeled and the volume occupied by each

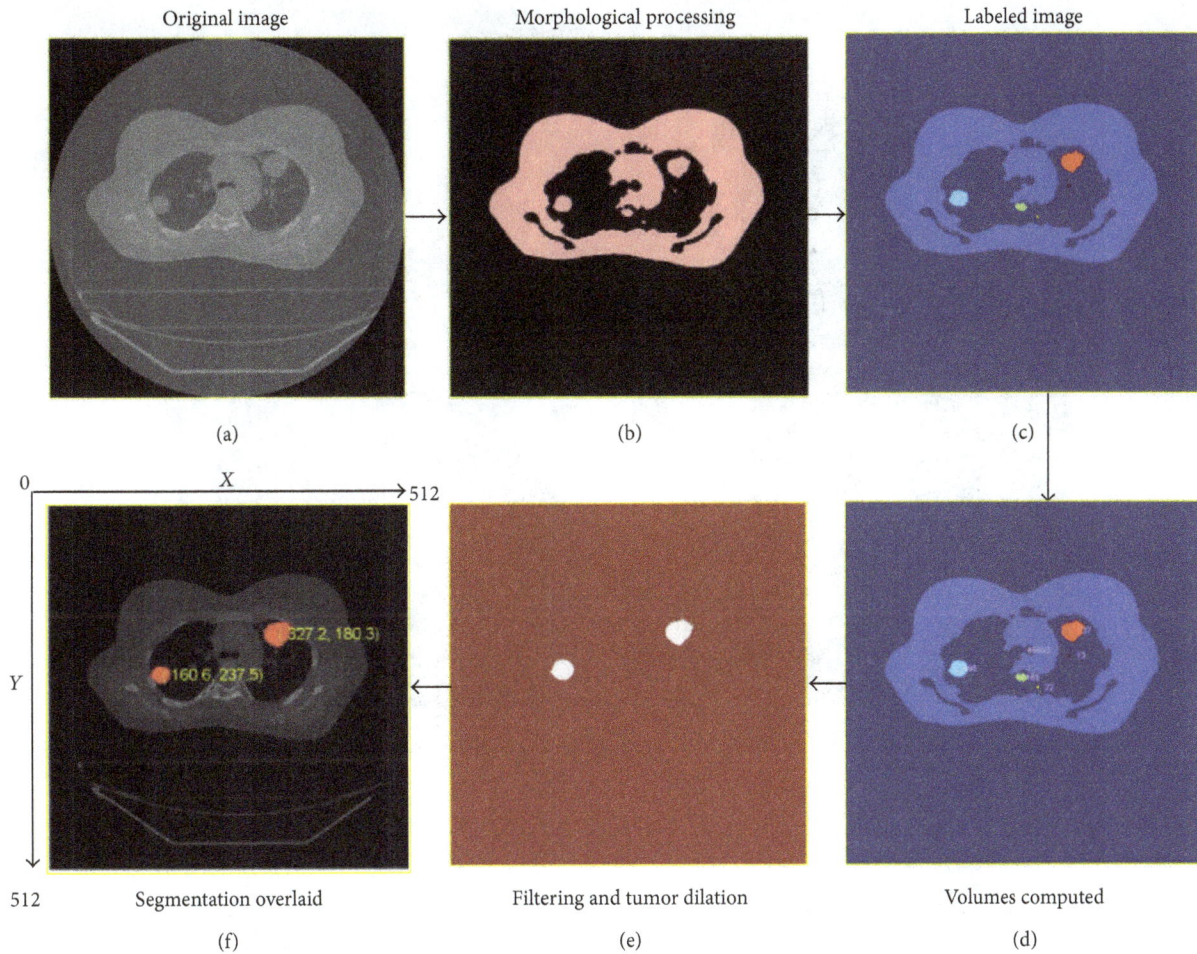

FIGURE 1: Morphological processing based automated segmentation approach for contouring the tumors. The center of geometry of the segmented tumors is useful for quantifying tumor motion between different phases.

labeled region was determined; that is, after morphologically separating the tumors using erosion, the different regions were labeled (using the union-find algorithm [13]) and then the morphologically connected regions and their volumes were calculated. The labeled regions were analyzed to identify the tumor region. This analysis process identifies regions with volumes close to the range of typical tumor volumes; that is, a limit on the maximum/minimum possible volume of the tumors was used as a filter to isolate the tumors. This filtering based on size removes nontumor regions. This identification can be supplemented with tumor location data if known.

The mask obtained above was dilated by the same amount as the prior erosion to obtain the tumor segmentation; that is, the erosion is reversed through a dilation to restore the tumors to their approximate original size.

The inputs needed for this algorithm are the minimum and maximum intensity threshold values for the tumor and surrounding regions (for generating a mask), the minimum and maximum limits for tumor volume, and the erosion/dilation radius (for morphological processing). The optimal input values for erosion/dilation radii and threshold ranges were empirically chosen. The algorithm was developed to work at both 2 and 3 dimensions.

Figure 1 shows the flowchart for the above described segmentation procedure in a specific example. The empirically chosen threshold ranges create a binary image, including the tumor and surrounding tissue with a direct connection between them. Image erosion (shown in Figure 1(b)) removes the connection between the tumor and the lung wall. The result is a postmorphologically processed image with separated tumors. All independent regions (nonconnected volumes) are labeled (Figure 1(c)) and the volume of each disconnected region was calculated (Figure 1(d)). The expected range of tumor volume provided as input allows for localizing the tumor among the labeled regions (Figure 1(e)). Morphological dilation restores tumors to the original size after tumor identification (Figure 1(f)).

2.1.2. Phantom Validation. The MPSL algorithm was validated using a phantom experiment. The LUNGMAN anthropomorphic chest phantom (Figure 2) was used for the validation. A 6-cm diameter sphere of virtual water was used to simulate the GTV. The Washington University 4D Motion system [14] generated realistic motion profiles, while 4DCT scans were acquired. Figure 2 shows the experimental setup.

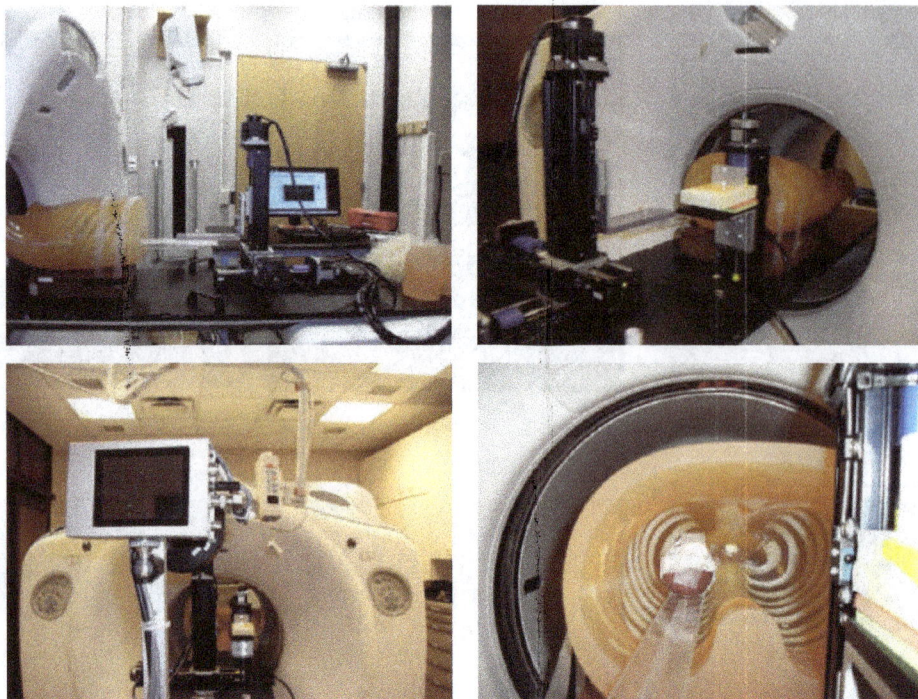

FIGURE 2: Experimental setup for validating MPSL-based motion and volume quantification using anthropomorphic chest phantom and the Washington University 4D motion system.

2.2. Ground-Truth Generation via Manual Contouring. The GTV contours generated by the MPSL algorithm were compared with the contours manually drawn on the different phases of the 4D data, considering the manual contours as "ground-truth." ITK-SNAP [15] was used to generate manual contours. Manual contours took 1–5 minutes per phase to complete depending on the size of the GTV. The manual contours were generated by one of the investigators (DS). Interobserver variation in generation of manual contours is expected, as shown in other studies [16, 17].

2.3. Deformable Registration Based GTV Segmentation. Deformable image registration (DIR) based GTV contours were generated using Elastix© software (a toolbox for deformable image registration) and MIMVista software for comparison with the results from our algorithm. Manual contours were drawn on the first phase of 4DCT data and were then propagated to the other phases using DIR. Elastix© used a b-spline transformation based DIR algorithm with a mutual information similarity metric and rigid penalty described by Staring in 2007 [18]. MIMVista used intensity-based free-form VoxAlign Deformation Engine, previously used in the literature, for propagating manually drawn contours on one phase to the remaining phases in the dynamic study [19, 20].

2.4. Motion Estimation. The target volumes as well as the center of geometry (COG) positions were recorded by computing the GTV contour statistics. The COG of the segmented target was used as a measurement of the GTV position, so that

GTV trajectory can be estimated. The GTV trajectory (the trajectory of the COG of the GTV) was estimated using MPSL method and was compared with the trajectory generated using MIMVista.

When using MIMVista the GTV in one phase was contoured in a semiautomated manner and the GTV in the remaining phases was segmented using deformable registration. The semiautomated segmentation of the GTV on one phase was performed as follows. A threshold of −83 HU was initially used, allowing voxels with intensity values above that threshold to be included in the contours for the GTV. Next, manual adjustments were made to fill in holes that were erroneously excluded from the GTV and to delete parts of normal anatomy that were included. Then, MIMVista's 4DCT adaptive recontouring tool was used to propagate the contours to the other phases.

2.5. Statistics. The comparison between GTV contours generated using MPSL and deformable registration based segmentation were compared with ground-truth using Dice similarity coefficient. Sensitivity, positive-predictive value (PPV) and accuracy in volume quantification were also compared for the contouring methods. The sensitivity measured the fraction of the voxels in the ground-truth that the automatic contour (MPSL/DIR based) included. The PPV measured the fraction of voxels inside the automatic (MPSL/DIR based) contour that were "true positives" (points in the ground-truth contour).

TABLE 1: Dice similarity coefficients, sensitivity, and PPV between GTV contours generated with the proposed MPSL method and DIR based segmentation.

Case number	Dice				Sensitivity			PPV		
	MPSL versus manual	DIR versus manual	MPSL versus DIR	MPSL versus manual	DIR versus manual	MPSL versus DIR	MPSL versus manual	DIR versus manual	MPSL versus DIR	
1	0.882	0.984	0.885	0.836	0.979	0.843	0.933	0.988	0.931	
2	0.872	0.914	0.856	0.805	0.907	0.796	0.950	0.921	0.925	
3	0.860	0.915	0.877	0.801	0.878	0.850	0.929	0.955	0.906	
4	0.941	0.941	0.914	0.901	0.956	0.863	0.984	0.927	0.971	
5	0.825	0.949	0.823	0.723	0.963	0.711	0.962	0.935	0.975	
6	0.845	0.841	0.792	0.876	0.945	0.737	0.816	0.758	0.855	
7	0.854	0.929	0.830	0.775	0.926	0.755	0.951	0.931	0.921	
8	0.887	0.885	0.828	0.899	0.954	0.781	0.875	0.825	0.880	
9	0.819	0.826	0.785	0.830	0.932	0.713	0.809	0.742	0.873	
Average	0.865	0.909	0.843	0.827	0.938	0.783	0.912	0.887	0.915	
St. dev.	0.037	0.051	0.043	0.059	0.031	0.059	0.064	0.089	0.042	

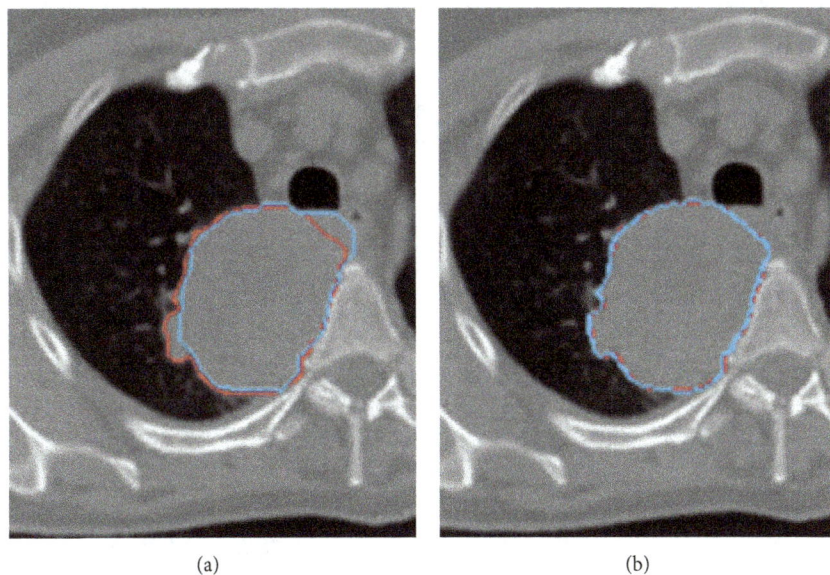

(a)   (b)

FIGURE 3: Comparison of automated contouring methods with ground-truth in case 1. (a) Manual contour (red) compared with MPSL (turquoise) based segmentation of GTV. (b) Manual contour (red) compared with DIR based contour (turquoise).

3. Results

3.1. Accuracy Comparison. In the phantom experiment, the volume and COG motion profiles estimated by the MPSL algorithm were within 5% error of the known ground-truth values.

The accuracy of the contours generated using MPSL and DIR based segmentation in patients was estimated by calculating the Dice similarity coefficient, as well as the sensitivity and PPV in comparison to the ground-truth.

Table 1 shows the results for the nine cases. The two-sided paired t-test for statistical difference between the Dice coefficients of MPSL and DIR methods resulted in a P value of 0.024. Similarly, the P values for statistical difference between

MPSL and DIR based methods for Sensitivity and PPV were 0.006 and 0.104, respectively.

Figures 3, 4, and 5 shows the GTV segmentation using MPSL algorithm and DIR based segmentation for three representative cases.

Segmentation methods based on thresholding and region-growing would fail in the case shown in Figure 3 due to large connection between GTV and the rest of the body.

3.2. Time Performance Comparison. The time for the automatic segmentation of the GTV using MPSL in the 9 cases considered in this study was 24.2 ± 6.1 seconds per phase. In the case of DIR based segmentation of GTV, the manual

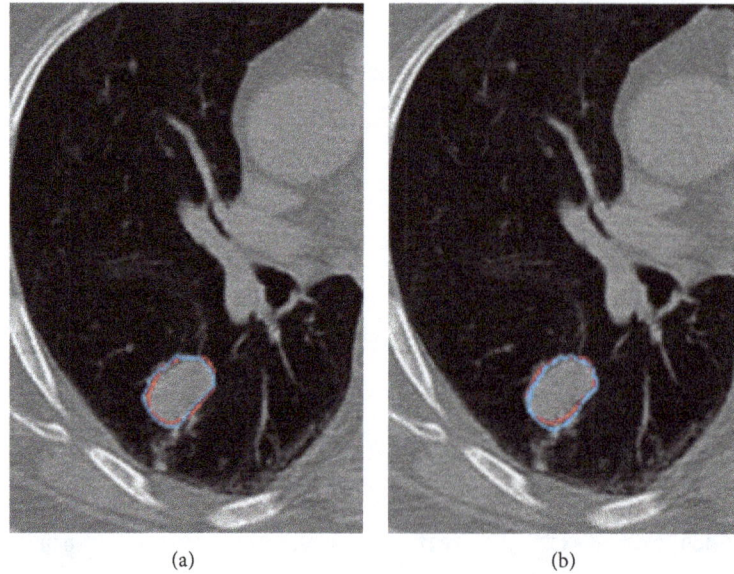

FIGURE 4: Comparison of automated contouring methods with ground-truth in case 2. (a) Manual contour (red) compared with MPSL (turquoise) based segmentation of GTV. (b) Manual contour (red) compared with DIR based contour (turquoise).

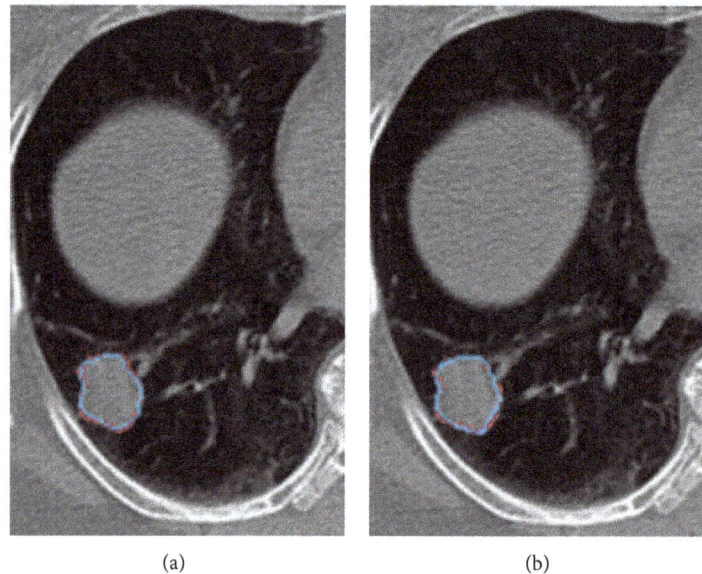

FIGURE 5: Comparison of automated contouring methods with ground-truth in case 3. (a) Manual contour (red) compared with MPSL (turquoise) based segmentation of GTV. (b) Manual contour (red) compared with DIR based contour (turquoise). Notice that diaphragm with similar intensity as that of the GTV was not included in the contour by the MPSL algorithm.

contouring on the first phase using ITK-SNAP took 153.4 ± 153.2 seconds (note that the large standard deviation in the time for manual contouring was due to one outlier case which had GTV spanning over many slices and it took 538 seconds to manually contour the GTV). The DIR based segmentation using Elastix© software took 142.3 ± 11.3 seconds to calculate the deformation map and then transform the contour from the first phase to one another phase.

3.3. Motion Quantification. Figures 6 and 7 show the quantification of GTV motion in x, y, and z directions using

MPSL for two representative cases. The MPSL based motion estimation was compared with motion estimation performed using ground-truth. In the result shown Figure 6 the ground-truth in all the different phase volumes was manually contoured, whereas, in Figure 7, the tumor in the volume corresponding to 40% phase was manually contoured and the contours were propagated to other phases using deformable registration. The figures show that MPSL segmentation based tumor position and volume quantification results are strongly correlated with the quantification results derived using MIMVista.

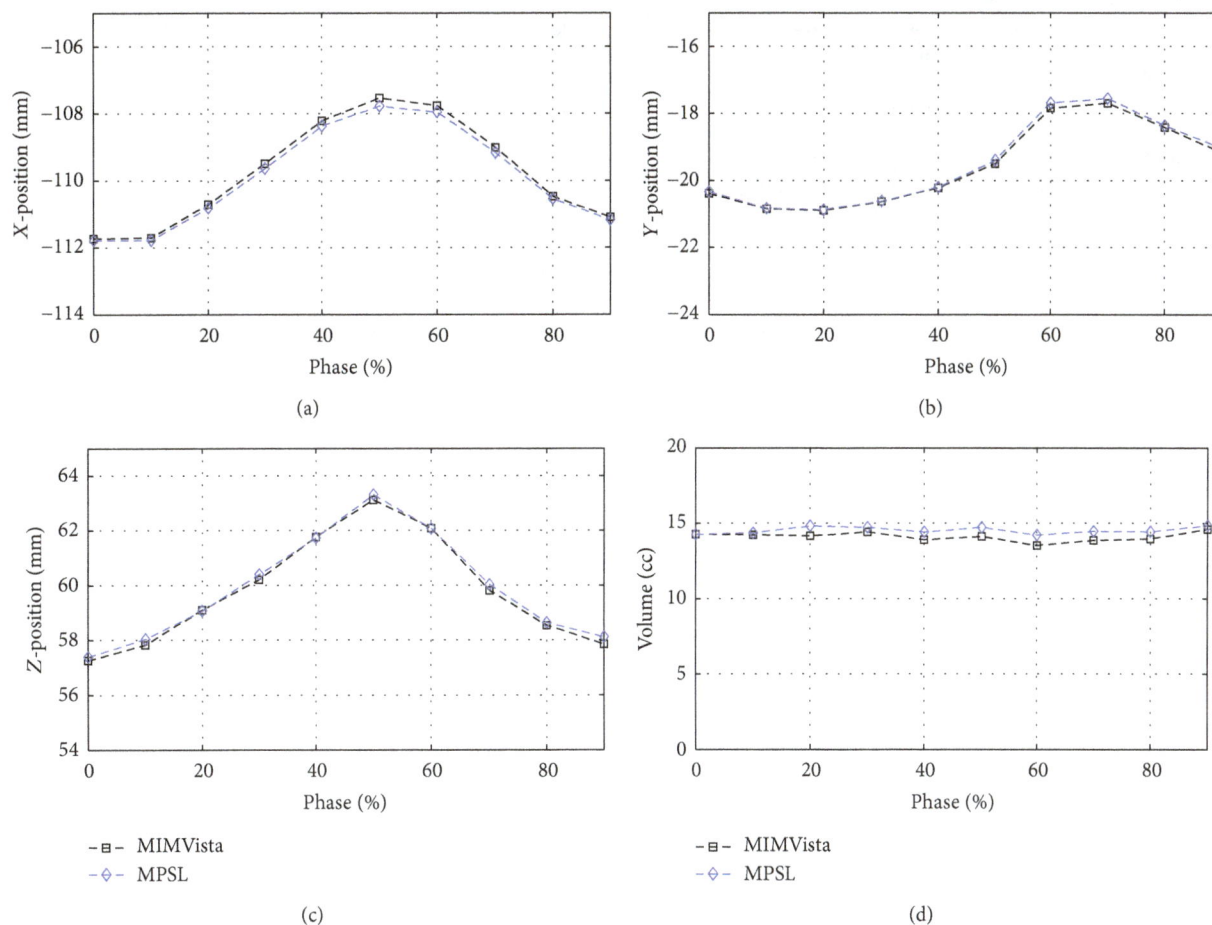

(a)

(b)

(c)

(d)

FIGURE 6: Good agreement of MPSL based estimation of GTV position and volume quantification with MIMVista based estimation for different phases of the 4DCT scan shown in a patient with 15cc GTV.

4. Discussion

MPSL-based segmentation was developed for rapid and accurate contouring of the GTV in different phases of 4D CT data. High Dice similarity (0.865 ± 0.037) with ground-truth and processing time of less than half a minute show the potential of MPSL for improving workflow in radiotherapy planning. MPSL method also achieved high sensitivity (0.827 ± 0.059) and PPV (0.912 ± 0.064). The MPSL algorithm achieved rapid segmentation in time scales shorter than the state-of-the-art deformable image registration based segmentation methods. In the case of a single 512 × 512 image, MPSL segmentation was achieved in time scale of a tenth of a second. For a 3D volume with in-plane resolution of 512 × 512 and 80–100 slices segmentation was achieved in less than 30 seconds. Furthermore, MPSL does not require manual contouring on one phase for propagating to other phases, facilitating efficient use without need for previous segmentation. The method is also less subjective. Therefore, the algorithm could be used in scenarios where fast contouring of the GTV is needed.

The paired t-test showed statistically significant difference for Dice coefficients and sensitivity between DIR and MPSL based segmentation methods. However, both had high values for Dice and sensitivity. DIR based segmentation was statistically closer to ground-truth as compared to MPSL based segmentation, but with nearly sixfold increase in the processing time. Furthermore, the cases with the greatest difference in the Dice similarity coefficient between MPSL and DIR based methods were the cases where a large region of the GTV was attached to the wall of the lung. In such cases, delineation of GTV in the "ground-truth" tends to be subjective. Hence, if the manual GTV contours on first phase are registered using deformable registration, higher agreement with ground-truth is expected as compared to MPSL because of the subjectivity propagated to the other phases. In those cases, the automatic segmentation algorithm makes morphological conclusion as to where the boundary will be, where the manual segmentation is bound to be subjective. In our data there were two such cases out of the nine. Omitting those two cases in the paired t-test analysis showed no statistical difference (P value of 0.09) between the Dice similarity coefficients from MPSL and DIR based methods.

In this work we have not used user-input to find the location of the GTV, which is attractive for ease and reproducibility. However, the algorithm could be modified to use input information regarding the location of GTV to

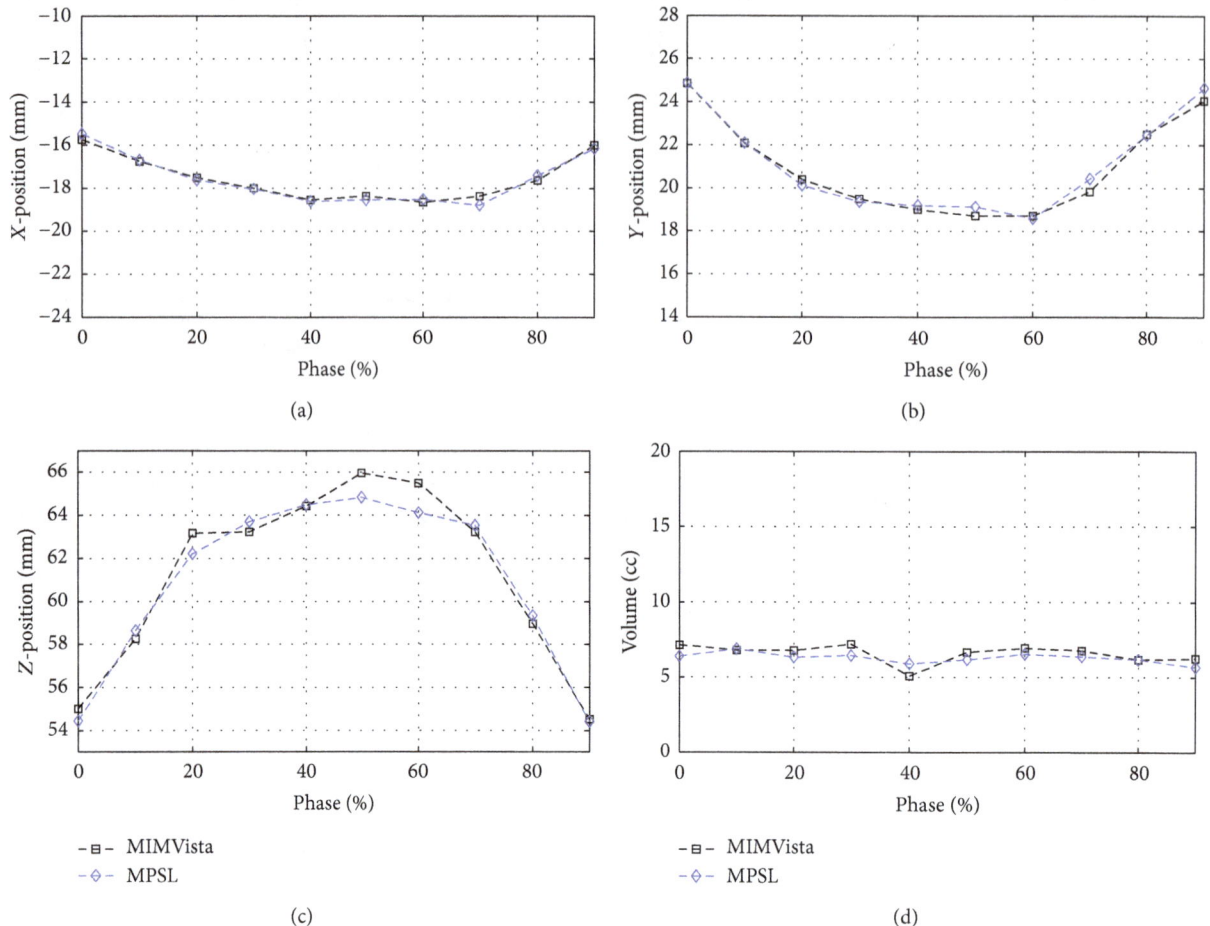

FIGURE 7: Good agreement of MPSL based estimation of GTV position and volume quantification with MIMVista based estimation for different phases of the 4DCT scan shown in a patient with 6cc GTV.

further improve the speed and accuracy. Hence, a tool has been implemented in the software for the user to provide a "click" inside the tumor as a starting point, which allows the algorithm the parallel ability to use the local neighborhood intensity values as a range for thresholding. Similarly, if preexisting GTV contours on earlier scans do exist, a rigid registration, which is much faster than DIR, could be applied to get input information about the target location.

The computation complexity of MPSL was compared with DIR based segmentation algorithms available in Elastix© and MIMVista software. There are other nonrigid registration algorithms such as diffeomorphic symmetric normalization (DSN). Comparison of DSN methods is beyond the scope of this work. Parallel processing and multithreaded approaches could be used to reduce the computational tim But we have not explored those approaches. The algorithms developed in this work are applicable to MR data and CBCT in addition to 4DCT data used in this work. Future work would explore the use of MPSL approach for real-time segmentation of GTV on MR and CBCT data.

5. Conclusion

Automated and rapid generation of GTV contours using the MPSL algorithm may be advantageous for a number of scenarios including adaptive radiotherapy planning. The MPSL method achieved similar segmentation accuracy as compared to state-of-the-art deformable registration based segmentation methods, but with significant reduction in the computation time.

References

[1] F. M. Kong, R. K. Ten Haken, M. J. Schipper et al., "High-dose radiation improved local tumor control and overall survival in patients with inoperable/unresectable non-small-cell lung cancer: long-term results of a radiation dose escalation study," International Journal of Radiation Oncology Biology Physics, vol. 63, no. 2, pp. 324–333, 2005.

[2] T. R. Mackie, T. Holmes, S. Swerdloff et al., "Tomotherapy: a new concept for the delivery of dynamic conformal radiotherapy," Medical Physics, vol. 20, no. 6, pp. 1709–1719, 1993.

[3] K. J. Ruchala, G. H. Olivera, E. A. Schloesser, and T. R. Mackie, "Megavoltage CT on a tomotherapy system," Physics in Medicine and Biology, vol. 44, no. 10, pp. 2597–2621, 1999.

[4] J. Pouliot, A. Bani-Hashemi, J. Chen et al., "Low-dose megavoltage cone-beam CT for radiation therapy," *International Journal of Radiation Oncology Biology Physics*, vol. 61, no. 2, pp. 552–560, 2005.

[5] J. J. Sonke, L. Zijp, P. Remeijer, and M. Van Herk, "Respiratory correlated cone beam CT," *Medical Physics*, vol. 32, no. 4, pp. 1176–1186, 2005.

[6] P. Giraud, S. Elles, S. Helfre et al., "Conformal radiotherapy for lung cancer: different delineation of the gross tumor volume (GTV) by radiologists and radiation oncologists," *Radiotherapy and Oncology*, vol. 62, no. 1, pp. 27–36, 2002.

[7] R. Speight, J. Sykes, R. Lindsay, K. Franks, and D. Thwaites, "The evaluation of a deformable image registration segmentation technique for semi-automating internal target volume (ITV) production from 4DCT images of lung stereotactic body radiotherapy (SBRT) patients," *Radiotherapy and Oncology*, vol. 98, no. 2, pp. 277–283, 2011.

[8] A. Al-Mayah, J. Moseley, M. Velec, S. Hunter, and K. Brock, "Deformable image registration of heterogeneous human lung incorporating the bronchial tree," *Medical Physics*, vol. 37, no. 9, pp. 4560–4571, 2010.

[9] Y. Yim, H. Hong, and Y. G. Shin, "Deformable lung registration between exhale and inhale CT scans using active cells in a combined gradient force approach," *Medical Physics*, vol. 37, no. 8, pp. 4307–4317, 2010.

[10] K. Wijesooriya, E. Weiss, V. Dill et al., "Quantifying the accuracy of automated structure segmentation in 4D CT images using a deformable image registration algorithm," *Medical Physics*, vol. 35, no. 4, pp. 1251–1260, 2008.

[11] V. V. Chebrolu, D. Tewatia, J. Dai et al., "Four-dimensional MRI/CT based auto-adaptive segmentation for real-time radiotherapy in lung cancer treatment," *Medical Physics*, vol. 38, p. 3846, 2011.

[12] V. V. Chebrolu, J. Dai, D. Tewatia et al., "Real-time automated target volume and motion quantification for adaptive four-dimensional MRI/CT guided radiation therapy," *International Journal of Radiation Oncology, Biology, Physics*, vol. 81, no. 2, p. S814, 2011.

[13] R. Sedgewick, *Algorithms in C*, Addison-Wesley, Reading, Mass, USA, 1998.

[14] K. Malinowski, K. Lechleiter, J. Hubenschmidt, D. Low, and P. Parikh, "Use of the 4D phantom to test real—time targeted radiation therapy device accuracy," *Medical Physics*, vol. 34, article 2611, 2007.

[15] P. A. Yushkevich, J. Piven, H. C. Hazlett et al., "User-guided 3D active contour segmentation of anatomical structures: significantly improved efficiency and reliability," *NeuroImage*, vol. 31, no. 3, pp. 1116–1128, 2006.

[16] C. B. Caldwell, K. Mah, Y. C. Ung et al., "Observer variation in contouring gross tumor volume in patients with poorly defined non-small-cell lung tumors on CT: the impact of 18FDG-hybrid PET fusion," *International Journal of Radiation Oncology Biology Physics*, vol. 51, no. 4, pp. 923–931, 2001.

[17] R. J. H. M. Steenbakkers, J. C. Duppen, I. Fitton et al., "Observer variation in target volume delineation of lung cancer related to radiation oncologist-computer interaction: a 'Big Brother' evaluation," *Radiotherapy and Oncology*, vol. 77, no. 2, pp. 182–190, 2005.

[18] M. Staring, S. Klein, and J. P. W. Pluim, "A rigidity penalty term for nonrigid registration," *Medical Physics*, vol. 34, no. 11, pp. 4098–4108, 2007.

[19] J. Piper, "Evaluation of an intensity-based free-form deformable registration algorithm," *Medical Physics*, vol. 34, no. 6, pp. 2353–2354, 2007.

[20] J. Piper, M. Duchateau, A. Nelson, D. Verellen, and M. De Ridder, "Characterizing Accuracy in 4DCT Deformable Registration Using the POPI Model," *Med Phys*, pp. 40–168, 2013.

9

Multidetector Computer Tomography: Evaluation of Blunt Chest Trauma in Adults

João Palas,[1] António P. Matos,[1] Vasco Mascarenhas,[2]
Vasco Herédia,[3] and Miguel Ramalho[1]

[1] Department of Radiology, Hospital Garcia de Orta, Avenida Torrado da Silva, Almada, 2801-951 Setúbal, Portugal
[2] Department of Radiology, Hospital da Luz, Avenida Lusíada 100, 1500-650 Lisbon, Portugal
[3] Department of Radiology, Hospital Espírito Santo, Largo do Senhor da Pobreza, 7000-811 Évora, Portugal

Correspondence should be addressed to Miguel Ramalho; miguel-ramalho@netcabo.pt

Academic Editor: Hoen-oh Shin

Imaging plays an essential part of chest trauma care. By definition, the employed imaging technique in the emergency setting should reach the correct diagnosis as fast as possible. In severe chest blunt trauma, multidetector computer tomography (MDCT) has become part of the initial workup, mainly due to its high sensitivity and diagnostic accuracy of the technique for the detection and characterization of thoracic injuries and also due to its wide availability in tertiary care centers. The aim of this paper is to review and illustrate a spectrum of characteristic MDCT findings of blunt traumatic injuries of the chest including the lungs, mediastinum, pleural space, and chest wall.

1. Introduction

In the United States and Western Europe, trauma is the fourth most common cause of death and the leading cause of death in the population with less than 45 years of age [1]. Thoracic injuries and related complications in the patient who has experienced blunt chest trauma have a mortality of 15.5% to 25% [2]. Traffic accidents are the major source of blunt chest trauma representing approximately two thirds of the cases [3].

Imaging studies play an essential part of thoracic trauma care. The information generated with different diagnostic imaging tools has a major role in management of chest trauma patients [4]. The ideal imaging technique should reach the correct diagnosis as fast as possible. Chest radiography (CXR) has been the traditional screening technique to evaluate thoracic trauma. However, the information obtained is suboptimal for the diagnosis of vascular and nonvascular thoracic injuries, as it underestimates the severity and extent of chest trauma and, in some cases, fails to detect the presence of injury [5]. There is growing evidence that multidetector computed tomography (MDCT) is more sensitive than CXR in the detection and characterization of thoracic injuries

after trauma [6, 7]. Traub et al. found that 42% patients had additional findings reported by MDCT scan beyond that found on their CXR [6]. Brink et al. [8] found additional findings in up to 59% of patients with MDCT compared with CXR and Trupka et al. reported clinical changes in management after CT scans in up to 70% of patients [9].

Due to its wide availability, speed, and ability to depict a variety of injuries, as well as being able to simultaneously evaluate other body regions (e.g., abdomen and pelvis), MDCT is now considered the gold standard imaging tool in the emergency department [4], particularly in trauma centers (level 1) and larger hospitals that have CT technologists and radiologists available 24 hours per day [7].

Optimal assessment requires careful technique, including the use of intravenous iodinated contrast media. MDCT's increasingly faster acquisition times as well as the significantly improved spatial resolution allow angiography, multiplanar reconstructions, and volume rendering techniques for clinical application. In severely injured patients and unstable patients, CXR remains the most used diagnostic modality, but it seems that in hemodynamically stable patients applying MDCT scan as the first-line diagnostic modality in blunt chest trauma can accelerate diagnosis as well as treatment, reduce costs, and result in better outcome [5]. Due to its high accuracy, and recent developments on dose reduction, MDCT is now being increasingly used in less severely injured trauma population.

Drawbacks of MDCT include the radiation exposure and the potential adverse effects related with the use of contrast media. Additionally, MDCT is also associated with higher costs and increasing time spent in the emergency department [10]. It is necessary to weigh a risk-benefit analysis taking into account the type of trauma (high energy versus low energy), patient's age, clinical parameters, and expected follow-up exams.

Most algorithms subsequently recommend selective MDCT; there is increasing evidence that, instead of selective MDCT of the chest, a routine thoracic and abdominal MDCT might be preferable as it reveals more injuries, with higher injury severity scores [1]. It should be noted that there is no clinical predictors that can rule out all important traumatic injuries and there is no clear evidence in which situation CT can be safely omitted without missing relevant injuries [8].

This paper reviews and illustrates a spectrum of characteristic MDCT findings of traumatic chest injuries.

2. CT Protocols

According to the type of MDCT available, a collimation of 1.25 mm (4-slice and 16-slice) or 0.6 mm (64-slice) is recommended. Usually we use a tube voltage of 120 kVp and a variable tube current time product (mAs), as Automatic Exposure Control (AEC) is regularly applied.

Our protocol includes injection of intravenous administration of contrast medium, many times only acquiring postcontrast imaging, so as not to miss any injury of the major mediastinal vessels and the heart. Optimal opacification may be obtained with injection of 100–120 mL of iodinated contrast medium at a flow rate of 3-4 mL/s and a delay of 25–40 s. If MDCT of the thorax is part of a whole body trauma CT, then a compromise can be made with a 60 s delay for the whole body.

When active bleeding is suspected, a delayed acquisition at 4-5 min is recommended, provided that the patient is hemodynamically stable [11, 12]. Due to time constraints we do not recommend the systematic use of ECG gating for chest trauma [13, 14]. Our standardized protocol includes reconstruction in a soft tissue, lung and bone windows. The axial thin slice acquisition can be used to create multiplanar reconstructions and volume-rendered images.

3. Lung Parenchymal Trauma

3.1. Pulmonary Contusion. Pulmonary contusion is the most common pulmonary lesion and is seen in 30%–70% of patients with blunt chest trauma [7, 15]. It is a focal parenchymal injury of the alveolar epithelium, with interstitial edema and alveolar hemorrhage, produced at the time of injury and usually adjacent to the area of trauma, but can also occur in a countercoup location [1, 3]. MDCT is precise in the diagnosis and quantification of the extent of pulmonary contusions. The appearance of pulmonary contusions depends on the severity of the parenchymal injury. In mild contusion, ill defined, patchy, "ground-glass" areas of heterogeneous opacities are generally seen and are related with interstitial or partial alveolar compromise (Figure 1). When alveolar injury is moderate to severe, it is seen as poorly defined areas of consolidation, with no air bronchogram sign, as a result of bronchial obstruction caused by secretions and/or blood. Massive pulmonary contusion may lead to the development of adult respiratory distress syndrome [7].

Pulmonary contusions may be associated with other lesions, such as chest wall contusions or fractures in the overlying area of impact, hemothorax (Figure 2), pneumothorax, or lacerations.

Resolution is usually rapid and the lung often returns to normal within a week. Failure of resolution usually suggests superimposed infection, atelectasis, aspiration, or a blood clot in a laceration.

3.2. Lung Laceration. Lung laceration refers to a traumatic disruption of alveolar spaces with cavity formation filled with blood (hematoma), air (pneumatocele), or, more frequently, a combination of both (hemato-pneumatocele) (Figure 3) [7, 15]. Lacerations are commonly solitary, but multiple lacerations may occur. Laceration was previously considered a rare finding. Nowadays, due to the broad use of MDCT, lacerations appear relatively common in blunt chest trauma [16]. Blunt chest trauma can produce substantial pulmonary lacerations; nevertheless they are most commonly caused by penetrating traumas such as stab or bullet wounds [17].

MDCT is superior to CXR to detect lacerations. The laceration may be lucent and filled with air, completely opacified as a result of blood accumulation within the cavity, or demonstrate an air-fluid level related to variable amounts of blood within its lumen [18]. The resultant pneumatocele has a variable course; it may persist for several weeks, although it usually resolves within one to three weeks, resulting in a pulmonary parenchymal scar [17].

Conservative treatment is the rule as most of these lesions usually resolve within weeks. Surgery is commonly indicated in cases of large parenchymal destruction, bleeding from a major vessel, or bronchovascular fistula [19].

4. Mediastinal Trauma

4.1. Pneumomediastinum. Pneumomediastinum is defined as free air collections surrounding mediastinal structures and dissecting along the mediastinal fat. Both overt and occult pneumomediastinum may occur in the setting of blunt chest trauma [20]. The presence of pneumomediastinum should raise suspicion for a tracheobronchial or esophageal rupture. Frequently it originates in an alveolar rupture. It fills the interstitium and then reaches the hilum and mediastinum, dissecting along the bronchovascular sheaths (Macklin effect) [3, 21]. If under pressure, air in the mediastinum might produce cardiovascular disturbance, which may be fatal if not treated immediately [17]. Pneumomediastinum may be mistaken for pneumothorax, but the presence of septa within it, delineated on lung window, helps in differentiating the two findings, especially if they coexist [3].

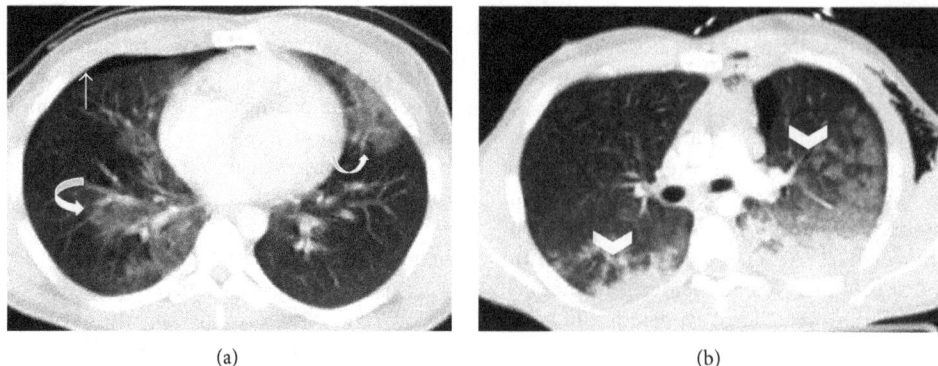

(a)   (b)

FIGURE 1: Bilateral pulmonary contusion. Axial MDCT in lung window reveals (a) ill-defined nonsegmental areas of "ground glass" attenuation in middle lobe, right inferior lobe, and lingula in a polytraumatized patient, consistent with bilateral contusion focus (curved arrows). Also note a small right pneumothorax (straight arrow). Axial MDCT of another patient (b) shows "ground glass" lung contusions (arrowheads) and bilateral nonsegmental air space consolidations with a posterior distribution due to blood filling of the alveolar spaces.

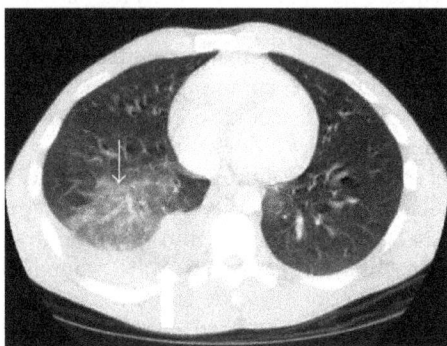

FIGURE 2: Pulmonary contusion and hemothorax in a patient who fell down of his bike. Axial MDCT in lung window at the level of left cardiac chamber shows right lower lung contusion (thin arrow) associated with ipsilateral hemothorax (thick arrow).

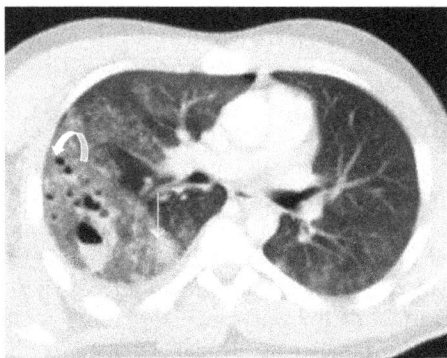

FIGURE 3: Pulmonary lacerations. Axial MDCT in lung window at the level of pulmonary trunk. Multiple focus of pulmonary lacerations can be depicted, some of them are filled with air (pneumatocele, curved arrow), others filled with blood (hematocele-straight arrow), and some filled with both, making an air-liquid level (pneumo-hematocele, arrowhead). Surrounding pulmonary contusions are appreciated. Associated left pulmonary contusions and a small right pneumothorax are also depicted.

4.2. Tracheobronchial Laceration.

Tracheobronchial injuries occur in less than 1.5% of blunt chest trauma patients. Bronchial tear is more common than tracheal tear and more often on the right side. Approximately 85% of tracheal lacerations occur 2 cm above the carina and are usually located at the cartilage-membranous junction [7]. Blunt trauma may cause an abrupt increase in intrathoracic airways pressure. If this happens against a closed glottis, a tracheobronchial laceration may occur [18, 22].

Discontinuity of the tracheal or bronchial wall may be seen, although infrequently, with air leaking around the airway (Figure 4). Other less specific signs of tracheobronchial tear include collapsed lung ("fallen lung" sign), persistent pneumothorax, and herniation or over distention of an endotracheal cuff in an intubated patient [7, 23, 24]. MDCT is also very effective in evaluating central airway permeability.

Repair of tracheobronchial lacerations should be performed promptly due to its high mortality rate and to avoid chronic pulmonary complications [18].

4.3. Esophageal Injury.

Blunt trauma of the esophagus is rare, due to its position in the mediastinum. Usually it is secondary to violent vomiting (Boerhaave's syndrome) or compressive bone forces [25]. The cervical esophagus has been reported as the most common site of injury. When esophageal rupture occurs, it is a nearly fatal condition and the associated mortality approaches 90% (almost always secondary to mediastinitis [17]).

MDCT findings that might suggest traumatic esophageal perforation include the presence of pneumomediastinum, mediastinitis, hydropneumothorax, or leakage of oral contrast material into the mediastinum or pleural space [26].

4.4. Large Chest Vessels Lesions.

The aorta is the most commonly affected vessel. Rarely, injuries of the aortic branches, pulmonary arteries, internal thoracic artery, or major mediastinal veins may occur [16]. Blunt traumatic aortic injury is associated with significant mortality. It was historically estimated that over 75% of patients experienced prehospital

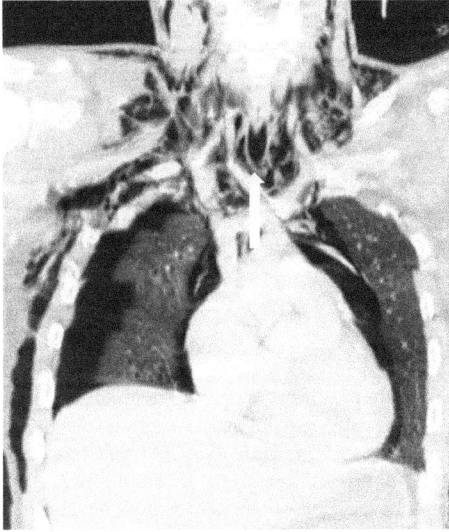

FIGURE 4: Tracheal rupture. Coronal reconstruction of axial MDCT in lung window. An extensive subcutaneous emphysema, bilateral pneumothorax, and pneumomediastinum are observed. Close attention to the tracheal wall depicted a small leak of air to the mediastinum (arrow).

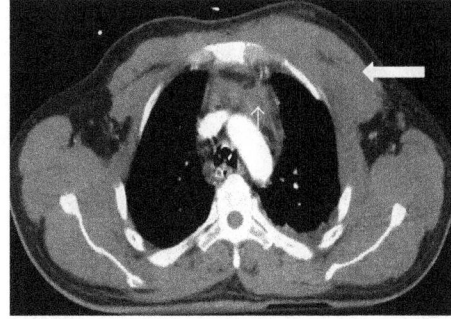

FIGURE 5: Polytraumatized patient who was hit by a car. Axial MDCT after intravenous contrast administration, at the level of aortic arch, demonstrates mediastinal hemorrhage (thin arrow) and left anterior chest muscle wall hematoma (pectoralis major, thick arrow).

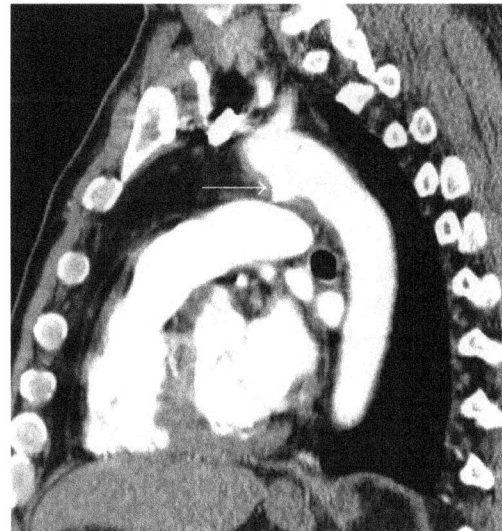

FIGURE 6: Thoracic aortic pseudoaneurysm in the context of blunt chest trauma. Sagittal reconstruction of arterial phase MDCT demonstrates an abnormal contour of the thoracic aorta. A sacculation filled with iodinated contrast material involving the anterior aspect of transition of the aortic arch with the descending aorta, immediately after the emergency of the left subclavian artery, consistent with aortic pseudoaneurysm (arrow).

mortality, and of those arriving to the hospital alive, up to 50% died within the first 24 hours following injury [27, 28]. Contemporary data suggest that approximately 4% of patients die during transport to the hospital and that 20% of these patients die early in their hospital course [29].

A blunt trauma can damage the thoracic aorta by several mechanisms (e.g., fracture dislocating thoracic vertebras; penetration of the first rib and clavicle), but the majority occurs after significant decelerating traumas, so that some authors believe that all victims of decelerating traumas, such as motor vehicle crashes, should be referred to an angiographic examination of the aorta [30].

The currently accepted grading system for these injuries was proposed in 2009 [31] and has been adopted by the Society for Vascular Surgery (SVS) in the clinical practice guidelines for management of thoracic blunt traumatic aortic injury [32]. In this grading system, injuries are assigned to one of four categories: grade I (intimal tear); grade II (intramural hematoma); grade III (pseudoaneurysm); and grade IV (rupture). Current guidelines from the SVS recommend endovascular repair of grade II–IV injuries of the thoracic aorta [32]. A recent investigation by Osgood et al. showed that injury progression in grade I-II is rare (≈5%) and did not cause death in their study cohort, proposing imaging follow-up for grade II [33]. The traumatic lesions of the thoracic aorta typically occur in the aortic isthmus, aortic arch, and descending aorta at the level of diaphragm [25]. Contrast enhanced MDCT of the chest has been promoted as an effective screening tool.

Findings associated with aortic lesions include mediastinal hemorrhage (Figure 5), aortic-contour deformity, intimal flap, intramural hematoma, direct evidence of a tear, thrombus into the aortic lumen, pseudoaneurysm (Figure 6),

abrupt tapering of the descending aorta relative to the ascending aorta ("pseudocoarctation"), and rupture with extravasation of contrast material [22, 25]. Injuries to the supra-aortic and pulmonary arteries and large venous vessels (vena cava, azygos) may be associated with cardiac tamponade or hypovolemic shock from massive hemorrhage [25].

4.5. Hemopericardium. Hemopericardium is a rare condition in the setting of blunt chest trauma, usually caused by venous hemorrhage but may also be caused by cardiac injury or secondary to ascending aorta rupture. MDCT can detect hemopericardium before the onset of pericardial tamponade [23]. MDCT findings include pericardial blood effusion (Figure 7), with or without dilation of the superior and inferior vena cava. Other findings include reflux of contrast material into the azygos vein and inferior vena cava,

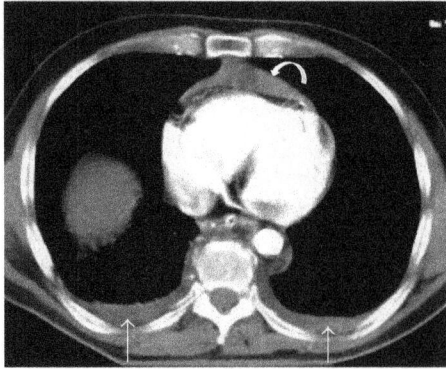

FIGURE 7: Hemopericardium and bilateral hemothorax. Postcontrast axial MDCT of a polytraumatized patient reveals a pericardial (curved arrow) and a bilateral pleural effusion (straight arrows), with high attenuation consistent with fresh blood content.

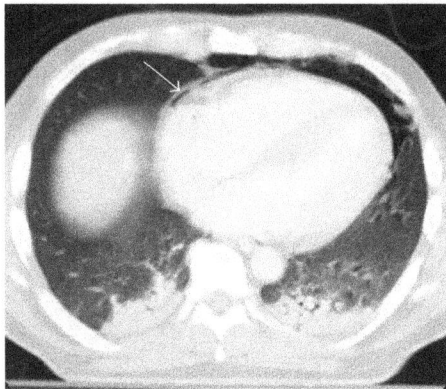

FIGURE 8: Pneumopericardium. A thin line of air is appreciated between the pericardium layers (arrow). Bilateral parenchymal contusions were also present.

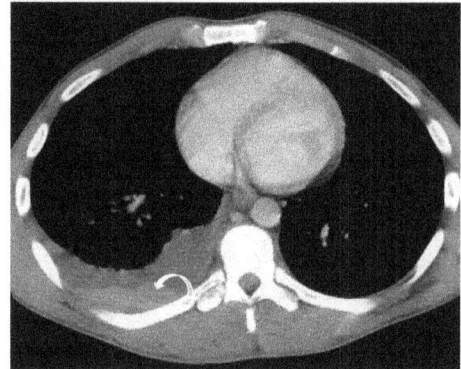

FIGURE 9: Right hemothorax with the "hematocrit sign." Postcontrast axial MDCT at the level of ventricular chambers demonstrates a right pleural effusion with a liquid-liquid level (curved arrow), giving an aspect of layered effusion, consistent with right hemothorax with different degrees of blood coagulation ("hematocrit sign").

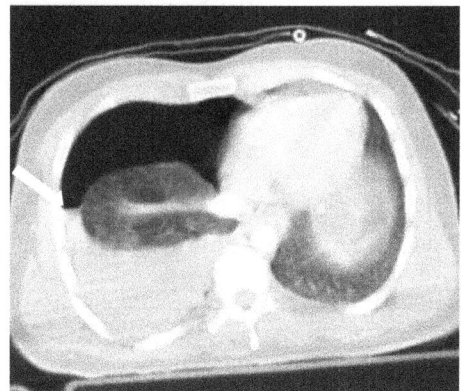

FIGURE 10: Right hemothorax and pneumothorax. Postcontrast axial MCDT shows a right hemopneumothorax creating an air-liquid level (arrow).

deformation and compression of cardiac chambers and other intrapericardial structures, and bulging of the interventricular septum [34].

4.6. Pneumopericardium. Esophageal ruptures or pleuropericardial fistulas may initiate air into the pericardial cavity [25]. It is a very rare finding, but if large, it may result in cardiac tamponade [16].

Findings include air around the heart that does not rise above the level of pericardial reflection at the root of the great vessels (Figure 8).

5. Injuries of the Pleural Space

5.1. Hemothorax. Hemothorax is defined as a collection of blood in the pleural space, usually due to lesions of the lung parenchyma, pleura, chest wall, mediastinum, or abdomen (liver and splenic injuries with diaphragmatic rupture). It occurs in 30%–50% of patients who suffer blunt chest trauma [7].

MDCT easily characterizes the pleural fluid and determines the value of attenuation (typically presents with an attenuation of 35–70 H.U.) [26]. Blood can be seen in the pleural space at different degrees of coagulation, giving rise to a layered appearance, called the "hematocrit sign" (Figure 9). MDCT is also more sensitive than CXR in detecting small hemothoraces [2]. The combination of pneumothorax and hemothorax is common (Figure 10) [19].

5.2. Pneumothorax. Pneumothorax occurs in 30–39% of cases of blunt chest trauma [35–37]. It represents an abnormal collection of air in the pleural space between the visceral and parietal pleura. Mechanisms include broken alveoli due to sudden increase in the intrathoracic pressure, chest deceleration (with or without rib fractures), ruptured emphysematous bulla, pulmonary laceration, or tracheobronchial injury or due to the "Macklin effect" [38].

MDCT has higher sensitivity than CXR in the detection of pneumothorax, particularly in the supine trauma patient [25, 39]. Pneumothoraces that are not apparent on the supine chest radiograph have been shown on CT in 10% to 50% of patients [25]. The detection of small volume pneumothorax has clinical importance, since artificial ventilation may worsen this condition.

Tension pneumothorax develops when air enters the pleural space but cannot leave and progressively accumulates as a result of a one-way valve mechanism. It expands the ipsilateral hemithorax, collapses the associated lung, depresses the associated hemidiaphragm, displaces the mediastinum to the opposite side, produces atelectasis in the contralateral lung, and prevents adequate diastolic filling of the heart, by compressing of the vena cava. These imaging features might be depicted with MDCT (Figure 11). The cardiorespiratory distress caused by tension pneumothorax might be severe [17].

The treatment of choice is pleural drainage. If hemodynamic impairment is suspected, prompt decompression with a thoracostomy tube while the patient is in the CT suite is possible [1], as well as immediate replacement of eventual malpositioned chest tubes [39]. Surgery is usually indicated when there is a persistent or massive air leak or lack of lung reexpansion [19].

6. Chest Wall and Diaphragm Trauma

6.1. Rib Fractures. Rib fractures are the most common lesion occurring in the setting of blunt chest trauma. They are usually identified on MDCT scans obtained following blunt chest trauma, being observed in 50% of patients (Figure 12) [3]. The fourth to the eighth arches are the most commonly affected ribs [3]. Fractures involving the first through the third ribs are a marker of high-energy trauma, as they are mostly protected by the clavicle, scapula, and upper chest wall musculature. Injury to the brachial plexus and subclavian vessels may be seen in 3% to 15% of patients who have upper rib fractures [40]. Fractures of the eighth to eleventh ribs should prompt careful evaluation for upper abdominal organ injuries [7, 26].

Flail chest is a traumatic condition in which there are three or more consecutive ribs with fractures in two or more places, often requiring surgical treatment (Figure 13) [7, 16].

Many of these rib fractures are not shown on the initial CXR. MDCT can determine the site and number of fractures, as well as other associated injuries (hemothorax, pneumothorax, subcutaneous emphysema, and pulmonary contusion) [23].

Treatment should be aimed to maintain a good respiratory function and control the pain. If required, mechanical ventilation for pneumatic stabilization of the chest can be performed. Adequate results have been reported with noninvasive mechanical ventilation in CPAP (Continuous Positive Airway Pressure) mode [19, 41]. Chest surgical stabilization is only indicated when the patient requires a thoracotomy for other reasons or has massive flail chest that might not be solved with mechanical ventilation [19].

6.2. Sternal Fractures. Sternal fractures have been reported in approximately 8% of blunt chest trauma patients [42]. Approximately 90% of such fractures are secondary to motor vehicle accident (due to seat belt or air bag trauma) [7]. They usually involve the sternal body and manubrium (Figure 14) and are often associated with mediastinal hematoma, lung

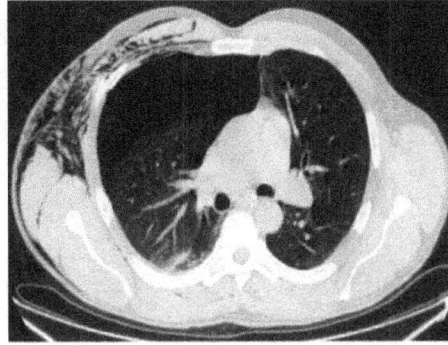

FIGURE 11: Tension pneumothorax. Axial MDCT in lung window at the level of the pulmonary trunk shows increased volume of the right hemithorax due to a large pneumothorax. This finding reduces the ipsilateral pulmonary volume and shifts the mediastinum to the left. A small contusion focus in the posterior segment of the right upper lobe and subcutaneous emphysema are also seen. This is an indication for immediate chest drainage.

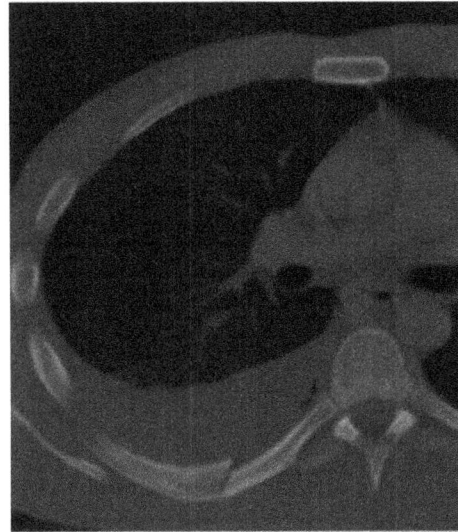

FIGURE 12: Rib fracture. Axial MDCT in bone window at the level of pulmonary trunk clearly demonstrates a fracture bone line of 8th posterior right arch associated with ipsilateral hemothorax.

lesions, and cardiac or spinal injuries. If vascular compromise or impingement is a concern, intravenous contrast should be administered.

The fracture is usually obvious at MDCT, often with an associated retrosternal mediastinal hematoma [15]. Multiplanar and three-dimensional reconstructions greatly improve accuracy and diagnostic confidence. In this setting, sagittal images are particularly helpful for the detection of sternal fractures; however, stair-step artifacts of the sternum may be seen on sagittal reformations due to respiration. Another common pitfall is the presence of constitutional abnormalities of the sternum segmentation, mimicking sternal fractures. Treatment is usually based on pain control and chest physical therapy [19].

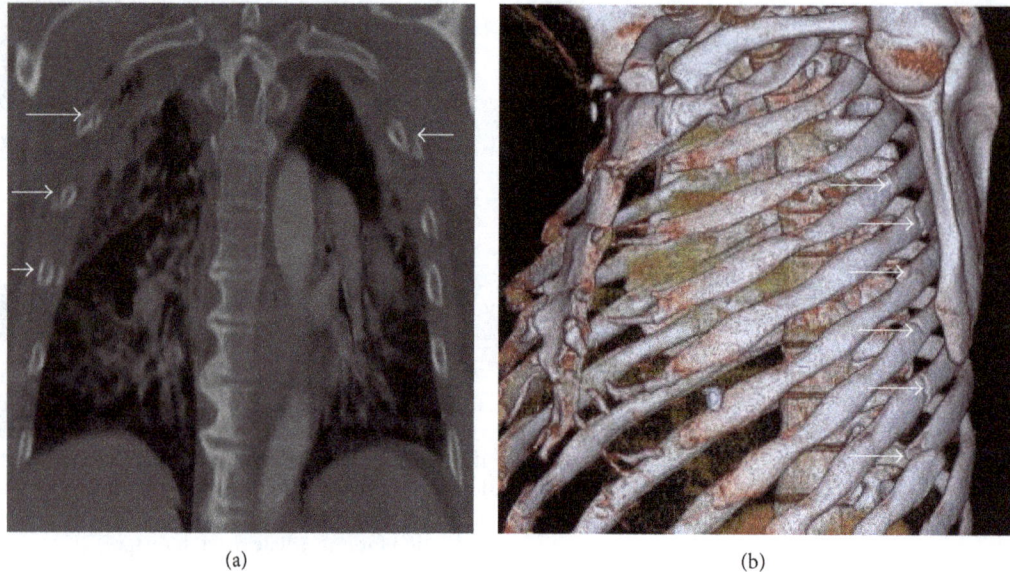

(a)   (b)

FIGURE 13: Rib fractures in 2 polytraumatized patients. Coronal MDCT in bone window (a) in a case of "flail chest" with four displaced rib fractures (straight arrows) in three consecutive right costal arches and in one left costal arc. Note the associated pulmonary contusions. Another patient (b) presenting with multiple left rib fractures (arrows), shown with oblique sagittal volume-rendering reconstruction.

6.3. Clavicle Fractures. Clavicle fractures are usually obvious on the clinical examination. The most important role of MDCT in clavicle fracture evaluation relies in the assessment of medial fractures and injuries affecting the sternoclavicular joint, especially in the diagnosis of sternoclavicular dislocation [16]. Anterior sternoclavicular dislocation is more common and it is a marker for high-energy trauma as patients usually have other chest injuries (Figure 15). A posterior sternoclavicular dislocation may be a cause of serious morbidity, but it is often clinically and radiographically occult, only being detected on chest CT [7]. Impingement of the underlying mediastinal vessels and nerves, such as the brachial plexus and recurrent laryngeal nerve, esophagus, and trachea, can occur by the displaced clavicle [2, 3]. If vascular compromise or impingement is a concern, the study should be performed with intravenous contrast enhancement. Treatment often requires open reduction [2].

6.4. Scapular Fracture. Scapular fractures are relatively common. Usually it is necessary a significant force for it to occur because the scapula is protected by the large muscle masses of the posterior thorax (Figure 16) [2]. Although most scapular fractures are treated nonoperatively, any fracture involving the glenoid or scapular neck requires open reduction and internal fixation to allow normal scapulothoracic motion and stabilization of the shoulder girdle [2]. They are often associated with pulmonary contusion, rib, clavicle, and vertebral fractures and arterial injuries (subclavian, axillary, or brachial) [3]. These injuries are usually well seen in MDCT and multiplanar reconstructions are helpful.

6.5. Thoracic Spine Fractures. Fractures of the thoracic spine occur in 3% of patients with blunt thoracic trauma [43]; a high percentage is associated with spinal cord injury. The most common site in this setting is the thoracoabdominal junction at the level of T9–T11 vertebral bodies [15].

MDCT is the modality of choice in the evaluation of spinal fractures. Signs of vertebral body fractures include disruption or fracture of the vertebral body, pedicle, and/or spinous processes, paraspinal hematoma, and confined posterior mediastinum hematoma (Figure 17) [22].

MDCT shows the presence and extent of a spinal injury, predicts the degree of instability produced, and can show bony fragments in the neural canal. Reconstructed sagittal and coronal multiplanar images are often useful [15, 23].

6.6. Chest Wall Hematoma. Chest wall hematoma is a relatively infrequent complication of a chest wall injury or of dedicated chest interventions, including drainage or insertion of a central venous catheter [16].

Hematomas may be of arterial or venous origin (Figure 5). Extrapleural hematomas are commonly associated with rib fractures that injure the intercostal, internal mammary, or subclavian arteries [7]. Blood accumulates between the parietal pleura and endothoracic fascia. Larger hematomas have a biconvex shape. Active bleeding may be seen [16].

6.7. Subcutaneous Emphysema. Air can spread through the fascial planes to the remainder of the chest wall, abdomen, or even into the head, neck, and extremities (Figure 18) [25]. Most of the times it has a tracheobronchial tear origin, but it can also be a consequence of esophageal rupture.

6.8. Lung Herniation. Lung herniation is a rare complication of blunt chest trauma where pleural-covered lung extrudes through a defect in the thoracic wall [7]. It occurs at the site of an inherited or acquired defect of the chest wall with a significant increase in intrathoracic pressure. The acquired

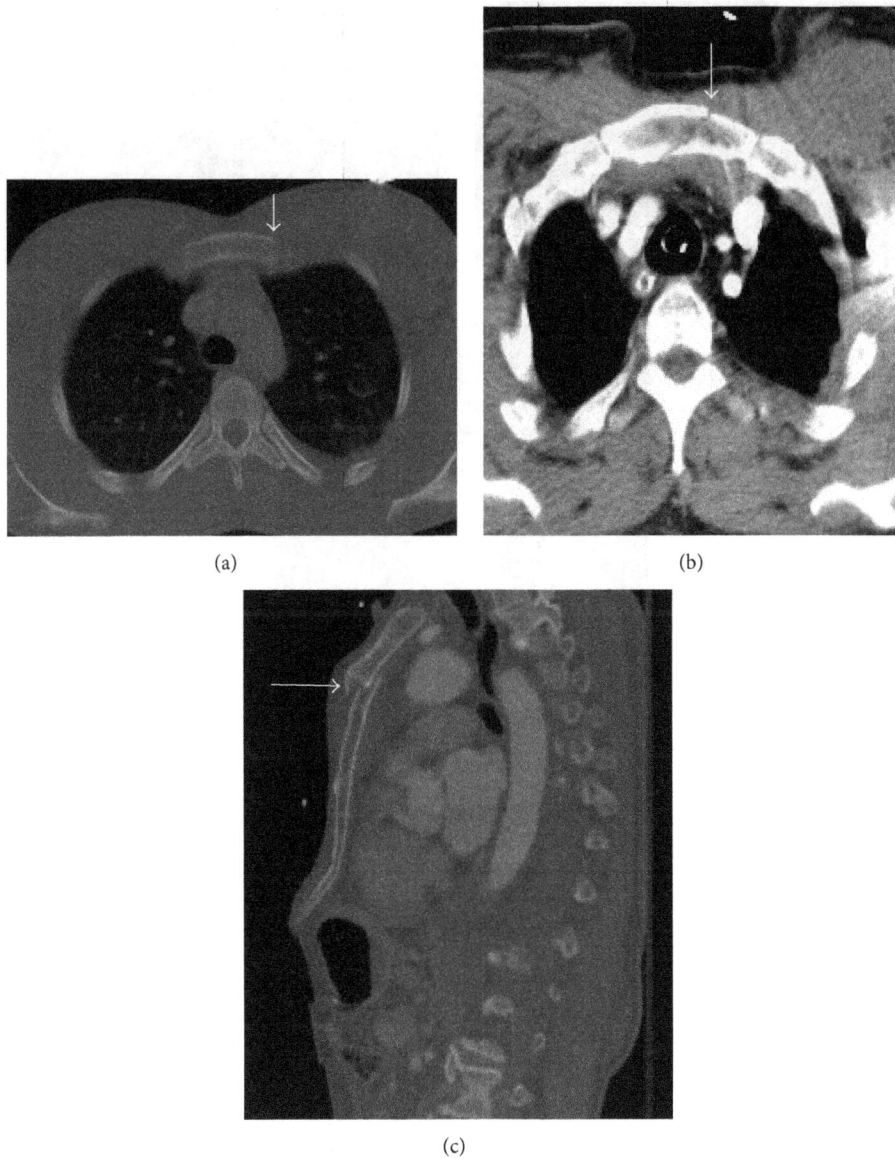

(a)

(b)

(c)

FIGURE 14: Sternum fracture in two different patients. Axial MDCT (bone window) in patient one (a) shows a complete sternum fracture at the level of the body, without displacement of the fragments (arrow). Axial MDCT (b) and sagittal reconstruction in bone window (c) in a second patient show a displaced sternal body fracture (arrows). A small retrosternal hematoma is also seen (b).

chest wall defects can be caused by multiple fractures of the ribs or by sterno- and costoclavicular dislocation [3].

The diagnosis is commonly achieved with MDCT, demonstrating the extent of chest wall injury and the amount of herniated lung. The anterolateral chest wall is more susceptible to traumatic lung herniation, because of the minimal soft tissue support (intercostal muscles) compared to the posterior wall. Supraclavicular hernias have also been reported. Treatment is required when lung herniation is symptomatic, usually by surgical reduction [7].

6.9. Diaphragmatic Trauma. Diaphragmatic rupture occurs in 0.8–7% of patients hospitalized with a blunt trauma [44]. It is a frequently overlooked injury but it is clinically very serious. Mechanisms of diaphragmatic rupture after blunt

trauma include a sudden increase in intrathoracic or intra-abdominal pressure while the diaphragm is immovable by a crushing force [18].

MDCT not only detects small diaphragmatic discontinuities, but also identifies the herniated fat or viscera. Usually there is a waist like constriction of the herniated stomach or bowel (collar sign) or lack of visualization of the hemidiaphragm [18, 25]. Coronal and sagittal reformations are essential in detecting diaphragmatic rupture (Figure 19).

Most diaphragmatic ruptures originate in the posterolateral portion of the diaphragm at the site of embryonic diaphragmatic fusion [3] and it is more common on the left side (77–90%), presumably because the liver protects the right hemidiaphragm [18]. Notably, the stomach is the most common herniated abdominal organ.

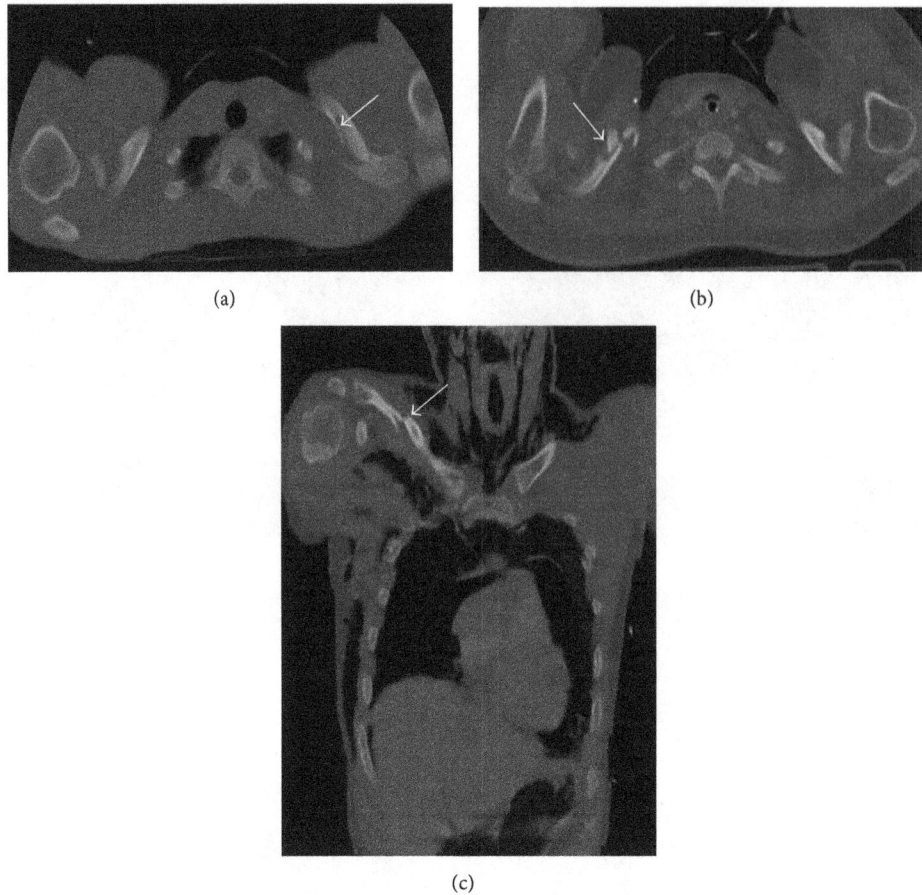

(a)

(b)

(c)

FIGURE 15: Three cases of clavicle fractures. Axial MDCT reconstruction in bone window ((a), (b)) and coronal reconstruction in bone window (c). A two-fracture line is seen in the left clavicle (a); a comminuted fracture is seen in the right clavicle, with multiple fragments (b); and a middle third fracture with dislocation is seen in the right clavicle (c). In (c) there are associated left anterior costal arc fracture, right pneumothorax, pneumomediastinum, and subcutaneous emphysema.

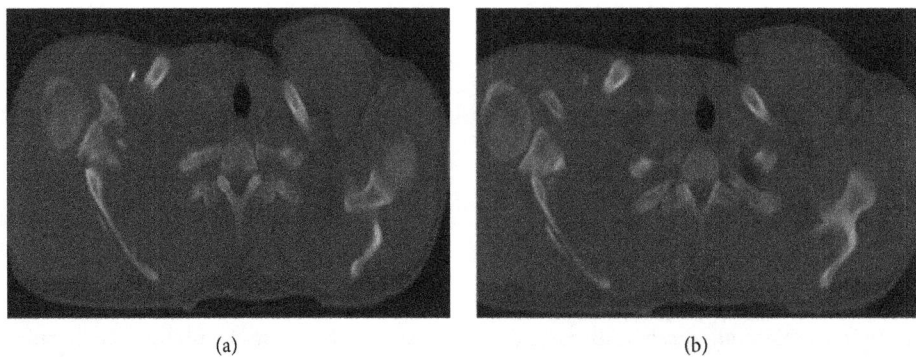

(a)

(b)

FIGURE 16: Right scapular fracture. Axial MDCT in bone window ((a), (b)). Comminuted right scapular fracture involving the scapular neck and spine is clearly observed.

False-positive interpretations are usually due to the loss of continuity of the diaphragm seen in older patients with incidental Bochdalek hernias [15].

Surgical repair is necessary to prevent late complications such as bowel incarceration or strangulation, thoracic organ compression, and diaphragmatic paralysis [25].

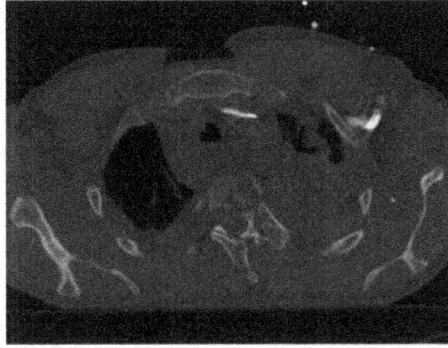

FIGURE 17: Thoracic vertebral fracture in a patient who suffered a car crash. Axial MDCT in bone window. A comminuted thoracic vertebral fracture is depicted with multiple fragments of the body and spinous processes of the third thoracic vertebra. Hemomediastinum, hemothorax, and pulmonary contusions are also associated.

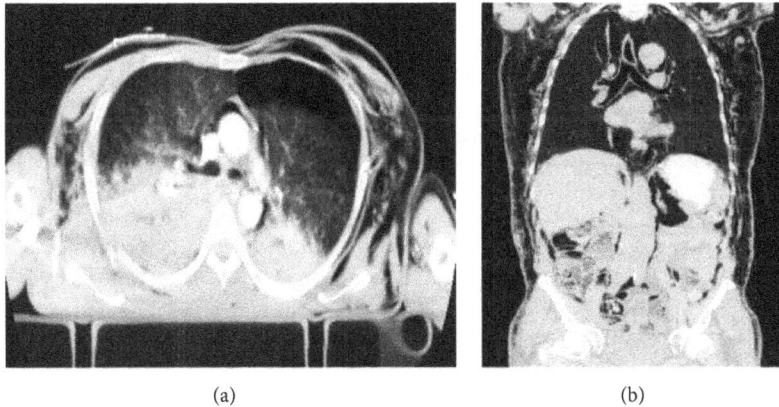

| (a) | (b) |

FIGURE 18: Subcutaneous emphysema. Axial MDCT (a) and coronal reconstruction (b) in lung window. An extensive subcutaneous emphysema is observed. A pneumomediastinum and retropneumoperitoneum are also associated.

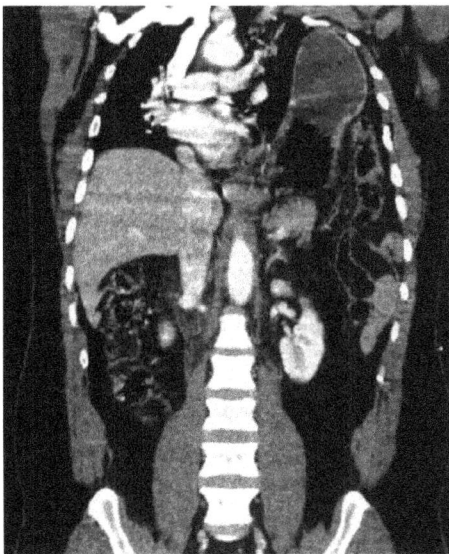

FIGURE 19: Signs of rupture of the diaphragm. Coronal MDCT reconstruction. A massive left diaphragmatic hernia with herniation of the stomach and left colon content is seen in a patient who suffered a car accident. It decreases left pulmonary volume and shifts the mediastinum towards right.

7. Conclusion

This paper reviewed a broad spectrum of characteristic MDCT findings of traumatic chest injuries. Although conventional radiography plays an important role in the initial emergency room setting in patients with chest trauma, MDCT has clearly established itself as the principal imaging method for this patient group, owing to its wide availability, rapid access, quick implementation, use of standardized protocols, and the possibility of generating multiplanar and three-dimensional reconstructions. The information provided by MDCT may lead to critical changes in patients' management; thus we believe that clinicians, radiologists, and radiology residents should be familiar with the different aspects of MDCT evaluation of this subset of patients.

References

[1] A. J. Mullinix and W. D. Foley, "Multidetector computed tomography and blunt thoracoabdominal trauma," *Journal of*

Computer Assisted Tomography, vol. 28, supplement 1, pp. S20–S27, 2004.

[2] L. A. Miller, "Chest wall, lung, and pleural space trauma," *Radiologic Clinics of North America*, vol. 44, no. 2, pp. 213–224, 2006.

[3] A. Oikonomou and P. Prassopoulos, "CT imaging of blunt chest trauma," *Insights Imaging*, vol. 2, pp. 281–295, 2011.

[4] M. Scaglione, A. Pinto, I. Pedrosa, A. Sparano, and L. Romano, "Multi-detector row computed tomography and blunt chest trauma," *European Journal of Radiology*, vol. 65, no. 3, pp. 377–388, 2008.

[5] M. Chardoli, T. Hasan-Ghaliaee, H. Akbari, and V. Rahimi-Movaghar, "Accuracy of chest radiography versus chest computed tomography in hemodynamically stable patients with blunt chest trauma," *Chinese Journal of Traumatology*, vol. 16, no. 6, pp. 351–354, 2013.

[6] M. Traub, M. Stevenson, S. McEvoy et al., "The use of chest computed tomography versus chest X-ray in patients with major blunt trauma," *Injury*, vol. 38, no. 1, pp. 43–47, 2007.

[7] G. P. Sangster, A. González-Beicos, A. I. Carbo et al., "Blunt traumatic injuries of the lung parenchyma, pleura, thoracic wall, and intrathoracic airways: multidetector computer tomography imaging findings," *Emergency Radiology*, vol. 14, no. 5, pp. 297–310, 2007.

[8] M. Brink, J. Deunk, H. M. Dekker et al., "Added value of routine chest MDCT after blunt trauma: evaluation of additional findings and impact on patient management," *The American Journal of Roentgenology*, vol. 190, no. 6, pp. 1591–1598, 2008.

[9] A. Trupka, C. Waydhas, K. K. J. Hallfeldt, D. Nast-Kolb, K. J. Pfeifer, and L. Schweiberer, "Value of thoracic computed tomography in the first assessment of severely injured patients with blunt chest trauma: results of a prospective study," *Journal of Trauma and Acute Care Surgery*, vol. 43, no. 3, pp. 405–411, 1997.

[10] B. Kea, R. Gamarallage, H. Vairamuthu et al., "What is the clinical significance of chest CT when the chest x-ray result is normal in patients with blunt trauma?" *The American Journal of Emergency Medicine*, vol. 31, no. 8, pp. 1268–1273, 2013.

[11] L. A. Rivas, J. E. Fishman, F. Múnera, and D. E. Bajayo, "Multislice CT in thoracic trauma," *Radiologic Clinics of North America*, vol. 41, no. 3, pp. 599–616, 2003.

[12] R. Novelline, "Imaging chest trauma," in *Diseases of the Heart, Chest & Breast. Part 1*, Springer, Milan, Italy, 2007.

[13] T. Schertler, T. Glücker, S. Wildermuth, K.-P. Jungius, B. Marincek, and T. Boehm, "Comparison of retrospectively ECG-gated and nongated MDCT of the chest in an emergency setting regarding workflow, image quality, and diagnostic certainty," *Emergency Radiology*, vol. 12, no. 1-2, pp. 19–29, 2005.

[14] J. F. Bruzzi, M. Rémy-Jardin, D. Delhaye, A. Teisseire, C. Khalil, and J. Rémy, "When, why, and how to examine the heart during thoracic CT: part I, basic principles," *The American Journal of Roentgenology*, vol. 186, no. 2, pp. 324–332, 2006.

[15] M. L. van Hise, S. L. Primack, R. S. Israel, and N. L. Müller, "CT in blunt chest trauma: indications and limitations," *Radiographics*, vol. 18, no. 5, pp. 1071–1084, 1998.

[16] H. Mirka, J. Ferda, and J. Baxa, "Multidetector computed tomography of chest trauma: indications, technique and interpretation," *Insights into Imaging*, vol. 3, no. 5, pp. 433–449, 2012.

[17] A. V. Moore, C. E. Putnam, and C. E. Ravin, "The radiology of thoracic trauma," *Bulletin of the New York Academy of Medicine*, vol. 57, no. 4, pp. 272–292, 1981.

[18] E.-Y. Kang and N. L. Müller, "CT in blunt chest trauma: pulmonary, tracheobronchial, and diaphragmatic injuries," *Seminars in Ultrasound CT and MRI*, vol. 17, no. 2, pp. 114–118, 1996.

[19] J. Gilart, M. Gil, G. Valera, and P. Casado, "Traumatismos torácicos," *Archivos de Bronconeumología*, vol. 47, supplement 3, pp. 9–14, 2011.

[20] J. B. Rezende-Neto, J. Hoffmann, M. Al Mahroos et al., "Occult pneumomediastinum in blunt chest trauma: clinical significance," *Injury*, vol. 41, no. 1, pp. 40–43, 2010.

[21] M. Wintermark and P. Schnyder, "The Macklin effect: a frequent etiology for pneumomediastinum in severe blunt chest trauma," *Chest*, vol. 120, no. 2, pp. 543–547, 2001.

[22] J. E. Kuhlman, M. A. Pozniak, J. Collins, and B. L. Knisely, "Radiographic and CT findings of blunt chest trauma: aortic injuries and looking beyond them," *RadioGraphics*, vol. 18, no. 5, pp. 1085–1106, 1998.

[23] S. Kerns and S. Gay, "CT of blunt chest trauma," *The American Journal of Roentgenology*, vol. 154, no. 1, pp. 55–60, 1990.

[24] J.-D. Chen, K. Shanmuganathan, S. E. Mirvis, K. L. Killeen, and R. P. Dutton, "Using CT to diagnose tracheal rupture," *American Journal of Roentgenology*, vol. 176, no. 5, pp. 1273–1280, 2001.

[25] M.-L. Ho and F. R. Gutierrez, "Chest radiography in thoracic polytrauma," *American Journal of Roentgenology*, vol. 192, no. 3, pp. 599–612, 2009.

[26] R. Kaewlai, L. L. Avery, A. V. Asrani, and R. A. Novelline, "Multidetector CT of blunt thoracic trauma," *Radiographics*, vol. 28, no. 6, pp. 1555–1570, 2008.

[27] T. Fabian, J. Richardson, M. Croce, J. Smith, G. Rodman, and P. Kearney, "Prospective study of blunt aortic injury. Multicenter Trial of the American Association for the Surgery of Trauma," *Journal of Trauma and Acute Care Surgery*, vol. 42, no. 3, pp. 374–383, 1997.

[28] W. R. E. Jamieson, M. T. Janusz, V. M. Gudas, L. H. Burr, G. J. Fradet, and C. Henderson, "Traumatic rupture of the thoracic aorta: third decade of experience," *The American Journal of Surgery*, vol. 183, no. 5, pp. 571–575, 2002.

[29] Z. M. Arthurs, B. W. Starnes, V. Y. Sohn, N. Singh, M. J. Martin, and C. A. Andersen, "Functional and survival outcomes in traumatic blunt thoracic aortic injuries: an analysis of the National Trauma Databank," *Journal of Vascular Surgery*, vol. 49, no. 4, pp. 988–994, 2009.

[30] S. Beslic, N. Beslic, S. Beslic, A. Sofic, M. Ibralic, and J. Karovic, "Diagnostic imaging of traumatic pseudoaneurysm of the thoracic aorta," *Radiology and Oncology*, vol. 44, no. 3, pp. 158–163, 2010.

[31] A. Azizzadeh, K. Keyhani, C. C. Miller III, S. M. Coogan, H. J. Safi, and A. L. Estrera, "Blunt traumatic aortic injury: initial experience with endovascular repair," *Journal of Vascular Surgery*, vol. 49, no. 6, pp. 1403–1408, 2009.

[32] W. A. Lee, J. S. Matsumura, R. S. Mitchell et al., "Endovascular repair of traumatic thoracic aortic injury: clinical practice guidelines of the Society for Vascular Surgery," *Journal of Vascular Surgery*, vol. 53, no. 1, pp. 187–192, 2011.

[33] M. Osgood, J. Heck, E. Rellinger et al., "Natural history of grade I-II blunt traumatic aortic injury," *Journal of Vascular Surgery*, vol. 59, no. 2, pp. 331–341, 2014.

[34] C. S. Restrepo, D. F. Lemos, J. A. Lemos et al., "Imaging findings in cardiac tamponade with emphasis on CT," *Radiographics*, vol. 27, no. 6, pp. 1595–1610, 2007.

[35] R. M. Shorr, M. Crittenden, M. Indeck, S. L. Hartunian, and A. Rodriguez, "Blunt thoracic trauma. Analysis of 515 patients," *Annals of Surgery*, vol. 206, no. 2, pp. 200–205, 1987.

[36] C. Tekinbas, A. Eroglu, I. Kurkcuoglu, A. Turkyilmaz, E. Yekeler, and N. Karaoglanoglu, "Chest trauma: analysis of 592 cases," *Ulus Travma Acil Cerrahi Dergisi*, vol. 9, no. 4, pp. 275–280, 2003.

[37] U. Farooq, W. Raza, N. Zia, M. Hanif, and M. M. Khan, "Classification and management of chest trauma," *Journal of the College of Physicians and Surgeons Pakistan*, vol. 16, no. 2, pp. 101–103, 2006.

[38] G. Gavelli, R. Canini, P. Bertaccini, G. Battista, C. Bnà, and R. Fattori, "Traumatic injuries: imaging of thoracic injuries," *European Radiology*, vol. 12, no. 6, pp. 1273–1294, 2002.

[39] L. Omert, W. W. Yeaney, and J. Protetch, "Efficacy of thoracic computerized tomography in blunt chest trauma," *American Journal of Surgery*, vol. 67, no. 7, pp. 660–664, 2001.

[40] G. Fermanis, S. Deane, and P. Fitzgerald, "The significance of first and second rib fractures," *Australian and New Zealand Journal of Surgery*, vol. 55, no. 4, pp. 383–386, 1985.

[41] C. T. Bolliger and S. F. van Eeden, "Treatment of multiple rib fractures. Randomized controlled trial comparing ventilatory with nonventilatory management," *Chest*, vol. 97, no. 4, pp. 943–948, 1990.

[42] K. Shanmuganathan and S. E. Mirvis, "Imaging diagnosis of nonaortic thoracic injury," *Radiologic Clinics of North America*, vol. 37, no. 3, pp. 533–551, 1999.

[43] M. Costantino, M. V. Gosselin, and S. L. Primack, "The ABC's of thoracic trauma imaging," *Seminars in Roentgenology*, vol. 41, no. 3, pp. 209–225, 2006.

[44] B. Meyers and C. McCabe, "Traumatic diaphragmatic hernia: occult marker of serious injury," *Annals of Surgery*, vol. 218, no. 6, pp. 783–790, 1993.

10

Intraoperative Myelography in Cervical Multilevel Stenosis Using 3D Rotational Fluoroscopy: Assessment of Feasibility and Image Quality

Thomas Westermaier, Stefan Koehler, Thomas Linsenmann, Michael Kiderlen, Paul Pakos, and Ralf-Ingo Ernestus

Department of Neurosurgery, University Hospital Wuerzburg, Josef-Schneider-Strasse 11, 97080 Wuerzburg, Germany

Correspondence should be addressed to Thomas Westermaier; westermaier.t@nch.uni-wuerzburg.de

Academic Editor: Ali Guermazi

Background. Intraoperative myelography has been reported for decompression control in multilevel lumbar disease. Cervical myelography is technically more challenging. Modern 3D fluoroscopy may provide a new opportunity supplying multiplanar images. This study was performed to determine the feasibility and image quality of intraoperative cervical myelography using a 3D fluoroscope. *Methods.* The series included 9 patients with multilevel cervical stenosis. After decompression, 10 mL of water-soluble contrast agent was administered via a lumbar drainage and the operating table was tilted. Thereafter, a 3D fluoroscopy scan (O-Arm) was performed and visually evaluated. *Findings.* The quality of multiplanar images was sufficient to supply information about the presence of residual stenosis. After instrumentation, metal artifacts lowered image quality. In 3 cases, decompression was continued because myelography depicted residual stenosis. In one case, anterior corpectomy was not completed because myelography showed sufficient decompression after 2-level discectomy. *Interpretation.* Intraoperative myelography using 3D rotational fluoroscopy is useful for the control of surgical decompression in multilevel spinal stenosis providing images comparable to postmyelographic CT. The long duration of contrast delivery into the cervical spine may be solved by preoperative contrast administration. The method is susceptible to metal artifacts and, therefore, should be applied before metal implants are placed.

1. Introduction

Patients with multilevel spinal stenosis present a diagnostic and operative challenge. If surgery is indicated, the necessary decompression has to be weighed up against the loss of stability [1]. In these patients, intraoperative control of appropriate surgical decompression is of interest and intraoperative imaging may be helpful for this purpose. In lumbar spinal procedures, decompression control has previously been assessed by intraoperative myelography [2]. Cervical myelography is technically more challenging and there have been no reports about its intraoperative use. In the last years, intraoperative 3D imaging has been introduced in surgical operating theaters. It has mainly been used for osteosynthesis control [3, 4]. However, its ability to acquire good quality multiplanar images may also be useful for decompression control when combined with intrathecal contrast agent.

This study investigated the feasibility, image quality, and diagnostic value of intraoperative 3D fluoroscopic myelography for decompression control in patients with multilevel stenosis of the cervical spine.

2. Materials and Methods

This retrospective analysis was in accordance with the guidelines of the institutional ethics committee. Before surgery, the option of intraoperative decompression control had been discussed with the patients. They were distinctly informed about the potential risks of lumbar puncture and placement of a lumbar drainage, including the risk of nerve root injury, the risks of administration of an iodine contrast agent, and radiation exposure, and a possible prolongation of the surgical procedure caused by intraoperative myelography. All patients gave informed consent.

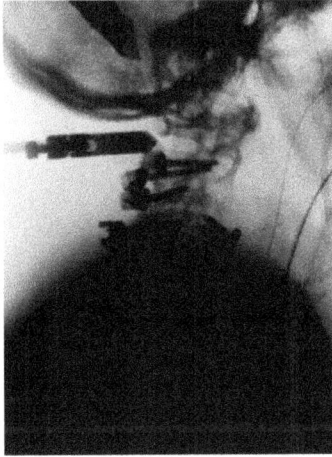

FIGURE 1: Lateral fluoroscopic view depicting the contrast delivery into the cervical spinal canal.

2.1. Inclusion Criteria.

Patients met the inclusion criteria if they were over 18 years and had stenosis of the cervical or upper thoracic vertebral canal with the indication for surgical treatment. Patients were excluded if they had a history of allergy **or intolerance** against iodine contrast agent or renal insufficiency or if the serum creatinine value was above $100\,\mu$mol/L (1.2 mg/100 mL).

2.2. Patient Positioning and Image Acquisition.

Prior to surgery, a lumbar drainage was implanted under general anesthesia. If posterior decompression was performed, the patient's head was fixed in a radiolucent carbon Mayfield clamp and positioned on a radiolucent operating table in a prone position. In case of anterior decompression, the patients were positioned on the radiolucent operating table in a supine position.

After decompression, 10 mL of iodine contrast agent (Isovist 240) was administered via the lumbar drainage. Then, the operating table was tilted head down in order to allow the contrast agent to flow into the cervical canal until serial lateral or anteroposterior fluoroscopy using the 3D fluoroscope (O-Arm, Medtronic) showed the intrathecal contrast flow (Figure 1). When the cervical canal was filled with contrast agent, a 3D rotational fluoroscopy scan was performed. Thereafter, the table was readjusted and the operation continued. For 3D image acquisition, the following O-Arm settings were used: "High Definition Mode"; gantry tilt 0 degrees; gantry rotation 360 degrees; image acquisition time 24 seconds; reconstruction time 24 seconds; standard O-Arm collimator thickness without additional collimation; digital flat panel detector 40×30 cm, camera resolution 2000×1500 (3 megapixels); pixel pitch 0.194 mm; reconstruction matrix $512 \times 512 \times 192$).

2.3. Evaluation of Images.

The images were visually assessed during the operation by the surgical team. Sufficient decompression was usually assumed if a continuous contrast-enhanced layer of cerebrospinal fluid (CSF) surrounded the spinal cord. In case of residual stenosis decompression was continued. For analysis of image quality, images were transferred to an Apple PowerMac workstation using OsiriX freeware and reassessed by two of the coauthors (Thomas Linsenmann, Stefan Koehler) using the following four-grade scale: −: spinal canal and cord not visible/assessable; (+): spinal canal and contrast agent poorly visible/assessable; +: spinal canal and contrast filling clearly visible/assessable. Postoperative CT and/or MRI was assessed by the same persons for residual stenosis. The clinical course after surgery was assessed using the European Myelopathy Score (EMS).

3. Results

3.1. Patient Characteristics.

Ten surgical procedures in the cervical spine were performed in $n = 9$ patients using intraoperative myelography. All patients had cervical, cervicothoracic, or upper thoracic spinal stenosis. Patient characteristics are depicted in Table 1. In six patients, a posterior approach was performed, and in two patients an anterior approach was performed. One patient underwent both anterior and posterior surgery.

3.2. Side Effects.

The implantation of lumbar drainage and the administration of intrathecal contrast agent were not followed by any unwanted side effects. In particular, no anaphylactic reaction or seizures occurred. No patient developed meningitis or other infectious complications and no symptoms due to a possible loss of CSF were recorded after surgery. Furthermore, there were no complications secondary to the implantation of a lumbar drainage.

3.3. Workflow and "Time-to-Arrival".

The 3D fluoroscope was positioned during preoperative preparation (shaving, disinfection). The contrast agent was administered after decompression was apparently completed. The time until the contrast agent arrived in the cervical spinal canal was 15 ± 12 min in posterior approaches and 25 ± 8 min in anterior approaches.

3.4. Image Quality.

Image quality was excellent if 3D scans were acquired prior to metal implantation (Figures 2(a) and 2(b)). Contrast enhancement was better in posterior approaches than in anterior approaches. Metal artifacts considerably reduced image quality, especially in posterior procedures (Figures 3(a) and 3(b)). Caspar-pins used for vertebral distraction in anterior approaches also caused strong metal artifacts and reduced image quality (Figures 4(a)–4(d)). The results of the assessment of image quality and the operative consequences drawn from intraoperative myelography are depicted in Table 1. In four of the 10 procedures, the operative strategy was changed after the evaluation of intraoperative myelograms.

3.5. Clinical and Radiological Follow-Up.

Of all patients, postoperative radiological follow-up examinations were available. Seven patients were followed up by MRI, and two patients by CT. In all cases, an excellent decompression without

TABLE 1: Characteristics and surgical approach in $n = 9$ patients undergoing intraoperative myelography. One of the patients had upper thoracic stenosis due to osteomyelitic vertebral body fracture. Myelography was performed to evaluate if the extent of decompression was sufficient. Image quality largely depends on metal artifacts and if the thoracic kyphosis can be overcome (OPLL = ossification of the posterior longitudinal ligament, VA = vertebral artery, CSM = cervical spondylotic myelopathy, f = female, m = male, CT = computed tomography, MRI = magnetic resonance imaging, and EMS = European Myelopathy Score).

Patient number	Name, sex, age	Pathology	Approach	Procedure	Image quality	Change of operative strategy	Residual stenosis in postoperative imaging	Clinical result (EMS before/after surgery)
1	D.N., m, 76 y	OPLL (after corpectomy C4–6)	Posterior	Spondylodesis C3–C7	+	Additional laminectomy C4	No (MRI)	12/14
2	K.S., m, 70 y	OPLL	Posterior	Laminectomy C1–C3 Spondylodesis C1–C3	(+)	—	No (MRI)	16/18
3	G.P., f, 69 y	Osteomyelitic fracture T3 and T4	Posterior	Costotransversectomy and vertebrectomy T3 and T4 ventrodorsal spondylodesis	– (metal artifacts)	—	No (MRI)	6/died 6 weeks after surgery due to peritonitis
4	E.M., f, 76 y	CSM, increasing dislocation of C2 fracture 3 months earlier	Posterior	Laminectomy C3–C5 Spondylodesis C2–C6	(+)	—	No (MRI)	17/18
5	W.S., f, 68 y	CSM, aggravated after laminectomy C5	Anterior	Corpectomy C4/5	–	—	No (MRI)	7/12
5	W.S., f, 68 y	CSM, aggravated after laminectomy C5 VA injury during corpectomy	Posterior	Laminectomy C4–C7 Spondylodesis C2–T2	+	Extension of posterior decompression	No (MRI)	7/12
6	E.N., m, 70 y	CSM, discectomy C4/5 1 year earlier	Anterior	Corpectomy C5	+	—	No (MRI)	15/16
7	W.S., m, 62 y	Dislocated C1/2 fracture	Posterior	Spondylodesis C1–3	+	—	No (CT)	17/18
8	R.M., m, 74 y	CSM	Posterior	Laminectomy C3 and C4 Spondylodesis C2–C6	+	Extension of decompression	No (MRI)	13/13
9	M.K., f, 73 y	CSM	Anterior	Discectomy C4/5 and 5/6	+	2-level discectomy instead of corpectomy	No (CT)	11/13

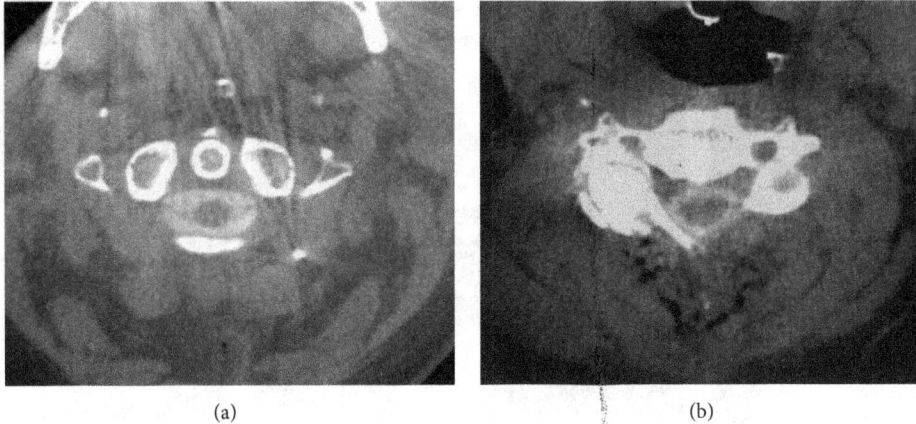

FIGURE 2: Without metal artifacts, good quality images can be obtained comparable to CT myelography. Transverse views of case 4 (a) and case 8 (b).

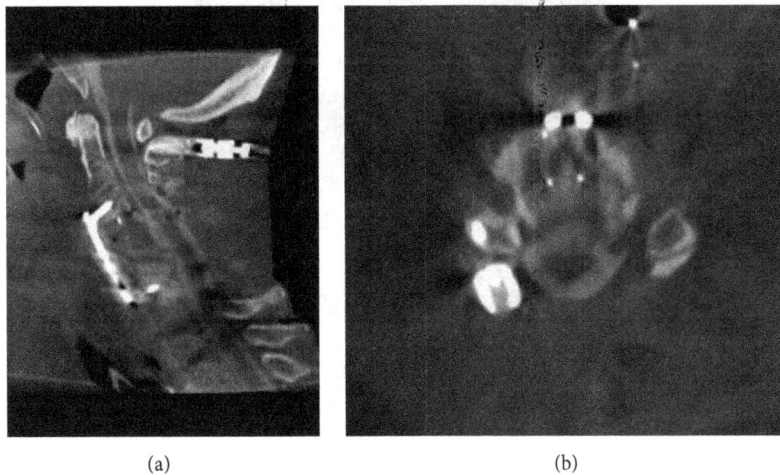

FIGURE 3: Sagittal (a) and transverse (b) view of intraoperative myelography after anterior and posterior decompression. The images were acquired after posterior instrumentation and depict the susceptibility to metal artifacts.

residual stenosis was found. Seven patients showed neurological improvement after surgery, and one patient remained unchanged. One patient died from peritonitis 6 weeks after surgery (Table 1).

4. Discussion

To the best of our knowledge, this is the first report about the use of intraoperative contrast-enhanced 3D fluoroscopy for cervical myelography. The results of this series show that intraoperative 3D fluoroscopic myelography can generate images of good quality comparable to CT myelography (CTM). Similar to computed tomography (CT), however, the technology is rather susceptible to metal artifacts. The interval between administration of the contrast agent via lumbar drainage and its arrival interrupts surgery and is a further drawback to be eliminated.

The general value of myelography as a diagnostic method for the evaluation of spinal diseases has been much disputed

in the recent years. Since magnetic resonance imaging (MRI) has become the standard examination for the diagnosis of spinal diseases, the role of myelography combined with CTM, a standard procedure in the pre-MRI era, has decreased. Its use for diagnostic purposes varies significantly depending on surgeon and department. Classical indications are patients carrying pacemakers and multilevel spinal stenosis with incongruent clinical and radiological findings.

For intraoperative use, the situation is different. Intraoperative MRI is poorly practicable for the control of operative results in spine surgery. Fluoroscopy is the gold standard for this purpose, particularly for the control of implant positions. Intraoperative myelography using biplanar fluoroscopy, in contrast, has long been used for particular cases of lumbar spinal diseases [5, 6]. Intraoperative 3D fluoroscopy is novel technique which provides good quality images and better comparability with preoperative tomographic examinations. Mauer and coworkers detected residual stenosis in 2 of 10 patients who underwent unilateral laminotomy for the treatment of lumbar degenerative disease using intraoperative 3D

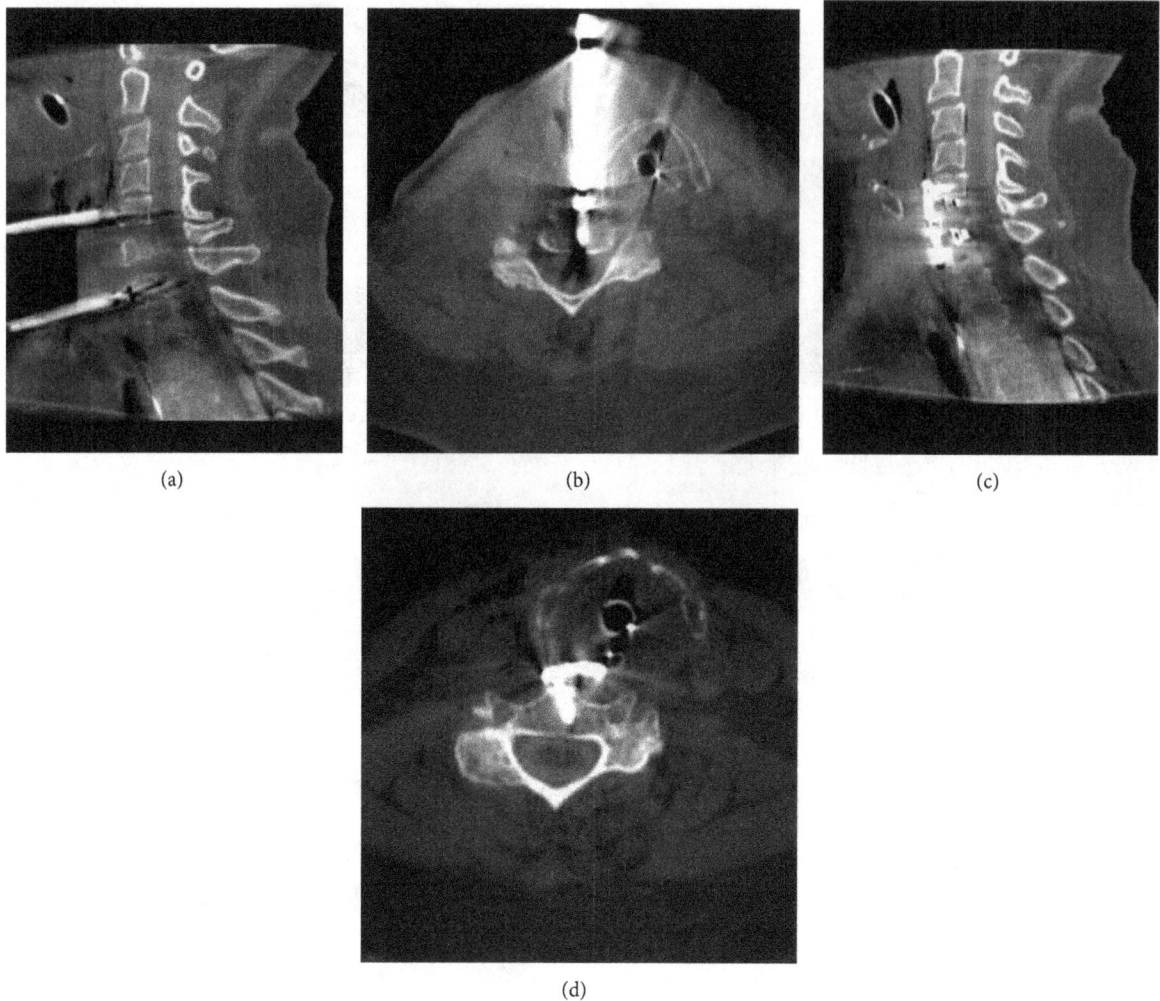

(a)   (b)   (c)

(d)

FIGURE 4: Intraoperative myelogram obtained for the purpose of decompression control. Vertebral bodies were distracted with Caspar-pins ((a) and (b)) which caused a considerable artifact making the assessment of sufficient decompression difficult. After removal of the Caspar-pins and implantation of intervertebral cages at the disc levels C5/6 and C6/7 and instrumentation with a plate screw osteosynthesis ((c) and (d)), the assessment of the extent of decompression is better with reduced metal artifacts.

fluoroscopy for decompression control [7]. The authors further concluded that intraoperative myelography, which had been performed in 5 of 10 patients, gave no additional information. However, in at least one patient, residual stenosis had been detected using contrast-enhanced 3D fluoroscopy. Unfortunately, there is no information whether the second patient with residual stenosis had also received contrast agent. Thus, the benefit of additional myelography to 3D fluoroscopy cannot be extracted from this series. Myelography provides direct information about the compression of neural structures in the spinal canal. Spinal stenosis is caused not only by bony structures but also by hypertrophic ligaments and facet joint capsules and prolapsed disk material which are unlikely to be detected by nonenhanced 3D fluoroscopy [8–11]. Therefore, it is likely that myelography may change the operative strategy in a number of patients as compared to nonenhanced 3D fluoroscopy. Patel et al. reported intraoperative myelography for the control of adequate decompression in a series of 10 patients. Three patients required further

decompression. The authors reported a delay of surgery between 10 and 20 minutes and considered the technique to be safe and efficient [12].

Sembrano and coworkers recently reported intraoperative 3D fluoroscopy in 100 thoracic and lumbar spine procedures [13]. In a part of their patients collective decompression control was the target of intraoperative imaging. 19 of these patients received intrathecal contrast agent for this purpose. In 6 patients, decompression was extended after an initial 3D rotational scan, which underlines the usefulness of intraoperative imaging in complex cases. Altogether, the authors reported a 20% rate of change of the surgical procedure after intraoperative image control. The numbers of patients in the abovementioned reports are small. However, the rate of residual stenosis seems to be between 20 and 30% in the lumbar spine if assessed by intraoperative myelography using 3D fluoroscopy. On first sight, these numbers seem to be rather high. Apparent residual stenosis, as depicted by 3D fluoroscopy or myelography, might not absolutely correlate with postoperative complaints. Evaluating the clinical benefit of decompression control by intraoperative imaging in terms of postoperative pain or neurological recovery requires a prospective study design and a large number of patients. However, incomplete decompression has been reported to be one reason for poor results after spinal decompression [14]. The present series is a technical report of 10 operations in patients with cervical stenosis. In 4 patients, the operative strategy was changed after intraoperative myelography. Structures in the cervical spine are smaller and a pronounced cervical lordosis bears the risk of under- or overestimation of the width of the spinal canal on the upper or lower limit of decompression and, therefore, intraoperative imaging may detect an even higher rate of residual stenosis in cervical stenosis, particularly in limited decompression surgery.

4.1. Technical Pitfalls and Limitations. Cervical myelography differs from the lumbar myelography in that the distance the contrast agent needs to be delivered is longer and includes the thoracic kyphosis. For that reason, diagnostic cervical myelography is usually performed in a lateral position. Contrast delivery to the cervical canal is challenging in the intraoperative setting when patients are in a prone or supine position. The operating table must be sharply tilted and the patient firmly fixed to maintain his position. During these 10 intraoperative myelographies, we noticed a learning effect, which especially concerned the sufficient tilting of the operating table and the implementation of myelography into the operative workflow and which reduced the prolongation of surgery. This is in accordance with the findings of Patel et al. who also reported a steep learning curve using intraoperative lumbar myelography in 10 patients with lumbar stenosis [12]. After a more frequent use, a further marked acceleration of the procedure can be expected. As the patient characteristics illustrate, all patients of this series were older than 60 years. Although we did not perform a systematic correlation of contrast delivery time and changes in the lumbar spine, older patients have an increasing natural risk to develop degenerative lumbar stenosis. This may have additionally prolonged the contrast delivery into the cervical region, a phenomenon which is well known from diagnostic myelography.

In anterior approaches, it may be particularly difficult to surmount the thoracic kyphosis and shift the contrast agent into the cervical canal. Therefore, its delivery into the region of interest takes markedly longer in supine than in prone position and the amount of contrast agent arriving in the cervical canal is lower. This is likely to be the reason for a poorer contrast enhancement in anterior approaches. Earlier administration of the contrast agent via the lumbar drainage, for example, at the beginning of decompression or even prior to surgery in a lateral position, will possibly solve this problem.

This series demonstrates that in the presence of osteosynthesis material image quality decreases due to metal artifacts. After anteroposterior instrumentation, the spinal canal may be not assessable at all. Therefore, decompression control before instrumentation must be recommended when using 3D fluoroscopy. Alternatively, image subtraction of native and contrast-enhanced images may solve this problem. Particular attention must be given to Caspar-pins used for vertebral distraction in anterior approaches. The way they are usually placed causes a line-shaped artifact which covers the region that is meant to be assessed for intraoperative decompression control.

5. Conclusions

The number of changes of the operative strategy secondary to intraoperative myelography in our series underlines that this technique is useful for the intraoperative assessment of residual stenosis. Myelography not only directly visualizes the compression of neural structures but also depicts the intraspinal anatomic conditions after patient positioning which is particularly valuable in patients planned to receive spondylodesis. Metal artifacts seriously deteriorate image quality. Thus, myelography prior to the placement of osteosynthesis material must be recommended. Similarly, the removal of other metal devices like retractors or Caspar-pins should be advised. The rather long delay of surgery is mainly due to the interval between contrast administration and its arrival in the cervical canal. This patient collective predominantly consists of older patients who are likely to have concomitant lumbar stenosis. The presence of lumbar stenosis may be one reason for the delayed delivery of the contrast agent into the cervical spinal canal. The lack of experience using a novel technique is another reason and is likely to improve after repeated use and shorten the operative delay. Preoperative contrast administration in a lateral position, similar to diagnostic myelography, may further decrease the delay of surgery. However, this has to be weighed up against the wash-out time of the intrathecal contrast agent which might be more rapid than operative decompression. These issues will be investigated in a further prospective study.

Acknowledgments

This work was funded by the German Research Foundation (DFG) and the University of Wuerzburg in the funding program "Open Access Publishing."

References

[1] V. V. Patel, A. Dwyer, S. Estes, and E. Burger, "Intraoperative 3-dimensional reconstructed multiplanar fluoroscopic imaging for immediate evaluation of spinal decompression," *Journal of Spinal Disorders and Techniques*, vol. 21, no. 3, pp. 209–212, 2008.

[2] J.-L. Pao and J.-L. Wang, "Intraoperative myelography in minimally invasive decompression for degenerative lumbar spinal stenosis," *Journal of Spinal Disorders & Techniques*, vol. 25, no. 5, pp. E117–E124, 2012.

[3] F. Ringel, J. Villard, Y.-M. Ryang, and B. Meyer, "Navigation, robotics, and intraoperative imaging in spinal surgery," in *Advances and Technical Standards in Neurosurgery*, vol. 41 of *Advances and Technical Standards in Neurosurgery*, pp. 3–22, Springer, 2014.

[4] G. Rahmathulla, E. W. Nottmeier, S. M. Pirris, H. G. Deen, and M. A. Pichelmann, "Intraoperative image-guided spinal navigation: technical pitfalls and their avoidance," *Neurosurgical Focus*, vol. 36, no. 3, p. E3, 2014.

[5] E. B. Siqueira, L. I. Kranzler, and L. Schaffer, "Intraoperative myelography. Technical note," *Journal of Neurosurgery*, vol. 58, no. 5, pp. 786–787, 1983.

[6] W. Schlickewei and E. H. Kuner, "Enhancing the value of intraoperative myelography in dorsal spinal instrumentation," *Unfallchirurgie*, vol. 18, no. 3, pp. 182–185, 1992.

[7] U. M. Mauer and U. Kunz, "Introperative three-dimensional imaging to monitor selective decompression in lumbar spinal stenosis," *Orthopaede*, vol. 35, no. 12, pp. 1258–1260, 2006.

[8] J. A. Epstein, "The surgical management of cervical spinal stenosis, spondylosis, and myeloradiculopathy by means of the posterior approach," *Spine*, vol. 13, no. 7, pp. 864–869, 1988.

[9] M. Yoshida, K. Shima, Y. Taniguchi, T. Tamaki, and T. Tanaka, "Hypertrophied ligamentum flavum in lumbar spinal canal stenosis. Pathogenesis and morphologic and immunohisto-chemical observation," *Spine*, vol. 17, no. 11, pp. 1353–1360, 1992.

[10] S. D. Daffner and J. C. Wang, "The pathophysiology and nonsurgical treatment of lumbar spinal stenosis," *Instructional Course Lectures*, vol. 58, pp. 657–668, 2009.

[11] L. A. Saint-Louis, "Lumbar spinal stenosis assessment with computed tomography, magnetic resonance imaging, and myel-ography," *Clinical Orthopaedics and Related Research*, no. 384, pp. 122–136, 2001.

[12] V. V. Patel, A. Dwyer, S. Estes, and E. Burger, "Intraoperative 3-dimensional reconstructed multiplanar fluoroscopic imaging for immediate evaluation of spinal decompression," *Journal of Spinal Disorders & Techniques*, vol. 21, no. 3, pp. 209–212, 2008.

[13] J. N. Sembrano, E. R. G. Santos, and D. W. Polly Jr., "New generation intraoperative three-dimensional imaging (O-arm) in 100 spine surgeries: does it change the surgical procedure?" *Journal of Clinical Neuroscience*, vol. 21, no. 2, pp. 225–231, 2014.

[14] V. Rohde, D. Mielke, Y. Ryang, and J. M. Gilsbach, "The immediately failed lumbar disc surgery: incidence, aetiologies, imaging and management," *Neurosurgical Review*, vol. 38, no. 1, pp. 191–195, 2015.

11

Influenceable and Avoidable Risk Factors for Systemic Air Embolism due to Percutaneous CT-Guided Lung Biopsy: Patient Positioning and Coaxial Biopsy Technique

Gernot Rott and Frieder Boecker

Department of Radiology, Bethesda Hospital Duisburg, Heerstraße 219, 47053 Duisburg, Germany

Correspondence should be addressed to Gernot Rott; info@myom-therapie.de

Academic Editor: Andreas H. Mahnken

Following the first case of a systemic air embolism due to percutaneous CT-guided lung biopsy in our clinic we analysed the literature regarding this matter in view of influenceable or avoidable risk factors. A systematic review of literature reporting cases of systemic air embolism due to CT-guided lung biopsy was performed to find out whether prone positioning might be a risk factor regarding this issue. In addition, a technical note concerning coaxial biopsy practice is presented. Prone position seems to have relevance for the development and/or clinical manifestation of air embolism due to CT-guided lung biopsy and should be considered a risk factor, at least as far as lesions in the lower parts of the lung are concerned. Biopsies of small or cavitary lesions in coaxial technique should be performed using a hemostatic valve.

1. Introduction

Percutaneous computed tomography- (CT-) guided lung biopsy, an everyday practice in many institutions, has well-known potential complications, in numbers, mainly occurring as pneumothorax and pulmonary bleeding with both of them normally requiring little or no further treatment. Systemic air embolism is a feared and potentially fatal complication but with very low reported incidences ranging from 0,001% to 0,003% according to publications dealing with greater series of biopsies [1, 2]. Statistically, most radiologists performing percutaneous lung biopsies will never have to deal with this complication. On the other hand one study with a smaller patient population recently reported an incidence of 3,8% [3].

Risk factors for systemic air embolism have been speculated, postulated, and reported; these include use of a coaxial biopsy system, number of biopsies, needle path through a longer distance of ventilated lung, coughing during the procedure, positive pressure ventilation, location of lesion in the lower lobes or lower parts of the lung, location of the lesion above the level of the left atrium, vasculitis, and small or cavitary lesions with some of these being influenceable or even avoidable and others not [2–9].

Prone positioning as a truly influenceable factor has been considered a risk factor [3] but to our knowledge has never been evaluated systematically in a literature review.

Our very first case of systemic air embolism after CT-guided lung biopsy occurred at our institution after performing the procedure for much more than 10 years with a frequency of at least 50 cases per year. We are presenting this case, as we strongly believe that, in the light of the very low incidence of this complication, every single case should be published in detail in a medical journal.

The serious complication led us to consider whether there might be possibilities to improve safety of percutaneous lung biopsy in this regard. We investigated the factor of patient positioning during lung biopsy in form of a literature review and came across a technical solution to eliminate one main mechanism for air embolism, which is presented in an additional technical note.

2. Material and Methods

We performed a literature search in PubMed in May 2014 for reported cases of systemic air embolism due to CT-guided lung biopsy with regard to the subject patient positioning during biopsy using the search terms "lung," "biopsy," "air," and "embolism." Abstracts were read and all articles of potential relevance were read in full, if furthermore necessary and available for free. In addition the reference lists of identified articles were checked to identify further relevant articles. Articles published in English, German, and French were selected. "Systemic air embolism" was defined as evidence of air within the left heart or greater circulation proven on CT-images. "Due to CT-guided lung biopsy" was defined as during, immediately after, or at least in a clearly temporal coincidence with CT-guided lung biopsy. Excluded were cases of air embolism due to conventional fluoroscopic-guided lung biopsy, due to needle marking of lung lesions and due to radiofrequency ablation of the lung.

3. Case Report

A 57-year-old man with a large cavity of the right upper lobe of the lung was referred to our institution for further diagnostic, after a diagnosis had not been able to be made during a hospital stay in another clinic. Several noninvasive diagnostics for pulmonary tuberculosis were negative. A flexible bronchoscopy with bronchial wash cytology, an aspiration cytology, and an endobronchial forceps biopsy were performed and also revealed neither tuberculosis nor tumour.

A percutaneous lung biopsy was requested. For this purpose, the patient was positioned left-lateral, that is, on the contra-lateral side, and a percutaneous biopsy under CT guidance was performed using a core needle biopsy system with a 17/18-gauge sized coaxial needle (Bard Magnum Biopsy System, Bard TruGuide Disposable Coaxial Needle; C. R. Bard, Tempe, USA). The guiding needle was placed 17 mm intrapulmonarily in the dorsal cavity wall and four cutting biopsies in slightly different directions were performed, each with a penetration depth of 22 mm (Figure 1). During these procedures, a one-time coughing episode of the otherwise clinically unremarkable patient was noticed. After the biopsies control-scans were performed, as it was routinely done in our institution until the described case, that is, with only a few selected scans in the area of the lesion and the midfield of the lungs to rule out pneumothorax or relevant bleeding, failing to detect any complication. After this the patient was turned back into the supine position and put into his bed, where he sat up. This manoeuvre immediately made him become unconscious. A promptly performed cranial CT scan showed a cerebral air embolism (Figure 2). After being intubated and ventilated in a Trendelenburg position, as far as was practically possible on the CT table, a control-scan of the

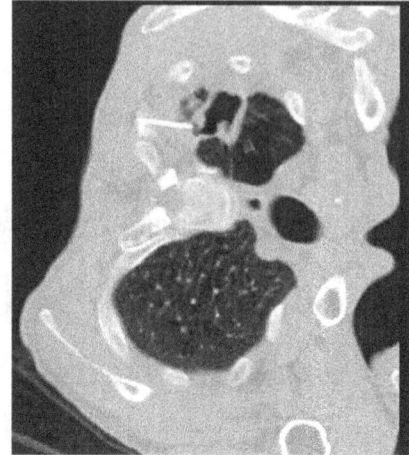

FIGURE 1: CT image obtained during lung biopsy with the patient in left lateral position and the tip of the guiding needle in the wall of a large cavitary lesion of the right upper lobe.

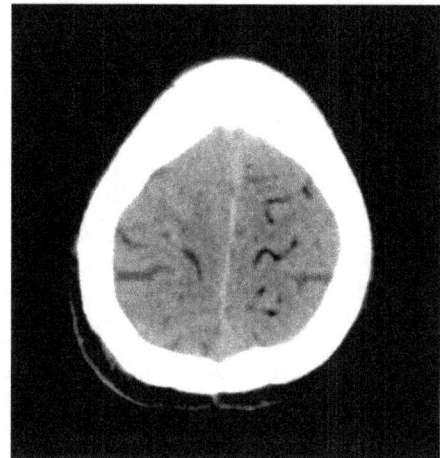

FIGURE 2: CT image of the brain after lung biopsy with signs of cerebral air embolism, typically visible as subcortical serpentiform formations with negative Hounsfield units.

entire thorax was performed to rule out air in the left heart or ascending aorta.

The patient was monitored in the intensive care unit and within few hours transferred to another facility where he received hyperbaric oxygen therapy. After five days, he was transferred back to our hospital. Follow-up cranial CT showed no signs of ischemia or cerebral infarction. Subjectively the patient became completely free of complaints, but neurological examination showed signs of a minor neurological deficit in the form of a pyramidal tract syndrome on the right side.

Lung biopsy specimens showed an inflammatory disorder but did not indicate presence of a tumour. The patient was dismissed 18 days after the incident.

Recapitulating this case, at least four risk factors for air embolism due to CT-guided lung biopsy can be pointed out: a cavitary lesion, coughing during the procedure, location of the lesion above the level of the left atrium, and use of

TABLE 1: Analysed publications with information about patient positioning.

Authors [references]	Number of cases	Patient positioning					
		P	S	L	R	Lat	N
36 [5, 6, 10–22, 25, 26, 28–45, *]	1	16	11	6	3	0	(0)
Kuo et al. [23]	2	0	2	0	0	0	(0)
Ibukuro et al. [24]	3	1	2	0	0	0	(0)
Hare et al. [2]	4	3	1	0	0	0	(0)
Um et al. [27]	4	1	2	0	0	0	(1)
Ishii et al. [4]	10	7	2	0	0	1	(0)
Freund et al. [3]	23	19	0	0	0	0	(4)
42	82	47	20	6	3	1	(5)

P: prone, S: supine, L: left-lateral, R: right-lateral, Lat: lateral but not specified, N: not mentioned.
*: own case report.

a coaxial needle in the conventional manner, that is, with opening the outer cannula to the atmosphere several times.

4. Results

4.1. Literature Review. Our literature search for reported cases of systemic air embolism due to CT-guided lung biopsy identified a total of 46 publications, which met our criteria as mentioned above, published between March 1988 and May 2014. Of these, one paper, whose results are included in another and four other papers, in which patient positioning is not mentioned or visible at all, were excluded, resulting in 41 publications [2–6, 10–45]. With our own case report included, a total of 42 papers were analysed. The number of cases reported per publication ranged from one to twenty-three with thirty-six 1-case reports, one 2-cases report, one 3-cases report, two 4-cases reports, one 10-cases report and one 23-cases report. In total, there were 82 case reports, but in 5 cases patient positioning was not precisely mentioned in a sufficient manner, so that 77 cases remained in the final analysis.

From the total of 77 cases of air embolism due to CT-guided lung biopsy 47 (61.0%) were performed in a prone position, 20 (26.0%) in a supine position, 3 (3.9%) in a right-lateral position, 6 (7.8%) in a left-lateral position and 1 (1.3%) in a lateral, but not otherwise specified position.

Data are illustrated and summarised in Table 1.

As our literature review investigated the technical aspect of patient positioning during biopsy, it is not surprising that the selected literature gives relatively imprecise information about other aspects of biopsy technique. These are briefly summarised in the following.

With respect to biopsy type 61 cases (74%) were performed as core biopsy, 9 cases (11%) as aspiration biopsy, and 4 cases (5%) as aspiration and core biopsy together (8 cases without precise information in this respect). As related to type of needle used 24 cases (29%) were performed as single-needle biopsy and 56 cases (68%) as coaxial biopsy (2 cases with no or imprecise information in this respect). Accurate information regarding needle size was available in 63 cases, with the most commonly used size in single-cannula technique being 18 gauge (12 cases), and in coaxial technique a needle combination of size 17/18 gauge (28 cases). Information concerning the number of conducted biopsies per case were available in 69 cases with more or less precise data. In the paper with by far the most noted cases [3], namely 23, the number of biopsies is described not entirely accurate as, "it was attempted to obtain at least 3 contiguous tissue cylinders". So in most cases the number of conducted biopsies would be "at least 3". Reviewing only the data naming the exact number of biopsies taken, in most cases (20) only one biopsy had been conducted.

4.2. Technical Note. Concerning the abovementioned potential risk factors for air embolism, coaxial biopsy technique has been the topic of commentaries in many papers but in our view thus far has surprisingly not received sufficient attention. Heretofore published strategies for preventing the exposure of the outer cannula of a coaxial biopsy needle to the atmosphere by removal of the internal stylet during lung biopsy include immediate occlusion of the guiding cannula with a saline drop, with the inner stylet, with a cap, or with the finger [46]. Even when valuable advice is given as "when performing the coaxial technique, never leave the outer cannula inside the patient without the inner stylet" [47], it is well-meaning, but technically unfeasible.

In coaxial biopsy technique, the outer cannula is opened to the atmosphere at least for a fraction of a second, when the mandrin is removed and each time the inner stylet is inserted into or removed out of the outer cannula. This means that a biopsy in usual coaxial technique with acquisition of, for example, three specimens, opens the outer cannula six times to the atmosphere, which in everyday practice probably adds up to a few seconds. For biopsies of relatively large lesions, where the guiding needle can be placed safely within the lesion, this is irrelevant, but of course things look quite different for small or cavitary lesions.

At least theoretically, this problem can be resolved with use of a hemostatic valve. A coaxial biopsy needle equipped with a hemostatic valve is not available in the open market, so it has to be assembled from separate existing components. The hemostatic valve connected should be short, lightweight, and, if possible, without additional components such as y-connector, connecting tube, or stopcock. For biopsy, we use a reusable core biopsy instrument and a disposable coaxial biopsy needle (Bard Magnum Biopsy System, Bard TruGuide Disposable Coaxial Needle; C. R. Bard, Tempe, USA). The guiding needle is available in four different lengths of 7 cm, 10 cm, 13 cm, and 17 cm, each one equipped with a flexible slip ring style depth stop for adjusting placement as necessary. For the hemostatic valve we use a simple selfadjusting hemostatic valve by Vygon (product code 1135.08; Vygon SA, Ecouen, France) with a male luer lock and just a short side outlet weighing only 3 grams, which fits perfectly to the Bard biopsy system, as its effective length when connected to the guiding needle measures exactly 3 cm. So the 7 cm guiding needle connected with the hemostatic valve can be handled with the inner cannula and the corresponding biopsy needle of the 10 cm device and the 10 cm guiding needle, as appropriate, with the 13 cm device, without any additional length compensation (Figure 3). Only the 13 cm guiding needle connected with the hemostatic valve needs a length compensation of 1 cm for use with the 17 cm inner cannula and 20 cm biopsy needle, for which the included depth stop is well-suited. The outer cannula of the guiding needle is connected with the hemostatic valve and flushed with saline solution over its side outlet, and the inner cannula of the one size larger coaxial needle is inserted.

The combination of materials as mentioned above reduces the maximal working length of the guiding cannula from 17 cm to 13 cm and increases material consumption, but it enables coaxial biopsy without opening the guiding needle to the atmosphere. Lung biopsies at our institution are performed both with 19/20-gauge and 17/18-gauge coaxial needles. Lesions with increased risk factors for systemic air embolism are biopsied with a 19/20-gauge device.

Based on our experience the combination of both products is quite feasible (Figure 4). Furthermore, the combined device makes the biopsy procedure more comfortable for the performing radiologist. Using a hemostatic valve for coaxial biopsy of lung lesions opens up the possibility to eliminate one risk factor for air embolism due to percutaneous lung biopsy.

5. Discussion

Risk factors for air embolism due to percutaneous lung biopsy can be subdivided into the following categories: patient factors, lesion factors, and technical factors. Since patient factors such as patient compliance, lung emphysema, or coughing during the procedure and lesion factors, in general, may be influenced only to a very certain degree, if at all, technical factors remain the key for resolving or at least reducing the problem.

Considering possible risk factors for air embolism due to percutaneous lung biopsy needs to begin with a look at the underlying mechanism. One mechanism is the creation of a fistula between air-containing space and a pulmonary blood vessel or vein with the biopsy needle. A second mechanism is opening the outer cannula of a coaxial biopsy needle to the atmosphere. The third mechanism occurs with one of the aforementioned mechanisms, but with transcapillary passage

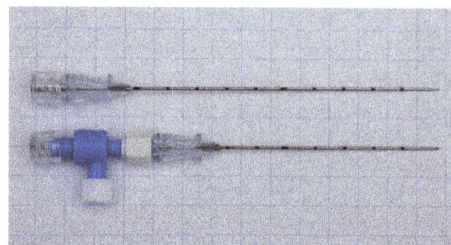

FIGURE 3: Combination of a coaxial biopsy guiding needle and a hemostatic valve for percutaneous lung biopsy. The 10 cm guiding needle connected with the hemostatic valve and closed with the inner cannula of the 13 cm device measures as much and can be handled according to the corresponding 13 cm device.

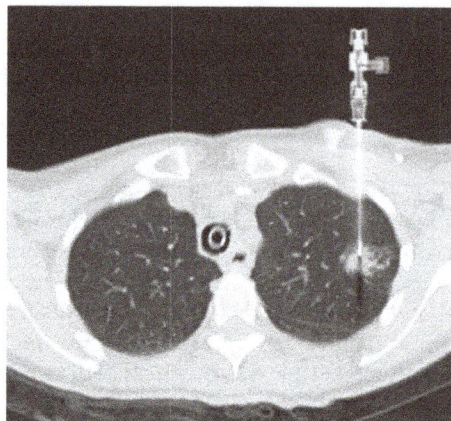

FIGURE 4: CT image during lung biopsy with guiding needle combined with hemostatic valve as described (under intubation anaesthesia at the explicit request of the patient, with venous port system visible in the edge region).

of air from a pulmonary artery, in the way of paradoxical air embolism [48]. The third mechanism of transcapillary route of embolism, however, occurs primarily, if not exclusively in other procedures where large amounts of gas or microbubbles caused by electrosurgical vapours enter the right heart, as, for example, in the case of so-called high-risk procedures in the context of central venous access, hysteroscopic surgery, or gastrointestinal endoscopy [49–51].

A fistula between air-containing space of the lung and a pulmonary vein causes an air embolism only in the presence of an additional positive pressure difference, in other words, when atmospheric pressure exceeds pulmonary venous pressure. This is the case, for example, in the event of coughing or deep breathing during and rarely even after the biopsy procedure.

From the facts listed so far, it is evident that needle path through ventilated lung, biopsy of small lesions, biopsy of a cavitary lesion, coughing during the procedure, positive pressure ventilation, or biopsy of a more vulnerable lesion as due to, for example, vasculitis obviously and without doubt can be considered risk factors for air embolism. From these, however, only the factor positive pressure ventilation can be regarded as essentially influenceable or avoidable.

Creation or, better said, widening of a fistula otherwise could be facilitated by other factors such as greater respiratory motion of the corresponding lung areas during lesion puncture with enlarging of the needle tract, which is more likely during procedures in the lower lobes. Here, greater respiratory motion may also make the procedure more difficult and necessitate a greater number of redirections of the needle [4]. Concerning the abovementioned correlations, the question of what the role of patient position during lung biopsy is up to this point, however, remains unanswered. In particular, whether prone position might be considered a risk factor for air embolism is a question of debate [3, 4] and for this reason was the subject of our literature review.

With respect to CT-guided lung biopsy in general, there is no overall strategy or recommendation concerning patient positioning. In many situations, the selected access route to the lesion with regard to the shortest needle track through the lung, avoiding fissures, large vessels, or bullae seems to be beyond question and determines the appropriate patient positioning. The latter allows various options for the radiologist. Many radiologists prefer, whenever possible, the supine or prone position to the lateral one as it is generally considered more stable and consistent [52]. A prone or supine position has also been recommended for the prevention of air embolism in the "Guidelines for radiologically guided lung biopsy" of the British Thoracic Society but significantly without any reasonable justification for this [53]. However, a lesion that can easily be reached from the back in a prone position usually can be reached from the back in a lateral position as well. In Rozenblit's investigation in this regard, he stated that in most cases (78%) transthoracic needle biopsy in an ipsilateral dependent position would be no more technically difficult than a routine chest biopsy [54]. Concerning preventive risk management when intrapulmonary hemorrhage with hemoptysis occurs, generally speaking the ipsilateral positioning during biopsy is the optimal position to avoid transbronchial spillage of blood in lung areas far apart from the lesion. So, all in all there is no compelling reason why prone positioning of the patient during a lung biopsy might be essential in general.

The two publications that have investigated most cases of air embolism due to CT-guided lung biopsy are those of Freund et al. [3] and Ishii et al. [4] with these also presenting the most compelling evidence. Both studies present level III evidence by using the Oxford Centre for Evidence-Based Medicine 2011 guidelines [55].

In the retrospective observational study of Freund, the publication with most of the cases of air embolism documented by far ever in a single institution, 19 of 23 (82,6%) cases of air embolism occurred in prone position and prone position turned out to be a significant risk factor for air embolism in both the univariate and the multivariate analysis. Consequently, Freund recommends avoiding prone position in CT-guided lung biopsy. Additional risk factors in Freund's analysis were the depth of the needle in the lesion, endotracheal anaesthesia, and the location of the lesion above the level of the left atrium. In the latter, the pulmonary venous pressure is reduced and the likelihood of a positive pressure

difference between air-containing space of the lung and a pulmonary vein is increased.

The conclusions of the recently published Japanese multicenter case-control study of Ishii et al. [4] stand in contrast to those of Freund. Although even here most cases of air embolism, seven out of ten, occurred in prone position, in the univariate and multivariate analysis of Ishii, patient positioning was not significantly associated with the occurrence of air embolism. However, a closer look at the investigation reveals two points of the analysis and interpretation which are at least disputable.

First, a detailed look at the data shows that the patient positioning factors compared were "supine" versus "prone and lateral" and not versus prone exclusively, which does not allow a clear statement regarding the inquiry of prone position being a possible risk factor.

Furthermore, in the point of view of Ishii, the true risk factor explaining his presented data was "location of the lesion in the lower lobe" and not prone position itself, as most of patients with a lesion in the lower lobe were positioned in prone. Ishii stated that location in the lower lobe would be an "inevitable" risk factor for air embolism, because of greater vessels in the lower parts of the lung and greater respiratory motion of the lower parts of the lung, the latter one resulting in enlargement of the needle tract and a more difficult procedure requiring a greater number of redirections of the needle. This view, however, does not consider that part of this, namely, a greater respiratory motion of the lung, is an influenceable risk factor that can widely or completely be eliminated if it is possible to carry out the biopsy from the back not in prone, but in ipsilateral dependent position. In lateral patient positioning the ipsilateral lung is compressed, its volume is reduced, and motions of the ipsilateral hemithorax and diaphragm are reduced resulting in an overall hypoinflation of the dependent lung, a fact well known from both lung biopsy and also, for example, adrenal biopsy [54, 56]. So the risk factors "greater vessels" and "greater respiratory motion" in the lower lobes can be, but do not necessarily have to be connected with each other. In other words, the probably minor risk factor "location in the lower lobe" due to greater vessels in the lower parts of the lung becomes a probably major one and is, respectively, potentiated by the risk factor "prone position" promoting greater respiratory motion of the lower parts of the lung, which can be minimised by using ipsilateral dependent position. This would also automatically fulfil the requirement of Freund concerning avoidance of the factor "lesion location above the left atrium" in lateral patient position.

Prone position also might be a risk factor for air embolism or better said for the clinical manifestation of air embolism for the following reasons.

Anatomically speaking, in a supine or lateral patient position air might be more likely to stay in a pocket in the left heart or ascending aorta before it gets further into the systemic circulation than air in a prone position. But, this is of course speculative.

Another similar explanation could be that when performing a CT-guided lung biopsy in a prone position the patient often is turned back to the supine position before a control-scan of the entire heart and ascending aorta has been conducted to rule out air embolism. This rotational manoeuvre of 180 degrees can cause the clinical manifestation of air embolism and is normally reduced to 90 degrees in a biopsy in lateral position and most often is totally prevented in a biopsy in supine position.

The papers of Freund and Ishii, supported by the data of our systematic literature review, provide important indications that lung biopsy of a lesion in the lower parts of the lung in prone position contains a combination of risk factors for the development of systemic air embolism based on the two single factors greater vessel calibre and greater respiratory motion of the lower parts of the lung with prone position being the influenceable and usually commonly avoidable risk factor.

One can statistically evaluate the data of our literature review with, on the one hand, far more than half of all air embolisms having occurred in prone position. However, on the other hand, most publications dealing only with one-case reports without information about data of the whole collective of biopsied patients are, quite naturally, without significance. Nevertheless we believe that our data has clinical relevance.

The practical conclusions from our point of view, however, are a bit different from those of Freund, who recommends that "whenever possible patients should be positioned on the back in such a way that the tumour is lower than the left atrium." We believe this requirement to be impractical. Beyond the general aspects of percutaneous lung biopsy, such as avoiding pleural fissures and avoiding long needle track through lung parenchyma, the two risk factors "lesion above the level of the left atrium" and "greater respiratory motion," in our opinion, have the following consequence: dorsal located lesions should be biopsied not in prone, but in ipsilateral dependent position. The question of whether all ventral located lesions should also be biopsied in an ipsilateral dependent position or in supine position is a bit more difficult to answer. A biopsy of a ventral lesion from an anterior or ventral access in an ipsilateral dependent position seems hardly feasible, at least in women and presumably also in men, due to compressed soft tissue of chest muscles, breast parenchyma, and subcutaneous fat in this position. From our point of view, ventral lesions should be biopsied in supine position for technical feasibility, ignoring the risk-factor "lesion above the level of the left atrium." Lateral lesions can be biopsied in supine position or from the back in ipsilateral dependent position.

The use of a hemostatic valve for coaxial biopsy of lung lesions as described in our technical note is a quite simple option to securely prevent opening the outer cannula to the atmosphere and thus eliminate one risk factor for air embolism due to percutaneous lung biopsy.

Not a risk factor for air embolism itself, but impacting its clinical consequences, is the correct way of handling the patient immediately after conducting the biopsy. In most current practice, the postprocedure CT scan only includes the target area of biopsy for the observation of pneumothorax and biopsy-tract haemorrhage. Early detection of air embolism in the left atrium or left ventricle, however, can prevent air embolism in the systemic circulation resulting from this. For this purpose, a CT scan of the whole aortocardiac region with the patient in an unaltered position as related to biopsy position should be performed to find any evidence of air embolism. If air embolism hereby can be ruled out, the patient position can be altered. If air embolism is recognised, any alteration of the patient position should be considered thoroughly to retain the air in the relative safe position of the left atrium or left ventricle. Repositioning the patient in the situation when air embolism has been detected might be a very critical point and should be decided on a case-by-case basis, perhaps only after transcatheter or even percutaneous-transcardial air-aspiration. This general advice has been given previously by several other investigators [23–25] but since now has not been established sufficiently in daily practice. The clearest example of this is the practice in our clinic, as it has been for many years before the event of the aforementioned case.

In conclusion, there is low-level evidence that possibly explains why prone position is a risk factor for the development and/or clinical manifestation of systemic air embolism due to CT-guided lung biopsy of lesions in the lower parts of the lung. Prone position, therefore, should be avoided for biopsy of lesions in the lower lobes or lower parts of the lung and replaced by ipsilateral dependent positioning of the patient, especially in situations where other risk factors for air embolism, such as small or cavitary lesions or needle path through longer distances of ventilated lung, are present.

For biopsies of small or cavitary lesions in coaxial technique, using a hemostatic valve is strongly recommended in general.

Furthermore, we recommend a control-scan of the entire thorax immediately after lung biopsy in an unaltered patient position before any repositioning of the patient, as has been previously recommended by several other investigators.

Recommendations for CT-guided lung biopsy should be propagated among radiologists in national or international guidelines.

References

[1] N. Tomiyama, Y. Yasuhara, Y. Nakajima et al., "CT-guided needle biopsy of lung lesions: a survey of severe complication based on 9783 biopsies in Japan," *European Journal of Radiology*, vol. 59, no. 1, pp. 60–64, 2006.

[2] S. S. Hare, A. Gupta, A. T. C. Goncalves, C. A. Souza, F. Matzinger, and J. M. Seely, "Systemic arterial air embolism after percutaneous lung biopsy," *Clinical Radiology*, vol. 66, no. 7, pp. 589–596, 2011.

[3] M. C. Freund, J. Petersen, K. C. Goder, T. Bunse, F. Wiedermann, and B. Glodny, "Systemic air embolism during percutaneous core needle biopsy of the lung: frequency and risk factors," *BMC Pulmonary Medicine*, vol. 12, article 2, 2012.

[4] H. Ishii, T. Hiraki, H. Gobara et al., "Risk factors for systemic air embolism as a complication of percutaneous CT-guided lung biopsy: multicenter case-control study," *CardioVascular and Interventional Radiology*, vol. 37, no. 5, pp. 1312–1320, 2014.

[5] J. Lorenz, "Systemic air embolism," *Seminars in Interventional Radiology*, vol. 28, no. 2, pp. 267–270, 2011.

[6] R. Thomas, B. Thangakunam, R. A. Cherian, R. Gupta, and D. J. Christopher, "Cerebral air embolism complicating CT-guided trans-thoracic needle biopsy of the lung," *Clinical Respiratory Journal*, vol. 5, no. 2, pp. e1–e3, 2011.

[7] W. M. Al-Ali, T. Browne, and R. Jones, "A case of cranial air embolism after transthoracic lung biopsy," *American Journal of Respiratory and Critical Care Medicine*, vol. 186, no. 11, pp. 1193–1195, 2012.

[8] P. Cianci, J. P. Posin, R. R. Shimshak, and J. Singzon, "Air embolism complicating percutaneous thin needle biopsy of lung," *Chest*, vol. 92, no. 4, pp. 749–751, 1987.

[9] T. Hiraki, H. Fujiwara, J. Sakurai et al., "Nonfatal systemic air embolism complicating percutaneous CT-guided transthoracic needle biopsy: four cases from a single institution," *Chest*, vol. 132, no. 2, pp. 684–690, 2007.

[10] M. Franke, H. C. Reinhardt, and M. von Bergwelt-Baildon, "Massive air embolism after lung biopsy," *Circulation*, vol. 129, no. 9, pp. 1046–1047, 2014.

[11] H. K. Kok, S. Leong, U. Salati, W. C. Torreggiani, and P. Govender, "Left atrial and systemic air embolism after lung biopsy: Importance of treatment positioning," *Journal of Vascular and Interventional Radiology*, vol. 24, no. 10, pp. 1587–1588, 2013.

[12] D. R. Smit, S. A. Kleijn, and W. G. de Voogt, "Coronary and cerebral air embolism: a rare complication of computed tomography-guided transthoracic lung biopsy," *Netherlands Heart Journal*, vol. 21, no. 10, pp. 464–466, 2013.

[13] K. Suzuki, M. Ueda, K. Muraga et al., "An unusual cerebral air embolism developing within the posterior circulation territory after a needle lung biopsy," *Internal Medicine*, vol. 52, no. 1, pp. 115–117, 2013.

[14] T. Kawaji, H. Shiomi, Y. Togashi et al., "Coronary air embolism and cardiogenic shock during computed tomography-guided needle biopsy of the lung," *Circulation*, vol. 126, no. 13, pp. e195–e197, 2012.

[15] Y.-F. Wu, T.-W. Huang, C.-C. Kao, and S.-C. Lee, "Air embolism complicating computed tomography-guided core needle biopsy of the lung," *Interactive Cardiovascular and Thoracic Surgery*, vol. 14, no. 6, pp. 771–772, 2012.

[16] O. Bylicki, V. Zarza, A. Marfisi-Dubost et al., "Embolie gazeuse de révélation tardive après ponction tranpariétale pulmonaire," *La Revue de Médecine Interne*, vol. 33, no. 4, pp. 223–226, 2012.

[17] G. R. Shroff, M. Sarraf, M. D. Sprenkle, and R. M. Karim, "Air embolism involving the coronary and pulmonary circulation: an unusual cause of sudden cardiac death," *Circulation*, vol. 124, no. 25, pp. 2949–2950, 2011.

[18] W. Lederer, C. J. Schlimp, B. Glodny, and F. J. Wiedermann, "Air embolism during CT-guided transthoracic needle biopsy," *BMJ Case Reports*, 2011.

[19] A. Singh, A. Ramanakumar, and J. Hannan, "Simultaneous left ventricular and cerebral artery air embolism after computed tomographic-guided transthoracic needle biopsy of the lung," *Texas Heart Institute Journal*, vol. 38, no. 4, pp. 424–426, 2011.

[20] D. Mokart, A. Sarran, A. Barthélémy et al., "Systemic air embolism during lung biopsy," *The British Journal of Anaesthesia*, vol. 107, no. 2, pp. 277–278, 2011.

[21] W. Bou-Assaly, P. Pernicano, E. Hoeffner et al., "Systemic air embolism after transthoracic lung biopsy: a case report and review of literature," *World Journal of Radiology*, vol. 2, no. 5, pp. 193–196, 2010.

[22] H.-M. Cheng, K.-H. Chiang, P.-Y. Chang et al., "Coronary artery air embolism: a potentially fatal complication of CT-guided percutaneous lung biopsy," *The British Journal of Radiology*, vol. 83, no. 988, pp. e83–e85, 2010.

[23] H. L. Kuo, L. Cheng, T. J. Chung, and et al, "Systemic air embolism detected during percutaneous transthoracic needle biopsy: report of two cases and a proposal for a routine postprocedure computed tomography scan of the aorto-cardiac region," *Clinical Imaging*, vol. 34, no. 1, pp. 53–56, 2010.

[24] K. Ibukuro, R. Tanaka, T. Takeguchi, H. Fukuda, S. Abe, and K. Tobe, "Air embolism and needle track implantation complicating CT-guided percutaneous thoracic biopsy: single-institution experience," *American Journal of Roentgenology*, vol. 193, no. 5, pp. W430–W436, 2009.

[25] S. Bhatia, "Systemic air embolism following CT-guided lung biopsy," *Journal of Vascular and Interventional Radiology*, vol. 20, no. 6, pp. 709–711, 2009.

[26] Y. Ishikawa, H. Matsuguma, R. Nakahara, A. Ui, H. Suzuki, and K. Yokoi, "Arterial air embolism: a rare but life-threatening complication of percutaneous needle biopsy of the lung," *Annals of Thoracic Surgery*, vol. 87, no. 5, p. 1622, 2009.

[27] S. J. Um, S. K. Lee, K. Y. Doo et al., "Four cases of a cerebral air embolism complicating a percutaneous transthoracic needle biopsy," *Korean Journal of Radiology*, vol. 10, no. 1, pp. 81–84, 2009.

[28] S. Hirasawa, H. Hirasawa, A. Taketomi-Takahashi et al., "Air embolism detected during computed tomography fluoroscopically guided transthoracic needle biopsy," *CardioVascular and Interventional Radiology*, vol. 31, no. 1, pp. 219–221, 2008.

[29] D. H. Hsi, T. N. Thompson, A. Fruchter, M. S. Collins, O. U. Lieberg, and H. Boepple, "Simultaneous coronary and cerebral air embolism after CT-guided core needle biopsy of the lung," *Texas Heart Institute Journal*, vol. 35, no. 4, pp. 472–474, 2008.

[30] M. Tomabechi, K. Kato, M. Sone et al., "Cerebral air embolism treated with hyperbaric oxygen therapy following percutaneous transthoracic computed tomography-guided needle biopsy of the lung," *Radiation Medicine*, vol. 26, no. 6, pp. 379–383, 2008.

[31] E. Foert, B. B. Frericks, and M. Klambeck, "Arterielle Gasembolie während CT-gestützter Lungenbiopsie: Behandlung mit hyperbarer Sauerstofftherapie," *Rofo*, vol. 180, no. 7, pp. 672–673, 2008.

[32] T. Kau, E. Rabitsch, S. Celedin, S. M. Habernig, J. R. Weber, and K. A. Hausegger, "When coughing can cause stroke - A case-based update on cerebral air embolism complicating biopsy of the lung," *CardioVascular and Interventional Radiology*, vol. 31, no. 5, pp. 848–853, 2008.

[33] M. Ghafoori and P. Varedi, "Systemic air embolism after percutaneous transthorasic needle biopsy of the lung," *Emergency Radiology*, vol. 15, no. 5, pp. 353–356, 2008.

[34] A. Khalil, H. Prigent, A. Parrot, and M.-F. Carette, "Systemic air embolism complicating percutaneous transthoracic needle biopsy," *The American Journal of Roentgenology*, vol. 187, no. 2, pp. W242–W243, 2006.

[35] G. Lattin Jr., W. O'Brien, B. McCrary, P. Kearney, and D. Gover, "Massive systemic air embolism treated with hyperbaric oxygen therapy following CT-guided transthoracic needle biopsy of a pulmonary nodule," *Journal of Vascular and Interventional Radiology*, vol. 17, no. 8, pp. 1355–1358, 2006.

[36] K. I. Timpert, J. Schmutz, and K. Steinke, "Massive zerebrale Luftembolie nach Computertomographie-gesteuerter Lungenbiopsie," *Fortschritte auf dem Gebiet der Röntgenstrahlen*, vol. 178, no. 4, pp. 441–443, 2006.

[37] A. Mansour, S. AbdelRaouf, M. Qandeel, and M. Swaidan, "Acute coronary artery air embolism following CT-guided lung biopsy," *CardioVascular and Interventional Radiology*, vol. 28, no. 1, pp. 131–134, 2005.

[38] K. Ashizawa, H. Watanabe, H. Morooka, and K. Hayashi, "Hyperbaric oxygen therapy for air embolism complicating CT-guided needle biopsy of the lung," *The American Journal of Roentgenology*, vol. 182, no. 6, pp. 1606–1607, 2004.

[39] B. W. Arnold and W. J. Zwiebel, "Percutaneous transthoracic needle biopsy complicated by air embolism," *American Journal of Roentgenology*, vol. 178, no. 6, pp. 1400–1402, 2002.

[40] S. Ohashi, H. Endoh, T. Honda, N. Komura, and K. Satoh, "Cerebral air embolism complicating percutaneous thin-needle biopsy of the lung: complete neurological recovery after hyperbaric oxygen therapy," *Journal of Anesthesia*, vol. 15, no. 4, pp. 233–236, 2001.

[41] B. Mokhlesi, I. Ansaarie, M. Bader, M. Tareen, and J. Boatman, "Coronary artery air embolism complicating a CT-guided transthoracic needle biopsy of the lung," *Chest*, vol. 121, no. 3, pp. 993–996, 2002.

[42] F. Kodama, T. Ogawa, M. Hashimoto, Y. Tanabe, Y. Suto, and T. Kato, "Fatal air embolism as a complication of CT-guided needle biopsy of the lung," *Journal of Computer Assisted Tomography*, vol. 23, no. 6, pp. 949–951, 1999.

[43] D. Regge, T. Gallo, J. Galli, A. Bertinetti, C. Gallino, and E. Scappaticci, "Systemic arterial air embolism and tension pneumothorax: two complications of transthoracic percutaneous thin-needle biopsy in the same patient," *European Radiology*, vol. 7, no. 2, pp. 173–175, 1997.

[44] B. K. Baker and E. E. Awwad, "Computed tomography of fatal cerebral air embolism following percutaneous aspiration biopsy of the lung," *Journal of Computer Assisted Tomography*, vol. 12, no. 6, pp. 1082–1083, 1988.

[45] T. L. Tolly, J. E. Fedlmeier, and D. Czarnecki, "Air embolism complicating percutaneous lung biopsy," *The American Journal of Roentgenology*, vol. 150, no. 3, pp. 555–556, 1988.

[46] C. C. Wu, M. M. Maher, and J.-A. O. Shepard, "Complications of CT-guided percutaneous needle biopsy of the chest: prevention and management," *American Journal of Roentgenology*, vol. 196, no. 6, pp. W678–W682, 2011.

[47] I.-C. Tsai, W.-L. Tsai, M.-C. Chen et al., "CT-guided core biopsy of lung lesions: a primer," *American Journal of Roentgenology*, vol. 193, no. 5, pp. 1228–1235, 2009.

[48] D. R. Aberle, G. Gamsu, and J. A. Golden, "Fatal systemic arterial air embolism following lung needle aspiration," *Radiology*, vol. 165, no. 2, pp. 351–353, 1987.

[49] The Royal College of Radiologists, *Protocol for Prevention of and Management of Vascular Air Embolism during Interventional Radiological Procedures*, The Royal College of Radiologists, London, UK, 2011, BFCR(11)7.

[50] B. M. P. Rademaker, F. A. Groenman, P. A. van der Wouw, and E. A. Bakkum, "Paradoxical gas embolism by transpulmonary passage of venous emboli during hysteroscopic surgery: a case report and discussion," *The British Journal of Anaesthesia*, vol. 101, no. 2, pp. 230–233, 2008.

[51] S. Donepudi, D. Chavalitdhamrong, L. Pu, and P. V. Draganov, "Air embolism complicating gastrointestinal endoscopy: a systematic review," *World Journal of Gastrointestinal Endoscopy*, vol. 5, no. 8, pp. 359–365, 2013.

[52] M. M. Maher, M. K. Kalra, R. L. Titton et al., "Percutaneous lung biopsy in a patient with a cavitating lung mass: indications, technique, and complications," *American Journal of Roentgenology*, vol. 185, no. 4, pp. 989–994, 2005.

[53] A. Manhire, M. Charig, C. Clelland et al., "Guidelines for radiologically guided lung biopsy," *Thorax*, vol. 58, no. 11, pp. 920–936, 2003.

[54] A. M. Rozenblit, J. Tuvia, G. N. Rozenblit, and A. Klink, "CT-guided transthoracic needle biopsy using an ipsilateral dependent position," *The American Journal of Roentgenology*, vol. 174, no. 6, pp. 1759–1764, 2000.

[55] Oxford Centre for Evidence-Based Medicine, The Oxford 2011 Levels of Evidence, http://www.cebm.net/index.aspx?o=5653.

[56] B. C. Odisio, A. L. Tam, R. Avritscher, S. Gupta, and M. J. Wallace, "CT-guided adrenal biopsy: comparison of ipsilateral decubitus versus prone patient positioning for biopsy approach," *European Radiology*, vol. 22, no. 6, pp. 1233–1239, 2012.

12

Differential Diagnoses of Overgrowth Syndromes: The Most Important Clinical and Radiological Disease Manifestations

Letícia da Silva Lacerda,[1] **Úrsula David Alves,**[1] **José Fernando Cardona Zanier,**[1]
Dequitier Carvalho Machado,[1,2] **Gustavo Bittencourt Camilo,**[1,2] **and Agnaldo José Lopes**[2]

[1] *Department of Radiology, State University of Rio de Janeiro, 20551-030 Rio de Janeiro, RJ, Brazil*
[2] *Postgraduate Programme in Medical Sciences, State University of Rio de Janeiro, 20550-170 Rio de Janeiro, RJ, Brazil*

Correspondence should be addressed to Agnaldo José Lopes; agnaldolopes.uerj@gmail.com

Academic Editor: Andreas H. Mahnken

Overgrowth syndromes comprise a heterogeneous group of diseases that are characterized by excessive tissue development. Some of these syndromes may be associated with dysfunction in the receptor tyrosine kinase (RTK)/PI3K/AKT pathway, which results in an increased expression of the insulin receptor. In the current review, four overgrowth syndromes were characterized (Proteus syndrome, Klippel-Trenaunay-Weber syndrome, Madelung's disease, and neurofibromatosis type I) and illustrated using cases from our institution. Because these syndromes have overlapping clinical manifestations and have no established genetic tests for their diagnosis, radiological methods are important contributors to the diagnosis of many of these syndromes. The correlation of genetic discoveries and molecular pathways that may contribute to the phenotypic expression is also of interest, as this may lead to potential therapeutic interventions.

1. Introduction

Longitudinal growth results from multifactorial and complex processes that take place in the broader context of different genetic traits and environmental influences [1, 2]. Overgrowth syndromes comprise a heterogeneous group of disorders that lead to excessive tissue proliferation, which is characterized by a phenotype of excessive somatic and visceral growth [1–3]. A myriad of syndromes are characterized by substantial localized or asymmetric tissue overgrowth, represented by Beckwith-Wiedemann syndrome, Sotos syndrome, Proteus syndrome, Klippel-Trenaunay-Weber syndrome, Madelung's disease, neurofibromatosis type I, Weaver syndrome, Nevo syndrome, Simpson-Golabi-Behmel syndrome, Bannayan-Riley-Ruvalcaba syndrome, Perlman syndrome, Pallister-Killian syndrome, and many other conditions. The Beckwith-Wiedemann and Sotos syndromes are the most frequent [1–4]. Overgrowth syndromes can be localized or diffuse and often manifest at birth or in the postnatal period [4].

Though most growth syndrome have a genetic basis, others such as Madelung's disease have unknown etiology

[4]. Genetic associations are already well established for some conditions including Weaver, Perlman, and Proteus syndromes [2]. The fact that Madelung's disease tends to occur in older males and is often associated with heavy alcohol consumption in 60–90% of cases suggests that it is an acquired abnormality or more susceptible to environmental modifiers [5, 6]. Importantly, most of these syndromes lead to increased risks of cognitive disorders and cancers [7]. The frequency of cancer is well documented in some syndromes such as Proteus (20%), Sotos (2–4%), and Perlman (65%) [2]. In some overgrowth syndromes, such as Beckwith-Wiedemann and Perlman syndromes, tumors appeared mostly in the abdomen; conversely, in other overgrowth syndromes, such as Sotos syndrome, the most frequent type of overgrowths is extra-abdominally located lymphohematological tumors [8].

A dysfunction in the receptor tyrosine kinase (RTK)/PI3K/AKT pathway that specifically promotes a rapid increase in insulin receptor expression is most likely the pathophysiological basis of some overgrowth syndromes [4]. Insulin receptor stimulation leads to an increase in PI3-kinase activity, which thereby generates PIP3 and leads to the activation of PKB/Akt [4]. This pathway plays an important role in the activation of somatic mutations in various tumors as well as in apoptosis, angiogenesis, and brain development [9–11]. A dysfunction in the (RTK)/PI3K/AKT pathway has been described in some conditions such as Proteus syndrome [4]. The genetic factor is intrinsically involved in some overgrowth syndromes. It is noteworthy to highlight the imprinted growth regulatory genes on chromosome 11p15.5. In this region, there is one domain in which the *H19* expression from the maternal allele is thought to protect against the tall stature. There is also a second domain that consists of the *CDKN1C* gene, which acts as an in-utero negative regulator of cell growth. Heritable forms of Beckwith-Wiedemann syndrome have been attributed mainly to mutations in the growth suppressor gene *CDKN1C* [2, 12]. There are some reports of *NSD-1* mutations in individuals with Sotos and Weaver syndromes and more recently mutations in the *EZH2* gene in three families with Weaver syndrome have been identified [13]. A previously unknown susceptibility locus was mapped and germline mutations in *DIS3L2* identified in individuals with Perlman syndrome. Functional studies demonstrated that underexpression of the *DIS3L2* gene was associated with cellular growth enhancement [14].

Several classifications have been developed in an attempt to facilitate the diagnosis of these syndromes, but these attempts have been hindered by the syndromes' several overlapping clinical manifestations [1, 15]. Neylon et al. [2] proposed a classification of overgrowth syndromes by ordering them according to their typical timing of clinical presentation as follows: (a) syndromes exhibiting overgrowth in the neonatal period, including Beckwith-Wiedemann syndrome, Sotos syndrome, Weaver syndrome, and Perlman syndrome and (b) overgrowth syndromes usually identified in childhood, including Klinefelter syndrome and Proteus syndrome. Major progress such as the identification of genetic causes has recently enhanced the knowledge of the underlying pathophysiological mechanisms, the delineation of the genotype-phenotype relationships, and the establishment of the main characteristics for each condition [1]. As a consequence, the possibilities for distinguishing between different overgrowth syndromes have increased. Several studies are currently underway to organize these types of disorders according to a molecular classification system for overgrowth syndromes in order to assist the practicing clinician [16–18]. Radiological abnormalities are increasingly important for the clinical differentiation between overgrowth syndromes, making those abnormalities valuable diagnostic criteria for some of these conditions.

In this review, four overgrowth syndromes—Proteus syndrome, Klippel-Trenaunay-Weber syndrome, Madelung's disease, and neurofibromatosis type I—are described. The main clinical and imaging features these syndromes are highlighted using clinical cases evaluated in our institution. Although they are not the most common overgrowth syndromes, manifestations of these four syndromes overlap with other more prevalent overgrowth syndromes. Thus, it is of interest to present these cases which were diagnosed from the suspicion caused by imaging findings.

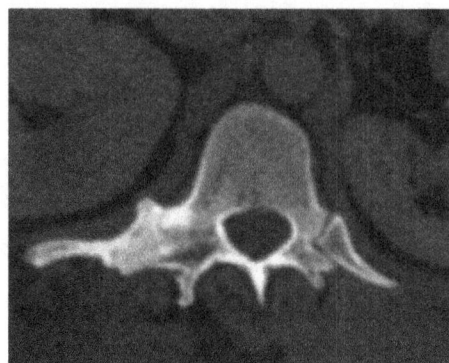

FIGURE 1: The right costovertebral joint space is fused. The T12 vertebra shows disproportionate asymmetric overgrowth which is characteristic for the Proteus syndrome.

2. Proteus Syndrome

Proteus syndrome is a congenital disorder of unknown etiology, and it is the prototype of overgrowth syndromes. It was first described in 1979 and is characterized by multisystem involvement and clinical variability [19]. This disorder became prominent in 1980 after being depicted in the movie *The Elephant Man* [19, 20]. Proteus syndrome is a rare condition with an estimated prevalence of one in 1 million people worldwide [21]. A study showed a somatic activating mutation of the *AKT1* oncogene kinase, an enzyme involved in cell proliferation, in this disorder [22]. This finding implies the activation of the *PI3K-AKT* pathway in the characteristic clinical findings of overgrowth and tumor susceptibility in patients with Proteus syndrome [22].

Proteus syndrome can affect all three germ lineages. Abnormal asymmetric growth and hemihypertrophy are its typical clinical manifestations, though overgrowth of the long bones, macrodactyly, asymmetric macrocephaly, plantar or palmar hyperplasia, vertebral abnormalities, lipoma, hemangioma, connective tissue nevi, lymphangiomas, and vascular malformations can also be observed in this syndrome [7, 23–25]. Because there is no specific genetic testing, the diagnosis of this syndrome is based on clinical data and radiological evolutions according to the criteria formulated in 1998 by the National Institutes of Health [19, 23]. The primary hallmark of Proteus syndrome is a mosaic or random distribution of lesions throughout the body that develop gradually during childhood, after which point the disease can stabilize or continue to slowly progress [23]. Some authors believe that the disease becomes stable at approximately 15–17 years of age [21, 26].

Skeletal changes are the most frequently expressed manifestations of Proteus syndrome and include kyphoscoliosis, macrodactyly, hyperostosis, asymmetric overgrowth of limbs, abnormal vertebral bodies (Figure 1), craniofacial abnormalities, and focal calvarial thickening [19, 23, 25]. Among the soft tissue manifestations, asymmetric growth of the subcutaneous tissue (Figure 2) is common and may be associated with exacerbated muscle development and the proliferation of lymphatic channels and vascular malformations [19, 23]. Connective tissue nevi may also

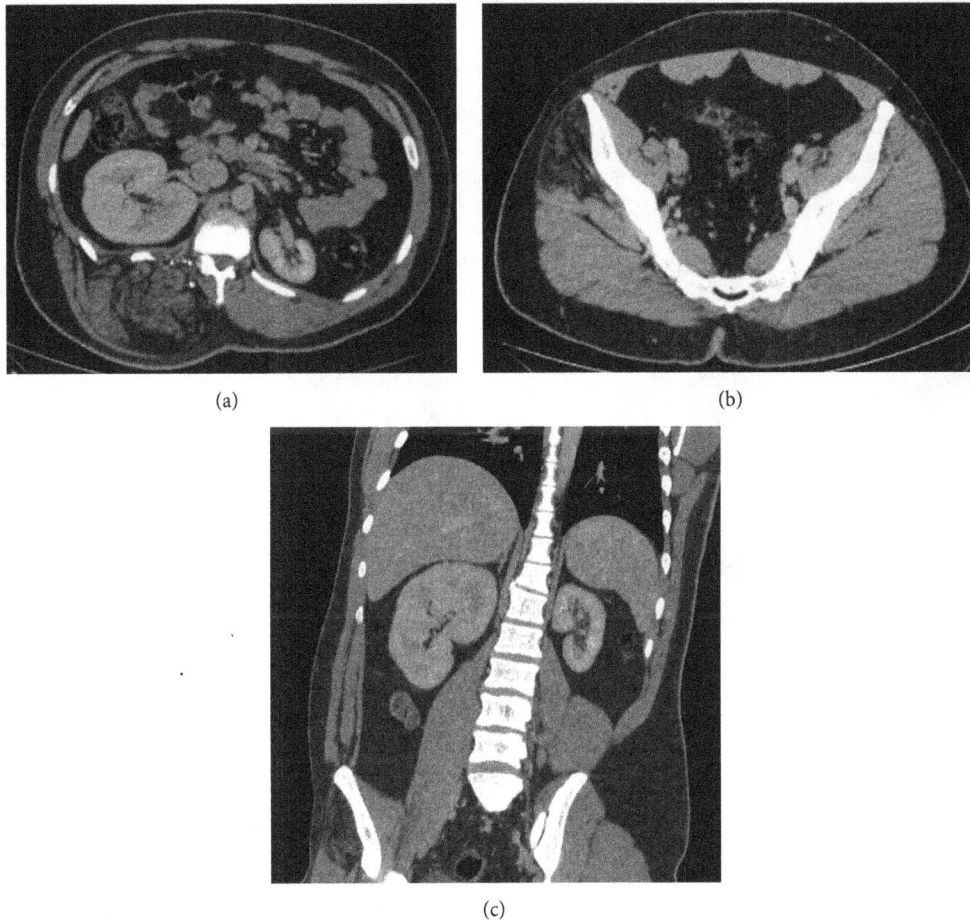

FIGURE 2: A 21-year-old man with Proteus syndrome presenting asymmetric lower limbs and epidermal nevus. CT of the abdomen showed tissue with a fat density infiltrating the right paraspinal musculature, with increased local volume extending from T7 to L5, in addition to an enlargement of the right kidney (a). The scan also noted fatty replacement in right gluteal muscles (b). Coronal CT showed asymmetry of the kidneys (c).

be observed, particularly in the plantar region, as well as cerebriform nevi [23]. Cerebral arteriovenous malformations, abnormal grey-white matter differentiation, and hydrocephalus are also common findings. Visceral changes, such as splenomegaly or nephromegaly (Figure 2), hydronephrosis, pancreatic lipomas, colonic polyps, emphysema, and lung cysts are less common findings [19, 23, 24]. All of these conditions aid in the differential diagnosis of Proteus Syndrome, which can be challenging because Klippel-Trenaunay-Weber syndrome, Maffucci's syndrome, enchondromatosis, neurofibromatosis type I, Bannayan-Zonana syndrome, hemihyperplasia, and Madelung's disease can also cause overgrowth [24, 27]. Importantly, disproportionate asymmetric overgrowth can be a clue to the differential diagnosis of other diseases of osseous overgrowth in which the enlarged bones retain their normal proportional relationships [24–26].

3. Klippel-Trenaunay-Weber Syndrome

Klippel-Trenaunay-Weber syndrome is rare and has an uncertain origin with an incidence of approximately 1 : 100,000 live births [28]. It appears to have no predilection for gender or race, and most of the cases are sporadic and appear at birth [29, 30]. The French physicians Maurice Klippel and Paul Trenaunay first described this syndrome in 1900 when they associated vascular malformations with hypertrophy in the affected limb. Subsequently, arteriovenous fistulas in these patients were described by Parkes Weber [30–32]. Several theories attempt to elucidate the etiology of this syndrome, such as multifactorial, paradominant inheritance, or mosaic mutation [33]. Some authors state that a deep venous obstruction or atresia can lead to swelling and limb hypertrophy [30]. Others state that the disease symptoms are caused by a change in the angiopoietin-2 antagonist, which determines the maintenance of small arteriovenous communications in the limbs [34]. However, further experts argue that the hypertrophy observed in soft tissues is a primary occurrence that occurs independently of fistulas [35].

Klippel-Trenaunay-Weber syndrome is characterized by the presence of capillary malformations associated with venous malformations or varicose veins (Figure 3) and with bone or tissue hypertrophy; a diagnosis of this syndrome is based on the presence of at least two of these three categories [29, 36]. 63% of diagnosed patients present

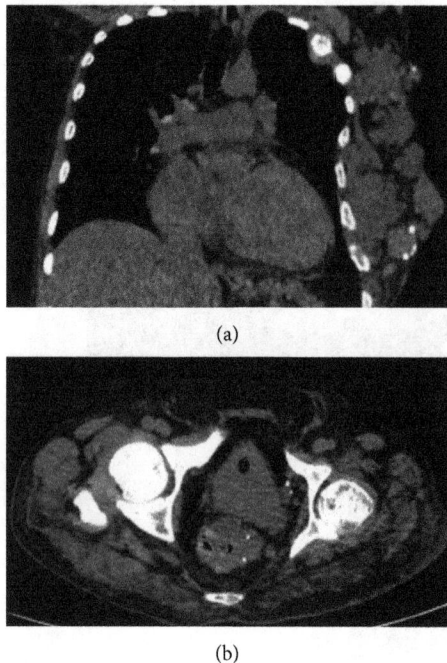

(a)

(b)

FIGURE 3: A 60-year-old man with Klippel-Trenaunay-Weber syndrome presenting asymmetric growth of the lower limbs. CT of the chest showed increased soft tissue as well as extensive vascular malformations in the left hemithorax wall with intermingled phleboliths, causing multiple lytic lesions with enlargement in the ipsilateral ribs (a). CT of the abdomen showed a thick-walled rectum intermingled with phleboliths, denoting varicose veins (b).

all three symptoms [35]. The most common manifestation, present in 98% of patients, is capillary malformation, which is represented by cutaneous hemangiomas or a port-wine stain [29, 36]. These lesions usually affect the hypertrophied limb, and when they occur in the trunk region, they rarely cross the midline [29, 37–39]. Varicose veins are also present in most patients with Klippel-Trenaunay-Weber syndrome, and they are more evident during adolescence and affect both the superficial and deep venous systems [26, 29]. The varicose veins may remain stable or progress, causing pain, lymphedema, thrombophlebitis, and ulcers [30]. Hypertrophy, usually resulting from venous ectasia, is always secondary to issues involving bone, soft tissue, or both, which distinguishes this syndrome from Proteus syndrome, in which bone and tissue overgrowth can occur independently of vascular malformations [23, 30, 35, 40].

Other features also differentiate these two syndromes. Klippel-Trenaunay-Weber syndrome is bilateral and less frequently involves the upper limbs [23]. Some authors believe that in Proteus syndrome, the limb overgrowth is usually mild or absent at birth, while in Klippel-Trenaunay-Weber syndrome it is present and severe at birth. Other authors have stated that limb hypertrophy is the latest indicator of Klippel-Trenaunay-Weber syndrome [30]. Bone overgrowth, which is dysplastic, progressive, and irregular, is typical of Proteus syndrome and not observed in Klippel-Trenaunay-Weber syndrome; thus, its detection is an important tool in differentiating between the diseases [23].

4. Madelung's Disease

Madelung's disease is also known as multiple symmetric lipomatosis, benign symmetric lipomatosis, or Launois-Bensaude adenolipomatosis. It is a rare condition that is possibly related to alcohol consumption and leads to denervation and subsequent adipocyte hypertrophy [41, 42]. Alcohol appears to play a role in the adipocyte hyperplasia process in genetically susceptible individuals through the prolipogenesis and antilipolytic effects [43]. However, other studies have also suggested the presence of mitochondrial inheritance through mutation of the maternal gene [44, 45]. Madelung's disease is most common in adult males of Mediterranean descent [46], with an estimated incidence of 1 : 25,000 in Italy [47].

It is manifested by the painless deposition of multiple nonencapsulated masses of fatty tissue, which are symmetrically distributed in the cervical and upper thoracic regions over a period of months to years. The face, hands, and feet are usually unaffected. A Madelung's disease diagnosis is based on an ectoscopy as well as additional tests that rule out the skin, vascular, and bone changes present in other diseases [48]. This disease often leads to aesthetic complaints, but it is rarely associated with complications such as dyspnea (caused by upper airway compression) or dysphonia (caused by an involvement of the recurrent laryngeal nerve). Madelung's disease is classified as type I when lipomatous masses are observed in the parotid, cervical, suprascapular, or deltoid regions and classified as type II when the lipomatosis is diffuse, resembling simple obesity [48].

Computed tomography (CT) is important for a Madelung's diagnosis because it can identify the key symptoms, such as lipomatosis in the characteristic regions (Figure 4), the calcification of lipomas, tracheal narrowing, and venous stasis in the chest wall, while confirming the absence of masses in other sites [46]. When performing a differential diagnosis, diseases in addition to other overgrowth syndromes must be considered. When there are similar cases in the family, familial lipomatosis is an option, and Dercum's disease (adiposis dolorosa) is a possibility if the fat accumulation is accompanied by pain [23].

5. Neurofibromatosis Type I

Neurofibromatosis type I, also known as von Recklinghausen's disease, was first described in 1882 by Friedrich Daniel von Recklinghausen. Neurofibromatosis type I is the most common type of phakomatosis or neurocutaneous syndrome, occurring in one out of every 2000 live births with no predilection for gender or race [49, 50]. It is an autosomal dominant disorder caused by heterozygous mutations of the NF-1 gene, located at chromosome 17q11.2 [51]. The NF1 gene encodes a large cytoplasmic protein called neurofibromin, which is a major negative regulator of *Ras* protooncogene, a key protein in a major signal transduction pathway [50, 52]. In half of the cases, however, this disease occurs sporadically via spontaneous mutations that cause abnormal growth in nervous and fibrous tissues [49, 50].

(a)

(b)

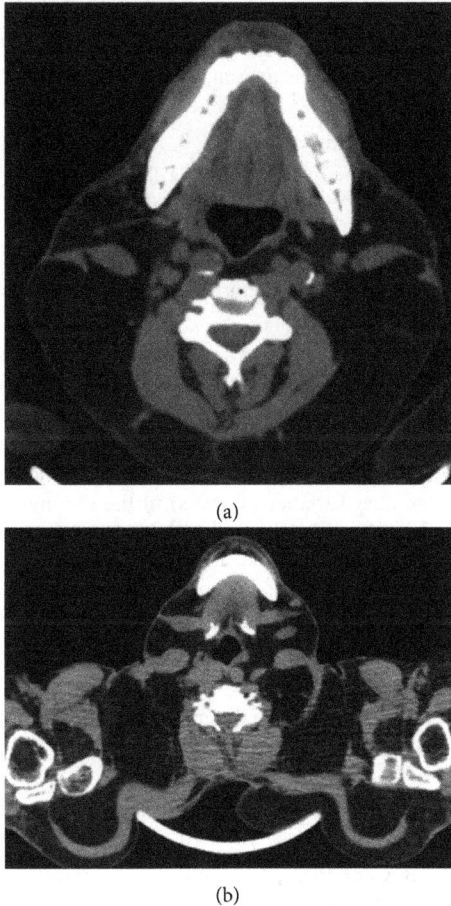

FIGURE 4: A 53-year-old man with Madelung's disease presenting a progressive painless increase of the cervical region. CT of the neck and chest showed fat deposition occurring predominantly in the posterior subcutaneous region of the neck (a) and in the supraclavicular and upper regions of the chest (b).

FIGURE 5: A 53-year-old man with neurofibromatosis type I. A morphostructural abnormality in the spine is characterized by significant dorsolumbar scoliosis with right convexity, as observed in his CT scan (coronal section).

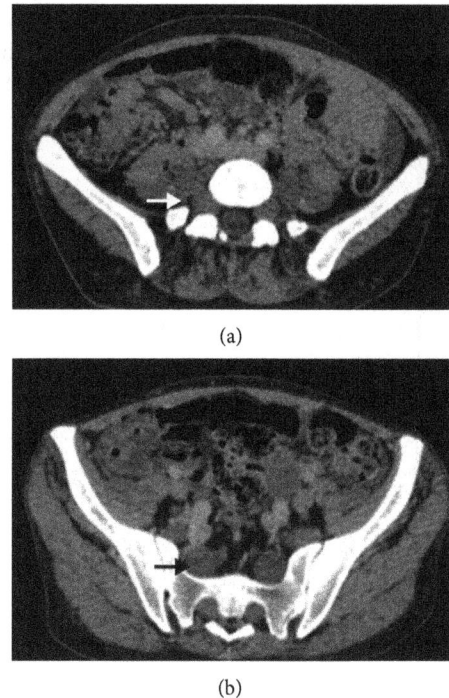

(a)

(b)

FIGURE 6: A 34-year-old woman with neurofibromatosis type I. Axial CT show plexiform neurofibromas of lumbar and sacral nerve roots.

Clinical symptoms are usually observed in childhood, though in approximately 10% of cases they occur later in life and are atypical [48, 53]. Neurofibromatosis type I can exhibit different clinical manifestations, which makes a diagnosis more difficult. Generally, the disease affects the skin, nervous system, bones, and endocrine glands by causing benign tumors [49]. The diagnostic criteria for this disease were developed in 1987 and redefined in 1997 [50], and they are based on the presence of two or more of the following findings: a first-degree relative who has neurofibromatosis type I, "café-au-lait" spots, neurofibromas, freckles in the axillary or inguinal regions, optic gliomas, iris hamartomas, and distinctive bone lesions.

The "café-au-lait" spots are present in approximately 95% of diseased patients and are usually congenital; they occur in different sizes and are distributed throughout the body surface [50, 54]. Among the most frequent skeletal abnormalities observed in neurofibromatosis type I are scoliosis (Figure 5), kyphosis, growth disorders, pseudarthrosis of long bones, and sphenoid wing dysplasia [55]. Over time, patients with neurofibromatosis type I may experience abnormalities of the skeleton (thinning or overgrowth of the bones in the arms or lower leg) [50, 55].

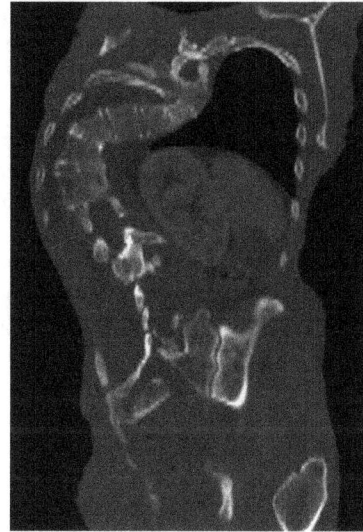

Neurofibromas are the tumors of the peripheral nervous system typically observed in this disease, particularly plexiform neurofibromas [49], which are derived from Schwann cells and fibroblasts. Approximately 30% of patients with a single neurofibroma will develop neurofibromatosis type I, and virtually all patients with multiple neurofibromas, especially of the plexiform type (Figure 6), have the disease [49].

Iris hamartomas (Lisch nodules) are bilateral and asymptomatic hamartomatous lesions on the surface of the iris. Multiple hamartomas are unique to neurofibromatosis type I.

Several of the diagnostic criteria are confirmed by radiological examinations. Tomographic findings depend on the histological features of the tumors and may exhibit soft tissue density. More commonly (in 73% of cases) there is low attenuation due to cystic degeneration, confluent areas of hypocellularity, or lipid abundance [49]. Neurofibromatosis is distinguished by its typical symptoms including neurofibromas, Lisch nodules, axillary freckles, and "café-au-lait" spots, which are absent in other overgrowth syndromes [23].

6. Conclusion

Overgrowth syndromes are characterized by diffuse or localized tissue proliferation and they may originate in a dysfunctional receptor tyrosine kinase (RTK)/PI3K/AKT pathway. These syndromes represent a heterogeneous group of diseases with manifestations that often overlap each other, requiring the use of preestablished diagnostic criteria in most cases.

In this review, four overgrowth syndromes were characterized according to their primary clinical and radiological features. Identifying these features is important for making the correct diagnosis and to appropriately monitor the patient's health because no specific genetic tests for these syndromes are available.

References

[1] R. Visser, S. G. Kant, J. M. Wit, and M. H. Breung, "Overgrowth syndromes: from classical to new," *Pediatric Endocrinology Reviews*, vol. 6, no. 3, pp. 375–394, 2009.

[2] O. M. Neylon, G. A. Werther, and M. A. Sabin, "Overgrowth syndromes," *Current Opinion in Pediatrics*, vol. 24, no. 4, pp. 505–511, 2012.

[3] I. Bentov and H. Werner, "IGF, IGF receptor and overgrowth syndromes," *Pediatric Endocrinology Reviews*, vol. 1, no. 4, pp. 352–360, 2004.

[4] K. T. Barker and R. S. Houlston, "Overgrowth syndromes: is dysfunctional PI3-kinase signalling a unifying mechanism?" *European Journal of Human Genetics*, vol. 11, no. 9, pp. 665–670, 2003.

[5] A. Tufan, R. Mercan, A. Kaya et al., "An unusual case of Madelung's disease with multiple atypical fractures," *Case Reports in Orthopedics*, vol. 2012, Article ID 180506, 3 pages, 2012.

[6] E. Mevio, M. Sbrocca, M. Mullace, S. Viglione, and N. Mevio, "Multiple symmetric lipomatosis: a review of 3 cases," *Case Reports in Otolaryngology*, vol. 2012, Article ID 910526, 4 pages, 2012.

[7] M. M. Cohen Jr., "Overgrowth syndromes: an update," *Advances in Pediatrics*, vol. 46, pp. 441–491, 1999.

[8] R. Gracia Bouthelier and P. Lapunzina, "Follow-up and risk of tumors in overgrowth syndromes," *Journal of Pediatric Endocrinology and Metabolism*, vol. 18, no. 1, pp. 1227–1235, 2005.

[9] G. M. Mirzaa, J. Rivière, and W. B. Dobyns, "Megalencephaly syndromes and activating mutations in the PI3K-AKT pathway: MPPH and MCAP," *American Journal of Medical Genetics C: Seminars in Medical Genetics*, vol. 163, no. 2, pp. 122–130, 2013.

[10] T. L. Yuan and L. C. Cantley, "PI3K pathway alterations in cancer: variations on a theme," *Oncogene*, vol. 27, no. 41, pp. 5497–5510, 2008.

[11] K. C. Kurek, V. L. Luks, U. M. Ayturk et al., "Somatic mosaic activating mutations in PIK3CA cause CLOVES syndrome," *American Journal of Human Genetics*, vol. 90, no. 6, pp. 1108–1115, 2012.

[12] B. Baskin, S. Choufani, Y. A. Chen et al., "High frequency of copy number variations (CNVs) in the chromosome 11p15 region in patients with Beckwith-Wiedemann syndrome," *Human Genetics*, vol. 133, no. 3, pp. 321–330, 2014.

[13] W. T. Gibson, R. L. Hood, S. H. Zhan et al., "Mutations in EZH2 cause weaver syndrome," *American Journal of Human Genetics*, vol. 90, no. 1, pp. 110–118, 2012.

[14] D. Astuti, M. R. Morris, W. N. Cooper et al., "Germline mutations in DIS3L2 cause the Perlman syndrome of overgrowth and Wilms tumor susceptibility," *Nature Genetics*, vol. 44, no. 3, pp. 277–284, 2012.

[15] G. Neri and M. Moscarda, "Overgrowth syndromes: a classification," *Endocrine Development*, vol. 14, pp. 53–60, 2009.

[16] D. Melis, R. Genesio, E. Del Giudice et al., "Selective cognitive impairment and tall stature due to chromosome 19 supernumerary ring," *Clinical Dysmorphology*, vol. 21, no. 1, pp. 27–32, 2012.

[17] S. C. Elalaoui, I. Garin, A. Sefiani, and G. Perez de Nanclares, "Maternal hypomethylation of KvDMR in a monozygotic male twin pair discordant for Beckwith-Wiedemann syndrome," *Molecular Syndromology*, vol. 5, no. 1, pp. 41–46, 2014.

[18] S. Senniappan, D. Ismail, C. Shipster, C. Beesley, and K. Hussain, "The heterogeneity of hyperinsulinaemic hypoglycaemia in 19 patients with Beckwith-Wiedemann syndrome due to KvDMR1 hypomethylation," *Journal of Pediatric Endocrinology & Metabolism*, 2014.

[19] M. J. Kaduthodil, D. S. Prasad, A. S. Lowe, A. S. Punekar, S. Yeung, and C. L. Kay, "Imaging manifestations in Proteus syndrome: an unusual multisystem developmental disorder," *British Journal of Radiology*, vol. 85, no. 1017, pp. e793–e799, 2012.

[20] H. Hamm, "Cutaneous mosaicism of lethal mutations," *American Journal of Medical Genetics*, vol. 85, no. 4, pp. 342–345, 1999.

[21] M. J. Lindhurst, J. C. Sapp, J. K. Teer et al., "A mosaic activating mutation in AKT1 associated with the proteus syndrome," *New England Journal of Medicine*, vol. 365, no. 7, pp. 611–619, 2011.

[22] C. Alves, A. X. Acosta, and M. P. Toralles, "Proteus syndrome: clinical diagnosis of a series of cases," *Indian Journal of Endocrinology and Metabolism*, vol. 17, no. 6, pp. 1053–1611, 2013.

[23] C. A. Jamis-Dow, J. Turner, L. G. Biesecker, and P. L. Choyke, "Radiologic manifestations of Proteus syndrome," *Radiographics*, vol. 24, no. 4, pp. 1051–1068, 2004.

[24] L. Biesecker, "The challenges of Proteus syndrome: diagnosis and management," *European Journal of Human Genetics*, vol. 14, no. 11, pp. 1151–1157, 2006.

[25] L. G. Biesecker, R. Happle, J. B. Mulliken et al., "Proteus syndrome: diagnostic criteria, differential diagnosis, and patient evaluation," *American Journal of Medical Genetics*, vol. 84, no. 5, pp. 389–395, 1999.

[26] C. Y. Li, Y. L. Chang, W. C. Chen, and Y. C. Lee, "Pulmonary manifestations and management of proteus syndrome," *Journal of the Formosan Medical Association*, vol. 109, no. 5, pp. 397–400, 2010.

[27] K. M. Elsayes, C. O. Menias, J. R. Dillman, J. F. Platt, J. M. Willatt, and J. P. Heiken, "Vascular malformation and hemangiomatosis syndromes: spectrum of imaging manifestations," *American Journal of Roentgenology*, vol. 190, no. 5, pp. 1291–1299, 2008.

[28] I. Lorda-Sanchez, L. Prieto, E. Rodriguez-Pinilla, and M. L. Martinez-Frias, "Increased parental age and number of pregnancies in Klippel-Trenaunay-Weber syndrome," *Annals of Human Genetics*, vol. 62, no. 3, pp. 235–239, 1998.

[29] S. H. Cha, M. A. Romeo, and J. A. Neutze, "Visceral manifestations of Klippel-Trénaunay syndrome," *Radiographics*, vol. 25, no. 6, pp. 1694–1697, 2005.

[30] C. A. De Leon, L. R. Braun Filho, M. D. Ferrari, B. L. Guidolin, and B. J. Maffessoni, "Klippel-Trenaunay syndrome: case report," *Anais Brasileiros de Dermatologia*, vol. 85, no. 1, pp. 93–96, 2010.

[31] M. Servelle, "Klippel and Trenaunay's syndrome. 768 operated cases," *Annals of Surgery*, vol. 201, no. 3, pp. 365–373, 1985.

[32] L. A. Favorito, "Vesical hemangioma in patient with Klippel-Trenaunay-Weber syndrome," *International Braz J Urol*, vol. 29, no. 2, pp. 149–150, 2003.

[33] N. Revencu, L. M. Boon, A. Dompmartin et al., "Germline mutations in RASA1 are not found in patients with Klippel-Trenaunay syndrome or capillary malformation with limb overgrowth," *Molecular Syndromology*, vol. 4, no. 4, pp. 173–178, 2013.

[34] P. Gloviczki and D. J. Driscoll, "Klippel-Trenaunay syndrome: current management," *Phlebology*, vol. 22, no. 6, pp. 291–298, 2007.

[35] R. L. G. Flumignan, D. G. Cacione, S. I. Lopes et al., "Klippel-Trenaunay-Weber syndrome: association of operative treatment with foam sclerotherapy," *Jornal Vascular Brasileiro*, vol. 10, no. 1, pp. 77–80, 2011.

[36] A. G. Jacob, D. J. Driscoll, W. J. Shaughnessy, A. W. Stanson, R. P. Clay, and P. Gloviczki, "Klippel-Trénaunay syndrome: spectrum and management," *Mayo Clinic Proceedings*, vol. 73, no. 1, pp. 28–36, 1998.

[37] M. M. Al-Salman, "Klippel-Trenaunay Syndrome: clinical features, complications, and management," *Surgery Today*, vol. 27, no. 8, pp. 735–740, 1997.

[38] K. T. Delis, P. Gloviczki, P. W. Wennberg, T. W. Rooke, and D. J. Driscoll, "Hemodynamic impairment, venous segmental disease, and clinical severity scoring in limbs with Klippel-Trenaunay syndrome," *Journal of Vascular Surgery*, vol. 45, no. 3, pp. 561–567, 2007.

[39] M. C. Garzon, J. T. Huang, O. Enjolras, and I. J. Frieden, "Vascular malformations. Part II: associated syndromes," *Journal of the American Academy of Dermatology*, vol. 56, no. 4, pp. 541–564, 2007.

[40] V. Latessa and K. Frasier, "Case study: a minimally invasive approach to the treatment of Klippel-Trenaunay syndrome," *Journal of Vascular Nursing*, vol. 25, no. 4, pp. 76–84, 2007.

[41] G. Enzi, "Multiple symmetric lipomatosis: an updated clinical report," *Medicine*, vol. 63, no. 1, pp. 56–64, 1984.

[42] G. Enzi, C. Angelini, P. Negrin, M. Armani, S. Pierobon, and D. Fedele, "Sensory, motor, and autonomic neuropathy in patients with multiple symmetric lipomatosis," *Medicine*, vol. 64, no. 6, pp. 388–393, 1985.

[43] Í. I. Shibasaki, H. I. Shibasaki, T. S. Nakamoto, F. S. Baccan, and L. S. Raposo, "Multiple symmetrical lipomatosis (Madelung's disease)," *Brazilian Journal of Otorhinolaryngology*, vol. 80, no. 1, pp. 90–91, 2014.

[44] F. Y. Lin and T. L. Yang, "Madelung disease," *Canadian Medical Association Journal*, vol. 185, no. 1, p. E79, 2013.

[45] C. Plummer, P. J. Spring, R. Marotta et al., "Multiple symmetrical lipomatosis: a mitochondrial disorder of brown fat," *Mitochondrion*, vol. 13, no. 4, pp. 269–276, 2013.

[46] M. V. Vieira, R. U. Grazziotin, M. Abreu et al., "Multiple symmetrical lipomatosis (Madelung's disease): a case report," *Radiologia Brasileira*, vol. 34, no. 2, pp. 119–121, 2001.

[47] M. S. Landis, R. Etemad-Rezai, K. Shetty, and M. Goldszmidt, "Case 143: Madelung disease," *Radiology*, vol. 250, no. 3, pp. 951–954, 2009.

[48] L. P. Rodrigues and E. L. A. Melo, "Madelung's disease: a case report and literature review," *Radiologia Brasileira*, vol. 43, no. 2, pp. 275–276, 2012.

[49] B. J. Fortman, B. S. Kuszyk, B. A. Urban, and E. K. Fishman, "Neurofibromatosis type 1: a diagnostic mimicker at CT," *Radiographics*, vol. 21, no. 3, pp. 601–612, 2001.

[50] E. N. Washington, T. P. Placket, R. A. Gagliano, J. Kavolius, and D. A. Person, "Diffuse plexiform neurofibroma of the back: report of a case," *Hawaii Medical Journal*, vol. 69, no. 8, pp. 191–193, 2010.

[51] V. C. Williams, J. Lucas, M. A. Babcock, D. H. Gutmann, B. Bruce, and B. L. Maria, "Neurofibromatosis type 1 revisited," *Pediatrics*, vol. 123, no. 1, pp. 124–133, 2009.

[52] K. A. Diggs-Andrews, J. A. Brown, S. M. Gianino, J. B. Rubin, D. F. Wozniak, and D. H. Gutmann, "Sex is a major determinant of neuronal dysfunction in neurofibromatosis type 1," *Annals of Neurology*, vol. 75, no. 2, pp. 309–316, 2014.

[53] P. R. Biondetti, M. Vigo, D. Fiore, D. De Faveri, R. Ravasini, and L. Benedetti, "CT appearance of generalized von Recklinghausen neurofibromatosis," *Journal of Computer Assisted Tomography*, vol. 7, no. 5, pp. 866–869, 1983.

[54] K. P. Boyd, B. R. Korf, and A. Theos, "Neurofibromatosis type 1," *Journal of the American Academy of Dermatology*, vol. 61, no. 1, pp. 1–14, 2009.

[55] A. Ferrari, G. Bisogno, A. Macaluso et al., "Soft-tissue sarcomas in children and adolescents with neurofibromatosis type 1," *Cancer*, vol. 109, no. 7, pp. 1406–1412, 2007.

13

The Features of Extrahepatic Collateral Arteries Related to Hepatic Artery Occlusion and Benefits in the Transarterial Management of Liver Tumors

Lin Yang, Xiao Ming Zhang, Yong Jun Ren, Nan Dong Miao, Xiao Hua Huang, and Guo Li Dong

Sichuan Key Laboratory of Medical Imaging, Department of Radiology, Affiliated Hospital of North Sichuan Medical College, Nanchong, Sichuan 637000, China

Correspondence should be addressed to Lin Yang; linyangmd@163.com

Academic Editor: Andreas H. Mahnken

Purpose. To investigate the extrahepatic collateral arteries related to hepatic artery occlusion (HAO) and to determine its benefits in the transarterial management of liver tumors. *Methods and Findings.* Eleven patients (7 hepatocellular carcinomas, 3 liver metastases, and 1 with hemangioma) with HAO confirmed with digital subtraction angiography (DSA) were admitted to our hospital. Of the 11 patients, 7 were men and 4 were women, with an average age of 41.5 ± 15.5 years (range: 29 to 70 years). DSA was performed to evaluate the collateral routes to the liver. In the 11 patients with HAO, DSA showed complete occlusion of the common hepatic artery in 9 patients and the proper hepatic artery (PHA) in 2 patients. Extrahepatic collateral arteries supplying the liver were readily evident. The collateral arteries originated from the superior mesenteric artery (SMA) in 8 patients, from the gastroduodenal artery in 2 patients, and from the left gastric artery (LGA) in 1 patient. Transcatheter treatment was successfully performed via the collateral artery in all patients except the one who had hemangioma. *Conclusions.* DSA is an effective method for detecting collateral circulation related to HAO and may provide information to guide transcatheter management decisions.

1. Introduction

Transarterial chemoembolization and infusion chemotherapies have been widely used to treat liver neoplasms [1–5]. However, certain complications following transarterial treatment, such as femoral nerve injury, liver cancer rupture, duodenum perforation, liver abscesses, and hepatic artery occlusion (HAO), were sometimes reported [6, 7]. Above all, HAO is a serious complication because it prevents continuation of transarterial therapy.

It was previously reported that the collateral arterial supply to the liver was evident immediately after HAO [8–10]. It is essential to study the collateral circulation related to HAO in transcatheterization procedures for liver tumor management [11]. Previous reports have indicated that computed tomography (CT) and computed tomography angiography (CTA) could reveal the arterial collateral system in patients with HAO [12, 13]; however, to the best of our knowledge, few studies have addressed the features of extrahepatic collateral routes related to HAO by using digital subtraction angiography (DSA) and benefits in the transarterial management of liver tumors.

In our practice, we primarily found that the collateral pathways after HAO were different from those reported in the literature [12, 13], and the details of the extrahepatic collateral routes to the liver in patients with HAO based on using DSA are unclear. We therefore conducted this study to investigate the extrahepatic collateral routes related to HAO and to determine its benefits in the transarterial management of liver tumors.

2. Methods

2.1. Objectives. We conducted this study to investigate anatomical changes to the extrahepatic collateral arteries related to HAO based on DSA and to determine the benefits of this method in the transarterial management of liver tumors.

2.2. Participants. From November, 2003 to May, 2011, a total of 431 transarterial procedures were performed in 348 patients with liver tumors at our hospital. The patients with complete occlusion of the common hepatic artery (CHA) or the proper hepatic artery (PHA) related to interventional procedures were included in this study. A total of 11 cases (7 hepatocellular carcinomas, 3 liver metastases, and 1 hemangioma) with HAO were retrospectively studied. Of the 11 patients, 7 were men and 4 were women, with an average age of 41.5 ± 15.5 years (range: 29 to 70 years).

2.3. Angiography and Transcatheterization Procedures. Two radiologists, one with more than 20 years of experience and the other with 8 years of experience in interventional radiology, performed the angiography and transcatheterization procedures. Angiography was performed in a DSA unit (LCV plus, GE Medical Systems) with the use of a 5-F RH angiographic catheter (Terumo, Japan) in all eleven patients to study the collateral arteries related to HAO, to assess the location and vessels feeding the tumors, and to determine the optimal catheter position for chemoembolization or infusion chemotherapy. Sometimes, a 3-F SP microcatheter (Terumo, Japan) was also used to perform the catheterization. The celiac axis and SMA were evaluated in all the patients, and the LGA was evaluated in onepatient. In all the patients except one patient with hemangiomas, DSA was followed by hepatic arterial infusion chemotherapy or chemoembolization (the patient with hemangiomas was scheduled to undergo liver resection). For the hepatic arterial infusion chemotherapy, 5-fluorouracil (1000 mg to 1500 mg), hydroxycamptothecin (30 mg to 40 mg), and adriamycin (40 mg to 50 mg) were administered. Chemoembolization was performed with the administration of the antitumor drugs mentioned above, followed by lipiodol. The volume of the embolus was determined by considering the hepatic serum functional indices (serum albumin level, serum bilirubin level, and prothrombin time ratio) and the diameter of the lesion. The chemoembolization procedure was stopped when the tumor stain disappeared or decreased or when the patient could no longer tolerate the procedure.

2.4. Ethics. This study was approved by our institutional review board, and patient informed consent (written consent) was obtained.

3. Results

In all eleven patients, there were good ratings of DSA acquisition. DSA showed complete occlusion of the CHA in 9 patients (81.8%) and the PHA in 2 patients (18.2%). Extrahepatic collateral arteries supplying the liver were readily evident. The collateral arteries originated from the SMA in 8 patients (72.7%), from the gastroduodenal artery in 2 patients (18.2%) and from the LGA in 1 patient (9.1%). The pancreaticoduodenal arcade, gastroduodenal artery, and the

LGA were dilated on celiac axis angiograms. Angiography showed good opacification of the portal vein in this group. Transcatheter treatment was successfully performed in all patients except the one who had hemangiomas. Three of the patients underwent chemoembolization, and seven of the patients underwent hepatic arterial infusion chemotherapy via the collateral artery. Four weeks later, the transarterial procedure was performed for the patient whose collateral artery originated from the LGA. DSA showed complete occlusion of the LGA and the CHA, and the new collateral artery originated from the SMA. Chemoembolization was performed via the new collateral artery. All eleven patients (100%) had a normal outcome and did not develop any complications on follow-up (Table 1) (Figures 1 and 2).

4. Discussion

The main cause of extrahepatic collateral vessel development was believed to be hepatic artery occlusion by postinterventional dissection or embolization. Some authors advocate that hepatic artery interruption by repeated TACE or arterial dissection is the primary cause [14]. Kim et al. [15] demonstrated that only about 4% of patients with extrahepatic collateral vessel development had proximal hepatic artery occlusion, and most patients with a collateral supply had a widely patent hepatic artery. In this study, all the 11 patients with extrahepatic collateral vessel had proximal hepatic artery (CHA or PHA) occlusion related to interventional procedures.

There have been a few CT-, and CTA-based studies that evaluated the collateral routes related to HAO [12, 13]. Studies indicated that the collateral routes were immediately evident during HAO and that most collateral arteries originated from the inferior phrenic artery (IPA), the SMA, celiac axis, LGA, or the dorsal pancreatic artery [11–13, 15, 16]. Tohma et al. [13] studied the arterial collateral system of 13 patients with various cancers (6 hepatocellular carcinomas, 4 metastatic liver tumors from colorectal cancer, 2 distal common duct tumors, and 1 pancreatic cancer) at the hepatic hilum by using CT and CTA during temporary balloon occlusion of the right or left hepatic artery. They found that during temporary occlusion of the right or left hepatic artery, the communicating arcade between the right and left hepatic arteries was immediately evident in all patients. Their results indicated that the communicating arcade played an important role in the interlobar arterial collateral system. Takeuchi et al. [12] used CTA to evaluate the routes of potential extrahepatic arteries (supplying to the liver) of 23 patients with liver tumors before and after temporary balloon occlusion of the PHA. They found that during temporary balloon occlusion of the PHA, extrahepatic arterial supply was immediately evident in 22 of the 23 patients. The liver was supplied by the right IPA in 17 of 20 patients, by the left IPA in five of six, by the SMA in 8 of 16, by the celiac axis in 2 of 10, and by the LGA in 1 of 6. Murata et al. [11] reported 14 patients with liver tumors and HAO following reservoir placement. They found that the main collateral pathway of the feeding artery on angiography was the IPA in 7 patients (50%), the dorsal pancreatic artery in 4 patients (29%), and the anastomotic branch of the celiac axis in 1 patient (7%). The main collateral

TABLE 1: Baseline patient demographics and collateral artery characteristics.

Patient no.	Age (y)	Sex	Primary	Occlusion of hepatic artery	Collateral pathways	Therapeutic method
1	56	Male	Colon cancer	Common hepatic artery	Superior mesenteric artery	Hepatic arterial infusion chemotherapy
2	46	Male	Colon cancer	Common hepatic artery	Superior mesenteric artery	Hepatic arterial infusion chemotherapy
3	53	Male	Hepatocellular carcinoma	Common hepatic artery	Superior mesenteric artery	Transarterial chemoembolization
4	36	Male	Hepatocellular carcinoma	Common hepatic artery	Superior mesenteric artery	Hepatic arterial infusion chemotherapy
5	37	Male	Hepatocellular carcinoma	Common hepatic artery	Left gastric artery	Transarterial chemoembolization
6	59	Male	Hepatocellular carcinoma	Common hepatic artery	Superior mesenteric artery	Transarterial chemoembolization
7	29	Female	Hepatocellular carcinoma	Common hepatic artery	Superior mesenteric artery	Hepatic arterial infusion chemotherapy
8	60	Female	Hemangiomas	Common hepatic artery	Superior mesenteric artery	Resection
9	50	Female	Stomach cancer	Common hepatic artery	Superior mesenteric artery	Hepatic arterial infusion chemotherapy
10	70	Female	Hepatocellular carcinoma	Proper hepatic artery	Gastroduodenal artery	Hepatic arterial infusion chemotherapy
11	70	Male	Hepatocellular carcinoma	Proper hepatic artery	Gastroduodenal artery	Hepatic arterial infusion chemotherapy

pathway could not be detected in 2 patients (14%). Kim et al. [15] demonstrated that extrahepatic collateral arteries commonly supply hepatocellular carcinomas if the tumors are large or peripherally located. They observed 2104 extrahepatic collateral vessels in 860 patients. The extrahepatic collateral vessels observed originated from the IPA, omental branch, adrenal artery, intercostal artery, cystic artery, internal mammary artery, renal or renal capsular artery, branch of the SMA, gastric artery, and lumbar artery. The right IPA was found to be the most common extrahepatic collateral vessel that supplies HCC [15, 17]. Kim et al. [15] indicated that when the tumor is located in liver segment S7 and is in contact with the right hemidiaphragm, selective angiography of the right IPA is mandatory. When the tumor is located in liver segments S2 or S3 and abuts the left hemidiaphragm, the possibility of a collateral blood supply from the left IPA should be kept in mind. In the present study, we found that the majority of collateral arteries originated from the SMA and that the most important and frequently encountered collateral vessels are the pancreaticoduodenal arcades. The collateral artery originated from the LGA in one patient, and angiography showed complete occlusion of the LGA; in addition, the new collateral arteries originated from the SMA four weeks later. Although we sometimes detected the right IPA as an extrahepatic collateral vessel that supplies HCC,

we did not found it in this patient population. One reason maybe is that the tumors of this group were not located in liver segment S7 and were not in contact with the right hemidiaphragm. The other reason maybe is that the IPA was not evaluated in this group. Because selective angiography of individual collateral vessels is tedious and time consuming, it is essential to try to determine first whether collateral blood supply is present. The initial CT scan provides useful information, and CT signs of direct invasion into adjacent organs or extracapsular infiltration indicate the presence of extrahepatic collateral vessels [15]. In the future, we should review the preinterventional CT images to study the tumor scans and observe if there is the collateral blood supply and routinely do an angiographic workup including selective angiogram of the phrenic artery.

It has been shown that hepatic arterial infusion chemotherapy or chemoembolization is effective and significantly improves survival of patients with liver tumors [3–5]. However, HAO can disrupt transcatheter management of liver tumors. There have been a few reports about successful transcatheter management through the collateral arteries, which is a promising trend [11, 16–18]. Ikeda et al. [18] provide several tips on surmounting these difficulties in interventional radiology including transcatheter arterial chemoembolization for hepatocellular carcinoma and an implantable

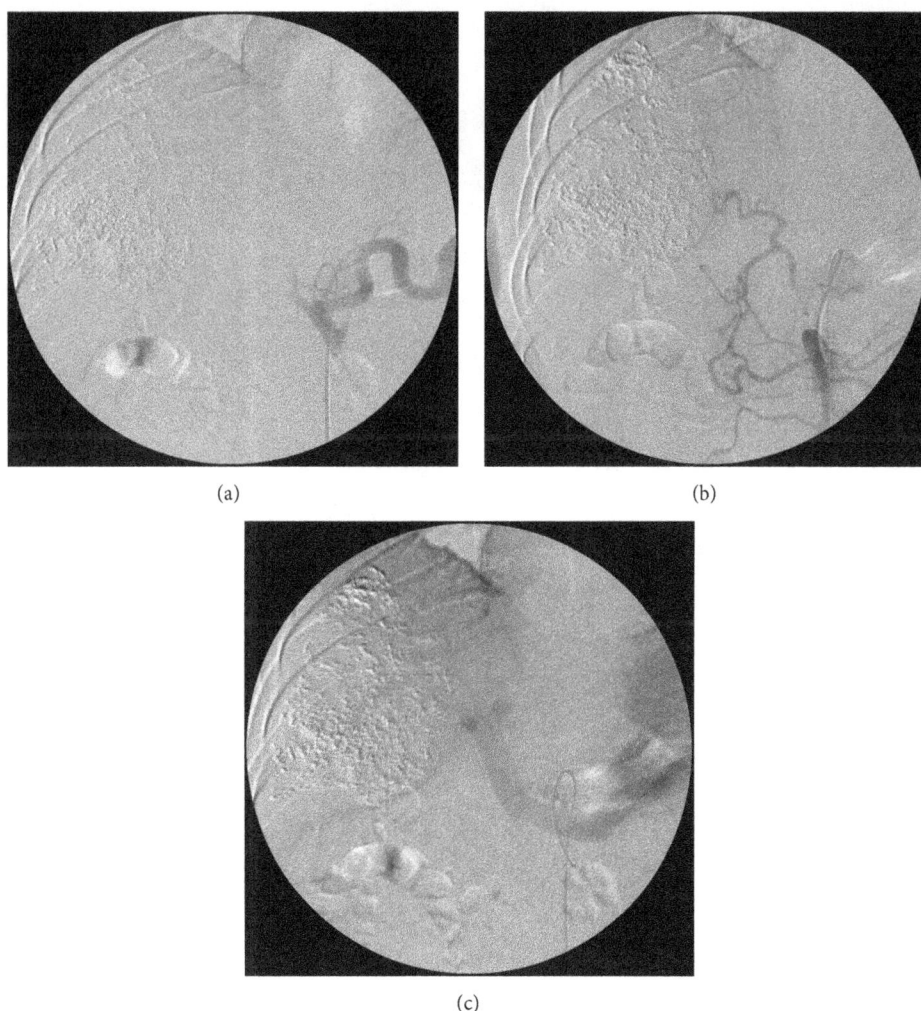

FIGURE 1: A 46-year-old man with hepatocellular carcinoma. (a) Four weeks after chemoembolization, digital subtraction angiography via the celiac axis showed complete occlusion of the common hepatic artery. (b) Angiography demonstrated the collateral arteries that originated from the superior mesenteric artery. (c) Angiography showed good opacification of the portal vein.

port system for hepatic arterial infusion chemotherapy to treat metastatic liver tumors. Chung et al. [17] reported that fifty patients with HCC underwent a total of 82 procedures of transcatheter oily chemoembolization therapy of the IPA, as well as of the hepatic artery. In 16 patients, additional extrahepatic collaterals were depicted and were also embolized in 10 patients. Their results indicated the efficacy and safety of transcatheter chemoembolization therapy via the extrahepatic collateral arteries in HCC. Murata et al. [11] performed transcatheter management in 14 patients for liver tumors after hepatic artery obstruction via the collateral pathway, and suggested that transcatheter treatment may be possible in patients with HAO. In the present study, transcatheter treatment was successfully performed via the collateral arteries in all patients except the one with hemangiomas.

Occlusion of the hepatic artery combined with concomitant portal vein occlusion leads to sharp segmental liver necrosis without formation of significant collaterals [19]. Vaidya et al. [20] studied adult orthotopic liver transplantation patients who underwent an angiography for suspected hepatic arterial abnormalities over an approximately 10-year period. They found that of the 129 angiographies, 24 (19.4%) were found to have collaterals on angiography, and eleven patients (41.7%) had complications related to the liver ischemia on follow-up. In this limited group, good portal venous inflow and collateral arterial flowto the liver prevented liver ischemia and infarction. There were no symptoms of liver ischemia or infarction in all the patients.

In summary, our results indicate that extrahepatic collateral arteries supplying the liver were readily evident in patients with HAO. They are important alternative routes for continuous transcatheter management of hepatic neoplasms following HAO. DSA is an effective method to detect collateral circulation related to HAO and may provide information to guide management decisions.

Acknowledgments

This work is supported by the projects of the Department of Education (07ZA030) and the Health of Sichuan Province (060072).

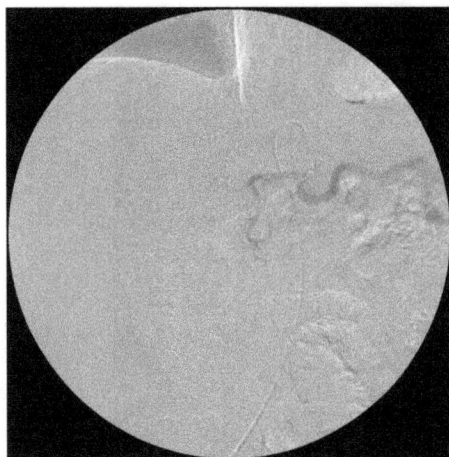

(a)

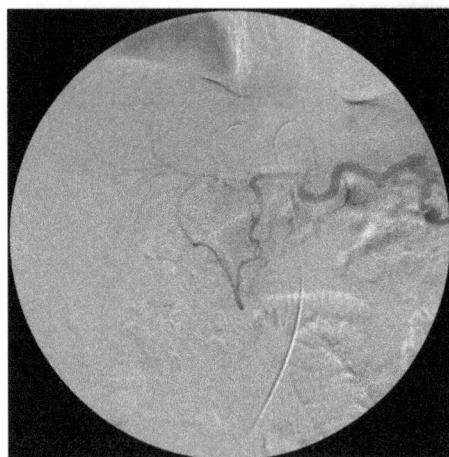

(b)

FIGURE 2: A 70-year-old man with hepatocellular carcinoma. (a) Angiography via the celiac axis showed complete occlusion of the proper hepatic artery. (b) Angiography demonstrated the collateral arteries originated from the gastroduodenal artery.

References

[1] W. Y. Lau and E. C. H. Lai, "Hepatocellular carcinoma: current management and recent advances," *Hepatobiliary and Pancreatic Diseases International*, vol. 7, no. 3, pp. 237–257, 2008.

[2] L. Marelli, R. Stigliano, C. Triantos et al., "Transarterial therapy for hepatocellular carcinoma: which technique is more effective? A systematic review of cohort and randomized studies," *CardioVascular and Interventional Radiology*, vol. 30, no. 1, pp. 6–25, 2007.

[3] J. M. Llovet, M. I. Real, X. Montaña et al., "Arterial embolisation or chemoembolisation versus symptomatic treatment in patients with unresectable hepatocellular carcinoma: a randomised controlled trial," *The Lancet*, vol. 359, no. 9319, pp. 1734–1739, 2002.

[4] Y. Arai, T. Endo, Y. Sone et al., "Management of patients with unresectable liver metastases from colorectal and gastric cancer employing an implantable port system," *Cancer Chemotherapy and Pharmacology*, vol. 31, pp. S99–S102, 1992.

[5] A. Harmantas, L. E. Rotstein, and B. Langer, "Regional versus systemic chemotherapy in the treatment of colorectal carcinoma metastatic to the liver.Is there a survival difference? Meta-analysis of the published literature," *Cancer*, vol. 78, no. 8, pp. 1639–1645, 1996.

[6] J. Xia, Z. Ren, S. Ye et al., "Study of severe and rare complications of transarterial chemoembolization (TACE) for liver cancer," *European Journal of Radiology*, vol. 59, no. 3, pp. 407–412, 2006.

[7] N. Maeda, K. Osuga, K. Mikami et al., "Angiographic evaluation of hepatic arterial damage after transarterial chemoembolization for hepatocellular carcinoma," *Radiation Medicine*, vol. 26, no. 4, pp. 206–212, 2008.

[8] Y. Sakamoto, Y. Harihara, T. Nakatsuka et al., "Rescue of liver grafts from hepatic artery occlusion in living-related liver transplantation," *British Journal of Surgery*, vol. 86, no. 7, pp. 886–889, 1999.

[9] T. Sakaguchi, S. Yoshimatsu, K. Sagara, Y. Yamashita, and M. Takahashi, "Evaluation of hepatic artery occlusion after intra-arterial infusion of SMANCS in patients with hepatocellular carcinoma," *Nippon Acta Radiologica*, vol. 58, no. 12, pp. 700–704, 1998.

[10] K. Yagihashi, K. Takizawa, Y. Ogawa et al., "Clinical application of a new indwelling catheter with a side-hole and spirally arranged shape-memory alloy for hepatic arterial infusion chemotherapy," *CardioVascular and Interventional Radiology*, vol. 33, no. 6, pp. 1153–1158, 2010.

[11] S. Murata, H. Tajima, Y. Abe et al., "Transcatheter management for multiple liver tumors after hepatic artery obstruction following reservoir placement," *Hepato-Gastroenterology*, vol. 52, no. 63, pp. 852–856, 2005.

[12] Y. Takeuchi, Y. Arai, Y. Inaba, K. Ohno, T. Maeda, and Y. Itai, "Extrahepatic arterial supply to the liver: observation with a unified CT and angiography system during temporary balloon occlusion of the proper hepatic artery," *Radiology*, vol. 209, no. 1, pp. 121–128, 1998.

[13] T. Tohma, A. Cho, S. Okazumi et al., "Communicating arcade between the right and left hepatic arteries: evaluation with CT and angiography during temporary balloon occlusion of the right or left hepatic artery," *Radiology*, vol. 237, no. 1, pp. 361–365, 2005.

[14] T. Shibata, N. Kojima, T. Tabuchi, K. Itoh, and J. Konishi, "Transcatheter arterial chemoembolization through collateral arteries for hepatocellular carcinoma after arterial occlusion," *Radiation Medicine*, vol. 16, no. 4, pp. 251–256, 1998.

[15] H.-C. Kim, W. C. Jin, W. Lee, J. J. Hwan, and H. P. Jae, "Recognizing extrahepatic collateral vessels that supply hepatocellular carcinoma to avoid complications of transcatheter arterial chemoembolization," *Radiographics*, vol. 25, pp. S25–S39, 2005.

[16] M. Nonokuma, M. Okazaki, H. Higashihara et al., "Successful embolization of pancreaticoduodenal artery pseudoaneurysm in a patient with common hepatic arterial occlusion after modified pancreatoduodenectomy with preservation of arteries in the head of pancreas," *Hepato-Gastroenterology*, vol. 56, no. 89, pp. 245–248, 2009.

[17] J. W. Chung, J. H. Park, J. K. Han et al., "Transcatheter oily chemoembolization of the IPA in hepatocellular carcinoma: the safety and potential therapeutic role," *Journal of Vascular and Interventional Radiology*, vol. 9, no. 3, pp. 495–500, 1998.

[18] O. Ikeda, Y. Tamura, Y. Nakasone, and Y. Yamashita, "Celiac artery stenosis/occlusion treated by interventional radiology," *European Journal of Radiology*, vol. 71, no. 2, pp. 369–377, 2009.

[19] C. A. Maurer, P. Renzulli, H. U. Baer et al., "Hepatic artery embolisation with a novel radiopaque polymer causes extended liver necrosis in pigs due to occlusion of the concomitant portal vein," *Journal of Hepatology*, vol. 32, no. 2, pp. 261–268, 2000.

[20] S. Vaidya, M. Dighe, P. Bhargava, and A. A. Dick, "Chronic hepatic artery occlusion with collateral formation: Imaging findings and outcomes," *Transplantation Proceedings*, vol. 43, no. 5, pp. 1770–1776, 2011.

14

Aortoenteric Fistula as a Complication of Open Reconstruction and Endovascular Repair of Abdominal Aorta

Marek Tagowski, Hendryk Vieweg, Christian Wissgott, and Reimer Andresen

Institute of Diagnostic and Interventional Radiology and Neuroradiology, Westkuestenklinikum Heide,
Academic Teaching Hospital of the Universities of Kiel, Luebeck and Hamburg, Esmarchstraße 50, 25746 Heide, Germany

Correspondence should be addressed to Hendryk Vieweg; hendryk.vieweg@googlemail.com

Academic Editor: Henrique M. Lederman

The paper intends to present a review of imaging characteristics of secondary aortoenteric fistula (AEF). Mechanical injury, infection, and adherence of a bowel segment to the aorta or aortic graft are major etiologic factors of AEF after open aortic repair. The pathogenesis of AEF formation after endovascular abdominal aortic repair is related to mechanical failure of the stent-graft, to stent graft infection, and to persistent pressurization of the aneurysmal sac. The major clinical manifestations of AEF comprise haematemesis, melaena, abdominal pain, sepsis, and fever. CT is the initial diagnostic modality of choice in a stable patient. However, the majority of reported CT appearances are not specific. In case of equivocal CT scans and clinical suspicion of AEF, scintigraphy, ^{67}Ga citrate scans or ^{18}F-FDG PET/CT is useful. Diagnostic accuracy of endoscopy in evaluation of AEF is low; nevertheless it allows to evaluate other than AEF etiologies of gastrointestinal bleeding. Without adequate therapy, AEF is lethal. Conventional surgical treatment is associated with high morbidity and mortality. The endovascular repair may be an option in hemodynamically unstable and high-risk surgical patients. We also illustrate an example of a secondary AEF with highly specific albeit rare radiologic picture from our institution.

1. Introduction

Secondary aortoenteric fistula (AEF) is a rare but potentially lethal complication of aortic surgery first reported by Brock in 1953. This currently better-known pathology still poses considerable diagnostic difficulties due to its unspecific clinical and radiologic manifestations. The aim of this paper is to present the current diagnostic approach to secondary AEF taking into account its complex and heterogeneous pathogenesis as a cause of the broad spectrum of its radiologic manifestations.

For a better understanding of the subject, we commence the paper by presenting a secondary AEF with highly specific albeit rare radiologic picture from our institution.

A 73-year-old man was referred to our emergency department with severe hematemesis and melena, suggestive of gastrointestinal bleeding. Low blood pressure and tachycardia indicated circulatory shock; laboratory results revealed anemia and elevated inflammatory markers (leukocytes 16.8/nL, CRP 14.5 mg/dL). In the medical history it was noted that he survived a covered perforation of an abdominal aortic aneurysm 2 months earlier. The incident was treated in another hospital with an open surgical approach, using a rifampicin-soaked Dacron Y-prosthesis. No complications occurred during the hospitalization but the patient refused to undergo follow-up examinations.

We performed a CT angiography of the abdominal aorta without oral or rectal contrast. The scans revealed a narrow fistulous communication between aorta and the third part of the duodenum with active extravasation of contrast-enhanced blood from the aortic to the duodenal lumen (Figures 1, 2, and 3).

Only a few minutes later the patient passed away due to uncontrollable blood loss.

In Figures 1–3, CT scans show extravasation of contrast material from the aorta into the third part and second part of the duodenum, perigraft gas collections, and increased soft tissue and fluid between the stent-graft and aortic wall and in the periaortic location.

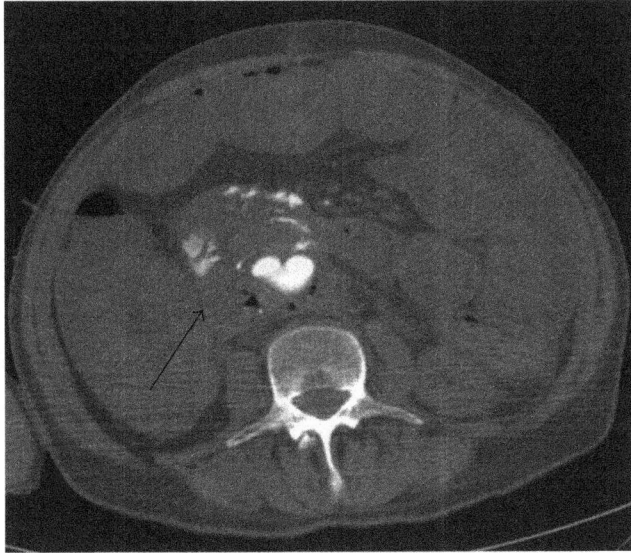

FIGURE 1: Axial contrast-enhanced CT scan of AEF.

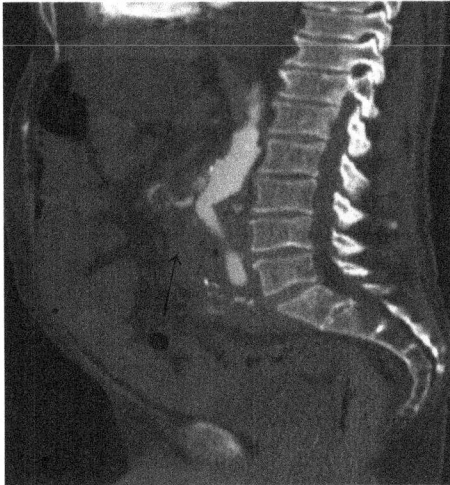

FIGURE 2: Sagittal contrast-enhanced CT scan of AEF.

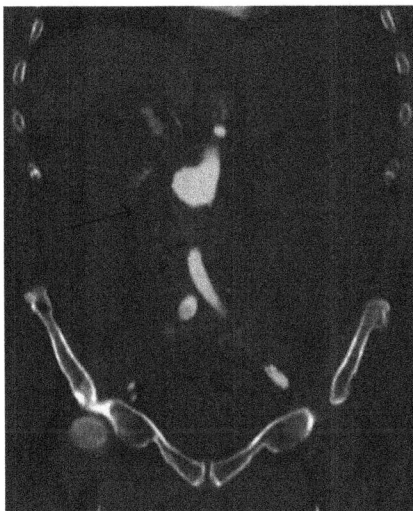

FIGURE 3: Coronal contrast-enhanced CT scan of AEF.

2. Review

Secondary aortoenteric fistula may be a complication of open surgical repair as well as endovascular interventions of the aorta. It consists in development of communication between aortic lumen and the gastrointestinal tract.

The age distribution of the reported patients with diagnosed secondary AEF is broad with the median around 65 years [1]. The majority of afflicted patients are male [1].

Its annual incidence approximates 1% [1] after elective procedures and 14% [2] after emergency repair of ruptured aneurysm, which corresponds to increased likelihood of microbiological contamination of the periaortic tissues and bowel trauma during hurried surgical dissection in the latter setting [1, 2].

The predominant original aortic procedures that can give rise to this complication are the elective abdominal aortic aneurysm resection, aortic replacement or bypass for aortoiliac occlusive disease, resection of ruptured aneurysm, and stent graft placement for aortic aneurysm [1, 2].

The most predisposed to fistula formation gut segments are the third and fourth portions of duodenum [2, 3] because of their retroperitoneal location and anatomic relationships with the graft. Less frequently other intestinal segments including stomach and appendix could also be involved in AEF formation [1, 2].

There were also reported rare cases with more than one simultaneous fistulization.

The AEF most frequently occurs at the proximal suture line (in the substantial number of patients with frank pseudoaneurysm formation), and graft body and distal anastomosis are less common locations [1, 2].

Median interval from the original operation to the formation of AEF is between 24 and 47 months with a broad time range from 2 days to 26 years [1].

Mechanical injury and infection may each act as a major etiologic factor of AEF.

Bowel trauma by surgical dissection or due to direct pressure of anastomotic pseudoaneurysm as well as direct pulsatile pressure by a graft predispose to focal necrosis and erosion of bowel wall. This enables local infection of adjacent graft material with resultant disruption of the vascular anastomosis and exsanguinating hemorrhage [3].

The infection may be caused by contamination from the environment at the time of the original operation, which is suggested by the presence of cutaneous flora (*S. aureus* or *S. epidermidis*) in the intraoperative cultures [3, 4].

By contrast, occurrence of Enterobacteriaceae and anaerobic bacteria is compatible with the secondary contamination of the graft material from the intestinal flora.

The third postulated source of infection may be postoperative bacteriemia from any cause (including transient bacteriemia from dental procedures or gastrointestinal endoscopy).

Graft susceptibility to bacteriemia is highest during the first postoperative months and decreases with formation of neointima and healing of the anastomotic sutures [2, 4].

Regardless of these factors adherence of a bowel segment to the aorta or aortic graft is essential for development of the aortoenteric communication [3, 4].

Therefore adequate tissue coverage and reperitonealization of the graft during the original operation are of utmost importance.

Relatively rare diagnosed fistulous communication between the bowel lumen and periaortic tissues is termed paraprosthetic-enteric fistula and is regarded as a step in the development of aortoenteric fistulization [3, 4].

The pathogenetic mechanism of AEF development after endovascular abdominal aortic repair may be related to mechanical failure of the stent-graft such as rupture or migration with kinking of the device in the aneurysmal sack, which leads to aortic graft erosion and pressure necrosis of the bowel wall [5–7].

AEF formation can also result from stent graft infection that predisposes to erosion of the adherent bowel wall [8, 9] as well as from persistent pressurization of the aneurysmal sack in the presence of endoleak or endotension [5, 10–12] (including endotension secondary to infection in an excluded aneurysm sac [10, 13]).

As holds true for the graft infection after surgical aortic repair, stent-graft infection may also be a result of AEF [14–16].

A rare cause of AEF development after endoleak embolization may be chronic injury of the aortic wall from metallic coils embedded in the aortic wall [17, 18].

In addition, aortoduodenal fistulization is precipitated by periaortic inflammatory tissue after endovascular repair of an inflammatory aortic aneurysm [15].

The major clinical manifestations of AEF are hematemesis (41%) and melena (54%) (with hemodynamic shock during the course of medical management in almost one third of cases) as well as abdominal pain, sepsis, and fever which occur, respectively, in 21%, 12%, and 11% of the afflicted patients [1].

Other less frequent presenting symptoms include back pain, pulsating tumor in abdomen, and anorexia [1].

Gastrointestinal herald bleeding which precedes the exsanguinating hemorrhage was reported in approximately 54% of cases [1].

It has been explained either as a result of a small fistulization temporarily sealed by thrombus or initial bowel wall ulceration.

Of particular importance is the fact that not every patient with AEF presents with detectable gastrointestinal bleeding.

Taking into consideration its devastating consequences there is no single, satisfyingly reliable diagnostic method of AEF. Even diagnostic laparotomy in a retrospective study has strikingly yielded an accuracy of "only" 91% [1], which underscores the importance of a strong clinical suspicion of possible aortoenteric fistulization in a patient after aortic procedures.

Nowadays computed tomography is regarded as the initial diagnostic modality of choice in a sufficiently stable patient, because of its high sensitivity and specificity (resp., 94% and 85% according to Low et al. [19]) in detecting perigraft infection with or without AEF and its wide availability in the emergency setting [19, 20].

The possible CT presentations of AEF are highly diverse. Therefore, the familiarity with the varied potential CT abnormalities reflecting this pathology is prerequisite for the prompt and accurate diagnosis.

Depicting of extravasation of contrast material from the aorta into the adjacent bowel lumen, leakage of gastrointestinal contrast agent into the periaortic space, and visualization of aortic graft in bowel lumen represent highly specific but very rare CT signs of AEF [21, 22].

The majority of its reported CT appearances are not specific. They are similar to those observed in perigraft infection (PGI) and include perigraft gas collections or gas in the graft lumen (>4–7 weeks following aortic reconstruction), focal thickening of the bowel wall adjacent to the aortic graft, periaortic soft tissue or fluid (>3 months following aortic reconstruction), focal disruption of the calcified aortic wrap, pseudoaneurysm formation, increased soft tissue between the graft and aortic wrap, and obliteration of the fat plane between the aorta and intestine. Additionally, rare reported CT findings of AEF are intramural duodenal hematoma and dystrophic vascular graft calcification in the bowel lumen [19–21, 23, 24].

According to Low et al. [19] the presence of ectopic gas collections and focal bowel wall thickening is more likely related to AEF than PGI without AEF.

In the postoperative period, periaortic hematoma should resolve within 3 months.

Ectopic gas collections are in most cases not detectable beyond the first postoperative week and should completely resolve within 4–7 weeks. After these periods any perigraft soft tissue, gas, or fluid should be presumed to be the sign of perigraft infection [25, 26].

In the first month following endovascular repair of abdominal aortic aneurysm perigraft gas within the aneurysmal sac may be a normal finding due to introduction of atmospheric air bubbles with the delivery system of the stent-graft [11, 27, 28].

Concurrent occurrence of these CT findings with fever and leukocytosis in the first days after stent-graft placement may result from local inflammatory response to the implanted stent-graft material without underlying infection, referred to as postimplantation syndrome.

During graft incorporation process after open aortic reconstruction hematoma between the graft and aneurysm wrap should gradually resolve. The study of Qvarfordt et al. presents its almost complete resolution in 7 weeks, with the aneurysm wall in close apposition to the graft [25]. Demonstration of increased soft tissue (>5 mm) between the graft and aortic wall can be the only CT finding suggesting graft infection.

The study of Hughes et al. [20] emphasizes the high diagnostic specificity related to the combination of gastrointestinal blood loss and the reported CT signs of AEF (periaortic fluid/soft tissue, breach of the aortic wall, pseudoaneurysm formation, loss of fat pad between aorta and intestine, ectopic gas, and intravasation of contrast material into the intestinal lumen).

Despite the limitation of this study due to absence of PGI cases without AEF in the control group, diagnostic significance of concomitant occurrence of gastrointestinal bleeding and CT characteristics of perigraft infection is unquestionable.

A significant number of surgically proven PGI (with or without AEF) demonstrates only subtle or no CT abnormalities [19]. This observation underscores the importance of meticulous evaluation of CT scans. In case of any doubt additional examinations including scintigraphy, MRI, or CT-guided percutaneous fine-needle aspiration biopsy may reveal the diagnosis.

Use of oral contrast material is frequently necessary to reliably assess the focal thickening of the bowel wall and allows to detect its extravasation into the periaortic space as a sign of AEF or paraprosthetic-enteric fistula [19, 20]. However, bowel opacification with positive contrast material is likely to obscure the intravasation of aortic contrast into the intestine.

Other conditions with overlapping CT features including retroperitoneal fibrosis and adenopathy should be also included in the differential diagnosis of secondary AEF.

Scintigraphy with autologous leukocytes labeled with ^{99m}Tc-HMPAO or ^{111}In and ^{67}Ga citrate scans may be useful in case of equivocal CT scans and clinical suspicion of perigraft infection, when subtle morphological changes (e.g., after surgery) are indistinguishable from low-grade inflammation on CT scans [29–31]. Scintigraphy with ^{99m}Tc-labeled autologous erythrocytes or ^{99m}Tc-HMPAO-labeled leukocytes enables to depict extravasation of tagged cells into the bowel loops, a finding highly suggestive of AEF [32, 33].

Compared to scintigraphy, ^{18}F-FDG PET/CT provides significantly more accurate anatomic localisation of infectious processes. It enables image acquisition within 1 hour after radiotracer administration in contrast to 24 hours in case of labeled leukocyte scan.

This is particularly advantageous in assessing the extent of retroperitoneal infection and its potential communication with the graft.

However, within the first months following graft implantation the specificity of ^{18}F-FDG PET is reduced due to increased ^{18}F-FDG uptake at sites of postoperative inflammatory changes. Further studies are needed for standardization of acquisition times and imaging interpretation criteria to establish the role of PET/CT in the diagnosis of graft infection [34–36].

The magnetic resonance imaging is not a first-line diagnosing tool of AEF because of its limited availability in the emergency setting and relatively long acquisition time.

In addition, signal voids resulting from periaortic gas collections and pulsation artifacts can cause considerable difficulties in image interpretation.

Transcutaneous ultrasonography has a very limited role in the diagnosis of AEF.

However, in hemodynamically unstable patients with a suitable body habitus it may enable fast detection of retroperitoneal hematoma or perigraft fluid.

According to the comprehensive literature review by Bergqvist and Björck the diagnostic accuracy of endoscopy in evaluation of AEF is low (30% accuracy of gastroscopy) [1].

Nevertheless endoscopy has its well established role as a primary tool in clinical management of gastrointestinal bleeding and allows to evaluate other than AEF etiologies of gastrointestinal hemorrhage [37–39]. Visualization of the third and fourth portions of duodenum is essential but frequently technically difficult.

At the present day conventional angiography is not a primary diagnostic modality in evaluation of AEF, but in certain clinical settings transcatheter arterial interventions may be useful in controlling the gastrointestinal hemorrhage related to AEF [39].

Without treatment, AEF has invariably catastrophic consequences with a mortality of virtually 100%. Conventional surgical treatment options are associated with high morbidity and mortality [40, 41] and include graft removal with primary or secondary axillobifemoral bypass as well as graft removal and in situ reconstruction, depending predominantly on the infection status of the surgical site [1, 42, 43].

The endovascular repair has emerged as a relatively new method of rapid hemorrhage control and restoration of peripheral perfusion in hemodynamically unstable patients. It can be regarded as a temporizing procedure prior to laparotomy, or a part of a long term palliation in high-risk surgical patients in whom the remained communication between the gut and aorta and the presence of infected prosthetic material preclude definitive eradication of infection [40, 41, 43].

3. Conclusion

The presence of aortoenteric fistula should be evaluated in any patient after conventional aortic reconstruction or endovascular aortic repair with gastrointestinal blood loss or with signs of graft infection.

Computed tomography is the most valuable diagnostic tool, although the observed abnormal CT findings are most frequently unspecific and similar to those secondary to perigraft infection. This fact underscores the importance of a strong clinical suspicion in management of this potentially lethal complication.

References

[1] D. Bergqvist and M. Björck, "Secondary arterioenteric fistulation—a systematic literature analysis," *European Journal of Vascular and Endovascular Surgery*, vol. 37, no. 1, pp. 31–42, 2009.

[2] S. E. Wilson, R. S. Bennion, A. I. Serota, and R. A. Williams, "Bacteriological implications in the pathogenesis of secondary aorto-enteric fistulas," *British Journal of Surgery*, vol. 69, no. 9, pp. 545–548, 1982.

[3] M. W. Flye and W. M. Thompson, "Aortic graft-enteric and paraprosthetic-enteric fisultas," *The American Journal of Surgery*, vol. 146, no. 2, pp. 183–187, 1983.

[4] G. D. Perdue Jr., R. B. Smith III, J. D. Ansley, and M. J. Costantino, "Impending aortoenteric hemorrhage. The effect of early recognition on improved outcome," *Annals of Surgery*, vol. 192, no. 3, pp. 237–243, 1980.

[5] D. Bergqvist, M. Björck, and R. Nyman, "Secondary aortoenteric fistula after endovascular aortic interventions: a systematic literature review," *Journal of Vascular and Interventional Radiology*, vol. 19, no. 2, pp. 163–165, 2008.

[6] B. J. D'Othée, P. Soula, P. Otal et al., "Aortoduodenal fistula after endovascular stent-graft of an abdominal aortic aneurysm," *Journal of Vascular Surgery*, vol. 31, no. 1, pp. 190–195, 2000.

[7] L. Norgren, B. Jernby, and L. Engellau, "Aortoenteric fistula caused by a ruptured stent-graft: a case report," *Journal of Endovascular Surgery*, vol. 5, no. 3, pp. 269–272, 1998.

[8] N. Saratzis, A. Saratzis, N. Melas, K. Ktenidis, and D. Kiskinis, "Aortoduodenal fistulas after endovascular stent-graft repair of abdominal aortic aneurysms: single-center experience and review of the literature," *Journal of Endovascular Therapy*, vol. 15, no. 4, pp. 441–448, 2008.

[9] M. A. Sharif, B. Lee, L. L. Lau et al., "Prosthetic stent graft infection after endovascular abdominal aortic aneurysm repair," *Journal of Vascular Surgery*, vol. 46, no. 3, pp. 442–448, 2007.

[10] F. J. Veith, R. A. Baum, T. Ohki et al., "Nature and significance of endoleaks and endotension: summary of opinions expressed at an international conference," *Journal of Vascular Surgery*, vol. 35, no. 5, pp. 1029–1035, 2002.

[11] S. Alankar, M. H. Barth, D. D. Shin, J. R. Hong, and W. R. Rosenberg, "Aortoduodenal fistula and associated rupture of abdominal aortic aneurysm after endoluminal stent graft repair," *Journal of Vascular Surgery*, vol. 37, no. 2, pp. 465–468, 2003.

[12] B. J. Ruby and T. H. Cogbill, "Aortoduodenal fistula 5 years after endovascular abdominal aortic aneurysm repair with the Ancure stent graft," *Journal of Vascular Surgery*, vol. 45, no. 4, pp. 834–836, 2007.

[13] J. R. Parra, C. Lee, K. J. Hodgson, and B. Perler, "Endograft infection leading to rupture of aortic aneurysm," *Journal of Vascular Surgery*, vol. 39, no. 3, pp. 676–678, 2004.

[14] R. Makar, J. Reid, A. D. Pherwani et al., "Aorto-enteric fistula following endovascular repair of abdominal aortic aneurysm," *European Journal of Vascular and Endovascular Surgery*, vol. 20, no. 6, pp. 588–590, 2000.

[15] D. J. Parry, A. Waterworth, D. Kessel, I. Robertson, D. C. Berridge, and D. J. Scott, "Endovascular repair of an inflammatory abdominal aortic aneurysm complicated by aortoduodenal fistulation with an unusual presentation," *Journal of Vascular Surgery*, vol. 33, no. 4, pp. 874–879, 2001.

[16] C. Schlensak, T. Doenst, M. Hauer et al., "Serious complications that require surgical interventions after endoluminal stent-graft placement for the treatment of infrarenal aortic aneurysms," *Journal of Vascular Surgery*, vol. 34, no. 2, pp. 198–203, 2001.

[17] D. J. Bertges, E. R. Villella, and M. S. Makaroun, "Aortoenteric fistula due to endoleak coil embolization after endovascular AAA repair," *Journal of Endovascular Therapy*, vol. 10, pp. 130–135, 2003.

[18] S. Elkouri, J.-F. Blair, E. Thérasse, V. L. Oliva, L. Bruneau, and G. Soulez, "Aortoduodenal fistula occurring after type II endoleak treatment with coil embolization of the aortic sac," *Journal of Vascular Surgery*, vol. 37, no. 2, pp. 461–464, 2003.

[19] R. N. Low, S. D. Wall, R. B. Jeffrey Jr., R. A. Sollitto, L. M. Reilly, and L. M. Tierney Jr., "Aortoenteric fistula and perigraft infection: evaluation with CT," *Radiology*, vol. 175, no. 1, pp. 157–162, 1990.

[20] F. M. Hughes, D. Kavanagh, M. Barry, A. Owens, D. P. MacErlaine, and D. E. Malone, "Aortoenteric fistula: a diagnostic dilemma," *Abdominal Imaging*, vol. 32, no. 3, pp. 398–402, 2007.

[21] K. D. Hagspiel, U. C. Turba, U. Bozlar et al., "Diagnosis of aortoenteric fistulas with CT angiography," *Journal of Vascular and Interventional Radiology*, vol. 18, no. 4, pp. 497–504, 2007.

[22] R. M. Peirce, R. H. Jenkins, and P. Maceneaney, "Paraprosthetic extravasation of enteric contrast: a rare and direct sign of secondary aortoenteric fistula," *The American Journal of Roentgenology*, vol. 184, no. 3, pp. S73–S74, 2005.

[23] Q. D. M. Vu, C. O. Menias, S. Bhalla, C. Peterson, L. L. Wang, and D. M. Balfe, "Aortoenteric fistulas: CT features and potential mimics," *Radiographics*, vol. 29, no. 1, pp. 197–209, 2009.

[24] S. P. Raman, A. Kamaya, M. Federle, and E. K. Fishman, "Aortoenteric fistulas: spectrum of CT findings," *Abdominal Imaging*, vol. 38, no. 2, pp. 367–375, 2013.

[25] P. G. Qvarfordt, L. M. Reilly, A. S. Mark et al., "Computerized tomographic assessment of graft incorporation after aortic reconstruction," *The American Journal of Surgery*, vol. 150, no. 2, pp. 227–231, 1985.

[26] P. J. O'Hara, G. P. Borkowski, N. R. Hertzer, P. B. O'Donovan, S. L. Brigham, and E. G. Beven, "Natural history of periprosthetic air on computerized axial tomographic examination of the abdomen following abdominal aortic aneurysm repair," *Journal of Vascular Surgery*, vol. 1, no. 3, pp. 429–433, 1984.

[27] O. C. Velázquez, J. P. Carpenter, R. A. Baum et al., "Perigraft air, fever, and leukocytosis after endovascular repair of abdominal aortic aneurysms," *The American Journal of Surgery*, vol. 178, no. 3, pp. 185–189, 1999.

[28] R. Kutlu and V. Nisanoğlu, "Air within the aneurysm sac following endovascular management of abdominal aortic aneurysm in a patient with acute pancreatitis," *Diagnostic and Interventional Radiology*, vol. 15, no. 2, pp. 153–156, 2009.

[29] E. Prats, J. Banzo, M. D. Abós et al., "Diagnosis of prosthetic vascular graft infection by technetium-99m-HMPAO-labeled leukocytes," *Journal of Nuclear Medicine*, vol. 35, pp. 1303–1307, 1994.

[30] M. R. Williamson, C. M. Boyd, R. C. Read et al., "111 In-labeled leukocytes in the detection of prosthetic vascular graft infections," *The American Journal of Roentgenology*, vol. 147, no. 1, pp. 173–176, 1986.

[31] I. Banzo, R. Quirce, J. Serrano, J. Jimenez, O. Tabuenca, and J. M. Carril, "Ga-67 citrate scan in vascular graft infection," *Annals of Nuclear Medicine*, vol. 6, no. 4, pp. 235–239, 1992.

[32] R. H. Ganatra, M. A. Haniffa, A. B. Hawthorne, and J. I. S. Rees, "Aortoenteric fistula complicating an infected aortic graft diagnosis by leukocyte scintigraphy," *Clinical Nuclear Medicine*, vol. 26, no. 9, pp. 800–801, 2001.

[33] N. P. Lenzo, T. A. Male, and J. H. Turner, "Aortoenteric fistula on (99 m)Tc erythrocyte scintigraphy," *The American Journal of Roentgenology*, vol. 177, no. 2, pp. 477–478, 2001.

[34] A. S. Krupnick, J. V. Lombardi, F. H. Engels et al., "18-Fluorodeoxyglucose positron emission tomography as a novel imaging tool for the diagnosis of aortoenteric fistula and aortic graft infection: a case report," *Vascular and Endovascular Surgery*, vol. 37, no. 5, pp. 363–366, 2003.

[35] Z. Keidar, A. Engel, A. Hoffman, O. Israel, and S. Nitecki, "Prosthetic vascular graft infection: the role of 18F-FDG PET/CT," *Journal of Nuclear Medicine*, vol. 48, no. 8, pp. 1230–1236, 2007.

[36] L. Burroni, C. D'Alessandria, and A. Signore, "Diagnosis of vascular prosthesis infection: PET or SPECT?" *Journal of Nuclear Medicine*, vol. 48, no. 8, pp. 1227–1229, 2007.

[37] J. M. van Baalen, A. B. Kluit, J. Maas, J. L. Terpstra, and J. H. van Bockel, "Diagnosis and therapy of aortic prosthetic fistulas: trends over a 30-year experience," *Teh British Journal of Surgery*, vol. 83, no. 12, pp. 1729–1734, 1996.

[38] M. P. Schenker, B. S. Majdalany, B. S. Funaki et al., *ACR Appropriateness Criteria Radiologic Management of Upper Gastrointestinal Bleeding*, American College of Radiology, Reston, Va, USA, 2010.

[39] M. D. Darcy, C. E. Ray Jr., J. M. Lorenz et al., *Acr Appropriateness Criteria Radiologic Management of Lower Gastrointestinal Tract Bleeding*, American College of Radiology, Reston, Va, USA, 2011.

[40] J. A. Burks Jr., P. L. Faries, E. C. Gravereaux, L. H. Hollier, and M. L. Marin, "Endovascular repair of bleeding aortoenteric fistulas: a 5-year experience," *Journal of Vascular Surgery*, vol. 34, no. 6, pp. 1055–1059, 2001.

[41] G. A. Antoniou, S. Koutsias, S. A. Antoniou, A. Georgiakakis, M. K. Lazarides, and A. D. Giannoukas, "Outcome after endovascular stent graft repair of aortoenteric fistula: a systematic review," *Journal of Vascular Surgery*, vol. 49, no. 3, pp. 782–789, 2009.

[42] J. H. Conn, J. D. Hardy, C. M. Chavez, and W. R. Fain, "Infected arterial grafts: experince in 22 cases with empsis on unusual bactia and technics," *Annals of Surgery*, vol. 171, no. 5, pp. 704–714, 1970.

[43] P. A. Armstrong, M. R. Back, J. S. Wilson, M. L. Shames, B. L. Johnson, and D. F. Bandyk, "Improved outcomes in the recent management of secondary aortoenteric fistula," *Journal of Vascular Surgery*, vol. 42, no. 4, pp. 660–666, 2005.

15

Soft Tissue Masses of Hand: A Radio-Pathological Correlation

Aditi Agarwal,[1] **Mahesh Prakash,**[1] **Pankaj Gupta,**[1] **Satyaswarup Tripathy,**[2] **Nandita Kakkar,**[3] **Radhika Srinivasan,**[4] **and Niranjan Khandelwal**[1]

[1]*Department of Radiodiagnosis and Imaging, Postgraduate Institute of Medical Education and Research (PGIMER), Chandigarh 160012, India*
[2]*Department of Plastic Surgery, Postgraduate Institute of Medical Education and Research (PGIMER), Chandigarh 160012, India*
[3]*Department of Histopathology, Postgraduate Institute of Medical Education and Research (PGIMER), Chandigarh 160012, India*
[4]*Department of Cytopathology, Postgraduate Institute of Medical Education and Research (PGIMER), Chandigarh 160012, India*

Correspondence should be addressed to Mahesh Prakash; image73@gmail.com

Academic Editor: Andreas H. Mahnken

Aim. To evaluate soft tissue masses of the hand with magnetic resonance imaging (MRI) and ultrasonography (USG) and to correlate imaging findings with pathological findings. *Material and Methods.* Thirty-five patients with soft tissue masses of the hand were evaluated with high resolution USG and contrast enhanced MRI of the hand, prospectively over a period of 2.5 years. The radiological diagnosis was then compared with cytology/histopathology. *Results.* There were a total of 19 (55%) females. The mean age was 27.45 ± 14.7 years. Majority (45%) of cases were heteroechoic. Four cases were predominantly hyperechoic. These were later diagnosed as lipomas. Four cases were anechoic (diagnosed as ganglions). Only four lesions showed hyperintense signal on T1-weighted images. Out of these, 3 were lipomas and one was cavernous haemangioma. Three lesions were hypointense on T2-weighted images. All these lesions were diagnosed as giant cell tumor of the tendon sheath. A correct diagnosis was possible on MRI in 80% of cases ($n = 28$). *Conclusion.* MRI provides specific findings for diagnosis of certain soft tissue lesions of the hand. Ultrasonography allows accurate diagnosis of hemangioma/vascular malformations. However, in most conditions, imaging findings are nonspecific and diagnosis rests on pathologic evaluation.

1. Introduction

Common soft tissue masses of hand include ganglia, giant cell tumor of tendon sheath (GCTTS), lipomas, nerve sheath tumors, glomus tumors, and hemangiomas [1]. High-resolution ultrasonography (USG) and magnetic resonance imaging (MRI) play an important role in characterisation of these masses. Besides, they provide information about the site, size, extent, and relation with surrounding structures. Previous studies have shown the efficacy of imaging in the characterisation of soft tissue masses in this location [1–6]. However, these studies have been limited by the patient number, variable sensitivity and specificity, and lack of uniform protocols. Besides, several advancements in imaging techniques particularly MRI are expected to have an impact on the evaluation of soft tissue masses. We conducted a prospective study to evaluate soft tissue masses in the hand using high resolution USG and MRI. A correlation with pathological diagnosis was also conducted.

2. Material and Methods

This prospective study was conducted over a period of 2.5 years from 1 July 2011 to 31 December 2014. The study was approved by institute ethics committee and informed written consent was obtained from all patients. A total of 35 patients presenting with soft tissue masses of the hand to the plastic surgery outpatient department were included. All patients underwent high resolution USG and contrast enhanced MRI of the hand. Patients with contraindication for MRI and those with history of previous MRI contrast reaction or renal failure and inconclusive histopathology/cytology were excluded from study.

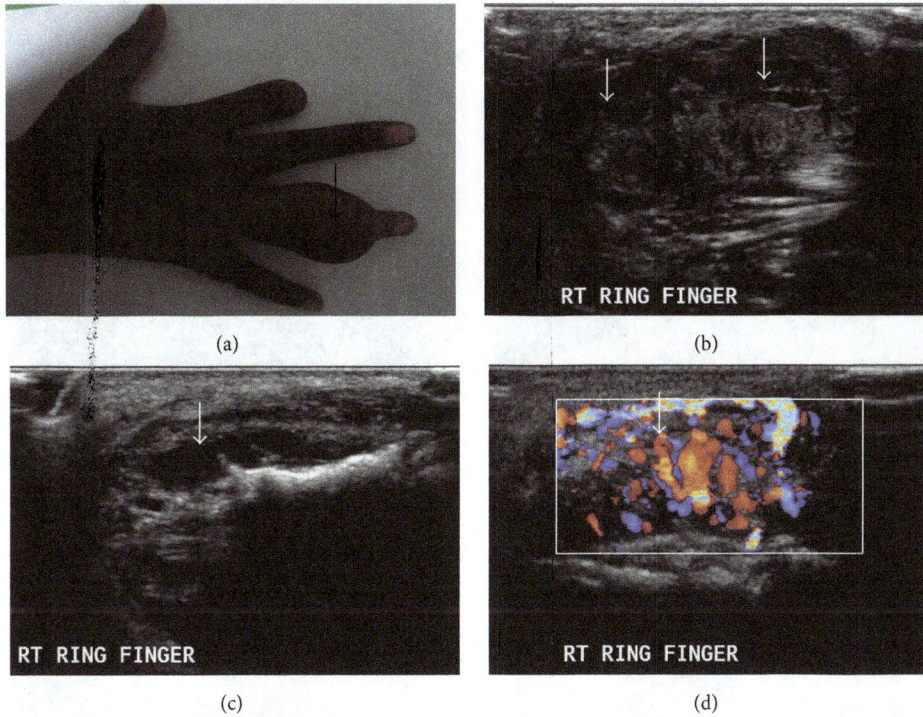

FIGURE 1: AVM. A 22-year-old female presented with compressible swelling involving middle phalanx of right ring finger ((a), arrow). Ultrasonography shows a heterogeneously hypoechoic lesion with multiple prominent linear hypoechoic channel (arrows) and irregularity of underlying bone ((b), (c)). Doppler showed markedly increased intralesional vascularity ((d), arrow).

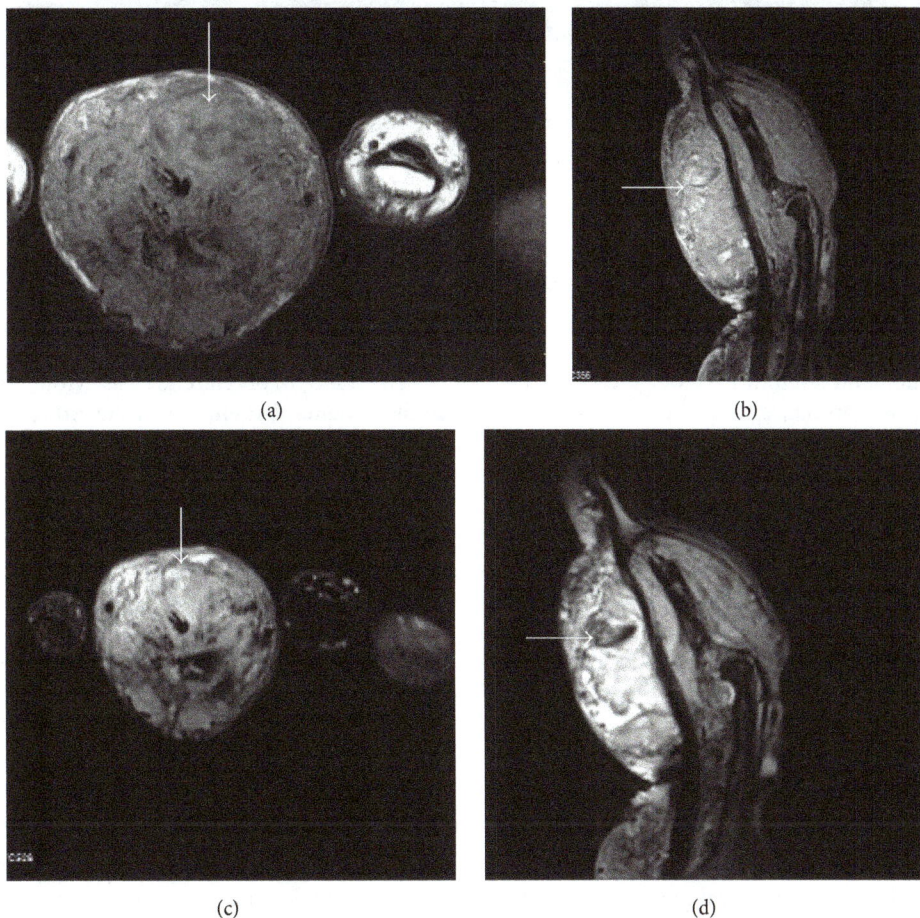

FIGURE 2: AVM. MRI (of the same patient as in Figure 1) shows a large heterogeneous T1W hypointense (a) and T2WFS hyperintense (b) lesion (arrows) showing few intralesional flow voids, marrow extension, and cortical breech. On post contrast T1WFS sequences ((c), (d)) the lesion shows intense heterogeneous postcontrast enhancement (arrows).

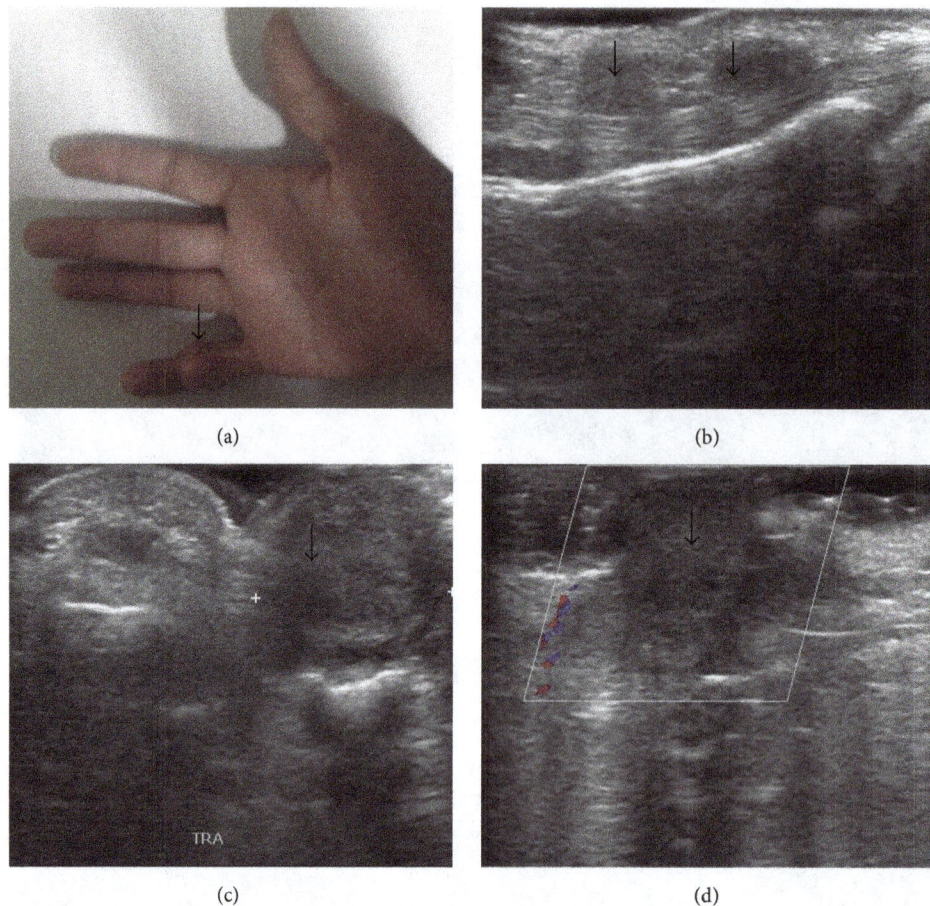

FIGURE 3: Giant cell tumor of tendon sheath. A 20-year-old female presented with swelling in right 5th finger over middle phalanx ((a), arrow). Ultrasonography and Doppler show multiple well-defined, hypoechoic, hypovascular lesions along the flexor tendons ((b)–(d), arrows).

2.1. Imaging. MRI was performed on a 3-Tesla scanner (Magnetom Verio, Siemens Medical Systems) using a dedicated wrist coil. The patients were scanned in the most comfortable position (as uniform positioning in each patient was not feasible in view of the hand swelling). T1-weighted (TR/TE, 650–1070/10–20), axial, coronal, and sagittal, T2-weighted (TR/TE, 3600–4324/80–98) axial, coronal and/or sagittal and axial, coronal, and sagittal gadolinium enhanced (following intravenous injection of 0.1 mL/kg of gadopentetate dimeglumine, maximum 10 mL) T1-weighted (TR/TE, 650–950/10–20) sequences were performed. Images were reviewed by two radiologists with 10 years and 3 years of experience in musculoskeletal MRI in consensus. The same radiologist performed B-mode as well as color Doppler USG of the masses using Philips HD 11 XE and iU22 machines equipped with a 3-to-12 MHZ linear transducer Doppler settings that were optimized to "low flow," with a medium wall filter (to minimize flash artifact) and a pulse repetition frequency of 700 Hz. The color gain was adjusted to just below the noise floor and maintained at this level throughout the scanning protocol. Each swelling was scanned in various planes. The correlation with pathological findings was performed only for MRI and ultrasonography was used as an adjunct imaging modality.

The radiologists were blinded to the clinical diagnosis/pathological findings. All patients underwent fine needle aspiration cytology (FNAC) and/or biopsy. The radiological diagnosis was then compared with cytology/histopathology.

The standard of reference was cytology/histopathology in all the patients. The efficacy of the radiological investigations was determined by comparing USG and MRI findings with the histopathological/cytological diagnosis.

2.2. Statistical Analysis. The statistical analysis was carried out using Statistical Package for Social Sciences (SPSS Inc., Chicago, IL, version 15.0 for Windows). All quantitative variables were estimated using measures of central location (mean and median) and measures of dispersion (standard deviation and standard error). Qualitative or categorical variables were described as frequencies and proportions (percentages).

3. Results

Out of the 35 patients in the study group, there were a total of 19 (55%) females and 16 (45%) male patients. The mean age of the sample population was 27.45 ± 14.7 years (range 3–61 years).

(a)

(b)

(c)

(d)

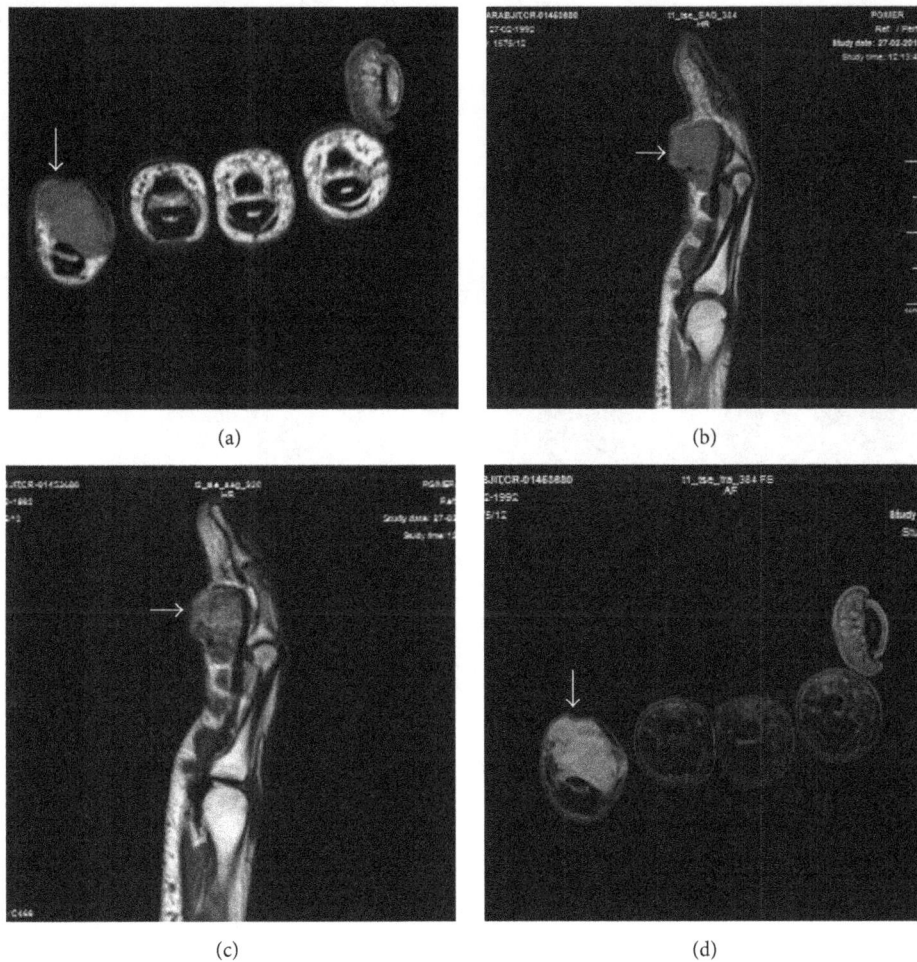

FIGURE 4: Giant cell tumor of tendon sheath. MRI (of the same patient as in Figure 3) show multiple, well-defined, lobulated, T1W, and T2W hypointense lesions ((a)–(c)) along the flexor tendons of right 5th finger. These lesions show mild enhancement seen on postgadolinium T1FS images (d).

3.1. Clinical Features.

All the patients (n = 35) presented with soft tissue swelling in the hand with mean size of 3.12±2.1 cms (range 0.5–8 cms). Ten (28.5%) patients had associated pain. Four of the thirty patients (11.5%) also had restriction of finger movement. There was a wide range of difference in the duration of the swelling in the study group. The mean duration of swelling was 3.5 years (range 2 months to 20 years). Four (11.5%) patients had swelling since birth which was gradually increasing in size. In 21 (60%) patients swelling was located of the ventral surface of the hand. Five (15%) had swelling on the dorsal aspect; in the rest of the 9 (25%) patients it involved both dorsal as well as the ventral aspect. In 16 (45%) patients it was located in the fingers, 12 (35%) had swelling in the palm, 5 (15%) involved both palm and wrist, and in 2 (5%) it was located in the web space. In 50% of the patients the swelling was well-defined. Twenty-five (70%) swellings were soft in consistency and the rest 10 (30%) were firm in nature. Twenty-one (60%) swellings were noncompressible while 14 (40%) were compressible. In 5 (15%) cases, swellings were found in relation to the tendons of the hand. Three of them were GCTTS and two were due to the presence of chronic tenosynovitis.

3.2. Imaging Findings.

The swellings included in this study demonstrated variable echogenicity on gray scale. The maximum number (45%) of cases was heteroechoic. Four cases included in the study were predominantly hyperechoic in echogenicity. These were later diagnosed as lipomas. Four cases were anechoic in appearance. These cases were diagnosed as ganglions. There was presence of increased color flow in 7 (20%) cases included in the study. These were either hemangioma or vascular malformations.

Majority of the cases (n = 31) included in the study showed hypointense signal on T1-weighted images. Only four lesions showed hyperintense signal on T1-weighted images. All these lesions show hypointensity on fat suppressed images. Out of these, 3 were lipoma of the thenar and hypothenar eminence; the fourth case was a cavernous haemangioma with predominant fatty component. T2-weighted hyperintensity was noted in 85% (n = 30) of the lesions. Three lesions were hypointense on T2-weighted images. All these lesions were diagnosed as GCTTS on histopathology. Rest of the lesions were isointense on T2-weighted images.

Only 7 (20%) of the cases were nonenhancing. Post-contrast enhancement was seen in the rest of them. It

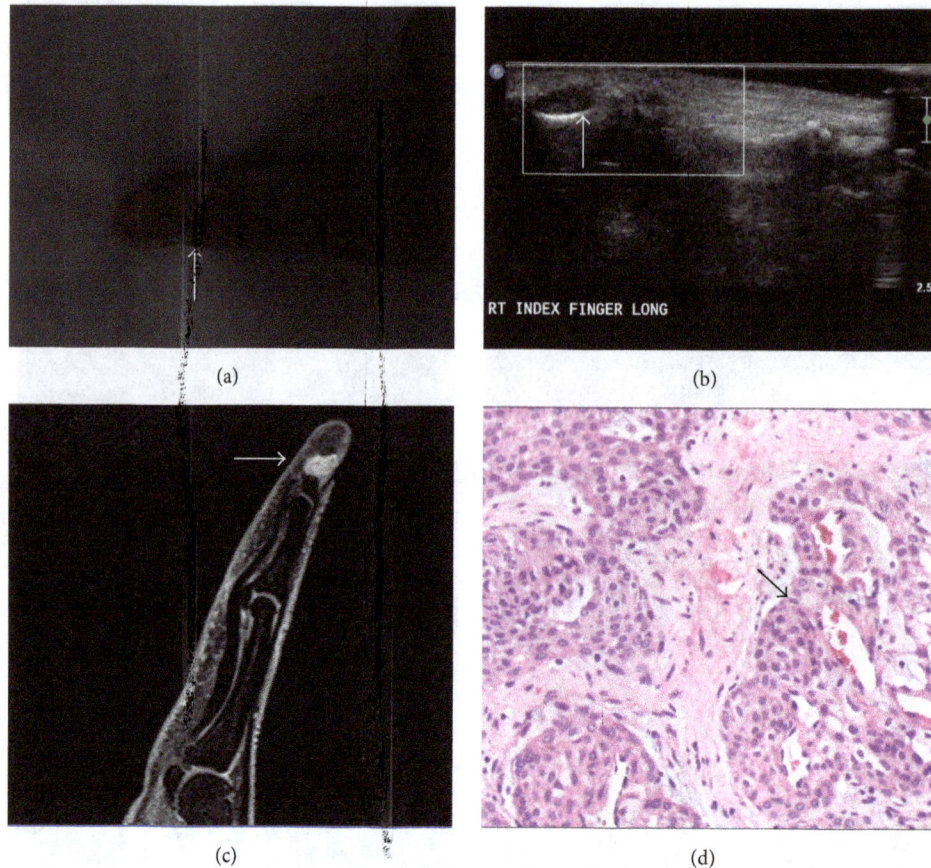

(a)

(b)

(c)

(d)

FIGURE 5: Glomus tumour. A 40-year-old female patient presented with painful, tender, and noncompressible swelling involving the region of distal phalanx of right index finger ((a), arrow). Ultrasonography (b) showed a well-defined, subcentimetric, hypoechoic, hypovascular soft tissue lesion (arrow). Postcontrast MRI (c) shows a small enhancing lesion along the flexor tendon sheath (arrow). Microphotograph (d) shows vascular lumina surrounded by a solid proliferation of glomus cells with perfectly round nuclei and acidophilic cytoplasm (arrow). H&E ×200.

was further divided into solid, peripheral enhancement and patchy enhancement. Most common pattern was patchy enhancement seen in 16 (45%) cases. Vascular lesions showed intense patchy progressive enhancement. The nonenhancing lesions consisted of lipomas ($n = 3$), ganglion ($n = 3$), and benign fibrous histiocytoma ($n = 1$). Glomus tumors and GCTTS showed solid enhancement. Peripheral enhancement was seen in chronic tenosynovitis and also in case of tubercular dactylitis with collection.

A correct diagnosis was possible on MRI in 80% of the cases ($n = 28$). The incorrect diagnosis included benign fibrous histiocytoma ($n = 2$), synovial sarcoma ($n = 2$), benign spindle cell tumor ($n = 2$), and hamartomatous lesions ($n = 1$).

3.3. Distribution of Cases according to Cytology/Histopathology. A total of 13 histologically different cases were included in the study (Table 1). The maximum number of cases comprised vascular malformations and hemagioma.

4. Discussion

Clinical assessment of the palpable lesions of hand is of utmost importance. Imaging is used for confirmation of

TABLE 1: Distribution of different types of tumors on HPE/FNAC.

Sr. number	Pathological diagnosis	Number of patients
1	Vascular malformation	5 (15%)
2	Haemangioma	4 (11.5%)
3	GCTTS	3 (8.5%)
4	Ganglion	3 (8.5%)
5	Glomus tumor	3 (8.5%)
6	Lipoma	3 (8.5%)
7	Schwannoma	2 (5.5%)
8	Hamartoma	2 (5.5%)
9	Neurofibroma	4 (11%)
10	Benign fibrous histiocytoma	2 (5.5%)
11	Synovial sarcoma	1 (2.7%)
12	TB	2 (5.5%)
13	Nonspecific inflammation	1 (2.7%)

the clinical diagnosis and delineation of lesion extent. The most common swellings are of ganglion, synovial, and peritendinous origin [5]. The imaging features of the ganglions are typical, therefore making MRI an important tool for

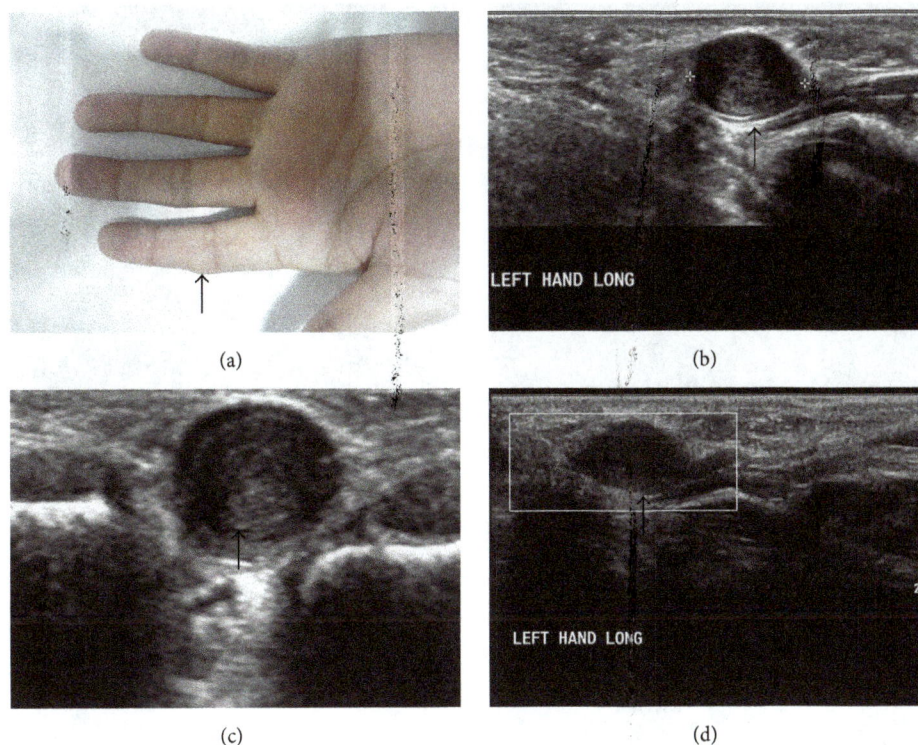

FIGURE 6: Schwannoma. A 25-year-old female patient presented with firm, noncompressible swelling over the radial aspect of the proximal interphalangeal joint of 2nd digit ((a), arrow). Ultrasonography ((b)–(d)) showed a well-defined, oval, hypoechoic, hypovascular lesion (arrow).

diagnosis. One has to look for the presence of soft tissue components and abnormal signal intensity to rule out other diagnoses. Many of the soft tissue masses have nonspecific appearance on imaging. However some of them like lipoma and GCTTS have typical imaging features.

In a study done by Capelastegui et al., MRI and case records of 134 patients presenting with swellings in the hand and wrist were reviewed [7]. In 126 cases, cause of the swelling could be demonstrated in the study. In 8 patients, no focal lesion was seen. In their study, ganglions were the most common cause of the swelling accounting for 36 (26.86%) cases. Vascular lesions were seen in 9 cases and were the most frequently encountered lesions among soft tissue tumors [7]. However in our study, the most common cases presenting with hand swellings were hemangiomas/vascular malformations.

Hemangiomas on USG show iso/hyperechoic well-defined lesions with anechoic areas in between with/without color flow [8]. The hyperechoic areas likely represent fatty component. Hemangiomas that usually have a well-defined margin but may show infiltrative margins [9]. They typically have intermediate signal intensity on T1-weighted images and high signal intensity on T2-weighted images [9, 10]. However, intralesional heterogeneity can be produced by reactive fatty tissue around the neoplastic vessels (hyperintense on T1W images), by blood vessels (hyperintense on T1W images) or by intralesional haemorrhage (variable signal intensity depending on the duration). In addition, phleboliths are seen as low signal intensity foci on both T1W and T2W images [10].

There is avid postcontrast enhancement with visualisation of feeding vessels. In a study by Theumann et al., MRI features were reported in 15 patients with hemagiomas of fingers [11]. Typical MRI findings were recorded in 10 patients and atypical findings in 5 patients. Atypical features included mass like appearance with homogeneous diffuse enhancement ($n = 2$) and poor heterogeneous enhancement ($n = 3$). We performed MRI in 4 lesions proven to be hemangiomas [11]. In one of the cases, there was fat component seen as T1W hyperintense component with suppression on fat suppressed images. In all the cases, patchy intense enhancement was seen.

Vascular malformations are classified into high flow and low flow [8, 12]. The latter is further classified into venous, lymphatic, capillary, and venocapillary forms based on the predominant component. Slow flow vascular malformations are usually septated and show intermediate to low signal intensity on T1W and high signal intensity on T2W images. The lymphatic malformation tends to be more infiltrative than the venous form and is more likely to demonstrate fluid-fluid levels [12]. The venous malformation is characterised by phleboliths seen as low signal foci on all pulse sequences. The lymphatic malformation shows no enhancement (microcystic) or septated enhancement (macrocystic). The venous form shows delayed venous enhancement. No arterial feeder (seen as flow voids), draining vein, and arterial or early venous enhancement are seen in low flow vascular malformation. The latter are the characteristics features of the high flow AVM [12]. The lesions can show intraosseous extension in either vascular malformation. In our study, we evaluated 5

(a)

(b)

(c)

(d)

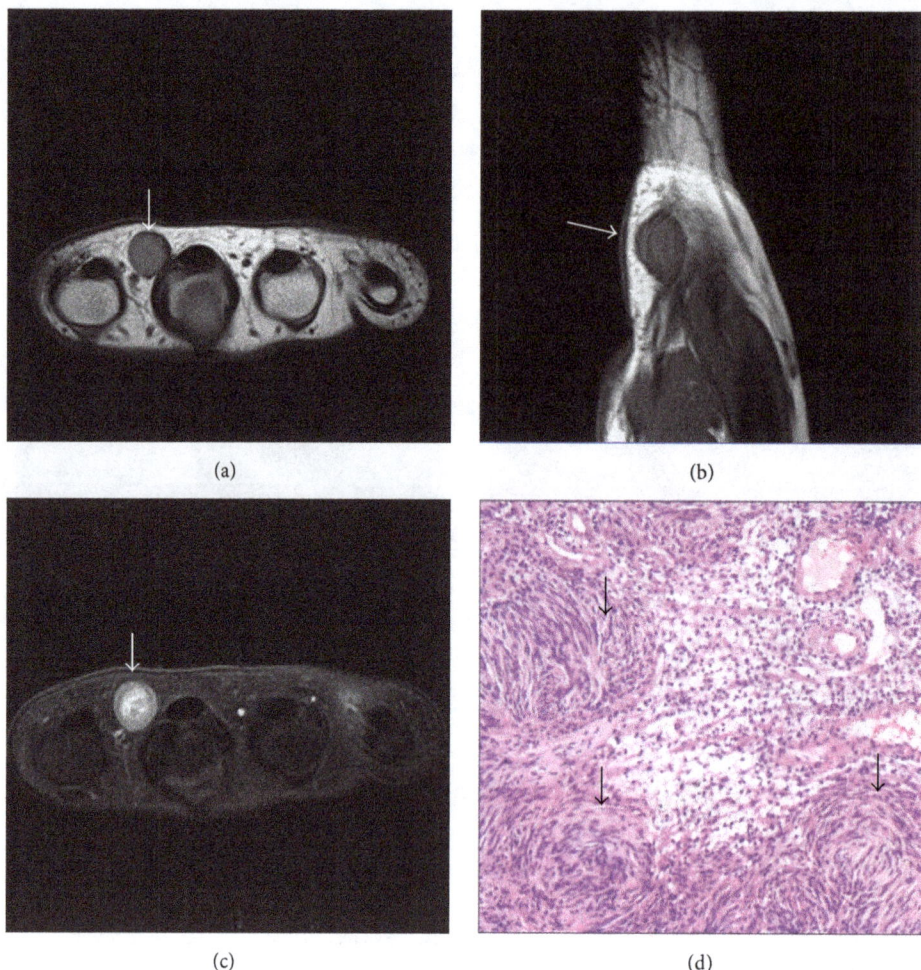

FIGURE 7: Schwannoma. MRI (of the same patient as in Figure 6) shows a well-defined T1W ((a), (b)) hypointense and T2WFS (c) hyperintense lesion in 2nd-3rd web space (arrows). Underlying bone shows normal cortical outline. Microphotograph (d) shows hypocellular and hypercellular areas with vessels showing perivascular hyalinization (arrows). H&E ×100.

vascular malformations in the hand. Flow voids were seen in three cases. All these cases also showed arterial feeders suggesting a diagnosis of high flow vascular malformation (Figures 1 and 2). Underlying bone changes were present in two cases. Two cases showed phleboliths. In all the cases included in our study the diagnosis of vascular malformation could be made on USG/Doppler alone; however MRI better defined the extent of the lesion, underlying bone changes, and involvement of marrow.

We encountered 3 cases of ganglions in our study. Imaging is important in some cases to look for atypical findings, solid components, heterogeneous contents, and abnormal SI, in the surrounding tissues [5]. De Flaviis et al. conducted a study on 14 patients presenting with soft tissue swellings of the hand [13]. Clinical diagnosis was kept as ganglion in 13 cases. High resolution USG was done in all the cases. Ganglions appeared as well-defined anechoic lesions with thin wall in recent cases. In older lesions, internal echoes and thicker walls were identified. Presence of a liquid filled duct directed towards articular surface is considered diagnostic [14]. A typical lesion on MRI shows fluid signal intensity with

subtle peripheral enhancement. Atypical findings presenting a diagnostic challenge include debris, haemorrhage, synovial thickening, or cyst rupture producing diverse MRI appearances [15]. In our study, no atypical findings were noted.

GCCTS are the second most common lesions of the hand and wrist. These present as slow growing, firm, nontender mass with a predilection for the radial three digits especially around the distal interphalangeal joint [16]. In a study by Capelastegui et al., GCTTS was the most frequent specific diagnosis [7]. These show characteristic imaging features, low signal on both T1 and T2 WI (due to fibrosis and hemosiderin deposition) with postcontrast enhancement. In 1 case it was located along the carpus [17]. In our study, 3 such cases were diagnosed. On gray scale imaging these were predominantly isoechoic with presence of heterogeneity in larger lesions. No increased vascularity was demonstrated on color flow imaging. MRI showed characteristic findings in relation to the flexor tendon (Figures 3 and 4).

Lipoma has characteristic signal intensity on MRI. It parallels that of subcutaneous fat on all pulse sequences [18]. On gray scale USG they are characteristically hyperechoic

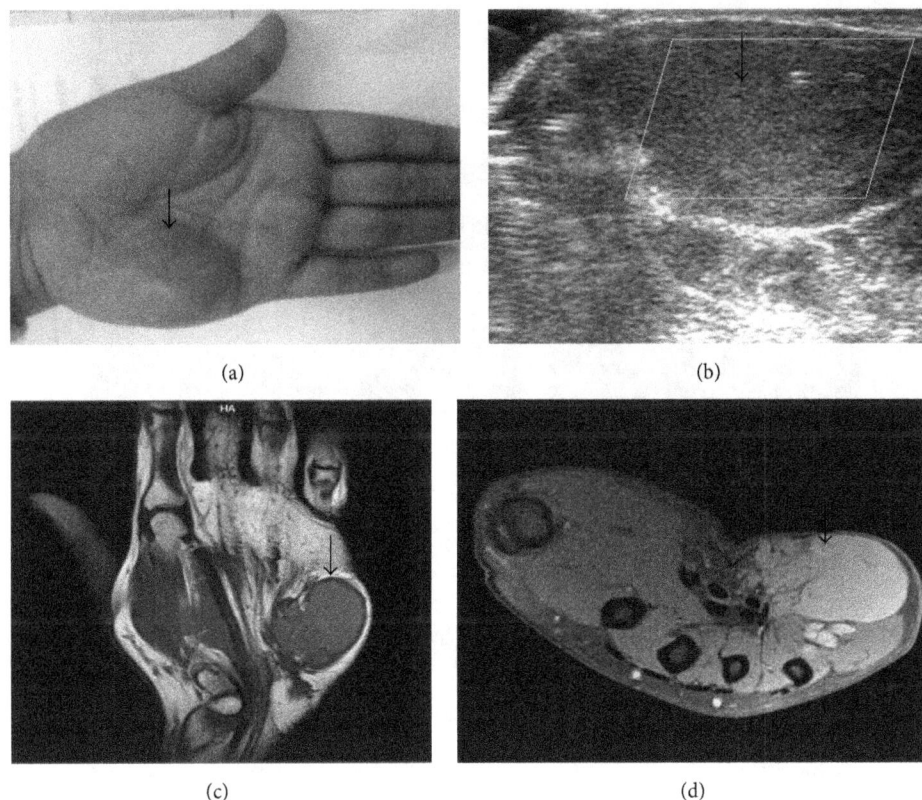

(a)

(b)

(c)

(d)

FIGURE 8: Synovial sarcoma. A 34-year-old female patient presented with noncompressible swelling involving hypothenar eminence of left hand ((a), arrow). Ultrasonography shows a hypoechoic lesion with absent color flow (b). MRI shows a large, lobulated T1W hypointense ((c), arrow) and T1WFS hyperintense ((d), arrow) lesion.

with no evidence of vascularity on color flow imaging. In MRI, the lesions show increased signal on all sequences with suppression on fat saturated images.

In a study by Montandon et al., imaging features in 8 cases of subungual glomus tumors were evaluated. Doppler ultrasonography was positive in five cases showing a hypoechoic nodule with internal vascularity [19]. Magnetic resonance imaging was positive in all of the cases. It showed solid nodule, hypointense on T1- and hyperintense on T2-weighted image, with homogeneous contrast enhancement [19]. In a study by Trehan et al., MRI findings in 36 of the 46 patients who had pathologically confirmed hand glomus tumor were analysed. A preoperative diagnosis could be established in 24 cases; 7 cases were indeterminate and 5 were negative [20]. Authors concluded that failure to diagnose glomus tumors on MRI could be attributed to atypical pathology, atypical location (i.e., not located in the subungual region), absence of bone erosion, and lack of clinical suspicion [20]. We evaluated 3 glomus tumors in our study (Figure 5). Atypical findings were recorded in none of the patients.

Neurogenic tumors (Figures 6 and 7), benign fibrous histiocytoma, hamartoma, synovial sarcoma (Figures 8 and 9), chronic nodular tenosynovitis, and tubercular dactylitis with abscess are rare lesions of the hand and their imaging characteristics are similar to those occurring elsewhere in the body [5, 21–25]. Diagnosis of neurogenic tumor on imaging is considered if relationship with a neurovascular bundle can

be demonstrated. Otherwise, the imaging can be nonspecific, however, important for delineating lesion extent. Similarly, the other lesions tend to have nonspecific imaging findings. The last two entities, however, have some features that can suggest the possible diagnosis. In nodular tenosynovitis, there is hypointense signal on T1W and T2W images. The bone lesion is the key to the diagnosis of the tubercular nature of the abscess in dactylitis.

5. Limitations of the Study

Our study population is small. There is diverse range of pathologies included in our study with insufficient number of cases of certain pathological entities in the included study population, for example, benign fibrous histiocytoma. Pathological confirmation was achieved by FNAC and not by histopathology in some cases.

6. Conclusion

Radiological investigations (USG and MRI) are important tools for the diagnosis of the soft tissue swellings of the hand. Relevant clinical history and examination play a pivotal role. Ultrasound is a widely available modality and can be diagnostic in certain entities like vascular malformations and ganglions. MRI can provide conclusive imaging findings in many

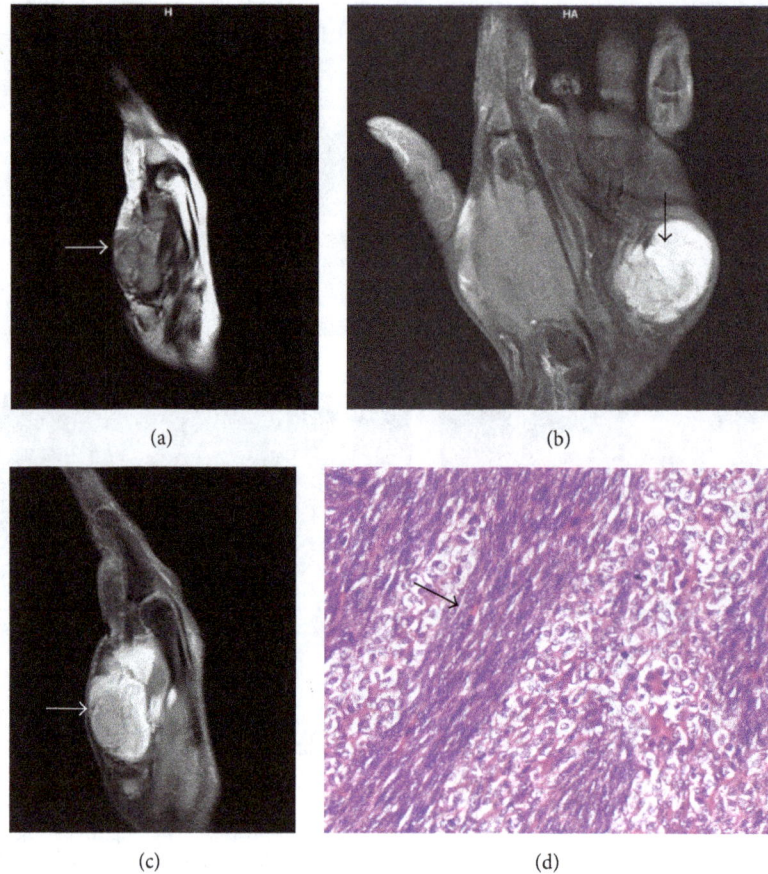

(a)

(b)

(c)

(d)

FIGURE 9: Synovial sarcoma. MRI (of the same patient as Figure 8). On T2W images ((a), (b)) the lesion is hyperintense (arrow). On postcontrast T1WFS images (c) the lesion shows heterogeneous postcontrast enhancement (arrow). Microphotograph (d) shows spindle shaped cells in fascicles (arrow) with intervening plump epithelial cells. H&E ×200.

pathological lesions (vascular lesions, lipomas, GCTTS, etc.) and is important for providing accurate anatomical extent. In certain lesions like glomus tumors, there is limited role of USG and patient can be directly subjected to MRI for the confirmation of the clinical diagnosis. However, pathologic confirmation of the diagnosis is important in some entities especially in absence of characteristic imaging findings.

Authors' Contribution

Aditi Agarwal and Mahesh Prakash contributed equally to this paper.

References

[1] S. Hasham and F. D. Burke, "Diagnosis and treatment of swellings in the hand," *Postgraduate Medical Journal*, vol. 83, no. 979, pp. 296–300, 2007.

[2] J. Teh and G. Whiteley, "MRI of soft tissue masses of the hand and wrist," *British Journal of Radiology*, vol. 80, no. 949, pp. 47–63, 2007.

[3] L. Gartner, C. J. Pearce, and A. Saifuddin, "The role of the plain radiograph in the characterisation of soft tissue tumours," *Skeletal Radiology*, vol. 38, no. 6, pp. 549–558, 2009.

[4] L. F. I. J. Oudenhoven, E. Dhondt, S. Kahn et al., "Accuracy of radiography in grading and tissue-specific diagnosis—a study of 200 consecutive bone tumors of the hand," *Skeletal Radiology*, vol. 35, no. 2, pp. 78–87, 2006.

[5] Y. Kuwano, K. Ishizaki, R. Watanabe, and H. Nanko, "Efficacy of diagnostic ultrasonography of lipomas, epidermal cysts, and ganglions," *Archives of Dermatology*, vol. 145, no. 7, pp. 761–764, 2009.

[6] J. Garcia and S. Bianchi, "Diagnostic imaging of tumors of the hand and wrist," *European Radiology*, vol. 11, no. 8, pp. 1470–1482, 2001.

[7] A. Capelastegui, E. Astigarraga, G. Fernandez-Canton, I. Saralegui, J. A. Larena, and A. Merino, "Masses and pseudomasses of the hand and wrist: MR findings in 134 cases," *Skeletal Radiology*, vol. 28, no. 9, pp. 498–507, 1999.

[8] J. B. Mulliken and J. Glowacki, "Hemangiomas and vascular malformations in infants and children: a classification based on endothelial characteristics," *Plastic and Reconstructive Surgery*, vol. 69, no. 3, pp. 412–422, 1982.

[9] L. F. Donnelly, D. M. Adams, and G. S. Bisset III, "Vascular malformations and hemangiomas: a practical approach in a multidisciplinary clinic," *American Journal of Roentgenology*, vol. 174, no. 3, pp. 597–608, 2000.

[10] K. I. Olsen, G. S. Stacy, and A. Montag, "Soft-tissue cavernous hemangioma," *Radiographics*, vol. 24, no. 3, pp. 849–854, 2004.

[11] N. H. Theumann, J. Bittoun, S. Goettmann, D. Le Viet, A. Chevrot, and J.-L. Drapé, "Hemangiomas of the fingers: MR imaging evaluation," *Radiology*, vol. 218, no. 3, pp. 841–847, 2001.

[12] C. S. P. van Rijswijk, E. van der Linden, H.-J. van der Woude, J. M. van Baalen, and J. L. Bloem, "Value of dynamic contrast-enhanced MR imaging in diagnosing and classifying peripheral vascular malformations," *American Journal of Roentgenology*, vol. 178, no. 5, pp. 1181–1187, 2002.

[13] L. De Flaviis, R. Nessi, P. Del Bo, G. Calori, and G. Balconi, "High-resolution ultrasonography of wrist ganglia," *Journal of Clinical Ultrasound*, vol. 15, no. 1, pp. 17–22, 1987.

[14] S. Bianchi, I. F. Abdelwahab, A. Zwass, and P. Giacomello, "Ultrasonographic evaluation of wrist ganglia," *Skeletal Radiology*, vol. 23, no. 3, pp. 201–203, 1994.

[15] S. Bianchi, I. F. Abdelwahab, A. Zwass et al., "Sonographic findings in examination of digital ganglia: retrospective study," *Clinical Radiology*, vol. 48, no. 1, pp. 45–47, 1993.

[16] L. De Beuckeleer, A. De Schepper, F. De Belder et al., "Magnetic resonance imaging of localized giant cell tumour of the tendon sheath (MRI of localized GCTTS)," *European Radiology*, vol. 7, no. 2, pp. 198–201, 1997.

[17] W. C. G. Peh, Y. Wong, T. W. H. Shek, and W.-Y. Ip, "Giant cell tumour of the tendon sheath of the hand: a pictorial essay," *Australasian Radiology*, vol. 45, no. 3, pp. 274–280, 2001.

[18] A. Laorr and A. Greenspan, "Hand lipomas: detection and characterization by magnetic resonance imaging," *Canadian Association of Radiologists Journal*, vol. 44, no. 1, pp. 14–18, 1993.

[19] C. Montandon, J. D. C. Costa, L. A. Dias et al., "Subungual glomus tumors: imaging findings," *Radiologia Brasileira*, vol. 42, no. 6, pp. 371–374, 2009.

[20] S. K. Trehan, E. A. Athanasian, E. F. DiCarlo, D. N. Mintz, and A. Daluiski, "Characteristics of glomus tumors in the hand not diagnosed on magnetic resonance imaging," *The Journal of Hand Surgery*, vol. 40, no. 3, pp. 542–545, 2015.

[21] M. D. Murphey, W. S. Smith, S. E. Smith, M. J. Kransdorf, and H. T. Temple, "From the archives of the AFIP. Imaging of musculoskeletal neurogenic tumors: radiologic-pathologic correlation," *Radiographics*, vol. 19, no. 5, pp. 1253–1280, 1999.

[22] E. Cerofolini, A. Landi, G. DeSantis, A. Maiorana, G. Canossi, and R. Romagnoli, "MR of benign peripheral nerve sheath tumors," *Journal of Computer Assisted Tomography*, vol. 15, no. 4, pp. 593–597, 1991.

[23] D. Mulkeen, J. Chin-Aleong, J. Callaghan, J. McCann, and P. J. Regan, "Fibrous histiocytoma of tendon sheath of the hand," *Irish Medical Journal*, vol. 93, no. 8, pp. 236–239, 2000.

[24] H. Nakajima, K. Matsushita, H. Shimizu et al., "Synovial sarcoma of the hand," *Skeletal Radiology*, vol. 26, no. 11, pp. 674–676, 1997.

[25] A. De Backer, F. Vanhoenacker, and D. Sanghvi, "Imaging features of extraaxial musculoskeletal tuberculosis," *Indian Journal of Radiology and Imaging*, vol. 19, no. 3, pp. 176–186, 2009.

16

Imaging Modalities to Identity Inflammation in an Atherosclerotic Plaque

Sunny Goel,[1] Avraham Miller,[1] Chirag Agarwal,[1] Elina Zakin,[2] Michael Acholonu,[1] Umesh Gidwani,[3] Abhishek Sharma,[4] Guy Kulbak,[5] Jacob Shani,[5] and On Chen[5]

[1]Department of Medicine, Maimonides Medical Center, Brooklyn, NY 11219, USA
[2]Department of Neurology, Icahn School of Medicine at Mount Sinai, New York, NY 10029, USA
[3]Department of Cardiology, Icahn School of Medicine at Mount Sinai, New York, NY 10029, USA
[4]Division of Cardiovascular Medicine, State University of New York Downstate Medical Centre, Brooklyn, NY 11203, USA
[5]Department of Cardiology, Maimonides Medical Center, Brooklyn, NY 11219, USA

Correspondence should be addressed to Sunny Goel; maverickmedico1985@gmail.com

Academic Editor: Paul Sijens

Atherosclerosis is a chronic, progressive, multifocal arterial wall disease caused by local and systemic inflammation responsible for major cardiovascular complications such as myocardial infarction and stroke. With the recent understanding that vulnerable plaque erosion and rupture, with subsequent thrombosis, rather than luminal stenosis, is the underlying cause of acute ischemic events, there has been a shift of focus to understand the mechanisms that make an atherosclerotic plaque unstable or vulnerable to rupture. The presence of inflammation in the atherosclerotic plaque has been considered as one of the initial events which convert a stable plaque into an unstable and vulnerable plaque. This paper systemically reviews the noninvasive and invasive imaging modalities that are currently available to detect this inflammatory process, at least in the intermediate stages, and discusses the ongoing studies that will help us to better understand and identify it at the molecular level.

1. Introduction

Atherosclerosis is a progressive inflammatory disease characterized by the accumulation of lipids in the walls of arteries, which over time can result in coronary artery disease, cerebrovascular disease, and peripheral arterial disease [1, 2]. Although there has been an overall increase in the awareness of its risk factors, cardiovascular disease still continues to be the leading cause of death worldwide [3]. Over the last three decades, much work has been done to develop imaging modalities which can diagnose atherosclerosis at least in its intermediate stages and visualize the stage of active inflammation within the vessel wall which converts a stable plaque into an unstable one. It is this process that generates erosion and plaque rupture with subsequent embolization and thrombosis, resulting in acute ischemic events [4]. Inflammation plays a critical role in the formation, progression, and rupture of the atherosclerotic plaque. The

hallmark characteristic of inflammation is the presence of macrophages within the plaque lipid core [4, 5]. Ongoing macrophage infiltration and cell death, along with accelerated lipid accumulation, contribute to an enlarging necrotic core that becomes progressively more inflamed, hypoxic, and unstable. Moreover, these cells secrete proinflammatory cytokines (including interleukin-1, monocyte chemotactic protein-1, and tumor necrosis factor-alpha) and matrix metalloproteinase, which actively weaken the fibrous cap, leading to plaque rupture [4]. Detection of atherosclerotic plaques at this inflammatory stage with the use of invasive and noninvasive imaging modalities could allow for the prevention of future cardiovascular events [6].

2. Noninvasive Imaging Modalities

Noninvasive imaging techniques do not only visualize the plaque but also could gather data on intraplaque hemorrhage

TABLE 1: Noninvasive imaging modalities to detect a vulnerable plaque.

Noninvasive imaging technique	Spatial resolution	Plaque characteristic identified	Advantages	Limitations
CT	50 micron	Plaque morphology (eccentric pattern, outward remodelling, and spotty calcifications), coronary plaque burden, cap thickness, and macrophages (N1177-specific contrast agent)	High spatial and temporal resolution, real time, quite fast, operator-independent, and excellent calcium detection	Radiation exposure, contrast, difficult to distinguish thrombus, blooming artefacts by calcium, and claustrophobia
MRI	10–100 micron	Plaque morphology, plaque composition, lipid-rich necrotic core, intraplaque haemorrhage, neoangiogenesis, macrophages, flow measurement, and quantification of stenosis	No radiation, high soft tissue contrast, can be repeated over time, functional, operator-independent, with or without contrast, and many plaque components detected	Low resolution, system fibrosis due to contrast agent, time-consuming, metal implants contraindicated, claustrophobia, cardiac motion artefact, and limited spatial resolution
Ultrasound	50 micron	Plaque morphology, intima media thickness, flow velocities, and neoangiogenesis (contrast US)	High temporal resolution, cheap, easy to use, no radiation, bedside/large availability, fastest, and functional	Limited sensitivity and specificity, interobserver variability, calcium and air artefacts, limited spatial resolution, and penetration
PET	1-2 millimeters	Plaque inflammation, macrophages, and neoangiogenesis	High sensitivity and specific targets are detected	Limited resolution, radiation exposure, expensive, limited availability, myocardial uptake of FDG, and cardiac motion artefact
SPECT	0.3–1 millimeters	Plaque inflammation, apoptosis, lipoprotein accumulation, chemotaxis, angiogenesis, proteolysis, and thrombogenicity.	High sensitivity, low cost, and more spatial resolution as compared with PET	Limited resolution, nonspecificity, radiation exposure, limited availability, and cardiac motion artefact

CT, computed tomography; MRI, magnetic resonance imaging; US, ultrasound; PET, positron emission tomography; SPECT, single positron emission computed tomography.

(IPH), plaque inflammation, calcification, and plaque remodelling, thus providing the examiner with information regarding the degree of plaque vulnerability [7]. The noninvasive modalities include computed tomography (CT), magnetic resonance imaging (MRI), ultrasound (US), positron emission tomography (PET), single positron emission computed tomography (SPECT), and microwave radiometry (Table 1).

2.1. Computed Tomography (CT). CT has excellent spatial and temporal resolution, which allows for detailed anatomical delineation of large and medium sized vessels. It is considered as one of the most accurate noninvasive studies for the evaluation of the coronary arteries [8]. With the recent introduction of 16-slice and 64-slice CT scan, enhanced temporal and spatial resolution, and decreased scans times and lower radiation exposure, CT imaging of the coronary tree has truly been revolutionized [9]. A recent study found that the pooled sensitivity and specificity for detecting a greater than 50% stenosis per arterial segment were 93% and 96% for a 64-slice CT, 83% and 96% for a 16-slice CT, and 84% and 93% for a 4-slice CT, respectively [10].

The coronary lesions detected by CT can be divided into calcified, noncalcified, or mixed plaques based on the attenuation of the calcified structures [11]. Detailed imaging of plaque morphology can also be performed when an appropriate contrast medium is used [12]. Contrary to popular belief, the lesions in patients with acute coronary syndrome (ACS) are composed mostly of mixed and noncalcified lesions, which might indicate that the amount of calcification is not an indicator of the vulnerability of the plaque. Studies show that the culprit lesions in acute myocardial infarction (AMI), unstable angina, and stable angina have different calcification patterns. With the help of iodinated contrast agents, even these noncalcified plaques can be detected by CT once the intima results in a 25% narrowing [13].

Although CT has evolved over the last decade, the hazards of radiation and the use of nephrotoxic contrast agents limit its usage on a large scale [14]. However, with recent technical advances, such as the use of volume scanning (as opposed to helical scanning), one can have a reduction in the effective radiation dose by 90% for the average examination [15]. Recent studies have shown promise with more novel agents, such as iodine-based compounds, gold nanorods with gadolinium, and nuclear tracers, as agents which can both reduce motion artefacts and acquire images with better resolution [16–19]. For example, N1177, a suspension composed of crystalline iodinated particles dispersed with surfactant that has high affinity to activated macrophages, is used, which can

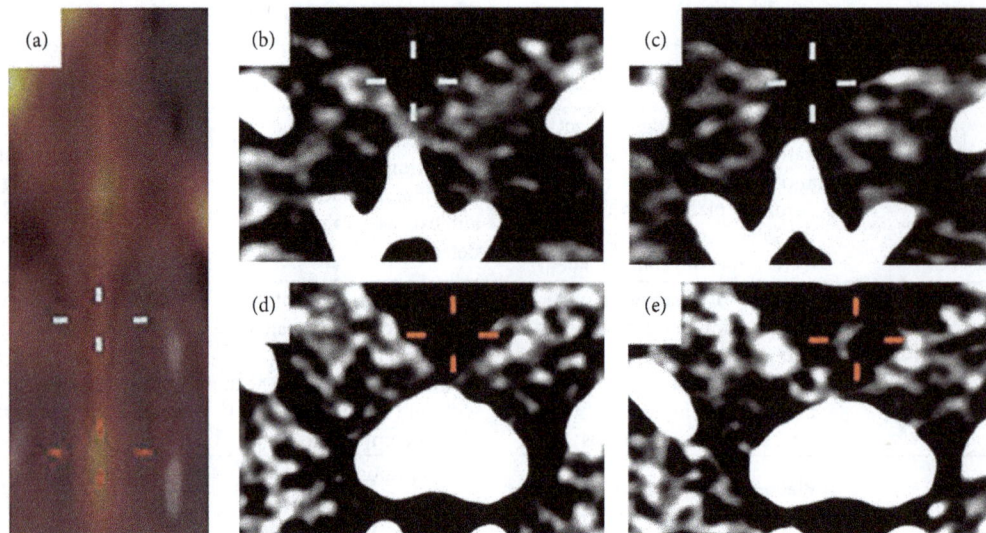

FIGURE 1: N1177-enhanced CT and corresponding FDG PET from atherosclerotic rabbit. Fused PET/CT coronal view of aorta obtained 3 hours after injection of 18F-labeled fluorodeoxyglucose (FDG) and corresponding axial aortic sections acquired before (b and d) and at 2 hours after injection of N1177, an iodine-based contrast agent that accumulates in macrophages (c and e). Aortic regions with high ((a), red cross) and low ((a), white cross) activities identified with PET at 3 hours after injection of FDG were associated with strong ((e), red cross) and weak ((c), white cross) intensities of enhancement detected in CT at 2 hours after injection of N1177 on corresponding axial views, respectively. Reprinted with permission from Hyafil et al. [20].

detect a vulnerable plaque, and is shown to correlate with FDG uptake (Figure 1) [20].

With the advent of the Coronary Artery Calcium (CAC) score coupled with new methods for decreasing one's exposure to radiation, the future of this imaging modality is promising. Recent studies have used CT imaging as baseline assessment in those about to begin statin therapy [21]. CT imaging is limited in its inability to differentiate stable versus unstable inflamed plaques. However, as this sophistication of this technique continues to improve, its ability to detect and predict atherosclerotic events will continue to advance and may become standard practice in the near future.

2.2. Magnetic Resonance Imaging (MRI). MRI is an accurate and noninvasive imaging modality used for the early detection of atherosclerotic burden in symptomatic patients especially in its intermediate stages when the luminal narrowing is sufficient enough to be detected by the MRI. What separates MRI from other imaging modalities is its ability to visualize plaques undergoing inflammatory changes [22]. It is possible to determine plaque anatomy and composition by using sequences such as T1-weighted, T2-weighted, and proton density-weighted imaging. Multiple imaging sequences may help identify certain plaque morphologies, such as the fibrous cap, the lipid rich necrotic core, intraplaque haemorrhage, neovascularization, and signs of vascular wall inflammation (Figure 2) [23]. Studies have shown that multicontrast magnetic resonance imaging of the human carotid arteries has a sensitivity of 85% and a specificity of 92% when detecting the lipid core and intraplaques haemorrhage [24, 25]. As previously mentioned, an ability to visualize plaques

undergoing inflammatory changes would enhance our ability to predict cardiovascular events.

Direct imaging of a thrombus in the coronary artery has been made possible with specially optimized T1-weighted imaging called magnetization-prepared 3-dimensional rapid acquisition gradient echo (MP-RAGE) sequences that are comprised of an inversion recovery radiofrequency (RF) pulse in place of the standard magnetization together with a fast gradient echo acquisition sequence [26]. With the inversion time properly selected, a strong T1-weighting can be achieved, thus effectively detecting haemorrhage inside of an atherosclerotic plaque. An innovative method called the Slab-Selective Phase-Sensitive Inversion-Recovery (SPI) technique is also a promising improvement used in detecting intraplaque haemorrhage [27]. SPI has better intraplaque haemorrhage identification accuracy ($P < 0.01$) and a significantly higher intraplaque haemorrhage-wall contrast-to-noise ratio than MP-RAGE, effectively producing a more enhanced image of what is truly going on inside the plaque [27, 28].

Studies have shown that MRI can detect features of the plaque associated with its vulnerability, including the lipid-rich necrotic core and the thin fibrous cap. An intact fibrous cap is generally seen as a continuous hypointense band against the bright lumen with a smooth surface during T1-weighted imaging, whereas an irregular surface or discontinuity of the hypointense band indicates recent haemorrhage and plaque rupture [29]. Contrast-enhanced MRI (CE-MRI) is typically used to perform magnetic resonance angiography (CE-MRA) and can be supplemented with time-resolved angiography, flow measurement, vessel wall imaging, and

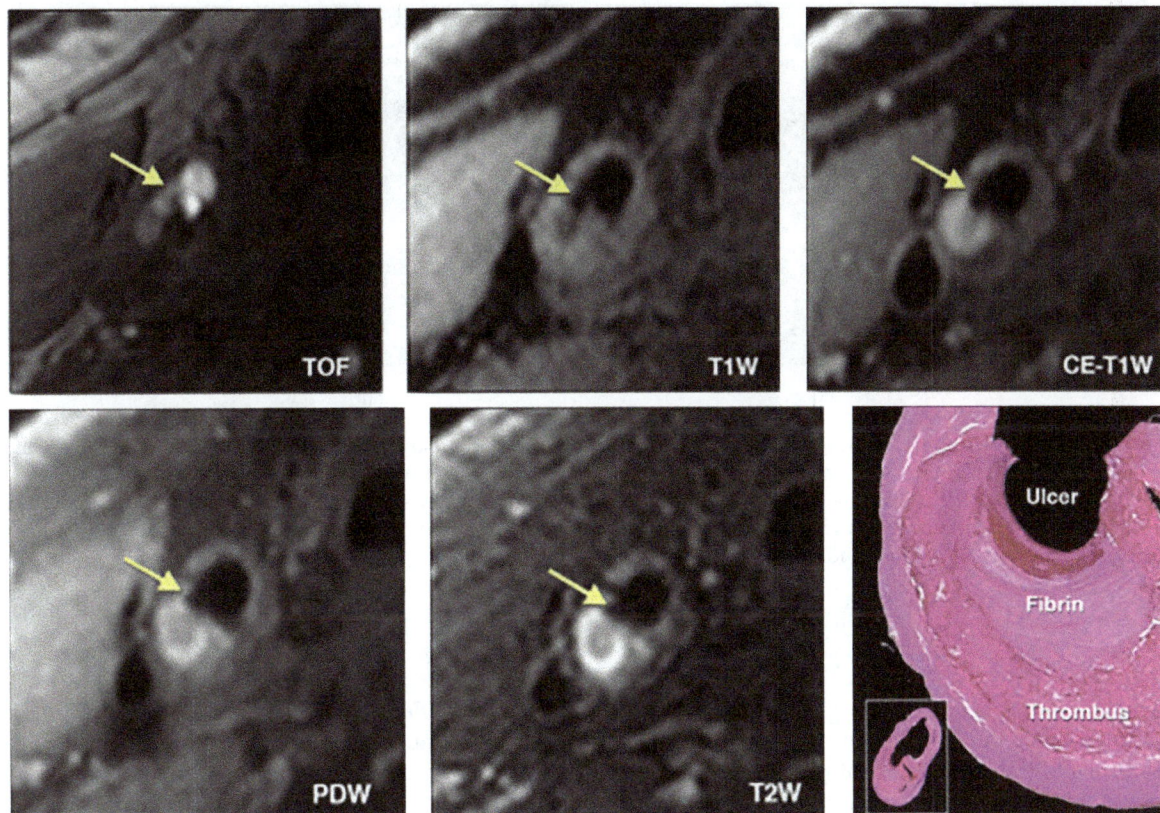

FIGURE 2: Morphologic characteristics of carotid artery atherosclerosis using MRI. 3-T magnetic resonance imaging (MRI) of a plaque in the right common carotid artery demonstrates fibrous cap rupture with ulcer formation (yellow arrows). The crescent-shaped high-signal region in the proton density-weighted (PDW), T2-weighted (T2W), and contrast enhanced T1-weighted (CE-T1W) images corresponds to a region of thrombus formation, shown on the matched histology section (hematoxylin and eosin stain). Reprinted with permission from Chu et al. [23].

plaque characterization for a more comprehensive assessment of vascular diseases [30].

Since the instability in an atherosclerotic lesion is promoted by the activation of mononuclear phagocytes, two MRI strategies have been used to detect this macrophage infiltration. The first technique uses gadolinium to detect the kinetics within the tissue that relate to phagocyte activation and mobilization. The other uses ultrasmall super paramagnetic particles of iron oxide (USPIO) to target macrophages in vivo [31, 32]. The ATHEROMA trial was conducted to test the ability of USPIO to detect plaques in forty asymptomatic patients, demonstrating a significant reduction in plaque uptake with high-dose statin over a 3-month period [33]. Although this trial did not show any significant association between USPIO signal intensity changes and subsequent cardiovascular and cerebrovascular events, it did show that USPIO was an effective method at detecting minute-to-minute changes in the cellular kinetics that were responsible for converting a stable plaque into an unstable one [34]. A recent study has shown that increased vascular permeability using an MR albumin-binding contrast agent and T1-mapping served as a surrogate measure of plaque progression and instability, which has the potential to help stratify atherosclerotic disease progression [35].

The MRI has higher spatial resolution when compared to other imaging modalities such as CT scanning and ultrasound, thus allowing for better tissue contrast. Many novel techniques are being developed at the present time using MRI-specific abilities that will allow us to not only visualize atherosclerotic plaque burden but also actually differentiate inflamed versus noninflamed plaques. This would greatly enhance our ability to determine those individuals who are at greater risk for significant cardiovascular events.

2.3. Ultrasound (US). Doppler ultrasound and high-resolution vascular B-mode ultrasound are widely available and have been shown to accurately depict flow-limiting stenosis in the large arterial circulation [36]. Ultrasound can provide useful information about vulnerable plaque components such as intraplaque haemorrhage, inflammation, lipid core, and vasa vasorum neovascularization, which are all related to plaque vulnerability [37]. However, ultrasound has a relatively poor sensitivity in its ability to detect ulcerations as compared to its ability to detect intravascular irregular borders (sensitivity of 97% and specificity of 81%) [38, 39]. The use of combined echolucency and heterogeneity scales, such as the Gray-Weal scale, may improve diagnostic accuracy but needs further development [40]. The new addition of gas

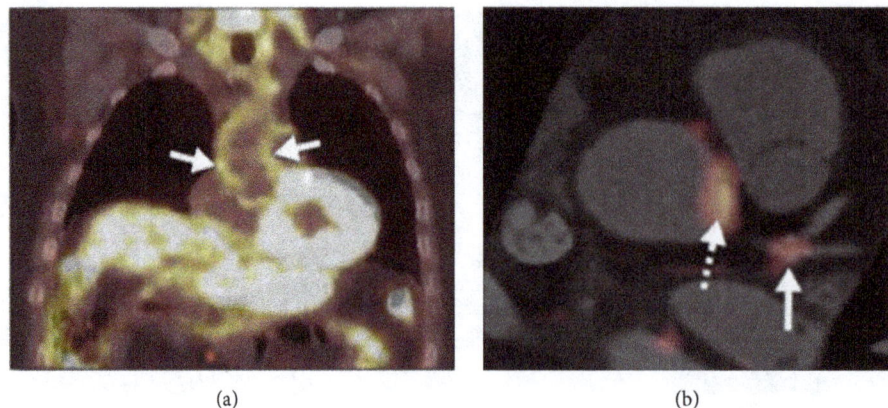

(a)   (b)

FIGURE 3: Imaging arterial inflammation using (a) FDG-PET patient demonstrating enhanced aortic uptake of FDG on PET scan, indicating inflammation in the arterial wall due to atherosclerosis. (b) Coregistered FDG-PET/computed tomography images showing FDG uptake at the left main coronary artery trifurcation (solid arrow) in a patient with acute coronary syndrome. Aortic FDG uptake is indicated by the dashed arrow. In such patients, both aortic and coronary artery FDG uptake was increased compared with patients with stable coronary artery disease. Reprinted with permission from Rudd et al. [47].

filled microspheres to ultrasound has given the technician the ability to visualize the vasa vasorum and its neovascularization, which are characteristics of vulnerable plaques. The use of microbubble contrast may improve the detection of ulcerations by enhancing the contrast between the lumen and the vessel wall, thus allowing the technician to visualize plaque hemorrhages [41].

Recent evidence suggests that Contrast Enhanced Ultrasonography (CEUS) can be used as a molecular imaging tool to target inflammation and visualize the associated neovascularization in a vulnerable plaque [42]. These two microvascular networks are both involved in the early process of plaque progression and vulnerability and may also be mutually linked with the development of plaque inflammation [42, 43]. CEUS medium consists of microbubbles of gas, enveloped by a shell of different substances (albumin, lipid, polymer, etc.). Gas microbubbles are strong reflectors of acoustic energy, thus increasing the return signal after tissue interrogation with ultrasound. Contrast microbubbles have a diameter of just a few microns (usually <5 micro meter) and have been shown to behave as a true intravascular tracer [44]. CEUS has the ability to image intraplaque neovessels that usually originate from the vasa vasorum in the adventitia which are linked to plaque vulnerability [42]. There have been multiple studies which have confirmed the utility of CEUS in the detection of intraplaque neovascularization with several clinical studies demonstrating that CEUS could help in the differentiation between stable and unstable plaques [42]. Additionally, plaque vascularization measured by CEUS has been shown to correlate positively with 18F-fluorodeoxyglucose (FDG) uptake measured by PET/CT in humans [45]. Although further prospective studies assessing the association of CEUS-detected neovascularization with future cardiovascular events are required, CEUS may represent a promising, safe, and widely available tool for detection of a vulnerable plaque.

2.4. Positron Emission Tomography (PET). The underlying principle of nuclear imaging techniques, such as PET, is the use of a radiotracer, which emits gamma rays that can be localized to a cell or receptor in an inflamed plaque. This allows for noninvasive detection of an inflamed and vulnerable plaque prone to rupture in the near future. Following the discovery of fluorine-18-flurodeoxyglucose (FDG), a radiotracer which has increased uptake in carotid plaques in patients with ischemic stroke, several studies have found an association between FDG uptake and vulnerable plaques (Figure 3) [46, 47]. Studies have proven that the amount of FDG uptake is directly proportional to the amount of inflammation in the plaque and that the use of statins reduces the inflammation as determined by the FDG uptake over time [48].

The disadvantage of FDG-PET is its limited spatial resolution when compared with MRI. Recently, this has been overcome with the use of hybrid imaging techniques such as PET-CT or PET-MRI, which can increase the spatial resolution [49]. Combined positron emission tomography and computed tomography, PET-CT, is a modern noninvasive imaging technique that combines functional information from PET with the fine anatomical detail provided by CT [50]. PET-CT has also been used to assess the efficacy of statin therapy in reducing the level of intravascular inflammation [51]. PET-CT can overcome the challenge of imaging the inflamed atheroma in the coronary vasculature with the use of 18F-FDG due to myocardial uptake of 18F-FDG in the smaller sized coronary arteries. PET-MRI has an advantage over PET-CT in that there is no radiation exposure, and it has a greater ability to differentiate between various plaque components (Figure 4) [52].

Although FDG-PET appears to provide a promising approach for the detection of inflammation in a vulnerable plaque, it does possess certain limitations. First, there are only a limited number of small prospective studies that have

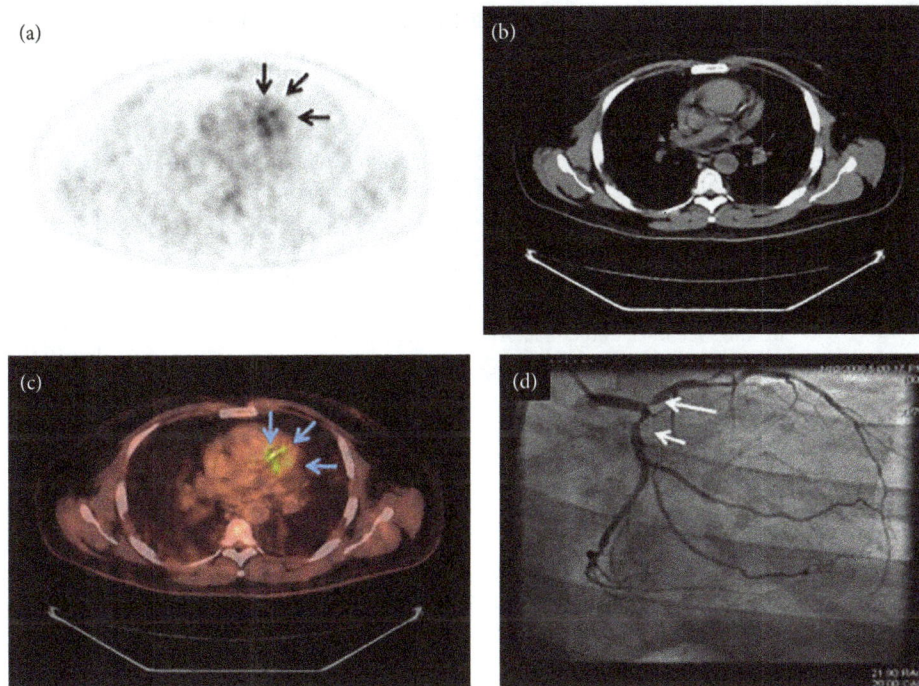

FIGURE 4: Representative images of coronary tree FDG uptake with corresponding angiographic images. Representative images of the coronary tree FDG uptake (arrows). FDG PET (a). CT (b). PET/CT (c) and coronary angiography (d) from patient with good myocardial uptake suppression with a low carbohydrate, high fat preparation. Reprinted with permission from Wykrzykowska et al. [52].

shown a correlation between adverse cardiovascular outcomes and increased FDG uptake in atherosclerotic plaque [53]. Second, FDG uptake in a plaque can be influenced by mechanisms other than inflammation such as hypoxia, which may give false positive results [52]. Therefore, even though FDG-PET seems to reliably detect an inflammatory plaque, it cannot currently be used as a predictor of outcome in a given atherosclerotic lesion.

2.5. Single Positron Emission Computed Tomography (SPECT). Both SPECT and PET work on the similar principle of radiofrequency signal uptake, but SPECT uses a different radiotracer which may be Iodine-123, Indium-111, or Technetium-99 [53]. Oxidized LDL labelled to Technetium-99 has been shown to have the greatest sensitivity in detecting vulnerable plaques [54]. Lecithin-like oxidized LDL receptor 1 (LOX-1) is a cell surface receptor for oxidized LDL that has been implicated in plaque instability and ^{99m}Tc-labeled anti-LOX 1 monoclonal IgG has been shown to have increasing accumulation in a vulnerable plaque, both of which can be detected by SPECT [55]. Another proposed mechanism for the detection of plaque instability with use of SPECT imaging is the detection of apoptotic cells in a plaque with Annexin A5 as the marker for apoptosis. Annexin A5 is a protein which targets the phosphatidylserine surface expression of cells (such as macrophages and platelets) during the apoptotic process. ^{99m}Tc-labelled Annexin A5 has been shown to have increased uptake in an inflamed atherosclerotic plaque [56, 57].

Despite these promising results, the use of SPECT in the detection of inflammation or plaque instability is limited due to the lack of resolution and low specificity. Additionally, this technique is not cost-effective [58].

2.6. Microwave Radiometry (MR). Microwave radiometry (MR) is a newly developed, noninvasive method, which possesses a high level of accuracy in the detection of the relative changes in temperature of human tissue, thus indicating degree of inflammation within an atherosclerotic plaque [59, 60]. Both experimental and clinical studies have proved the efficacy of microwave radiometry in the detection of vulnerable plaques, with recent studies also demonstrating the association of microwave radiometry with plaque neovascularization as assessed by contrast enhanced ultrasound (CEUS) [61]. After validation of MR in rabbit studies as test subjects, the first application of MR in human carotids was performed to demonstrate its utility in the detection of thermal heterogeneity [62]. Forty-four patients with significant carotid artery stenosis were included in the study. The primary outcomes of this study showed that MR can measure thermal heterogeneity of carotid atheromatic plaques in vivo and that in vivo temperature measurements by MR correlated well with the ultrasound findings of atherosclerotic plaque characteristics [62]. There is no gold standard method for the in vivo quantification of neovascularization and/or inflammation detected by MR; thus more clinical studies are needed.

TABLE 2: Invasive imaging modalities to detect a vulnerable plaque.

Invasive imaging techniques	Spatial resolution	Plaque characteristic identified	Advantages	Limitations
IVUS	150–250 micron	Plaque distribution, severity, cross-sectional area, and characterization of plaque (lipid core and spotty calcification)	High resolution images of vessel wall and plaque structure	Intra- and interobserver subjectivity, invasiveness, limited spatial resolution, and limited temporal resolution
OCT	4–20 micron	Plaque composition (fibrous, fibrofatty, and fatty), thin fibrous cap, macrophages, neoangiogenesis, and collagen formation	10 times higher image resolution compared to IVUS and greater tissue contrast	Requires blood-free imaging field, intra- and interobserver variation, invasiveness, and limited tissue penetration
IVMR	120 micron	Early atherosclerosis and more advanced plaque formations and plaque composition (lipid, fibrous, and calcified tissues)	High resolution of plaque structure and composition	Invasiveness and need for occlusion balloon
NIRS	NA	Thin fibrous cap, lipid core, and macrophages	High resolution of plaque structure with reliability	Invasiveness, limited tissue penetration, and cardiac motion artefact

IVUS, intravascular ultrasound; OCT, optical coherence tomography; IVMR, intravascular magnetic resonance; NIRS, near infrared spectroscopy.

3. Invasive Imaging Modalities

Invasive imaging techniques utilize intravascular catheters that are mounted with an imaging device and have revolutionized our understanding of the atherosclerotic plaque. Invasive imaging modalities are able to provide the highest resolution images with in-depth analysis about vessel wall and plaque morphology [63]. The current intravascular imaging techniques available to assess vulnerable plaques include intravascular ultrasound (IVUS), optical coherence tomography (OCT), intravascular magnetic resonance, and near infrared spectroscopy (NIRS) (Table 2).

3.1. Intravascular Ultrasound (IVUS). IVUS consists of an ultrasound unit mounted on the tip of an intravascular catheter, which consists of a piezoelectric material with either a single element or 64 elements. The difference between these units is the frequency range. The single unit frequency is 30–45 MHz and for 64 elements it is 20 MHz. These catheters can provide tomographic images of the vessel, vessel wall, and the atherosclerotic plaque [64]. Since its introduction in 1972, IVUS has advanced from its conventional grey-scale IVUS to its newest version of virtual histology intravascular ultrasound (VH-IVUS), which uses the same equipment and technology as the grey-scale IVUS but with the use of spectral analysis to interpret the back-scattered signals using power spectrum graph which plots the back-scattered US signals against the frequency [65]. Grey-scale IVUS is helpful in determining the vessel lumen size, distribution of the plaque, and severity of the plaque in addition to its ability to detect the plaque cross-sectional area, but it cannot determine the plaque histology [66]. Also, the detection of thin-cap lipid-rich vulnerable plaque (<65 micron) can be difficult to assess via grey-scale IVUS as its resolution is approximately 100 micron [67]. VH-IVUS allows for real time qualification of plaques into different subtypes and effectively overcomes the limitations of the grey-scale IVUS

[68]. VH-IVUS uses autoregressive modelling to convert the radiofrequency data into a power spectrum graph. The statistical classification system sorts the radiofrequency data based on the combination of spectral parameters into one of four subtypes: (1) fibrous plaque with a dark green spectral color code, (2) fibrofatty plaque with a yellow-green spectral color code, (3) necrotic core with a red spectral color code, and (4) dense calcium with a white spectral color code (Figure 5) [69].

Pathological studies have shown that the rupture of the thin-cap fibroatheroma (TCFA) is the most common cause of acute thrombotic coronary occlusion and VHIVUS has been able to identify this TCFA with a necrotic core of >10% and without evidence of overlying fibrous tissue [70, 71]. The biggest disadvantage of IVUS is its inability to detect inflammation within a plaque, especially as the inflammatory cells (i.e., macrophages) within the fibrous cap require a resolution of around 10–20 microns for detection, which is not possible using IVUS [72].

3.2. Optical Coherence Tomography (OCT). Optical coherence tomography is an intravascular invasive imaging modality that uses a similar principle as IVUS but instead implements near infrared light instead of ultrasound for imaging [73]. It has ten times higher image resolution and greater tissue contrast as compared to IVUS [74]. OCT is useful in the evaluation of plaque structure due to its resolution, providing the examiner with the ability to analyse various plaque components including fibrous cap thickness, the necrotic core, macrophage infiltration, plaque rupture/erosions, and plaque calcium content. It can also visualize calcified nodules, erosions, and microthrombi near the lumen [75].

Among all the available intravascular imaging modalities, OCT has been shown to have enough resolution to measure the thickness of the thin fibrous cap, which is the main characteristic of TCFA (Figure 6) [76].

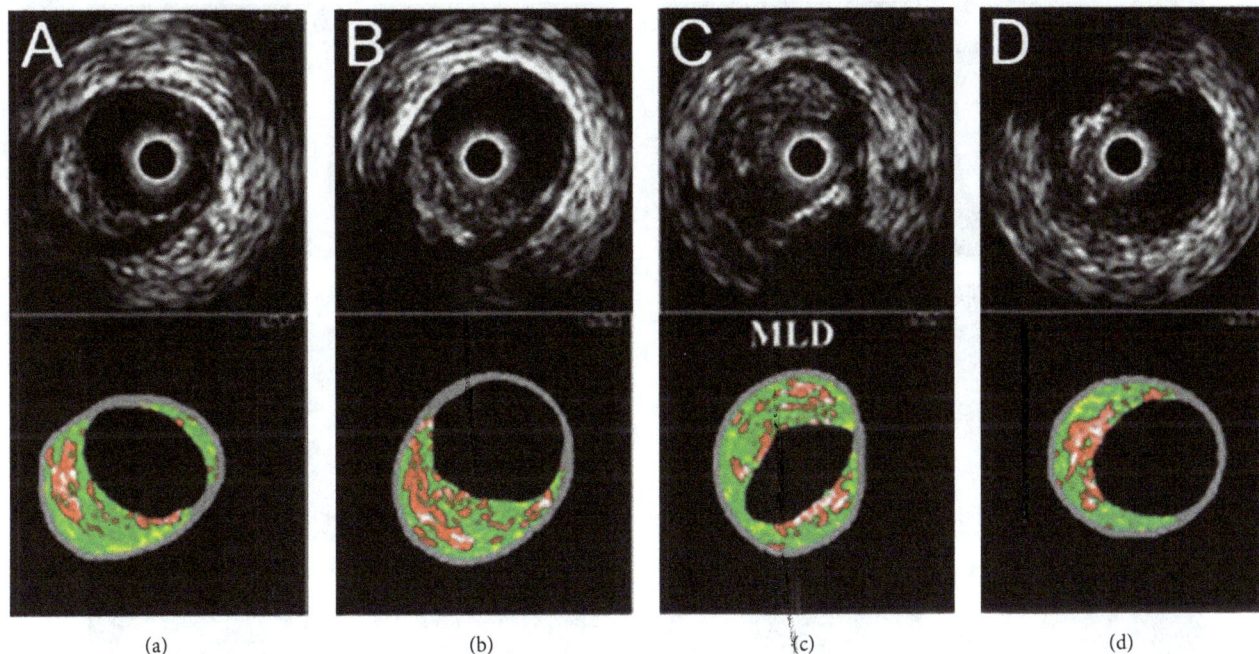

FIGURE 5: Four cross-sectional images from proximal to distal within the same patient coronary lesion obtained by IVUS and VH. In the upper panels we see grey-scale IVUS with reconstructed IVUS virtual histology in the lower panels. (a) A thick fibrous cap overlying a necrotic core. (b) A thick fibroma can be seen with the thick overlying fibrous cap containing small spots of necrotic core. (c) Minimal Lumen diameter site. (d) A thin-cap fibroatheroma can be seen. Reprinted with permission from Surmely et al. [69].

Studies show that OCT imaging provides an accurate measurement of fibrous cap thickness with a mean difference of $-24 + 44$ micron between the thicknesses measured by OCT versus that measured via digitalized histological images [77]. OCT allows for in-depth analysis of the distribution of inflammatory cells within a vulnerable plaque due to its excellent resolution. Macrophages appear as bright spots with high signal variance from the surrounding tissue because of their lipid content, which contains a high degree of optical contrast [78]. OCT together with ultrasmall super paramagnetic iron oxides [USPIO] can magnify the detection of inflammation in the plaque, thus distinguishing this imaging modality from IVUS [79]. OCT can also detect plaque rupture and erosion, the levels of which differ significantly in different types of unstable angina patients [80]. Additionally, the full extent of OCT imaging can be utilized in conjunction with the use of functionalized magnetofluorescent nanoparticles targeting endothelial markers, such as VCAM-1, which is a critical component of the leukocyte-endothelial adhesion cascade which regulates the atherogenic process [81].

One of the limitations of using short wavelength OCT is the reflection it produces off of the red blood cells, which can diminish the image quality during blood flow and requires frequent saline flushing from the guidewire to clear the image field [82]. This, together with the slow image acquisition speed of current OCT, makes it difficult to detect long arterial segments. However, recent improvements in OCT have rectified this issue, thus allowing for the creation of OFDI (Optical Frequency Domain Imaging) through which images can be obtained at a higher frame rate (>100 frames/sec) with faster 3D image of a long vessel in just one nonocclusive saline flush [83].

3.3. Intravascular Magnetic Resonance. The underlying principle in this technique is the utilization of pulsed field gradients together with magnetic resonance imaging, by which the water diffusion coefficient can be calculated. The diffusion coefficient D is equal to $0.26 \pm 0.13 \times 10^{-5}$ cm$^2 \cdot$s^{-1} in plaque lipid core, $1.45 \pm 0.41 \times 10^{-5}$ cm$^2 \cdot$s^{-1} in a collagenous cap, and $1.54 \pm 0.30 \times 10^{-5}$ cm$^2 \cdot$s^{-1} in normal media [84]. Water will diffuse less in lipid-rich plaques than in fibrous plaques, which allows us to determine the lipid content in atherosclerotic vessels. This technique can determine the composition of most plaques and could now be performed at the level of the aorta and coronary arteries [85].

Recent data has shown that this new method, when compared to ex vivo histology, showed a sensitivity of 100% and a specificity of 89%. Some of its limitations involve necessity of mechanically rotating the catheter within the vessel. However, much of the recent preliminary data shows that this new method may be superior to the IVUS, though its ability to detect inflammation in an atherosclerotic plaque is yet to be determined [86].

3.4. Near Infrared Spectroscopy (NIRS). This near infrared spectroscopy (NIRS) method is based on the concept of organic molecules absorbing and scattering light differently. As a result, different plaques made up of differing concentrations of lipids and proteins will scatter light differently,

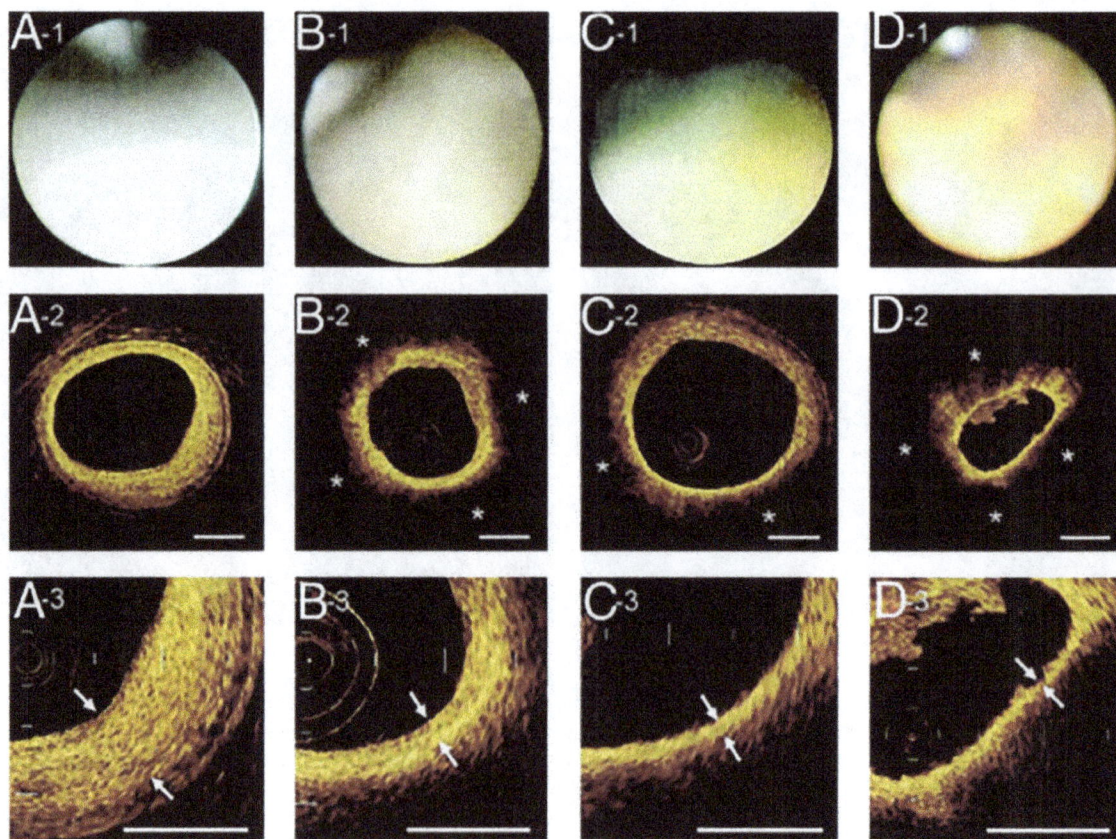

FIGURE 6: Angioscopic and corresponding OCT images obtained in patients presenting with acute coronary syndrome. In the angioscopic images, plaque color is graded as white (A-1), light yellow (B-1), yellow (C-1), or intensive yellow (D-1). In the optical coherence tomography (OCT) images, a lipid pool (*) is characterized by a signal-poor region (A-2, B-2, C-2, and D-2). The fibrous cap is identified as a signal-rich region between the coronary artery lumen and inner border of lipid pool in the OCT image, and its thickness is measured at the thinnest part (A-3, B-3, C-3, and D-3; arrows). Reprinted with permission from Kubo et al. [76].

thus allowing for a novel technique in which to differentiate atherosclerotic plaque makeup [87]. Recent work with explanted human aorta specimens shows NIRS ability to differentiate between a lipid pool, a thin cap, and inflammatory cells with sensitivity between 77% and 90% and specificity between 89% and 93% [88]. Further studies are needed to establish whether this method will be just as accurate in vivo, as well as its ability to detect inflammation.

4. Conclusion and Future Directions

Over the past thirty years, remarkable advances have been made in understanding the role of inflammation in a vulnerable plaque and the sequence of events that make a plaque vulnerable/prone to rupture. It is now widely accepted that inflammation plays a key role in plaque instability, conversion into a vulnerable plaque, and subsequent rupture, thus leading to ischemic events. A number of different novel imaging modalities have been investigated to define the specific characteristics of vulnerable plaque. However, most of these techniques are still undergoing constant refinement and cannot reliably identify vulnerable plaque in the clinical setting. It is important to realize that plaque composition is not equal to

plaque vulnerability. Most of the methodologies described in this review are able to detect particular components of plaque, for example, lipids and calcium. However, at present, there is no definitive evidence that in vivo plaque composition is directly related to plaque vulnerability or that the observed characteristics of a plaque are related to outcome. Further research is required to increase the sensitivity and specificity of these modalities to more accurately predict adverse events in the context of high-risk plaque.

Traditionally, scientists and clinicians have only been able to determine the molecular composition of some of the most devastating atherosclerotic plaques by observing and dissecting histological specimens. Currently this practice is changing. In the very near future, the possibility of performing high resolution imaging, both invasively and noninvasively, will allow us to effectively evaluate every component of an inflamed plaque in vivo. As it currently stands, we do possess the ability to invasively pursue certain plaques, but as we move along into the future, the practice will move towards acquisition of noninvasive mechanisms. Using noninvasive techniques and imaging modalities to determine which plaques have become significantly inflamed and unstable will allow the clinician to make real time decisions about what the next step should be to prevent an acute ischemic event.

Abbreviations

CT: Computed tomography
MRI: Magnetic resonance imaging
US: Ultrasound
PET: Positron emission tomography
SPECT: Single positron emission computed tomography
MR: Microwave radiometry
IVUS: Intravascular ultrasound
OCT: Optical coherence tomography
NIRS: Near infrared spectroscopy.

References

[1] A. J. Lusis, "Atherosclerosis," *Nature*, vol. 407, no. 6801, pp. 233–241, 2000.

[2] R. Ross, "The pathogenesis of atherosclerosis: a perspective for the 1990s," *Nature*, vol. 362, no. 6423, pp. 801–809, 1993.

[3] S. Sans, H. Kesteloot, and D. Kromhout, "The burden of cardiovascular diseases mortality in Europe: Task Force of the European Society of Cardiology on Cardiovascular Mortality and Morbidity Statistics in Europe," *European Heart Journal*, vol. 18, pp. 1231–1248, 1997.

[4] E. Falk, P. K. Shah, and V. Fuster, "Coronary plaque disruption," *Circulation*, vol. 92, no. 3, pp. 657–671, 1995.

[5] E. Falk, M. Nakano, J. F. Bentzon, A. V. Finn, and R. Virmani, "Update on acute coronary syndromes: the pathologists' view," *European Heart Journal*, vol. 34, no. 10, pp. 719–728, 2013.

[6] Z. A. Fayad and V. Fuster, "Clinical imaging of the high-risk or vulnerable atherosclerotic plaque," *Circulation Research*, vol. 89, no. 4, pp. 305–316, 2001.

[7] S. Waxman, F. Ishibashi, and J. E. Muller, "Detection and treatment of vulnerable plaques and vulnerable patients: novel approaches to prevention of coronary events," *Circulation*, vol. 114, no. 22, pp. 2390–2411, 2006.

[8] F. Moselewski, D. Ropers, K. Pohle et al., "Comparison of measurement of cross-sectional coronary atherosclerotic plaque and vessel areas by 16-slice multidetector computed tomography versus intravascular ultrasound," *The American Journal of Cardiology*, vol. 94, no. 10, pp. 1294–1297, 2004.

[9] S. Leschka, L. Husmann, L. M. Desbiolles et al., "Optimal image reconstruction intervals for non-invasive coronary angiography with 64-slice CT," *European Radiology*, vol. 16, no. 9, pp. 1964–1972, 2006.

[10] P. K. Vanhoenacker, M. H. Heijenbrok-Kal, R. Van Heste et al., "Diagnostic performance of multidetector CT angiography for assessment of coronary artery disease: meta-analysis," *Radiology*, vol. 244, no. 2, pp. 419–428, 2007.

[11] A. W. Leber, A. Knez, C. W. White et al., "Composition of coronary atherosclerotic plaques in patients with acute myocardial infarction and stable angina pectoris determined by contrast-enhanced multislice computed tomography," *American Journal of Cardiology*, vol. 91, no. 6, pp. 714–718, 2003.

[12] S. Motoyama, M. Sarai, H. Harigaya et al., "Computed tomographic angiography characteristics of atherosclerotic plaques subsequently resulting in acute coronary syndrome," *Journal of the American College of Cardiology*, vol. 54, no. 1, pp. 49–57, 2009.

[13] S. Ehara, Y. Kobayashi, M. Yoshiyama et al., "Spotty calcification typifies the culprit plaque in patients with acute myocardial infarction: an intravascular ultrasound study," *Circulation*, vol. 110, no. 22, pp. 3424–3429, 2004.

[14] A. J. Einstein and J. Knuuti, "Cardiac imaging: does radiation matter?" *European Heart Journal*, vol. 33, no. 5, pp. 573–578, 2012.

[15] A. J. Einstein, C. D. Elliston, A. E. Arai et al., "Radiation dose from single-heartbeat coronary CT angiography performed with a 320-detector row volume scanner," *Radiology*, vol. 254, no. 3, pp. 698–706, 2010.

[16] F. Hyafil, J.-C. Cornily, J. E. Feig et al., "Noninvasive detection of macrophages using a nanoparticulate contrast agent for computed tomography," *Nature Medicine*, vol. 13, no. 5, pp. 636–641, 2007.

[17] T. Luo, P. Huang, G. Gao et al., "Mesoporous silica-coated gold nanorods with embedded indocyanine green for dual mode X-ray CT and NIR fluorescence imaging," *Optics Express*, vol. 19, no. 18, pp. 17030–17039, 2011.

[18] H. Sun, Q. Yuan, B. Zhang, K. Ai, P. Zhang, and L. Lu, "Gd^{III} functionalized gold nanorods for multimodal imaging applications," *Nanoscale*, vol. 3, no. 5, pp. 1990–1996, 2011.

[19] Y. Xiao, H. Hong, V. Z. Matson et al., "Gold nanorods conjugated with doxorubicin and cRGD for combined anti-cancer drug delivery and PET imaging," *Theranostics*, vol. 2, no. 8, pp. 757–768, 2012.

[20] F. Hyafil, J.-C. Cornily, J. H. F. Rudd, J. Machac, L. J. Feldman, and Z. A. Fayad, "Quantification of inflammation within rabbit atherosclerotic plaques using the macrophage-specific CT contrast agent N1177: a comparison with ^{18}F-FDG PET/CT and histology," *Journal of Nuclear Medicine*, vol. 50, no. 6, pp. 959–965, 2009.

[21] K. Inoue, S. Motoyama, M. Sarai et al., "Serial coronary CT angiography-verified changes in plaque characteristics as an end point: evaluation of effect of statin intervention," *JACC: Cardiovascular Imaging*, vol. 3, no. 7, pp. 691–698, 2010.

[22] Z. A. Fayad, "The assessment of the vulnerable atherosclerotic plaque using MR imaging: a brief review," *International Journal of Cardiovascular Imaging*, vol. 17, no. 3, pp. 165–177, 2001.

[23] B. Chu, M. S. Ferguson, H. Underhill et al., "Detection of carotid atherosclerotic plaque ulceration, calcification, and thrombosis by multicontrast weighted magnetic resonance imaging," *Circulation*, vol. 112, no. 1, pp. e3–e4, 2005.

[24] C. Yuan, L. M. Mitsumori, K. W. Beach, and K. R. Maravilla, "Carotid atherosclerotic plaque: noninvasive MR characterization and identification of vulnerable lesions," *Radiology*, vol. 221, no. 2, pp. 285–299, 2001.

[25] C. Yuan, L. M. Mitsumori, M. S. Ferguson et al., "In vivo accuracy of multispectral magnetic resonance imaging for identifying lipid-rich necrotic cores and intraplaque hemorrhage in advanced human carotid plaques," *Circulation*, vol. 104, no. 17, pp. 2051–2056, 2001.

[26] A. R. Moody, R. E. Murphy, P. S. Morgan et al., "Characterization of complicated carotid plaque with magnetic resonance

direct thrombus imaging in patients with cerebral ischemia," *Circulation*, vol. 107, no. 24, pp. 3047–3052, 2003.

[27] J. Wang, M. S. Ferguson, N. Balu, C. Yuan, T. S. Hatsukami, and P. Bornert, "Improved carotid intraplaque hemorrhage imaging using a slab-selective phase-sensitive inversion-recovery (SPI) sequence," *Magnetic Resonance in Medicine*, vol. 64, no. 5, pp. 1332–1340, 2010.

[28] R. M. Kwee, R. J. van Oostenbrugge, M. H. Prins et al., "Symptomatic patients with mild and moderate carotid stenosis: plaque features at MRI and association with cardiovascular risk factors and statin use," *Stroke*, vol. 41, no. 7, pp. 1389–1393, 2010.

[29] L. M. Mitsumori, T. S. Hatsukami, M. S. Ferguson, W. S. Kerwin, J. Cai, and C. Yuan, "In vivo accuracy of multisequence MR imaging for identifying unstable fibrous caps in advanced human carotid plaques," *Journal of Magnetic Resonance Imaging*, vol. 17, no. 4, pp. 410–420, 2003.

[30] J. Bremerich, D. Bilecen, and P. Reimer, "MR angiography with blood pool contrast agents," *European Radiology*, vol. 17, no. 12, pp. 3017–3024, 2007.

[31] W. S. Kerwin, "Noninvasive imaging of plaque inflammation: role of contrast enhanced MRI," *Journal of the American College of Cardiovascular Imaging*, vol. 3, pp. 1136–1138, 2010.

[32] R. A. Trivedi, C. Mallawarachi, J.-M. U-King-Im et al., "Identifying inflamed carotid plaques using in vivo USPIO-enhanced MR imaging to label plaque macrophages," *Arteriosclerosis, Thrombosis, and Vascular Biology*, vol. 26, no. 7, pp. 1601–1606, 2006.

[33] T. Y. Tang, S. P. S. Howarth, S. R. Miller et al., "The ATHEROMA (atorvastatin therapy: effects on reduction of macrophage activity) study. Evaluation using ultrasmall superparamagnetic iron oxide-enhanced magnetic resonance imaging in carotid disease," *Journal of the American College of Cardiology*, vol. 53, no. 22, pp. 2039–2050, 2009.

[34] A. J. Degnan, A. J. Patterson, T. Y. Tang, S. P. S. Howarth, and J. H. Gillard, "Evaluation of ultrasmall superparamagnetic iron oxide-enhanced MRI of carotid atherosclerosis to assess risk of cerebrovascular and cardiovascular events: follow-up of the ATHEROMA trial," *Cerebrovascular Diseases*, vol. 34, no. 2, pp. 169–173, 2012.

[35] A. Phinikaridou, M. E. Andia, B. L. Plaza, P. Saha, A. Smith, and R. Botnar, "Increased vascular permeability is a surrogate marker of atherosclerotic plaque instability," *Journal of Cardiovascular Magnetic Resonance*, vol. 17, supplement 1, Article ID Q111, 2015.

[36] L. Esposito, T. Saam, P. Heider et al., "MRI plaque imaging reveals high-risk carotid plaques especially in diabetic patients irrespective of the degree of stenosis," *BMC Medical Imaging*, vol. 10, article no. 27, 2010.

[37] B. Widder, K. Paulat, J. Hackspacher et al., "Morphological characterization of carotid artery stenoses by ultrasound duplex scanning," *Ultrasound in Medicine & Biology*, vol. 16, no. 4, pp. 349–354, 1990.

[38] L. Saba, G. Caddeo, R. Sanfilippo, R. Montisci, and G. Mallarini, "CT and ultrasound in the study of ulcerated carotid plaque compared with surgical results: potentialities and advantages of multidetector row CT angiography," *American Journal of Neuroradiology*, vol. 28, no. 6, pp. 1061–1066, 2007.

[39] R. Kagawa, K. Moritake, T. Shima, and Y. Okada, "Validity of B-mode ultrasonographic findings in patients undergoing carotid endarterectomy in comparison with angiographic and clinicopathologic features," *Stroke*, vol. 27, no. 4, pp. 700–705, 1996.

[40] D. W. Droste, M. Karl, R. M. Bohle, and M. Kaps, "Comparison of ultrasonic and histopathological features of carotid artery stenosis," *Neurological Research*, vol. 19, no. 4, pp. 380–384, 1997.

[41] A. C. Gray-Weale, J. C. Graham, J. R. Burnett, K. Byrne, and R. J. Lusby, "Carotid artery atheroma: comparison of preoperative B-mode ultrasound appearance with carotid endarterectomy specimen pathology," *Journal of Cardiovascular Surgery*, vol. 29, no. 6, pp. 676–681, 1988.

[42] D. Staub, A. F. L. Schinkel, B. Coll et al., "Contrast-enhanced ultrasound imaging of the vasa vasorum: from early atherosclerosis to the identification of unstable plaques," *JACC: Cardiovascular Imaging*, vol. 3, no. 7, pp. 761–771, 2010.

[43] J. F. Granada and S. B. Feinstein, "Imaging of the vasa vasorum," *Nature Clinical Practice Cardiovascular Medicine*, vol. 5, supplement 2, pp. S18–S25, 2008.

[44] S. B. Feinstein, "The powerful microbubble: from bench to bedside, from intravascular indicator to therapeutic delivery system, and beyond," *The American Journal of Physiology—Heart and Circulatory Physiology*, vol. 287, no. 2, pp. H450–H457, 2004.

[45] O. Hjelmgren, L. Johansson, U. Prahl, C. Schmidt, J. Fredén-Lindqvist, and G. M. L. Bergström, "A study of plaque vascularization and inflammation using quantitative contrast-enhanced US and PET/CT," *European Journal of Radiology*, vol. 83, no. 7, pp. 1184–1189, 2014.

[46] Y. Kono, S. P. Pinnell, C. B. Sirlin et al., "Carotid arteries: contrast-enhanced US angiography—preliminary clinical experience," *Radiology*, vol. 230, pp. 561–568, 2004.

[47] J. H. F. Rudd, E. A. Warburton, T. D. Fryer et al., "Imaging atherosclerotic plaque inflammation with [^{18}F]-fluorodeoxyglucose positron emission tomography," *Circulation*, vol. 105, no. 23, pp. 2708–2711, 2002.

[48] J. H. F. Rudd, K. S. Myers, S. Bansilal et al., "^{18}Fluorodeoxyglucose positron emission tomography imaging of atherosclerotic plaque inflammation is highly reproducible: implications for atherosclerosis therapy trials," *Journal of the American College of Cardiology*, vol. 50, no. 9, pp. 892–896, 2007.

[49] P. G. Camici, O. E. Rimoldi, O. Gaemperli, and P. Libby, "Non-invasive anatomic and functional imaging of vascular inflammation and unstable plaque," *European Heart Journal*, vol. 33, no. 11, pp. 1309–1317, 2012.

[50] N. N. Mehta, D. A. Torigian, J. M. Gelfand, B. Saboury, and A. Alavi, "Quantification of atherosclerotic plaque activity and vascular inflammation using [18-F] fluorodeoxyglucose positron emission tomography/computed tomography (FDG-PET/CT)," *Journal of Visualized Experiments*, no. 63, Article ID e3777, 2012.

[51] N. Tahara, H. Kai, M. Ishibashi et al., "Simvastatin attenuates plaque inflammation: evaluation by fluorodeoxyglucose positron emission tomography," *Journal of the American College of Cardiology*, vol. 48, no. 9, pp. 1825–1831, 2006.

[52] J. Wykrzykowska, S. Lehman, G. Williams et al., "Imaging of inflamed and vulnerable plaque in coronary arteries with ^{18}F-FDG PET/CT in patients with suppression of myocardial uptake using a low-carbohydrate, high-fat preparation," *Journal of Nuclear Medicine*, vol. 50, no. 4, pp. 563–568, 2009.

[53] S. S. Silvera, H. E. Aidi, J. H. F. Rudd et al., "Multimodality imaging of atherosclerotic plaque activity and composition using FDG-PET/CT and MRI in carotid and femoral arteries," *Atherosclerosis*, vol. 207, no. 1, pp. 139–143, 2009.

[54] E. M. Laufer, M. H. M. Winkens, M. F. Corsten, C. P. M. Reutelingsperger, J. Narula, and L. Hofstra, "PET and SPECT

imaging of apoptosis in vulnerable atherosclerotic plaques with radiolabeled Annexin A5," *The Quarterly Journal of Nuclear Medicine and Molecular Imaging*, vol. 53, no. 1, pp. 26–34, 2009.

[55] S. Ishino, T. Mukai, Y. Kuge et al., "Targeting of lectinlike oxidized low-density lipoprotein receptor 1 (LOX-1) with 99mTc-labeled anti-LOX-1 antibody: potential agent for imaging of vulnerable plaque," *Journal of Nuclear Medicine*, vol. 49, no. 10, pp. 1677–1685, 2008.

[56] D. Li, A. R. Patel, A. L. Klibanov et al., "Molecular imaging of atherosclerotic plaques targeted to oxidized LDL receptor LOX-1 by SPECT/CT and magnetic resonance," *Circulation: Cardiovascular Imaging*, vol. 3, no. 4, pp. 464–472, 2010.

[57] D. Hartung, M. Sarai, A. Petrov et al., "Resolution of apoptosis in atherosclerotic plaque by dietary modification and statin therapy," *Journal of Nuclear Medicine*, vol. 46, no. 12, pp. 2051–2056, 2005.

[58] M. Elkhawad and J. H. F. Rudd, "Radiotracer imaging of atherosclerotic plaque biology," *Cardiology Clinics*, vol. 27, no. 2, pp. 345–354, 2009.

[59] A. H. Barrett, P. C. Myers, and N. L. Sadowsky, "Microwave thermography in the detection of breast cancer," *American Journal of Roentgenology*, vol. 134, no. 2, pp. 365–368, 1980.

[60] J. Shaeffer, A. M. El-Mahdi, and K. L. Carr, "Cancer detection studies using a 4.7 Gigahertz radiometer," *Cancer Detection and Prevention*, vol. 4, no. 1–4, pp. 571–578, 1981.

[61] K. Toutouzas, A. Synetos, C. Nikolaou, K. Stathogiannis, E. Tsiamis, and C. Stefanadis, "Microwave radiometry: a new noninvasive method for the detection of vulnerable plaque," *Cardiovascular Diagnosis and Therapy*, vol. 2, no. 4, pp. 290–297, 2012.

[62] K. Toutouzas, C. Grassos, M. Drakopoulou et al., "First in vivo application of microwave radiometry in human carotids: a new noninvasive method for detection of local inflammatory activation," *Journal of the American College of Cardiology*, vol. 59, no. 18, pp. 1645–1653, 2012.

[63] G. A. Beller, "Imaging of vulnerable plaques: will it affect patient management and influence outcomes?" *Journal of Nuclear Cardiology*, vol. 18, no. 4, pp. 531–533, 2011.

[64] A. Nair, B. D. Kuban, E. M. Tuzcu, P. Schoenhagen, S. E. Nissen, and D. G. Vince, "Coronary plaque classification with intravascular ultrasound radiofrequency data analysis," *Circulation*, vol. 106, no. 17, pp. 2200–2206, 2002.

[65] S. E. Nissen and P. Yock, "Intravascular ultrasound: novel pathophysiological insights and current clinical applications," *Circulation*, vol. 103, no. 4, pp. 604–616, 2001.

[66] J. Layland, A. M. Wilson, I. Lim, and R. J. Whitbourn, "Virtual histology: a window to the heart of atherosclerosis," *Heart Lung and Circulation*, vol. 20, no. 10, pp. 615–621, 2011.

[67] M. Yamagishi, M. Terashima, K. Awano et al., "Morphology of vulnerable coronary plaque: insights from follow-up of patients examined by intravascular ultrasound before an acute coronary syndrome," *Journal of the American College of Cardiology*, vol. 35, no. 1, pp. 106–111, 2000.

[68] G. A. Rodriguez-Granillo, E. P. Mc Fadden, J. Aoki et al., "In vivo variability in quantitative coronary ultrasound and tissue characterization measurements with mechanical and phased-array catheters," *International Journal of Cardiovascular Imaging*, vol. 22, no. 1, pp. 47–53, 2006.

[69] J.-F. Surmely, K. Nasu, H. Fujita et al., "Coronary plaque composition of culprit/target lesions according to the clinical presentation: a virtual histology intravascular ultrasound analysis," *European Heart Journal*, vol. 27, no. 24, pp. 2939–2944, 2006.

[70] A. Nair, B. D. Kuban, N. Obuchowski, and D. G. Vince, "Assessing spectral algorithms to predict atherosclerotic plaque composition with normalized and raw intravascular ultrasound data," *Ultrasound in Medicine & Biology*, vol. 27, no. 10, pp. 1319–1331, 2001.

[71] R. Virmani, A. P. Burke, A. Farb, and F. D. Kolodgie, "Pathology of the vulnerable plaque," *Journal of the American College of Cardiology*, vol. 47, no. 8, pp. C13–C18, 2006.

[72] R. Virmani, F. D. Kolodgie, A. P. Burke, A. Farb, and S. M. Schwartz, "Lessons from sudden coronary death: a comprehensive morphological classification scheme for atherosclerotic lesions," *Arteriosclerosis, Thrombosis, and Vascular Biology*, vol. 20, no. 5, pp. 1262–1275, 2000.

[73] G. A. Rodriguez-Granillo, H. M. García-García, E. P. Mc Fadden et al., "In vivo intravascular ultrasound-derived thin-cap fibroatheroma detection using ultrasound radiofrequency data analysis," *Journal of the American College of Cardiology*, vol. 46, no. 11, pp. 2038–2042, 2005.

[74] M. Vavuranakis, I. A. Kakadiaris, S. M. O'Malley et al., "A new method for assessment of plaque vulnerability based on vasa vasorum imaging, by using contrast-enhanced intravascular ultrasound and differential image analysis," *International Journal of Cardiology*, vol. 130, no. 1, pp. 23–29, 2008.

[75] I.-K. Jang, B. E. Bouma, D.-H. Kang et al., "Visualization of coronary atherosclerotic plaques in patients using optical coherence tomography: comparison with intravascular ultrasound," *Journal of the American College of Cardiology*, vol. 39, no. 4, pp. 604–609, 2002.

[76] T. Kubo, T. Imanishi, S. Takarada et al., "Implication of plaque color classification for assessing plaque vulnerability: a coronary angioscopy and optical coherence tomography investigation," *JACC: Cardiovascular Interventions*, vol. 1, no. 1, pp. 74–80, 2008.

[77] I.-K. Jang, G. J. Tearney, B. MacNeill et al., "In vivo characterization of coronary atherosclerotic plaque by use of optical coherence tomography," *Circulation*, vol. 111, no. 12, pp. 1551–1555, 2005.

[78] T. Kume, T. Akasaka, T. Kawamoto et al., "Measurement of the thickness of the fibrous cap by optical coherence tomography," *American Heart Journal*, vol. 152, no. 4, pp. 755.e1–755.e4, 2006.

[79] B. D. MacNeill, I.-K. Jang, B. E. Bouma et al., "Focal and multifocal plaque macrophage distributions in patients with acute and stable presentations of coronary artery disease," *Journal of the American College of Cardiology*, vol. 44, no. 5, pp. 972–979, 2004.

[80] M. Mizukoshi, T. Imanishi, A. Tanaka et al., "Clinical classification and plaque morphology determined by optical coherence tomography in unstable angina pectoris," *American Journal of Cardiology*, vol. 106, no. 3, pp. 323–328, 2010.

[81] K. A. Kelly, J. R. Allport, A. Tsourkas, V. R. Shinde-Patil, L. Josephson, and R. Weissleder, "Detection of vascular adhesion molecule-1 expression using a novel multimodal nanoparticle," *Circulation Research*, vol. 96, no. 3, pp. 327–336, 2005.

[82] B.-X. Chen, F.-Y. Ma, W. Luo et al., "Characterization of atherosclerotic plaque in patients with unstable angina pectoris and stable angina pectoris by optical coherence tomography," *Zhonghua Xin Xue Guan Bing Za Zhi*, vol. 37, no. 5, pp. 422–425, 2009.

[83] T. Kubo and T. Akasaka, "OCT-ready for prime time? Clinical applications of optical coherence tomography," *Cardiac Interventions Today*, vol. 4, pp. 35–37, 2009.

[84] J.-F. Toussaint, J. F. Southern, V. Fuster, and H. L. Kantor, "Water diffusion properties of human atherosclerosis and thrombosis measured by pulse field gradient nuclear magnetic resonance," *Arteriosclerosis, Thrombosis, and Vascular Biology*, vol. 17, no. 3, pp. 542–546, 1997.

[85] J. Schneiderman, R. L. Wilensky, A. Weiss et al., "Diagnosis of thin-cap fibroatheromas by a self-contained intravascular magnetic resonance imaging probe in ex vivo human aortas and in situ coronary arteries," *Journal of the American College of Cardiology*, vol. 45, no. 12, pp. 1961–1969, 2005.

[86] E. Larose, S. Kinlay, A. P. Selwyn et al., "Improved characterization of atherosclerotic plaques by gadolinium contrast during intravascular magnetic resonance imaging of human arteries," *Atherosclerosis*, vol. 196, no. 2, pp. 919–925, 2008.

[87] J. Wang, Y.-J. Geng, B. Guo et al., "Near-infrared spectroscopic characterization of human advanced atherosclerotic plaques," *Journal of the American College of Cardiology*, vol. 39, no. 8, pp. 1305–1313, 2002.

[88] P. R. Moreno, R. A. Lodder, K. R. Purushothaman, W. E. Charash, W. N. O'Connor, and J. E. Muller, "Detection of lipid pool, thin fibrous cap, and inflammatory cells in human aortic atherosclerotic plaques by near-infrared spectroscopy," *Circulation*, vol. 105, no. 8, pp. 923–927, 2002.

17

MR Micro-Neurography and a Segmentation Protocol Applied to Diabetic Neuropathy

P. F. Felisaz,[1] G. Maugeri,[1] V. Busi,[1] R. Vitale,[1] F. Balducci,[1] S. Gitto,[2] P. Leporati,[3] A. Pichiecchio,[4] M. Baldi,[5] F. Calliada,[1,6] L. Chiovato,[3] and S. Bastianello[4,7]

[1]*Radiology Department, University of Pavia, Pavia, Italy*
[2]*Postgraduation School in Radiodiagnostics, Università degli Studi di Milano, Milan, Italy*
[3]*Unit of Internal Medicine and Endocrinology, IRCCS Salvatore Maugeri Foundation, Scientific Institute of Pavia, Pavia, Italy*
[4]*Neuroradiology Department, C. Mondino National Neurological Institute, Pavia, Italy*
[5]*Radiology Department, IRCCS Salvatore Maugeri Foundation, Scientific Institute of Pavia, Pavia, Italy*
[6]*Institute of Radiology, IRCCS Fondazione Policlinico San Matteo, Pavia, Italy*
[7]*Department of Brain and Behavioral Sciences, University of Pavia, Pavia, Italy*

Correspondence should be addressed to P. F. Felisaz; paulfel@hotmail.it

Academic Editor: Rod Scott

The aim of this study was to assess with MRI morphometric ultrastructural changes in nerves affected by diabetic peripheral neuropathy (DPN). We used an MR micro-neurography imaging protocol and a semiautomated technique of tissue segmentation to visualize and measure the volume of internal nerve components, such as the epineurium and nerve fascicles. The tibial nerves of 16 patients affected by DPN and of 15 healthy volunteers were imaged. Nerves volume (NV), fascicles volume (FV), fascicles to nerve ratio (FNR), and nerves cross-sectional areas (CSA) were obtained. In patients with DPN the NV was increased and the FNR was decreased, as a result of an increase of the epineurium (FNR in diabetic neuropathy 0,665; in controls 0,699, $p = 0,040$). CSA was increased in subjects with DPN (12,84 mm^2 versus 10,22 mm^2, $p = 0,003$). The FV was increased in patients with moderate to severe DPN. We have demonstrated structural changes occurring in nerves affected by DPN, which otherwise are assessable only with an invasive biopsy. MR micro-neurography appears to be suitable for the study of microscopic changes in tibial nerves of diabetic patients.

1. Introduction

Diabetic peripheral neuropathy (DPN) affects approximately 50% of patients with long-standing type 1 or type 2 diabetes. The onset of DPN is related to the duration of diabetes, the levels of hyperglycemia, and additional risk factors such as smoking, high body mass index (BMI), and hypertension [1]. Symmetric distal polyneuropathy is the most common form of diabetic neuropathy, typically occurring first in the lower extremities and then extending upward with proximal progression. Symptoms include motor impairment such as weakness and clumsiness of movement and sensory loss with a "glove and stocking" pattern of distribution. Tenderness, dysesthesia, numbness, tingling, burning, sharp pain, and neuropathic pain may also be present, but about 50% of the patients remain asymptomatic [2–4].

In common practice, the diagnosis of DPN is based on physical examination and electrophysiology. Physical examination should include simple standardized tests such as the Quantitative Sensory Testing (QST) that explores touch-pressure, vibration (by tuning fork), coolness and warmth, pain (pinprick test), and evaluation of the ankle jerk reflex. Electrophysiology studies are more sensitive and provide quantitative information, but they are limited by interrater variability and lack of standardized techniques [5]. More invasive tests include skin biopsy and sural nerve biopsy. Skin biopsy with intraepidermal nerve fiber density (IENFD) measurements may provide additional information at earlier stages, since the small sensory fibers are the first to be involved [6]. Both metabolic and ischemic factors are involved in the disruption of small fibers, which directly mediate the neuropathic pain. In advanced stages blood flow alterations and inflammation may lead to foot ulceration and amputation [7]. The sural nerve biopsy is less frequently required but may help in the differential diagnosis with other types of neuropathy [8]. Nerve biopsies in diabetic subjects show thickening of the base membrane, degeneration of pericytes, and endothelial cell hyperplasia, secondary to microvascular disease [9]. The inflammatory response is localized around the vessels of epineurium and perineurium [10]. In both symmetric and asymmetric neuropathy axonal degeneration is associated with nerve fascicles atrophy and fatty infiltration of the epineurium [11].

Magnetic resonance imaging (MRI) is a noninvasive technique with promising applications for the study of neuropathies. The several techniques already used in common practice, or still in their development stage, are known under the name of MR neurography. Typical protocols include high-resolution axial planes of the nerve trunks based on conventional turbo-spin echo sequences, T1 and fluid-sensitive weighting with fat suppression obtained with chemical shift selective pulses (CHESS), inversion recovery (STIR), or the Dixon method [12]. Interpretation of MR neurography is based on signal changes and nerve enlargement. Typically, the affected nerve displays an increased overall T2 signal, reflecting the presence of edema, hyperemia, or increased cellularity [13]. However, subtle changes are difficult to detect, and the lack of spatial resolution does not allow a clear-cut separation of the internal nerve components, which may be distinctly and differently damaged. Further issues are related to the variable orientation of the nerve along its course, which may lead to partial volume effects and magic angle artifacts, secondary to the anisotropic architecture of the nerve fibers [14].

MR microscopic techniques are less commonly reported but may play a role in this field. MR micro-neurography is a developing technique that pushes ahead the limits of spatial resolution, still using clinical high field scanners and surface coils. Within a smaller field of view it is possible to visualize anatomical details, such as the epineurium, the perineurium, and single fascicles, which otherwise would require a biopsy to be detected [15, 16].

There are detailed morphometric studies demonstrating increased fascicular area in nerves with DPN [17] as perineurial sheath expansion due to increased perineurial lamellar area and interlamellar space [18]. Previous studies have described as well endoneurial and epineurial alterations due to microvascular damage [19] and thickening of the epineurial sheath due to increased amount of connective tissue [20].

Since MR micro-neurography is capable of depicting some components of the internal nerve architecture, the aim of our study was to assess micro-structural changes in nerves affected by DPN. We have examined the nerve volume (NV), fascicle volume (FV), epineurial volume (EV), fascicles to nerve volume ratio (FNR), and nerve cross-sectional areas (CSA), comparing a population of subjects affected by DPN with a group of sex/age matched healthy volunteers. We

have then assessed correlations of these parameters with the severity of neuropathy.

2. Materials and Methods

2.1. Patients. The procedures carried out in this study were in accordance with the ethical standards of the World Medical Association (Declaration of Helsinki). The ethical committee of our institution approved the study and examinations were performed after the acquisition of an informed consent from every subject. Inclusion criteria were as follows: age between 25 and 75 years, diagnosis of diabetes mellitus at least 5 years ago, and symmetric distal polyneuropathy confirmed by abnormal nerve conduction study. Exclusion criteria were as follows: unilateral neuropathy, compressive or posttraumatic radiculopathy, or the presence of other conditions that might be responsible for the neuropathy. Poor quality examinations were also excluded from the study after imaging acquisition (one subject was finally excluded due to the presence of obvious artifacts). The final study population included 16 patients (11 men and 5 women, age range 50–72, mean 60,9, and standard deviation 7,9). The severity of DPN was assessed using the revised Neuropathy Disability Score (NDS) [21] and two subgroups were created: mild neuropathy (NDS < 6) or moderate/severe neuropathy (NDS ≥ 6). We finally had 6 subjects with mild DPN and 10 with moderate/severe DPN. 15 healthy volunteers matched by age and sex (10 men and 5 women, age range 41–70, mean 54,9, and standard deviation 9,1) were evaluated by MRI as a control group.

2.2. Imaging Protocol. All images were acquired on a Discovery MR750 3 T scanner (GE Healthcare, Milwaukee, USA) [22] using a 6-channel carotid array coil, adapted for the study of the ankle region. The examinations were focused on the study of the tibial nerve at the medial aspect of the ankle, right above the tibial malleolus. Both sides were imaged in every subject. The protocol included a 3D SPGR sequence with standard fat suppression, short acquisition time (1-2 minutes), and anatomical coverage including the complete ankle region. Multiplanar reconstruction was used to select a perpendicular plane to the main axis of the tibial nerve and orient the next sequences. The second sequence was applied with a field of view located approximately 2 centimeters above the medial malleolus in a straight tract of the nerve, in order to obtain axial images to the nerve, minimizing partial volume effects. We used a higher resolution 3D SPGR with IDEAL (iterative decomposition of water and fat with echo asymmetry and least-squares estimation GE Healthcare, Milwaukee, USA) with an axial field of view of 5 × 5 cm and a longitudinal coverage of 2.8 cm. Details on the parameters that we used are listed in Table 1.

2.3. Postprocessing. One examiner performed the postprocessing blinded to the name of the subjects and their group (controls or neuropathic). The segmentation process used in the present study has been validated in a previous work [16]. The "in phase" and the "water" set of images were from the four sets obtained with the IDEAL sequence ("water," "fat," "in phase," and "out of phase").

TABLE 1: Parameters of the MR sequences.

	Localizer	Fluid sensitive HR	Fat sensitive HR	T1-weighted HR
Type	3D SPGR	3D SPGR IDEAL	3D SPGR IDEAL	2D FSE
TR (ms)	5,9	16,9	16,9	650
TE (ms)	Min	Min	Min	Min
Flip angle	10	10	10	90
FOV (cm)	8	6	6	6
Acquisition matrix	128×128	512×420	512×420	512×416
Number of slices	128	20	20	11
Slice thickness (mm)	2	2	2	2
Gap (mm)	0	0	0	1
ETL	—	—	—	5
NEX	1	1	1	3
BW (KHz)	15	35	35	31
Fat sup.	Yes	No	No	No

The operator manually outlined the tibial nerve in every axial image (in total 14 slices) into all the "in phase" images, using the proprietary software JIM (Xinapse Systems Ltd, Essex, UK). On these images the external epineurial sheath was hypointense over a hyperintense background and served as a reliable segmentation border. This region of interest was then applied to the corresponding "water" image. In the "water" set of images, the fascicles and the perineurium appeared hyperintense and we assumed that the overall fascicle volume would be hyperintense over a dark background including the epineurial collagen and fat. Segmentation was performed with FAST (FMRIB Automated Segmentation Tool, Analysis Group, Oxford, UK) with a two-class algorithm based on signal and spatial intensity variation. This technique separated the hyperintense voxels (considered the fascicles) from the hypointense voxels (considered the epineurium). We obtained measurements of the fascicles volume (FV), epineurial volume (EV), and total nerve volume (NV). Then we calculated the fascicles to nerve ratio (FNR). We measured the nerve CSA with OsiriX (Pixmeo, Geneva, Switzerland), manually outlining the boundaries of the nerve and calculating the mean of three measurements at three random levels of the tibial nerve.

2.4. *Statistical Analysis.* Statistical analysis was performed with SPSS (IBM Corp., Armonk, NY, USA). Homogeneity of the groups was investigated using an independent sample T-test. The means of the NV, EV, FNR, and CSA were compared using an independent sample T-test. Differences between subgroups of neuropathy were tested using the two-tailed Mann–Whitney U test. Pearson correlation coefficient was used to assess relationships between NV, FV, FNR, CSA, and age.

3. Results

Subjects with DPN controls were found to be fairly similar for number (16 cases, 15 controls) and gender (11 men and 5 women in the DPN group, 10 men and 5 women in the healthy group). T-test for independent samples showed that age and sex distribution were not significantly different between the two groups.

The acquired images demonstrated the neurovascular bundle of the tibial nerve at the level of the ankle, right above the tibial malleolus. The IDEAL sequence provided a four-set images: "water," "fat," "in phase," and "out of phase." The "fat" images and the TSE T1 allowed a better depiction of the intraepineurial fat, with poorer contrast between the fascicles (Figure 1). The "water" images allowed the best characterization of internal nerve aspects: the fascicles appeared bright over a dark background corresponding to epineurium. The perineurium was a very thin hyperintense rim surrounding the fascicles and it was inconstantly visualized since affected by partial volume effects that limited the spatial resolution. Therefore perineurium segmentation was not reliable and this data was not collected (Figure 2). A visual increase of the epineurium as compared with the fascicles was seen in some DPN nerves, as shown in Figures 3(A)-3(B).

The volumes measured with the segmentation technique are listed in Table 2. The total NV (considering 2.8 cm in the longitudinal axis of acquisition) was significantly higher in nerves with DPN than controls (361.9 versus 286.9 mm^3, $p = 0.028$) (Figure 4, Table 2). FV was also increased in patients with DPN, but the difference did not reach statistical significance. On the other hand, the FNR was significantly lower in DPN than controls (DPN 0,665, controls 0,699; $p = 0,040$). CSA was significantly higher in DPN than in the healthy group (12,84 versus 10,22 mm^2, $p = 0,003$).

Considering the subgroups on neuropathy, a statistical significant increase in NV and FV was only observed between the control group and the moderate/severe neuropathy. Similarly, the FNR was statistically decreased only between the control group and the moderate/severe neuropathy. CSA was significantly increased between the control and the mild neuropathy and between control and moderate/severe neuropathy, but not between mild and moderate/severe neuropathy (Table 3).

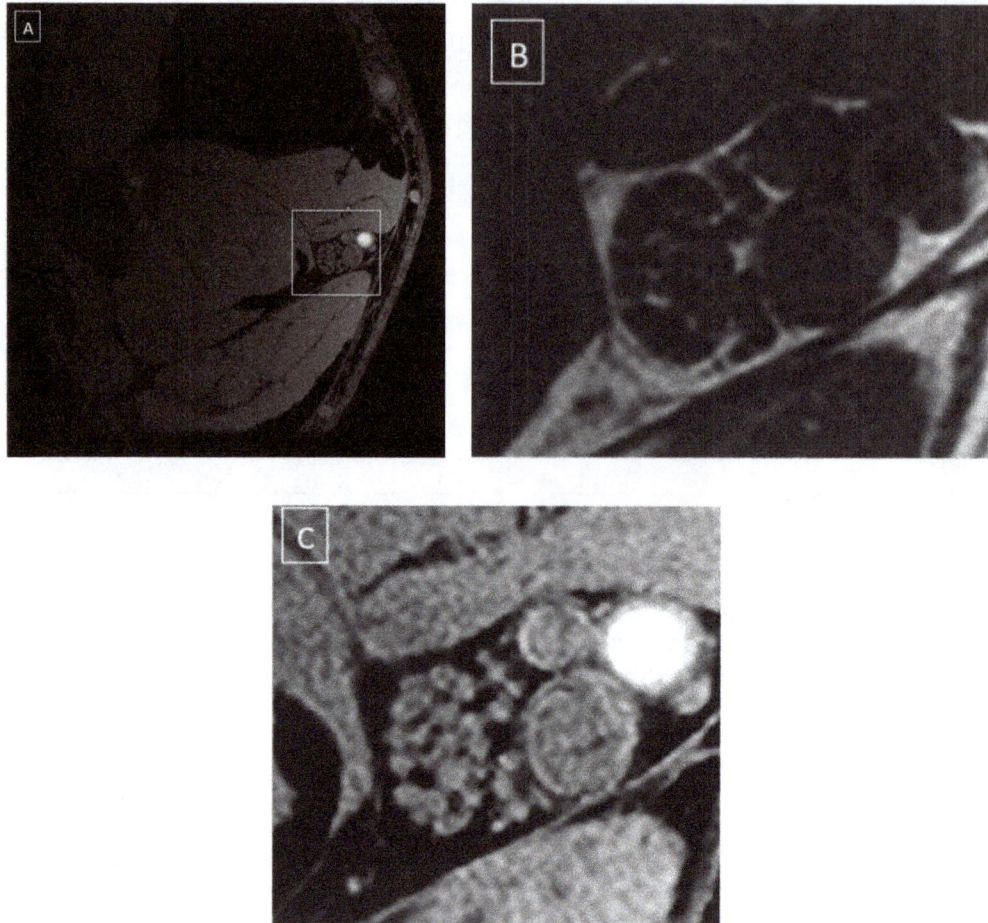

FIGURE 1: (A) Ankle, axial plane. Sequence: 3D SPGR IDEAL-water image. (B) Neurovascular bundle with the tibial nerve. Sequence: TSE T1 weighted. The nerve fascicles appear dark over a brighter background, corresponding to the epineurial fat. (C) Sequence: 3D SPGR-water image. The fascicles appear bright over a dark background corresponding to the epineurium. The perineurium can be seen surrounding some of the fascicles (see Figure 2).

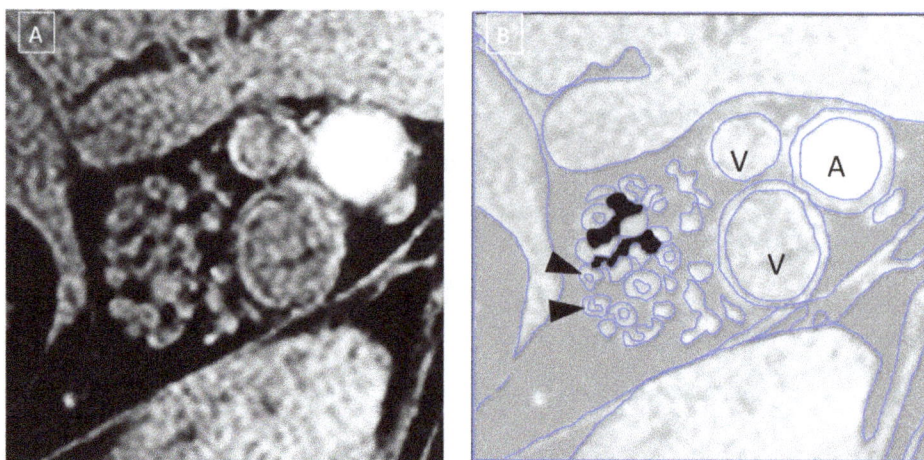

FIGURE 2: (A) Tibial nerve right above the level of the tibial malleolus, axial plane. Sequence: 3D SPGR IDEAL-water image. Voxel size is about $120 \times 140 \times 2000$ μm. (B) Diagram of the internal nerve aspect that is visualized. Arrowheads: two fascicles surrounded by the perineurium. Dark areas: epineurium. A: posterior tibial artery. V: posterior tibial veins.

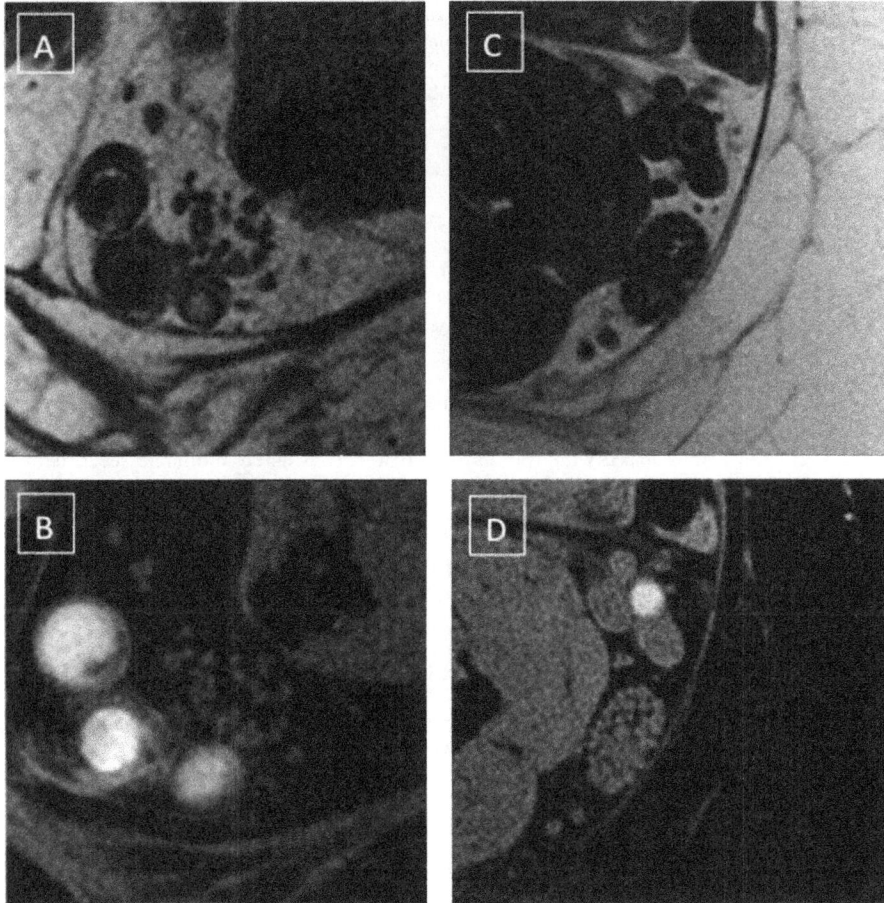

FIGURE 3: Tibial nerve with chronic degenerative changes (left (A, B)) compared with a volunteer (right (C, D)). The patient was in the group of the moderate/severe DPN and suffered from chronic pain and severe motor impairment. (A, C) Sequence: TSE T1. (B, D) Sequence: IDEAL-WATER. There is a visual increase of the interfascicular tissue (epineurium), while the fascicles appear reduced in number and area. Increase of fat and fibrous tissue within the epineurium is common in chronic stage of diabetic neuropathy.

No statistical significant correlation was found between age, sex, and the parameters NV, FV, FNR, and CSA.

4. Discussion

The MR technique described in the present study allowed the investigation of some internal nerve components such as the FV, EV, and FNR that are not usually detected using conventional MR neurography. In subjects with diabetic neuropathy the NV and the CSA were increased while the FNR was decreased. CSA is a well-known parameter that may be increased in some neuropathies such as diabetic [23]. FNR instead is a novel parameter that indicates changes within the nerve (e.g., reduction in nerve fascicles), adjusted for the nerve volume and thus more independent from typical sources of intersubject variability such as body weight and height.

We observed also an increase of the FV, but statistical significance was only observed between controls and patients with moderate/severe neuropathy. This observation is in agreement with previous morphometric studies [17].

The decrease of the FNR in patients with DPN may be interpreted as a net increase of the epineurial fraction (EV). Also these results are in agreement with histopathology [20, 24]. Chronic damage secondary to long-standing diabetes results in fascicles atrophy and axonal degeneration, fibrous connective tissue proliferation, and fat accumulation. These nerve alterations eventually lead to a thickening of the epineurial layer.

The perineurium, a hyperintense rim surrounding the nerve fascicles, was inconstantly seen and was not considered as a parameter in the present study, although a thickening of the perineurial sheath would be expected in DPN.

The role of imaging in DPN is limited, but it might be useful when clinical examination or conduction studies are inconclusive. Diagnostic application fields might be the occurrence of one-side symptoms dominance, a pattern of distribution affecting a single nerve territory, or a rapidly progressive neuropathy. One of the main indications of MRI is the exclusion of a mass or a thickening of osteofibrous tunnels that may cause hindering and compression of the nerve. T2 signal is one parameter commonly used to assess

TABLE 2: Comparison of parameters between subjects with diabetic neuropathy and controls. Data is expressed in mean ± SEM. Bold characters are used to enhance statistical significance. DPN = diabetic peripheral neuropathy. NV = mean of the nerve volumes (for a length of 28 mm). FV = mean of the fascicles volumes (for a length of 28 mm). FNR = fascicles to nerve ratio. CSA = mean of the cross-sectional areas. There is statistical difference ($p < 0,05$) in NV, FNR, and CSA between subjects with diabetic neuropathy and controls.

	DPN	Controls	p	Confidence interval (95%)	
				Inferior	Superior
NV (mm³)	361.85 ± 26.3	286.87 ± 18.0	**0.028**	−141.1	−8.87
FV (mm³)	239.12 ± 16.8	198.4 ± 12.8	0.065	−84.21	2.78
FNR	0.666 ± 0.011	0.699 ± 0.011	**0.040**	0.002	0.064
CSA (mm²)	12.84 ± 0.72	10.22 ± 0.45	**0.003**	−4.374	−0.854

TABLE 3: Test between the control group and the two subgroups of diabetic neuropathy. All data are expressed in mean ± SEM. All patients included in the diabetic neuropathy group had abnormal nerve conduction studies. Subjects with a neuropathy disability score of less than 6 points were considered "mild neuropathy," and subjects with 6 points or more were considered "moderate/severe neuropathy." Bold characters are used to enhance statistical significance. N.S. = Nonsignificant.

	Nondiabetic (A)	Mild neuropathy (B)	Moderate/severe (C)	A versus B	B versus C	A versus C
NV	286.8 ± 18.0	326.7 ± 48.4	383.0 ± 30.6	N.S.	N.S.	**<0.01**
FV	198.4 ± 12.8	218.7 ± 29.7	251.4 ± 20.3	N.S.	N.S.	**<0.03**
FNR	0.699 ± 0.011	0.677 ± 0.018	0.659 ± 0.014	N.S.	N.S.	**<0.03**
CSA	10.22 ± 0.45	12.62 ± 1.27	12.97 ± 0.91	**<0.04**	N.S.	**<0.01**

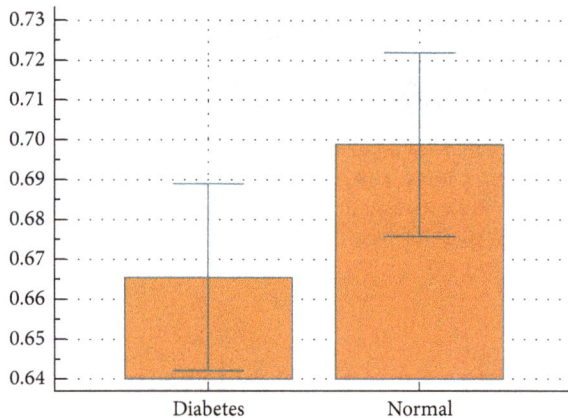

FIGURE 4: Data comparison graph for FNR in subjects with diabetic neuropathy (indicated with "diabetes") and controls (indicated with "normal"). There is a significant difference between the two populations. For more details see Table 2.

nerve damage since increased intensity may reflect axonal degeneration and the presence of fluid within the fascicles and the interstitium [25]. T2 quantification has been used to identify nerve damage in DPN and to track it along the nerve course, showing alterations predominant at the proximal thighs rather than distal legs [26]. However, segmentation of the volume of fascicles and of epineurium may provide more detailed information, for example, which of the internal nerve compartment is enlarged, whether the epineurium is thickened, and whether the fascicles are swelling or atrophic.

Limitations of the present study may be as follows. FSL FAST is routinely used as a brain segmentation tool but it has seldom applications outside the brain; as for brain plaques quantification, the described nerve segmentation technique shares similar limitations, such as spatial resolution, contrast resolution, and signal to noise ratio. Improvement of MRI technologies is likely to lead to better image quality with easier distinction of the internal nerve components. Second, we have analyzed the tibial nerve and not the sural nerve, although only the latter has been commonly subject to biopsy. We used the tibial nerve since it is easier to study with our technique. Compared to the sural nerve, the tibial nerve has a greater fascicular area (2 to 4 times), increasing the signal to noise ratio and providing best results of segmentation.

This study focused on the MRI signs of chronic neuropathy. However the development of techniques that might recognize early neuropathic changes in diabetic patients is crucial, because it might impact the course of the disease. First, nondiabetes-related neuropathies may be discovered, some of which can be treated. In addition, there is a variety of treatment options for symptomatic DPN that, even though not altering the underlying disease or the natural history of diabetes, may positively impact the quality of life of these patients.

In conclusion, MR micro-neurography was able to show chronic changes occurring in nerves affected by DPN. In the future, the development of more accurate MRI protocols might replace invasive biopsies, allowing early detection of the disease and supporting the follow-up and the response to therapy.

Abbreviations

BMI: Body mass index
QST: Quantitative Sensory Testing

IENFD: Intraepidermal nerve fiber density
MRI: Magnetic resonance imaging
EV: Epineurial volume
FV: Fascicles volume
NV: Nerve volume
FNR: Fascicles to nerve volumes ratio
CSA: Cross-sectional area
SPGR: Spoiled gradient echo
IDEAL: Iterative decomposition of water and fat with echo asymmetry and least-squares estimation
FAST: FMRIB Automated Segmentation Tool.

Competing Interests

The authors declare that they have no conflict of interests regarding the publication of this paper.

References

[1] E. Adeghate, P. Schattner, and E. Dunn, "An update on the etiology and epidemiology of diabetes mellitus," *Annals of the New York Academy of Sciences*, vol. 1084, pp. 1–29, 2006.

[2] M. Davies, S. Brophy, R. Williams, and A. Taylor, "The prevalence, severity, and impact of painful diabetic peripheral neuropathy in type 2 diabetes," *Diabetes Care*, vol. 29, no. 7, pp. 1518–1522, 2006.

[3] M. Pasnoor, M. M. Dimachkie, P. Kluding, and R. J. Barohn, "Diabetic neuropathy part 1: overview and symmetric phenotypes," *Neurologic Clinics*, vol. 31, no. 2, pp. 425–445, 2013.

[4] S. Tesfaye, "Recent advances in the management of diabetic distal symmetrical polyneuropathy," *Journal of Diabetes Investigation*, vol. 2, no. 1, pp. 33–42, 2011.

[5] P. J. Dyck, J. W. Albers, J. Wolfe et al., "A trial of proficiency of nerve conduction: greater standardization still needed," *Muscle and Nerve*, vol. 48, no. 3, pp. 369–374, 2013.

[6] M. E. Shy, E. M. Frohman, Y. T. So et al., "Quantitative sensory testing: report of the therapeutics and technology assessment subcommittee of the American academy of neurology," *Neurology*, vol. 60, no. 6, pp. 898–904, 2003.

[7] P. C. Johnson, S. C. Doll, and D. W. Cromey, "Pathogenesis of diabetic neuropathy," *Annals of Neurology*, vol. 19, no. 5, pp. 450–457, 1986.

[8] C. J. Sumner, S. Sheth, J. W. Griffin, D. R. Cornblath, and M. Polydefkis, "The spectrum of neuropathy in diabetes and impaired glucose tolerance," *Neurology*, vol. 60, no. 1, pp. 108–111, 2003.

[9] F. Behse, F. Buchthal, and F. Carlsen, "Nerve biopsy and conduction studies in diabetic neuropathy," *Journal of Neurology, Neurosurgery and Psychiatry*, vol. 40, no. 11, pp. 1072–1082, 1977.

[10] D. S. Younger, "Diabetic neuropathy: a clinical and neuropathological study of 107 patients," *Neurology Research International*, vol. 2010, Article ID 140379, 4 pages, 2010.

[11] G. Said, "Diabetic neuropathy—a review," *Nature Clinical Practice Neurology*, vol. 3, no. 6, pp. 331–340, 2007.

[12] W. T. Dixon, "Simple proton spectroscopic imaging," *Radiology*, vol. 153, no. 1, pp. 189–194, 1984.

[13] A. Chhabra, "Magnetic resonance neurography-simple guide to performance and interpretation," *Seminars in Roentgenology*, vol. 48, no. 2, pp. 111–125, 2013.

[14] K. E. Chappell, M. D. Robson, A. Stonebridge-Foster et al., "Magic angle effects in MR neurography," *American Journal of Neuroradiology*, vol. 25, no. 3, pp. 431–440, 2004.

[15] P. F. Felisaz, E. Y. Chang, I. Carne et al., "In vivo MR microneurography of the tibial and common peroneal nerves," *Radiology Research and Practice*, vol. 2014, Article ID 780964, 6 pages, 2014.

[16] P. F. Felisaz, F. Balducci, S. Gitto et al., "Nerve fascicles and epineurium volume segmentation of peripheral nerve using magnetic resonance micro-neurography," *Academic Radiology*, vol. 23, no. 8, pp. 1000–1007, 2016.

[17] R. A. Malik, P. G. Newrick, A. K. Sharma et al., "Microangiopathy in human diabetic neuropathy: relationship between capillary abnormalities and the severity of neuropathy," *Diabetologia*, vol. 32, no. 2, pp. 92–102, 1989.

[18] M. Ghani, R. A. Malik, D. Walker et al., "Perineurial abnormalities in the spontaneously diabetic dog," *Acta Neuropathologica*, vol. 97, no. 1, pp. 98–102, 1999.

[19] R. A. Malik, S. Tesfaye, S. D. Thompson et al., "Endoneurial localisation of microvascular damage in human diabetic neuropathy," *Diabetologia*, vol. 36, no. 5, pp. 454–459, 1993.

[20] B. Kundalić, S. Ugrenović, I. Jovanović et al., "Morphometric analysis of connective tissue sheaths of sural nerve in diabetic and nondiabetic patients," *BioMed Research International*, vol. 2014, Article ID 870930, 7 pages, 2014.

[21] M. J. Young, A. J. M. Boulton, A. F. Macleod, D. R. R. Williams, and P. H. Sonksen, "A multicentre study of the prevalence of diabetic peripheral neuropathy in the United Kingdom hospital clinic population," *Diabetologia*, vol. 36, no. 2, pp. 150–154, 1993.

[22] S. B. Reeder, C. A. McKenzie, A. R. Pineda et al., "Water-fat separation with IDEAL gradient-echo imaging," *Journal of Magnetic Resonance Imaging*, vol. 25, no. 3, pp. 644–652, 2007.

[23] A. Breiner, M. Qrimli, H. Ebadi et al., "Peripheral nerve high-resolution ultrasound in diabetes," *Muscle & Nerve*, 2016.

[24] R. A. Malik, "The pathology of human diabetic neuropathy," *Diabetes*, vol. 46, no. 2, pp. S50–S53, 1997.

[25] R. S. Thakkar, F. Del Grande, G. K. Thawait, G. Andreisek, J. A. Carrino, and A. Chhabra, "Spectrum of high-resolution MRI findings in diabetic neuropathy," *American Journal of Roentgenology*, vol. 199, no. 2, pp. 407–412, 2012.

[26] P. Bäumer, M. Weiler, M. Bendszus, and M. Pham, "Somatotopic fascicular organization of the human sciatic nerve demonstrated by MR neurography," *Neurology*, vol. 84, no. 17, pp. 1782–1787, 2015.

18

Contrast Induced Nephropathy with Intravenous Iodinated Contrast Media in Routine Diagnostic Imaging: An Initial Experience in a Tertiary Care Hospital

Shuchi Bhatt,[1] **Nipun Rajpal,**[1] **Vineeta Rathi,**[1] **and Rajneesh Avasthi**[2]

[1]*Department of Radiodiagnosis, University College of Medical Sciences and GTB Hospital, Dilshad Garden, Delhi 110095, India*
[2]*Department of Medicine, University College of Medical Sciences and GTB Hospital, Dilshad Garden, Delhi 110095, India*

Correspondence should be addressed to Shuchi Bhatt; drshuchi@hotmail.com

Academic Editor: Sotirios Bisdas

Background. Contrast induced nephropathy (CIN) is common cause of hospital acquired renal failure, defined as iatrogenic deterioration of renal function following intravascular contrast administration in the absence of another nephrotoxic event. *Objectives.* Objectives were to calculate incidence of CIN with routine IV contrast usage and to identify its risk factors. *Materials and Methods.* Study was conducted on 250 patients (having eGFR $\geq$ 45 mL/min/1.73 m^2) receiving intravenous contrast. Various clinical risk factors and details of contrast media were recorded. Patients showing 25% increase in postprocedural serum creatinine value or an absolute increase of 0.5 mg/dL (44.2 mmol/L) were diagnosed as having CIN. *Results and Conclusions.* Postprocedural serum creatinine showed significant increase from baseline levels. 25 patients (10%) developed CIN. CIN was transient in 21 (84%) patients developing CIN. One patient (4%) developed renal failure and another died due to unknown cause. Dehydration, preexisting renal disease, cardiac failure, previous contrast administration, and volume of contrast had significant correlation with development of CIN ($p < 0.05$); whereas demographic variables, baseline serum creatinine/eGFR, previous renal surgery, diabetes mellitus, hypertension, nephrotoxic drug intake, abnormal routine hematology, and contrast characteristics had no correlation with CIN. CIN is a matter of concern even in routine imaging requiring intravenous contrast media, in our set-up.

1. Introduction

Contrast induced nephropathy (CIN) is iatrogenic deterioration of renal function following intravascular contrast media (CM) administration in the absence of another nephrotoxic event. It is considered to be the third most common cause of hospital acquired acute renal failure [1]. Recently there also has been a controversy over the term CIN, and the Acute Kidney Injury Network (AKIN) has adopted "Acute Kidney Injury (AKI)" as a synonym of CIN when AKI occurs due to contrast administration [2]. However, the use of the term CIN is still popular among the radiologists and cardiologists dealing with contrast.

CIN in most cases goes undetected especially if the investigation is done in an outpatient setting. Most of the episodes of CIN are transient and resolution occurs within 1 to 3 weeks, but in a few cases permanent impairment of renal function

may occur, reflected as an increase in serum creatinine [3]. Though serum creatinine is a late and an insensitive marker, it remains the cornerstone for diagnosing CIN due to its low cost and ease of estimation.

CIN is associated with both short and long term adverse outcomes and therefore the recognition of this condition is necessary [3].

Till date no universally accepted definition of CIN exists and therefore a variable incidence has been reported in the literature ranging from 1.3 to 14.5% depending upon the criteria used [4]. The most accepted definition is that of the European Society of Urogenital Radiology (ESUR) which defines CIN as "an increase in serum creatinine by >25% or an absolute increase of 44.2 mmol/L [0.5 mg/dL] within 3 days after intravascular administration of contrast medium, without an alternative etiology" [5]. The magnitude of CIN risk has been evaluated more for intra-arterial contrast especially in patients undergoing cardiac angiography where the reported incidence of 3–16% is relatively higher [3, 6, 7].

In the recent times, with the development of multidetector CT technology allowing enhanced clinical applications of CT especially CT angiographies, the intravenous use of CM has increased many folds. This voluminous increase in the use of contrast has generated an interest among the investigators to assess its safe intravenous administration with respect to the renal status. CIN due to intravenous use of contrast has not been adequately evaluated and the existing studies too have contradictory results. An incidence of 11% had been reported with intravenous (IV) contrast in patients undergoing emergency Contrast Enhanced Computed Tomography (CECT) examination in a recent study [8]. However, in another study the occurrence of CIN with IV contrast media was only considered to be coincidental [9].

It is extremely important to study the risk factors in the target population and thus identify the high risk patients. Already established patient factors responsible for causing CIN are preexisting renal insufficiency, diabetes mellitus, dehydration before and after the contrast procedure, congestive cardiac failure, and advanced age. Certain contrast related risk factors like the volume and type of contrast administered have also been identified in the development of CIN [10–14].

There is a compelling need for the clinicians and the radiologists to recognize this definite risk associated with the intravenous contrast usage in the radiology department. This study was conducted with the aim to determine the incidence of contrast induced nephropathy (CIN) in low risk patients undergoing routine diagnostic imaging like Intravenous Urography (IVU) or Contrast Enhanced Computed Tomography (CECT) examination with intravenous administration of iodinated contrast media and to identify the patient and contrast related factors responsible for CIN. The secondary objectives of the study were to compare the incidence of contrast induced nephropathy between ionic and nonionic contrast media and to suggest guidelines for the routine working of the department to achieve safe intravenous contrast administration.

2. Materials and Methods

The study was a cross-sectional study conducted in the Department of Radiodiagnosis, University College of Medical Sciences and Guru Tegh Bahadur Hospital, Delhi, between November 2012 and April 2014.

After taking clearance from the institutional ethical committee, the study was carried along the following lines.

Sample size considering the incidence of CIN to be 11% as reported in a prospective study on CECT patients [8] and allowing an absolute error of 4% (11 ± 4%), a minimum sample size of 234 patients was required to achieve a confidence interval of 95% in the study.

We enrolled 390 unbiased samples of adult patients coming for Intravenous Urography (IVU) or Contrast Enhanced Computed Tomography (CECT) examination and requiring intravenous administration of contrast media. A written informed consent was obtained from the patients. The demographic details, suspected clinical diagnosis, and preliminary investigations were recorded on predesigned proforma. History of allergy to contrast media/any other drug was elicited and recorded. Alternative investigation was recommended to patients allergic to contrast to answer the clinical question. In case the contrast study was deemed necessary by the clinician, the contrast investigations were performed using low osmolal nonionic contrast media after premedication with steroids as per guidelines. These patients were excluded from the study population. Serum creatinine was repeated if the preprocedural report was more than 1 week old from the date of investigation.

Estimated Glomerular Filtration Rate (eGFR) of the patient was calculated by the resident (NR) using the Modification of Diet in Renal Disease (MDRD) equation [15]:

$$
\begin{aligned}
\text{eGFR} &\left(\text{mL/min/1.73 m}^2 \right) \\
&= 186 \times (\text{serum creatinine})^{1.154} \times (\text{Age})^{-0.203} \\
&\quad \times (0.742 \text{ if female}) \\
&\quad \times (1.210 \text{ if African American}).
\end{aligned}
\tag{1}
$$

Patients requiring preventive hydration therapy having eGFR < 45 mL/min/1.73 m^2 [16] were excluded from the study. Review for the need of the investigation was done in consultation with the concerned physician and the investigation performed in 14 such patients using preventive strategies as per Consensus Guidelines for the Prevention of Contrast Induced Nephropathy by Canadian Association of Radiologists [15] and were recorded separately.

Patients who refused to give consent were excluded. Patients who did not receive intravenous (IV) contrast or patients having an eGFR of less than 45 mL/min/1.73 m^2 were excluded. Patients whose postprocedural serum creatinine was not available were not included in the study. Therefore, the final study sample consisted of 250 patients comprised of 64.1% of the total enrolled patients.

Patients were interrogated regarding the presence of any known risk factor according to a predesigned questionnaire and their answers were recorded. Appropriate laboratory investigations were advised when history suggestive of one or more risk factors was present. The available clinical records of the patients were checked for the presence of any defined risk factor. Appropriate routine instructions were given to the patients for the prospective intravenous contrast investigation.

The following risk factors were identified representing a blend of available literature.

Dehydration. Patients having recent history of prolonged diarrhoea or vomiting or having limited oral intake in recent past with history of recent weight loss and lethargic look were clinically examined and labelled as dehydrated if dry mucous membranes and abnormal skin turgor were present.

Preexisting renal disease on basis of structural (e.g., single kidney and renal cell carcinoma) and functional abnormality (e.g., raised previous serum creatinine) of kidneys on previous investigations was identified as separate risk factor. Patients having only calculus or mild hydronephrosis but normal function of kidney were not included.

Previous Renal Surgery. History of previous renal surgery like nephrectomy, pyelolithotomy, and so forth was also identified as a separate risk factor.

Diabetes Mellitus. Patient who was a known case of diabetes mellitus on antidiabetic treatment (on oral hypoglycemic drugs or on insulin) or had recent fasting blood glucose >126 mg/dL was identified as a separate risk factor [17].

Hypertension. Patient is a known case of hypertension on antihypertensive drugs or has blood pressure >140/90 mm of Hg [18].

Cardiac Failure. Patients have a past or present documented history of cardiac failure.

Nephrotoxic Drug Intake. Patients use nephrotoxic drugs like NSAIDs, beta blockers, aminoglycosides, or amphotericin B.

Previous Contrast Use. Patients who had undergone previous contrast study were considered as a separate risk factor. Patients having history of intravascular iodinated contrast study within two weeks of the contrast investigation were included in this study.

Abnormal Routine Blood Investigations. Abnormal routine blood investigations were considered as separate risk factor which included anaemic patients (with haemoglobin level of less than 13 g/dL and less than 12 g/dL in women) [19] or laboratory findings suggestive of infection like leukocytosis (value greater than 11000/μL) or patients with elevated CRP [20].

Patients with history of gout, multiple myeloma, or hyperthyroidism were also considered to be risk factors. However, no such patient was present in our study.

The type and amount of contrast media given to the patient were decided as per standard protocol being followed routinely in the department.

After completion of the investigation (IVU or CECT), volume, and type of contrast media, the total iodine content or any reaction if occurred was recorded.

Contrast was subdivided on the basis of ionicity into ionic and nonionic; osmolarity into high osmolal contrast media (HOCM) and low osmolal contrast media (LOCM); structure into monomer and dimer. The Following contrasts were used in the study population: iohexol (nonionic, monomer, and LOCM); sodium meglumine diatrizoate (ionic, HOCM, and monomer); iopamidol (nonionic, monomer, and LOCM); and ioxaglate (Ionic, LOCM, and dimer).

Repeated serum creatinine estimation was done 48–72 hrs after contrast (IVP or CECT) investigation.

After the contrast administration, patients showing an increase in serum creatinine by 25% or an absolute increase of 0.5 mg/dL from preprocedural level were diagnosed as having contrast induced nephropathy [5].

In patients who were diagnosed as CIN, serum creatinine was repeated weekly till it reached the pre procedural values.

All patients with CIN were followed 4–6 weeks and were watched for features of renal deterioration like oliguria, symptoms related to pulmonary edema or any metabolic disturbances, and were recorded separately.

3. Outcome Measures

The primary end point of this study was CIN defined as an increase in the postprocedural serum creatinine value by 25% from the baseline or an absolute increase of 0.5 mg/dL (44.2 mmol/L) within three days to intravascular contrast administration [5]. This definition of CIN was chosen over the recently proposed relatively lower threshold of 0.3 mg/dL for defining AKI (due to contrast administration) by the AKIN [2]. The former is more specific and less likely to yield a false-positive result from cumulative biologic and assay variability and remains a more commonly used definition in current medical practice [21–23]. Thus, this has been used to define CIN in the present study.

3.1. Statistical Analysis. The collected data was entered into a spreadsheet format using Microsoft Office Excel. Data was processed using statistical software SPSS version 17.1.

The incidence of CIN was calculated in the study population and separately for nonionic and ionic contrast media groups. The calculated incidence was compared with previously reported incidence using tests of proportions, for which $p < 0.05$ was considered statistically significant.

The baseline preprocedural and postprocedural serum creatinine values were compared for any difference and evaluated whether the difference was significant using paired t-test.

For evaluation of eGFR, because of nonnormal distribution, a nonparametric method (Mann-Whitney U test) was used.

Risk factors responsible for CIN were identified by estimating their distribution in the CIN and the non-CIN groups. Continuous variables including age, weight, volume of contrast, and total iodine given to patient were presented as mean ± SD and compared using Student's t-test.

Categorical variables including dehydration, preexisting renal disease, history of renal surgery, diabetes mellitus, hypertension, nephrotoxic drug Intake, heart failure, previous contrast use, and the osmolarity of the contrast media were presented as counts and percentages and compared with Fisher's exact test. Categorical variables including sex, abnormal routine hematologic investigations, administered contrast volume subgroups, and the ionicity of the contrast were compared using chi-square tests.

Results of this model were presented as relative risk (RR) with 95% confidence intervals using univariate analysis.

4. Results

All 250 patients in our study were adults with age ranging from 18 to 86 years with the mean age of 41.41 ± 16.63 years. The sample size included 147 (58.8%) male and 103 (41.2%) female patients; 201 (80.4%) underwent contrast enhanced

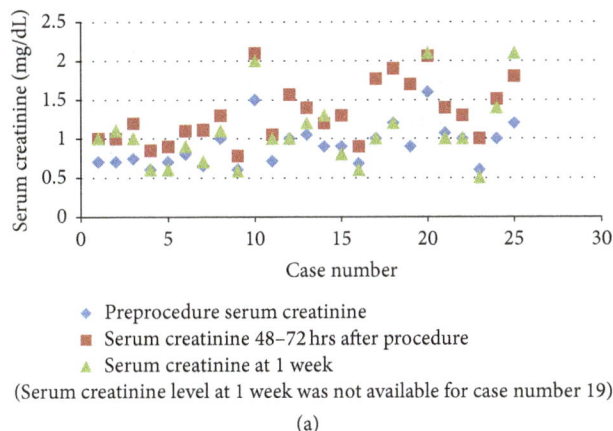

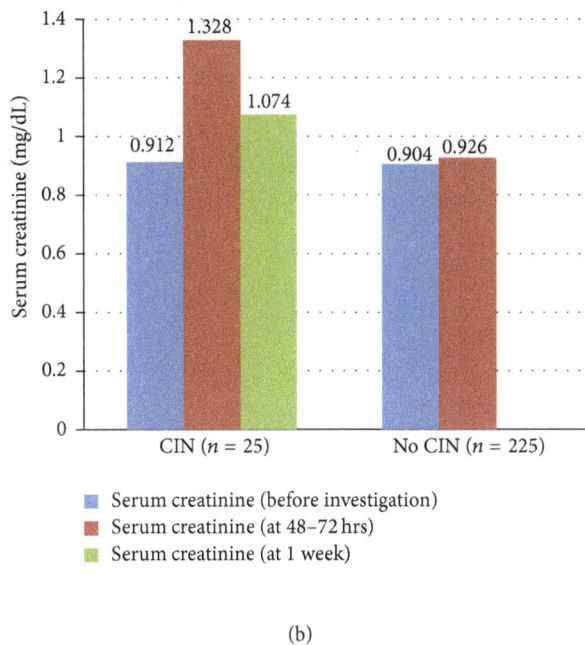

FIGURE 1: (a) Scatter diagram depicting serum creatinine levels at different time intervals in "CIN" patients. (b) represents the mean serum creatinine values in the pre- and post-IV iodinated contrast investigation in the CIN and the No CIN groups.

CT examination while in the rest 49 (19.6%) patients Intravenous Urography (IVU) was done. In these 250 patients, mean preprocedural serum creatinine was 0.905 ± 0.248 mg/dL which increased to 0.966 ± 0.300 mg/dL after 48–72 hours of the contrast investigation. This increase in serum creatinine was found to be statistically significant using paired t-test with p value < 0.001 (Figure 1).

A total of 25 (10%) of the 250 patients in sample group developed CIN as per the definition of European Society of Urogenital Radiology. Therefore, the incidence of CIN found to be 10% (95% CI 6.8% to 14.4%) in our study.

Out of a total of 187 patients who were given nonionic contrast medium, 20 satisfied the criteria of CIN; and 5 out of the total of 58 patients who were given ionic contrast medium developed CIN. The incidence of CIN is 10.7% in the nonionic group and 7.9% in the ionic group.

The patient sample was divided into 2 groups "CIN group" and "No CIN group," the distribution of the various risk factors studied in these two groups to calculate their association with CIN.

Following univariate analysis, analysis of different features revealed the CIN and No CIN groups to be homogeneous for the demographic characteristics including age, sex, and weight with $p > 0.05$ (Table 1).

Both the groups were not significantly different with respect to the age, sex, or weight of the patients and therefore these demographic factors were not found to affect the incidence of the occurrence of CIN with the IV contrast media.

Regarding clinical risk factors (Table 2), it was found that the CIN group had significantly higher proportion of patients with dehydration, preexisting renal disease, previous contrast

TABLE 1: Demographic distribution between "CIN group" and "No CIN group."

	CIN ($n = 25$)	No CIN ($n = 225$)	p value
Females	9 (36%)	94 (41.8%)	0.671
Males	16 (64%)	131 (58.2%)	
Age (years)	45.12 ± 17.82	41.00 ± 16.48	0.241
Weight (kg)	58.44 ± 13.00	55.00 ± 10.12	0.119

*p value calculated using chi-square test, correlation to be significant if $p < 0.05$.

administration, and cardiac failure ($p < 0.05$) with high relative risks. Previous renal surgery, diabetes mellitus, and hypertension were not statistically significantly different in both groups with $p > 0.05$ with relative risks of 3.02 (95% CI 0.88–10.37), 2.23 (95% CI 0.97–5.15), and 2.08 (95% CI 1.79–5.49), respectively (Figure 2).

Patients with history of nephrotoxic drug intake and abnormal routine blood investigations were found to be homogenously distributed in both CIN and No CIN groups with low relative risks.

4.1. Contrast Related Risk Factors. "CIN" and "No CIN" groups were homogenous in terms of ionicity, osmolarity, and molecular structure of contrast ($p > 0.05$) while mean volume of contrast administered was significantly higher in CIN group ($p < 0.05$). Mean total iodine given to patients in "CIN" group was higher which was the limit of significance ($p = 0.05$) (Table 3).

In the CIN group, renal function returned to normal within 3 weeks in 84% patients. Serum creatinine values returned to normal within one week in 11 (44%), while in 10

TABLE 2: Distribution of clinical risk factors between "CIN" group and "No CIN" group.

Risk factors	CIN (n = 25)	No CIN (n = 225)	p value	Relative risks	95% CI	
					Lower	Upper
Dehydration	8 (32%)	20 (8.9%)	0.003	3.73	1.78	7.84
Abnormal routine blood investigations	7 (29%)	48 (21.8%)	0.457	1.35	0.59	3.06
Preexisting renal disease	6 (24%)	13 (5.8%)	0.006	3.84	1.74	8.45
Diabetes mellitus	6 (24%)	25 (11.1%)	0.100	2.23	0.97	5.15
Previous contrast use	6 (24%)	2 (0.9%)	0.000	9.56	5.30	17.21
Hypertension	4 (16%)	17 (7.6%)	0.143	2.08	0.79	5.49
Previous renal surgery	2 (8%)	5 (2.2%)	0.148	3.02	0.88	10.37
Cardiac failure	2 (8%)	1 (0.4%)	0.027	7.16	2.94	17.43
Nephrotoxic drug intake	3 (12%)	19 (8.4%)	0.469	1.41	0.46	4.35

* p value calculated using Fisher's exact test or chi-square test wherever appropriate; correlation was considered significant if $p < 0.05$.

TABLE 3: Contrast characteristics in "CIN" and "No CIN" groups.

Contrast characteristics		CIN (n = 25)	No CIN (n = 225)	p value
Ionicity	Ionic	5 (20%)	58 (25.8%)	0.633
	Nonionic	20 (80%)	167 (74.2%)	
Osmolarity	HOCM	4 (16%)	43 (19.11%)	1.000
	LOCM	21 (84%)	182 (80.89%)	
Structure	Dimer	1 (4%)	15 (6.67%)	1.000
	Monomer	24 (96%)	210 (93.33%)	
Total iodine (g)		22.37 ± 5.312	20.21 ± 5.30	0.05
Volume (mL)		73.20 ± 18.19	65.11 ± 17.93	0.03

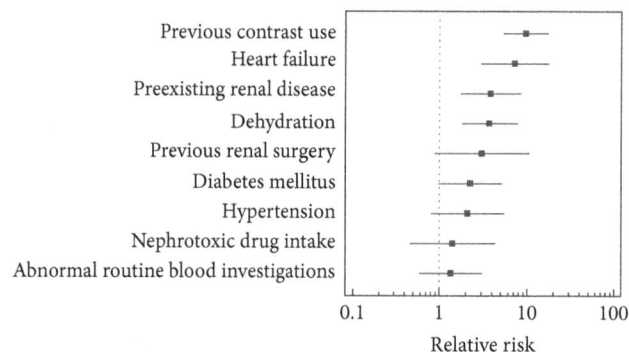

FIGURE 2: Forest plot depicting relative risk of clinical risk factors (result of univariate analysis).

(40%) patients it returned in 3-week time. Only one patient (4%) took a longer time (5 weeks) to attain the baseline levels. One female patient aged 49 years, with baseline serum creatinine of 1.2 mg/dL, had received 40 mL of 300 mg% of iohexol (12 g iodine) for a CECT head study. She developed acute renal failure and had to undergo dialysis. Another 55-year-old male patient with suspected renal cell carcinoma (pre-CT serum creatinine of 1.6 mg/dL) received 100 mL of 240 mg% of iohexol (24 g iodine), developed CIN (postprocedure serum creatinine 2.06 mg/dL), and died at home, and the cause of death could not be ascertained. Both these patients had mild dehydration and chronic kidney disease. One patient was lost to follow-up.

5. Discussion

This observational study was conducted in a hospital based radiology set-up which entertains both routine and emergency CT and IVU requisitions requiring intravenous CM administration. 250 patients constituted the final study group for determining the incidence of CIN and to identify various patients and contrast related risk factors.

As a routine practice, the baseline serum creatinine levels (done within a week for indoor patients) were estimated to screen patients with decreased eGFR calculated using MDRD formula before administering intravascular iodinated CM. Serum creatinine of 1.8 mg/dL corresponding to an eGFR of

$45\,\text{mL/min/1.73}\,\text{m}^2$ has been found to be significant for the development of AKI in patients receiving CM in comparison to the patients not receiving any contrast [24]. In our study sample, eGFR of less than $45\,\text{mL/min/1.73}\,\text{m}^2$ was used as an exclusion criterion and therefore patients did not carry any additional risk of developing CIN nor required any pre-imaging (CECT or IVU) hydration therapy. Thus, low risk patients not requiring any preventive therapy before administration of IV contrast were recruited for the study.

The preprocedural mean serum creatinine value of 0.905 ± 0.248 mg/dL was compared with the postprocedural mean serum creatinine value of 0.966 ± 0.300 mg/dL in the study sample. The postinvestigation increase in the serum creatinine levels was found to be statistically significant, suggesting a significant deterioration in renal function. Previous studies indicated a definite pathophysiological renal insult occurring due to administration of intravascular iodinated contrast because of an increased viscosity of blood leading to sluggish blood flow which induces local hypoxia [25–27]. Besides reducing the renal perfusion, it also causes direct toxicity to tubular cells resulting in deterioration of the renal function [25, 28].

Of the 250 patients, 25 patients satisfied the selected criteria for CIN, resulting in an incidence of 10% following intravenous contrast administration. This incidence of 10% is alarming in low risk (patients with eGFR of $45\,\text{mL/min/1.73}\,\text{m}^2$ or more) patients sample receiving contrast through the intravenous route which has been considered to be safe in most past studies [29]. However, in a recent study, incidence of AKI was calculated following noncontrast and contrast CT and concluded that it is inversely proportional to baseline eGFR and varies from 1.2% to 14% [30]. The incidence was not statistically different to a similar study conducted by Mitchell et al. on 633 patients undergoing emergency CECT examination ($p > 0.05$) [8]. On the contrary, our patients underwent routine IVU or CECT study. A varying incidence of CIN is present in the literature, ranging from 1.3 to 14.5% [4]. This wide range might be due to different criteria used for diagnosing CIN, wide variation in the study sample, and administration of intravascular contrast through varying routes. There is no consensus regarding the clinical significance of a mild but statistically significant increase in the serum creatinine following contrast administration. Hayman advocated that a change of 0.3 mg/dL of serum creatinine [31] has no clinical significance, whereas Levy et al. found that even a small increase in serum creatinine increases mortality by causing a significant decrease in GFR and thus the renal function [32].

In the CIN group of 25 patients, serum creatinine reached the baseline level within a week in a maximum of 44% patients, while in 40% baseline levels were obtained in up to 3-week time. One patient (4%) took longer to recover and one patient died due to unknown cause. One patient (4%) with known kidney disease (with preinvestigation serum creatinine of 1.2 mg/dL) developed acute renal failure requiring dialysis. Thus, most (84%) of the patients developing CIN had a full recovery in 3-week time postinvestigation. This reiterates the previous study which states that CIN is a transient process with serum creatinine levels rising within 24 hours of contrast administration, peaks within 3–5 days to return to the baseline levels within two weeks [7]. Some investigators believe that there is no biological significance of CIN whereas few are still unclear regarding its clinical significance. The CIN consensus working panel has found CIN to be responsible for 11% of all cases of kidney impairment requiring hospitalization, but with intra-arterial use of CM [33]. Some authors have estimated the incidence of renal failure to be less than 2% [34–36]. With intravenous contrast, Thomsen and Morcos [5] also found significant increase of mortality or renal failure in CIN patients. Our study did not focus on this aspect and hence the significance of mortality/morbidity due to CIN cannot be commented upon. But as the incidence of CIN is quite high for a routine setting as reflected by our work, it further requires an intensive study to study its clinical implications.

The study sample was divided into two groups: "CIN" and "No CIN" groups to see whether the distribution of the risk factors was significantly different in the two groups or not.

Demographic variables like age and weight were homogenous in both CIN and No CIN groups indicating no role in the occurrence of CIN. Sex ratio was also statistically similar in both the groups. Similar observation of no influence of gender was made by Evola et al. in their study [37]. Though the mean age was higher in "CIN group" as compared to "No CIN group," it was not found to be statistically significant ($p > 0.05$) in our study, whereas older age is considered to be an independent predictor of CIN [37–39]. Our results can be explained by the relatively younger population of mean age 41.41 ± 16.63 years constituting the study group in comparison to 65.32 ± 12.02 years for others [37]. Mean weight had no correlation to the occurrence of CIN and no reference exists in the literature.

Multiple factors have been identified for development of CIN, with reduction in renal function being the most significant, though not studied specifically in the past studies. Traditional risk factors of CIN like dehydration, preexisting renal disease, heart failure, and history of previous contrast administration were found to be significant in the development of CIN with a high relative risk. Dehydration increases the risk of developing CIN due to decreased intravascular volume resulting in decreased renal blood flow and ischemia and thus, exaggerating the renal insult [40, 41].

Preexisting renal disease is an independent risk factor of nephrotoxicity and development of CIN. It is the single greatest risk factor with the severity of CIN increasing in proportion to the baseline renal insufficiency [42]. The higher is the baseline serum creatinine value and the greater is the risk [29, 43], but not in patients with mild decrease in renal function (eGFR > 45 and < $90\,\text{mL/min/1.73}\,\text{m}^2$), not requiring prophylactic therapy.

The mean preprocedural serum creatinine was 0.912 ± 0.266 mg/dL in the "CIN" and 0.904 ± 0.246 mg/dL in the "NO CIN" group, corresponding to mean eGFR of 85 (68–108.5) $\text{mL/min/1.73}\,\text{m}^2$ and 88 (70.5–107.5) $\text{mL/min/1.73}\,\text{m}^2$, respectively. This difference was not found to be significant in our study. Despite all patients having eGFR >

$45 \, \text{mL/min/1.73} \, \text{m}^2$ (low risk patients), still incidence of CIN was quite high (10%), thus emphasizing the need for detection of risk factors which may independently or in conjunction with mild renal derangement cause significant renal deterioration and development of CIN.

There was a significant increase in the risk of CIN in patients of cardiac failure in our study. Previous researchers found that reduction in effective intravascular volume associated with reduced cardiac output decreases the renal perfusion and there is an increased risk of CIN [13, 40] as also found in our study.

Two doses given 24 to 48 hours apart increase the risk of CIN [44, 45]. But CIN was also found in patients who had received previous (within two weeks) intravenous contrast in our study raising the possibility of significant renal derangement for up to two weeks after injecting contrast, which may have been responsible for the finding in our study.

Past renal surgery, diabetes mellitus, and hypertension are found to have high relative risks but not significantly associated with the occurrence of CIN in the present study. Though an increased incidence of CIN is seen in diabetic patients in our study, comparison between the two groups failed to reach any statistical significance ($p > 0.05$), hence not being identified as a separate risk factor in our study, in contradiction to the available literature [11]. Hypertensive patients were found to have no statistical difference showing no correlation to development of CIN in our study sample. Most of the published studies and reviews did not find arterial blood pressure as a separate risk factor [31, 37, 46] although it is included in suggested list of risk factors in 2013 ACR Manual on Contrast Media [47].

The previous renal surgery was not qualified as a separate risk factor in our study as also in most studies and meta-analyses [26, 36]. Nephrotoxic drug intake and abnormal hematological findings are not related to the development of CIN and are not yet established as risk factors in existing literature.

Contrast of different types based on their physicochemical properties has conflicting reports, regarding its relation to the occurrence of CIN. Contrast related factors like ionicity, structure, and osmolality are not related to development of CIN with comparable incidence in ionic (7.9%) and nonionic (10.7%) CM groups in our study as well ($p = 0.63$). A meta-analysis contradicts our study by reporting significantly reduced incidence of CIN with use of "low osmolar" compared to "ionic high osmolar" CM, though in patients with preexisting CKD [48]. Volume of contrast administered intravenously was directly linked to the occurrence of CIN in the present study as already established [37, 49]. The total iodine received by patients may have a possible relation to the development of CIN as suggested by our study, with p value of 0.05 reaching the limit of significance. This could be likely due to the direct relation of total iodine content with the volume of CM. No literature is available in this context opening up future prospects for the same. This could prove to be significant in CT-angiographic and CT-perfusion studies requiring lower volume but a higher strength of contrast and thus higher iodine content.

Dehydration, preexisting renal disease, cardiac failure, previous contrast administration, and volume of contrast were identified as significant risk factors for the development of CIN in our study. These factors are quite similar to the risk factors identified by Mehran and Nikolsky [36]; however, diabetes, advanced age, and baseline renal function were not found to be significant in our study. This possibly occurred due to a relatively younger study population, exclusion of patients with poor baseline renal function, and limited sample size.

The statistically significant rise in serum creatinine levels after imaging requiring IV contrast successfully established the occurrence of a definite renal insult with incidence of CIN being 10%. The study design was able to recognize the important risk factors in the study and also suggest their relative risk of developing CIN.

Limitations of the study were that no control group was present. A relatively smaller sample size though statistically adequate resulted in inadequate number to study significance of few already known risk factors (like previous renal surgery, diabetes mellitus, and hypertension) for development of CIN. Only the "CIN" and not the "NO CIN" group of patients were followed up after the contrast procedure. Long term complications in patients developing CIN needs to be studied. Also, risk associated with presence of multiple risk factors needs to be investigated.

6. Conclusions

Incidence of CIN is 10% in patients undergoing CECT or IVU examinations with IV iodinated CM. However, no relationship could be established between the occurrence of CIN and the base line renal functions. There is a definite renal insult with IV iodinated CM showing significant increase in postinvestigation serum creatinine. CIN is transient in majority with recovery occurring in 84% patients within 3 weeks. Traditional risk factors of CIN including dehydration, preexisting renal disease, cardiac failure, and previous intravascular contrast administration are related to the development of CIN with a high relative risk. Previous renal surgery, diabetes mellitus, and hypertension have high relative risks but are not significantly associated with the occurrence of CIN. Volume of IV contrast is directly linked to occurrence of CIN. CIN is an important concern for radiologists with a high incidence in our set-up. The radiologists are advised to recognize this intrinsic risk to iodinated contrast media, identifying the patients at risk of developing CIN and those requiring hospital care.

Based on the study, a performa was developed to be used for IV administration of CM to identify "at risk patients" for developing CIN with routine use of intravenous contrast, detect CIN, and follow up these patients (Table 4). We suggest all the fellow radiologists to utilize this performa to address the sensitive issue of contrast induced nephropathy.

TABLE 4: Recommended requisition form for contrast enhanced investigations in our department.

Name	Consent*		
Age	Baseline (not more than 1 week old) serum creatinine (mg/dL) = eGFR calculated (mL/min/1.73 m^2) = If < 45 mL/min/1.73 m^2 defer CECT/IVP, take preventive measures		
Sex	H/o contrast allergy, drug allergy, or allergic condition; if yes, defer Ix and preventive measures taken		
Weight	(1) Preexisting renal disease	Y/N	Type of disease
Clinical indication for IVP/CECT	(2) Dehydration on history or clinical exam	Y/N	
Ix required IVP/CECT study and ID	(3) H/o previous contrast (within 2 wks)	Y/N	IV or IA, type of CM
Any significant past or present medical illness	(4) H/o heart failure	Y/N	Past/present
	(5) H/o renal surgery	Y/N	Type of surgery
Hb/TLC/CRP	(6) H/o diabetes mellitus	Y/N	Recent fasting blood sugar level
	(7) H/o hypertension	Y/N	Blood pressure = mm of Hg
	(8) H/o nephrotoxic drug intake	Y/N	Type of drug

If one of the risk factors 1–4 or two of risk factors 5–8 or subnormal renal function (eGFR 46 to 90 mL/min/1.73 m^2) or if volume of administered IV contrast is equal to or more than 100 mL

Repeat S creatinine after 2-3 days of Ix, postprocedural S. Creatinine level =

Postprocedural S. Creatinine raised Yes/No % increase =

If increase > 25% or is by an absolute value of 0.5 mg/dL, CIN is diagnosed; Group allotted: CIN or No CIN

If CIN present, serum creatinine is repeated weekly and refer to nephrologist if there is clinical deterioration

If not, send back to referring clinician

*Consent to be taken on separate form, Ix: investigation.

patients to be enrolled in the study and they were free to leave the study at any time. The research was approved by the ethical committee of institute "University College of Medical Sciences," University of Delhi.

Authors' Contribution

Shuchi Bhatt contributed to study concept and design, data interpretation, preparation of paper, and final revision. Nipun Rajpal collected the data and prepared the paper. Vineeta Rathi prepared the paper. Rajneesh Avasthi collected the data.

References

[1] K. Nash, A. Hafeez, and S. Hou, "Hospital-acquired renal insufficiency," American Journal of Kidney Diseases, vol. 39, no. 5, pp. 930–936, 2002.

[2] R. L. Mehta, J. A. Kellum, S. V. Shah et al., "Acute Kidney Injury Network: report of an initiative to improve outcomes in acute kidney injury," Critical Care, vol. 11, article R31, 2007.

[3] L. Gruberg, R. Mehran, G. Dangas et al., "Acute renal failure requiring dialysis after percutaneous coronary interventions,"

Catheterization and Cardiovascular Interventions, vol. 52, no. 4, pp. 409–416, 2001.

[4] P. A. McCullough, A. Adam, C. R. Becker et al., "Epidemiology and prognostic implications of contrast-induced nephropathy," The American Journal of Cardiology, vol. 98, no. 6, supplement 1, pp. 5–13, 2006.

[5] H. S. Thomsen and S. K. Morcos, "Contrast media and the kidney: European Society of Urogenital Radiology (ESUR) guidelines," British Journal of Radiology, vol. 76, no. 908, pp. 513–518, 2003.

[6] C. S. Rihal, S. C. Textor, D. E. Grill et al., "Incidence and prognostic importance of acute renal failure after percutaneous coronary intervention," Circulation, vol. 105, no. 19, pp. 2259–2264, 2002.

[7] P. A. McCullough, R. Wolyn, L. L. Rocher, R. N. Levin, and W. W. O'Neill, "Acute renal failure after coronary intervention: incidence, risk factors, and relationship to mortality," The American Journal of Medicine, vol. 103, no. 5, pp. 368–375, 1997.

[8] A. M. Mitchell, A. E. Jones, J. A. Tumlin, and J. A. Kline, "Incidence of contrast-induced nephropathy after contrast-enhanced computed tomography in the outpatient setting," Clinical Journal of the American Society of Nephrology, vol. 5, no. 1, pp. 4–9, 2010.

[9] R. J. McDonald, J. S. McDonald, J. P. Bida et al., "Intravenous contrast material-induced nephropathy: causal or coincident phenomenon?" Radiology, vol. 267, no. 1, pp. 106–118, 2013.

[10] A. S. Berns, "Nephrotoxicity of contrast media," Kidney International, vol. 36, no. 4, pp. 730–740, 1989.

[11] A. Kolonko, F. Kokot, and A. Wiecek, "Contrast-associated nephropathy—old clinical problem and new therapeutic perspectives," *Nephrology Dialysis Transplantation*, vol. 13, no. 3, pp. 803–806, 1998.

[12] S. T. Cochran, W. S. Wong, and D. J. Roe, "Predicting angiography-induced acute renal function impairment: clinical risk model," *American Journal of Roentgenology*, vol. 141, no. 5, pp. 1027–1033, 1983.

[13] M. R. Rudnick, J. S. Berns, R. M. Cohen, and S. Goldfarb, "Nephrotoxic risks of renal angiography: contrast media-associated nephrotoxicity and atheroembolism—a critical review," *American Journal of Kidney Diseases*, vol. 24, no. 4, pp. 713–727, 1994.

[14] R. Mehran, E. D. Aymong, E. Nikolsky et al., "A simple risk score for prediction of contrast-induced nephropathy after percutaneous coronary intervention: development and initial validation," *Journal of the American College of Cardiology*, vol. 44, no. 7, pp. 1393–1399, 2004.

[15] National Kidney Foundation, "K/DOQI clinical practice guidelines for chronic kidney disease: evaluation, classification, and stratification," *American Journal of Kidney Diseases*, vol. 39, no. 2, supplement 1, pp. S1–S266, 2002.

[16] R. J. Owen, S. Hiremath, A. Myers, M. Fraser-Hill, and B. Barrett, "Consensus guidelines for the the prevention of contrast induced nephropathy," *Canadian Association of Radiologists Journal*, vol. 58, no. 2, pp. 79–57, 2007.

[17] American Diabetes Association, "Report of the expert committee on the diagnosis and classification of diabetes mellitus," *Diabetes Care*, vol. 20, no. 7, pp. 1183–1197, 1997.

[18] A. Chobanian, G. L. Bakris, H. R. Black et al., "The seventh report of the Joint National Committee on Prevention, Detection, Evaluation and Treatment of high blood pressure: the JNC 7 report," *The Journal of the American Medical Association*, vol. 289, pp. 2560–2572, 2003.

[19] WHO, UNICEF, and UNU, *Iron Deficiency Anaemia: Assessment, Prevention and Control, a Guide for Programme Managers*, World Health Organization, Geneva, Switzerland, 2001.

[20] N. Abramson and B. Melton, "Leukocytosis: basics of clinical assessment," *American Family Physician*, vol. 62, no. 9, pp. 2053–2060, 2000.

[21] B. M. Elicker, Y. S. Cypel, and J. C. Weinreb, "IV contrast administration for CT: a survey of practices for the screening and prevention of contrast nephropathy," *American Journal of Roentgenology*, vol. 186, no. 6, pp. 1651–1658, 2006.

[22] C. Davidson, F. Stacul, P. A. McCullough et al., "Contrast medium use," *American Journal of Cardiology*, vol. 98, supplement 1, no. 6, pp. 42–58, 2006.

[23] S. S. Waikar and J. V. Bonventre, "Creatinine kinetics and the definition of acute kidney injury," *Journal of the American Society of Nephrology*, vol. 20, no. 3, pp. 672–679, 2009.

[24] R. J. Bruce, A. Djamali, K. Shinki, S. J. Michel, J. P. Fine, and M. A. Pozniak, "Background fluctuation of kidney function versus contrast-induced nephrotoxicity," *American Journal of Roentgenology*, vol. 192, no. 3, pp. 711–718, 2009.

[25] R. W. Katzberg, "Urography into the 21st century: new contrast media, renal handling, imaging characteristics, and nephrotoxicity," *Radiology*, vol. 204, no. 2, pp. 297–312, 1997.

[26] T. G. Gleeson and S. Bulugahapitiya, "Contrast-induced nephropathy," *American Journal of Roentgenology*, vol. 183, no. 6, pp. 1673–1689, 2004.

[27] P. P. Leyssac, N.-H. Holstein-Rathlou, and O. Skøtt, "Renal blood flow, early distal sodium, and plasma renin concentrations during osmotic diuresis," *The American Journal of Physiology—Regulatory Integrative and Comparative Physiology*, vol. 279, no. 4, pp. R1268–R1276, 2000.

[28] J. Tumlin, F. Stacul, A. Adam et al., "Pathophysiology of contrast-induced nephropathy," *The American Journal of Cardiology*, vol. 98, no. 6, pp. 14K–20K, 2006.

[29] R. D. Moore, E. P. Steinberg, N. R. Powe et al., "Nephrotoxicity of high-osmolality versus low-osmolality contrast media: randomized clinical trial," *Radiology*, vol. 182, no. 3, pp. 649–655, 1992.

[30] J. S. McDonald, R. J. McDonald, R. E. Carter, R. W. Katzberg, D. F. Kallmes, and E. E. Williamson, "Risk of intravenous contrast material-mediated acute kidney injury: a propensity score-matched study stratified by baseline-estimated glomerular filtration rate," *Radiology*, vol. 271, no. 1, pp. 65–73, 2014.

[31] L. A. Hayman, "Contrast-induced renal failure," *Radiology*, vol. 137, pp. 867–869, 1980.

[32] E. M. Levy, C. M. Viscoli, and R. I. Horwitz, "The effect of acute renal failure on mortality: a cohort analysis," *The Journal of the American Medical Association*, vol. 275, no. 19, pp. 1489–1494, 1996.

[33] P. A. McCullough, F. Stacul, C. R. Becker et al., "Contrast-induced nephropathy (CIN) consensus working panel: executive summary," *Reviews in Cardiovascular Medicine*, vol. 7, no. 4, pp. 177–197, 2006.

[34] O. Toprak and M. Cirit, "Risk factors and therapy strategies for contrast induced nephropathy," *Renal Failure*, vol. 28, no. 5, pp. 365–381, 2006.

[35] I. Goldenberg and S. Matetzky, "Nephropathy induced by contrast media: pathogenesis, risk factors and preventive strategies," *Canadian Medical Association Journal*, vol. 172, no. 11, pp. 1461–1471, 2005.

[36] R. Mehran and E. Nikolsky, "Contrast-induced nephropathy: definition, epidemiology and patients at risk," *Kidney International*, vol. 69, pp. S11–S15, 2006.

[37] S. Evola, M. Lunetta, F. Macaione et al., "Risk factors for contrast induced nephropathy: a study among italian patients," *Indian Heart Journal*, vol. 64, no. 5, pp. 484–491, 2012.

[38] M. J. E. Gussenhoven, J. Ravensbergen, J. H. van Bockel, J. D. M. Feuth, and J. C. N. M. Aarts, "Renal dysfunction after angiography; a risk factor analysis in patients with peripheral vascular disease," *Journal of Cardiovascular Surgery*, vol. 32, no. 1, pp. 81–86, 1991.

[39] A. S. Kini, C. A. Mitre, M. Kim, M. Kamran, D. Reich, and S. K. Sharma, "A protocol for prevention of radiographic contrast nephropathy during percutaneous coronary intervention: effect of selective dopamine receptor agonist fenoldopam," *Catheterization and Cardiovascular Interventions*, vol. 55, no. 2, pp. 169–173, 2002.

[40] B. J. Barrett and P. S. Parfrey, "Prevention of nephrotoxicity induced by radiocontrast agents," *The New England Journal of Medicine*, vol. 331, no. 21, pp. 1449–1450, 1994.

[41] O. Miettnen, "Design options in epidemiologic research. An update," *Scandinavian Journal of Work, Environment & Health*, vol. 8, supplement 1, pp. 7–14, 1982.

[42] M. R. Rudnick, J. S. Berns, R. M. Cohen, and S. Goldfarb, "Contrast media-associated nephrotoxicity," *Seminars in Nephrology*, vol. 17, no. 1, pp. 15–26, 1997.

[43] K. A. Hall, R. W. Wong, G. C. Hunter et al., "Contrast-induced nephrotoxicity: the effects of vasodilator therapy," *Journal of Surgical Research*, vol. 53, no. 4, pp. 317–320, 1992.

[44] H. Trivedi and W. D. Foley, "Contrast-induced nephropathy after a second contrast exposure," *Renal Failure*, vol. 32, no. 7, pp. 796–801, 2010.

[45] H. H. Abujudeh, M. S. Gee, and R. Kaewlai, "In emergency situations, should serum creatinine be checked in all patients before performing second contrast CT examinations within 24 hours?" *Journal of the American College of Radiology*, vol. 6, no. 4, pp. 268–273, 2009.

[46] E. M. Lautin, N. J. Freeman, A. H. Schoenfeld et al., "Radio-contrast-associated renal dysfunction: a comparison of lower-osmolality and conventional high-osmolality contrast media," *American Journal of Roentgenology*, vol. 157, no. 1, pp. 59–65, 1991.

[47] Contrast-Induced Nephrotoxicity, *ACR Manual on Contrast Media 2013*, 9th edition, 2013, http://geiselmed.dartmouth.edu/radiology/pdf/ACR_manual.pdf.

[48] B. J. Barrett, "Contrast nephrotoxicity," *Journal of the American Society of Nephrology*, vol. 5, no. 2, pp. 125–137, 1994.

[49] E. Nikolsky, R. Mehran, D. Turcot et al., "Impact of chronic kidney disease on prognosis of patients with diabetes mellitus treated with percutaneous coronary intervention," *The American Journal of Cardiology*, vol. 94, no. 3, pp. 300–305, 2004.

19

Application of Real-Time 3D Navigation System in CT-Guided Percutaneous Interventional Procedures

Priya Bhattacharji[1,2] and William Moore[1,2]

[1]Department of Radiology, State University of New York at Stony Brook University Hospital, HSC Level IV, Room 120, Stony Brook, NY 11794, USA
[2]Department of Radiology, New York University Medical Center, 650 First Avenue, Third Floor, Room 355, New York, NY 10016, USA

Correspondence should be addressed to William Moore; william.moore@nyumc.org

Academic Editor: Andreas H. Mahnken

Introduction. To evaluate the accuracy of a quantitative 3D navigation system for CT-guided interventional procedures in a two-part study. *Materials and Methods.* Twenty-two procedures were performed in abdominal and thoracic phantoms. Accuracies of the 3D anatomy map registration and navigation were evaluated. Time used for the navigated procedures was recorded. In the IRB approved clinical evaluation, 21 patients scheduled for CT-guided thoracic and hepatic biopsy and ablations were recruited. CT-guided procedures were performed without following the 3D navigation display. Accuracy of navigation as well as workflow fitness of the system was evaluated. *Results.* In phantoms, the average 3D anatomy map registration error was 1.79 mm. The average navigated needle placement accuracy for one-pass and two-pass procedures, respectively, was 2.0 ± 0.7 mm and 2.8 ± 1.1 mm in the liver and 2.7 ± 1.7 mm and 3.0 ± 1.4 mm in the lung. The average accuracy of the 3D navigation system in human subjects was 4.6 mm ± 3.1 for all procedures. The system fits the existing workflow of CT-guided interventions with minimum impact. *Conclusion.* A 3D navigation system can be performed along the existing workflow and has the potential to navigate precision needle placement in CT-guided interventional procedures.

1. Introduction

Precision placement of intervention instruments is critical for all procedures especially in percutaneous procedures such as biopsies and ablations in order to achieve diagnostic accuracy as well as accurate tumor targeting. Additionally, with the increasing importance of immune-histochemical markers and molecular markers in cancer patients, the need for larger and more accurate biopsy has become paramount [1, 2]. More recently, the use of minimally invasive treatments that require highly precise imaging guidance such as radiofrequency ablation (RFA), cryoablation, and microwave ablation (MWA) has become common place in cancer management because of their effectiveness and safety [3, 4].

Lesions in soft tissue organs, such as the liver and lung, present a unique challenge for radiologists to target in image guided interventions because of motion and deformation. The modality chosen for these procedures depends on the target of interest, its size, accessibility, and visibility all of which play a crucial role in increasing the complexity of diagnostic and therapeutic interventions.

Computed tomography (CT) and ultrasound (US) are the most commonly used modalities for interventional procedures in the liver and lung. US is of limited utility in the lung and can potentially be limited in the abdominal soft tissues specifically in the ability to detect small lesions, less than 1 cm in diameter [5]. Despite having high accuracy rates [6–8], CT is limited by the lack of real-time imaging which is often necessary for procedural guidance. CT fluoroscopy can result in improvement in needle/probe positioning at the cost of additional radiation exposure to the patient and operator. Additionally, CT fluoroscopy is still a subject of debate for

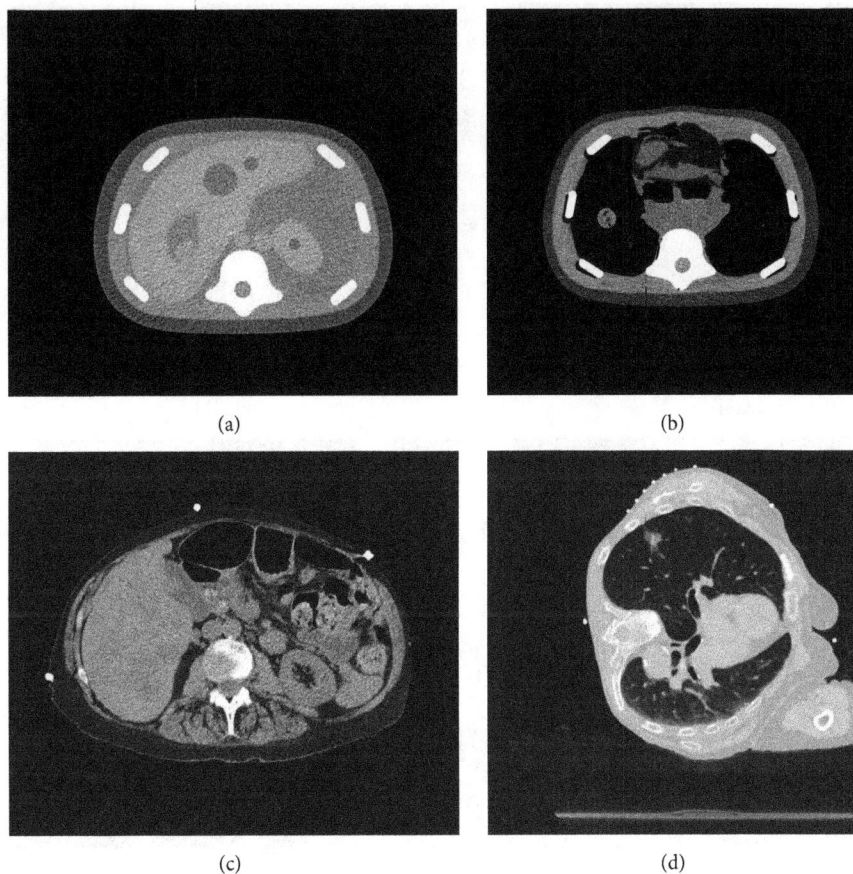

FIGURE 1: Sample of preprocedural CTs: (a) phantom abdominal scans; (b) phantom thoracic scans; (c) patient abdominal scan; (d) patient thoracic scan.

small lesions and lesions near vital anatomies [9, 10]. Cone Beam Computed Tomography (CBCT) allows for real-time visualization with CT imaging. Additionally, CBCT uses an open gantry and provides flexibility to the operator with needle positioning allowing for high accuracy rates even in technically challenging conditions [11]. However, currently, this technique can be labor intensive and slow compared to traditional CT scanners.

Electromagnetic tracking systems (EMTS) use electromagnetic navigation (EMN), an established method to improve accuracy using 3D spatial navigation information [12, 13]. These systems have the ability to fuse several imaging modalities (CT, PT, MRI, or US), thus combining the benefits of each of these modalities to optimize visualization during interventional procedures and providing the ability to approach lesions that were not well visualized on conventional imaging [14–18]. Given the increasing central role that imaging plays in the early detection and diagnosis of a variety of malignancies including lung cancer, colon cancer, and renal cell cancer, [19–21] these systems are emerging synergistically to allow for potential early detection initiatives and to provide support for precisely targeted lesions for diagnostic procedures and minimally invasive treatments.

We connected this investigational EMNTS system to patients who were having CT-guided biopsies to determine the accuracy of this navigational system. To our knowledge, this is the only EMTNS that can generate a 3D fully quantified anatomic map of the target and its surrounding vessels and structures from one preprocedural CT or MRI scan and plan a trajectory to the target lesion clear of vital anatomies. This small pilot study aims to assess the feasibility and accuracy of a 3D quantitative computer aided navigation system, for thoracic and abdominal biopsies as well as interventional oncologic procedures.

2. Materials and Methods

2.1. 3D Navigation System. The quantitative 3D navigation system (IQQA-Guide, EDDA Technology, Inc.) contains an electromagnetic tracking software package and tracks instrument position and orientation in a fully quantified 3D patient-specific anatomy map generated from one preprocedural CT (Figures 1(a)–1(d)) or MRI and its spatial relation to target. All procedures were performed with a Siemens Somatom (Erlangen, Germany) 16-detector CT scanner. CT images were taken with 2 mm thickness with a pitch of 1 : 1.1, 16×0.5 mm detector configuration, at 120 peak kilovoltage (kVp) and a variable milliamperage using an effective mAs of 100 mA.

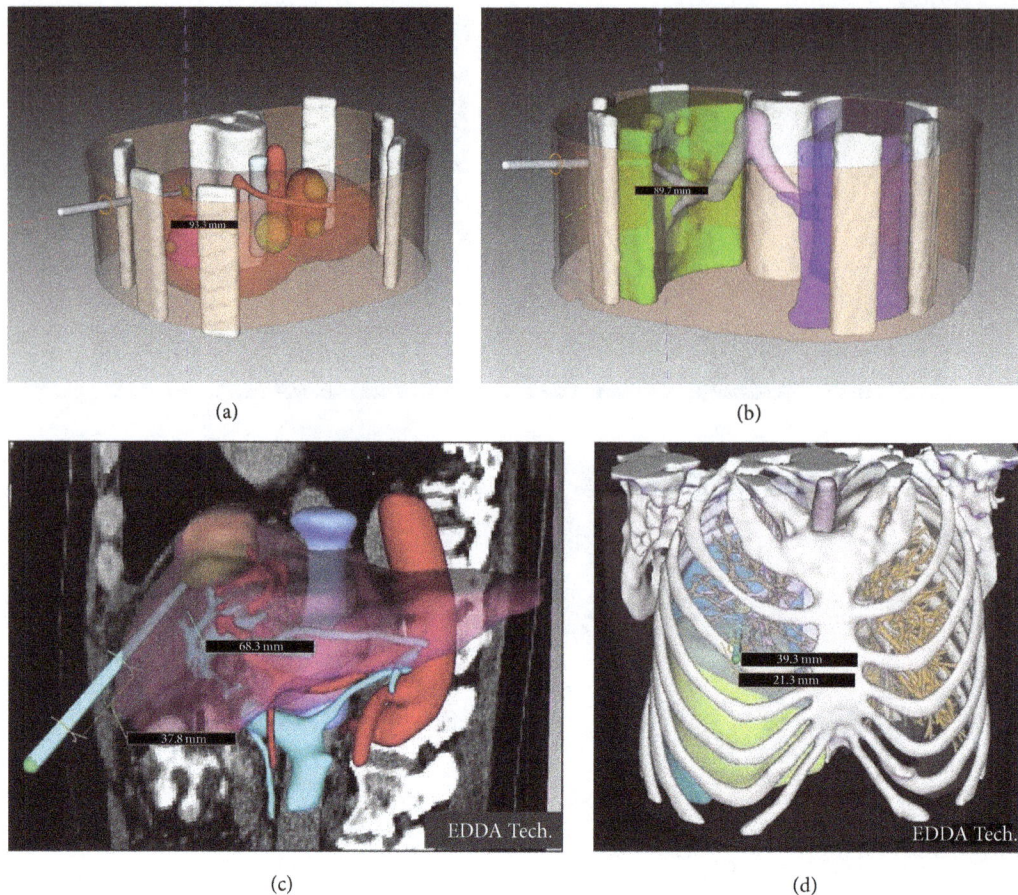

FIGURE 2: Fully quantified 3D anatomy generated from the CT scans with interactively planned and real-time depth. (a) Abdominal scan in phantom (b) Thoracic scan in phantom (c-d) 3D anatomic map in patients.

The navigation system has an extendable arm with an electromagnetic field generator attached. The generator, with a working distance of over 40 cm, was positioned facing the intervention area, (patient). CIVCO (Coralville, Iowa) eTRAX coaxial needle system (for liver biopsies) and CIVCO general purpose sensor together with virtuTRAX navigator (for lung biopsies and ablations) were used to acquire position and orientation tracking information of the needle. Tracked fiducial markers were placed on the patient. The electromagnetic- (EM-) tracked fiducial markers allow the "patient-space" to be registered with the 3D patient-specific anatomic map ("image-space"). This registration together with the EM tracking information from the sensor in the eTRAX/virtuTRAX allows the position and orientation of the instrument relative to the 3D anatomic map to be computed and displayed. The patient's registration can be updated with additional intraprocedural scans as needed.

2.2. Phantom Experiment. An abdominal phantom and a thoracic phantom (CIRS Inc. Norfolk, VA, USA) each with 6 small lesions were used in this study. Preprocedural CT images were sent over the hospital networked to a 3D quantitative navigation system (IQQA-Guide, EDDA technology, Inc., Princeton, NJ). Quantified 3D anatomic renderings of the liver and the lung inclusive of anatomic features (lesions,

ducts, skin, bone, etc.) were then generated using the navigation system (Figures 2(a)–2(d)), [22]. Accuracy of the 3D anatomic map registration (i.e., image registration between the initial CT from which the 3D anatomic map was generated and the final needle tip position based on the coregistration of anatomic landmarks such as the carina or major vascular structures and fiducial markers placed on the skin) was determined using final needle tip position on the final conformational CT compared to the expected location of the needle tip based on the 3D model. Initial CT images were performed at the time of the procedure not prior to the procedure.

All procedures with this system were performed by a radiologist with more than 15 years of experience in image guided intervention. The radiologist used either a one-pass or a two-pass method of accessing the specific lesion. In the one-pass needle placement, the physician inserted the needle directly to target using the quantitative 3D navigation system as a guide for appropriate needle positioning. A final conformational CT was performed, to determine final needle positioning; however, no additional imaging was performed during the needle placement to assist with the guidance. For the two-pass needle placement method, the radiologist inserted the needle part of the way to the target using the navigation system as guidance. Then, an intraprocedural

(a)

(b)

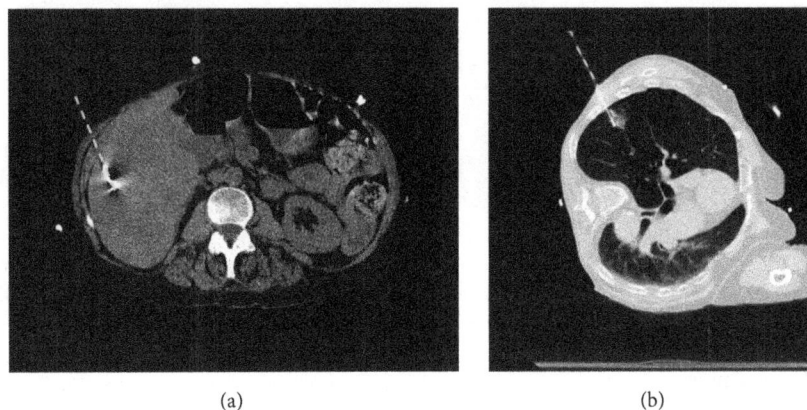

FIGURE 3: Sample of final confirmation CTs showing the actual needle positions and needle positions projected by the navigation system (dashed lines). (a) Patient abdominal scan; (b) patient thoracic scan.

CT scan was performed, confirming the location of the tip of the needle. The intraprocedural CT scan was used to update the "patient-space" with "image-space" alignment. The radiologist then inserted the needle to the target using the 3D navigational system and a final conformational CT scan was performed.

2.3. Feasibility in Patients.
From January 2014 to August 2014, patients with preprocedural CT imaging who were scheduled for a CT-guided biopsy or ablation of the liver or lung were recruited for participation in this IRB approved prospective pilot study. A total of 21 patients were included in this part of the study. During this part of the study the interventional radiologist did not use the navigational system. The system was used passively; that is, the guidance system was not shown to the radiologist during the procedure, and the radiologist was required to perform the procedure as he normally would. The navigational system collected all data and was reviewed for accuracy after the procedure was complete.

2.4. Biopsy Procedure.
The patient or phantom was positioned on the CT table. All biopsy patients received sedation specifically titrated to moderate sedation using intravenous versed and fentanyl. Both ablation patients received general anesthesia. Five EM-tracked fiducial marks were placed on the phantom or patient in order to create the "patient-space." In patients, the fiducial markers were placed on the patients' skin outside of the sterile field. An initial CT exam was then performed as part of standard of care and the 3D anatomic map was generated from this dataset. The procedure proceeded as was planned by the radiologist. The radiologist adjusted the needles as was his practice and performed CT scans to verify the needle trajectory and lesion position for targeting purposes. During the biopsy procedure, the navigational system was monitored in order to determine the registration accuracy of the needle tracked comparing the 3D anatomic map and the actual path as seen in the CT images. This was specifically performed by comparing the actual needle tip position based on CT with the

computer generated 3D map anticipated needle tip position. The interventional radiologist specifically looked at the actual needle path confirmed by CT as part of the standard of care. The radiologist was not allowed to see the 3D navigational system. With each of the CT scans taken during the procedure, the navigation system registration was updated allowing for continued refinement of needle position.

2.5. Accuracy and Workflow Fitness.
Accuracy of the system was defined as the distance between the final needle tip position on the conformational CT scan and the anticipated needle tip position predicted by the navigation system (Figures 3(a) and 3(b)). Workflow of the system was also evaluated by the interventional radiologist. Setup time for the system and each of the additional steps necessary to use the navigation system were noted and the time to complete each step was recorded.

2.6. Statistical Analysis.
All statistical analysis was performed using Graphpad Prism Version 6.0f (La Jolla, CA). All data was analyzed using two-tailed Student's t-test. Statistical significance was set at $p < 0.05$.

3. Results

3.1. Evaluation in Phantoms.
In the phantom experiment, a total of 6 thoracic lesions and 6 liver lesions were biopsied with the guidance of the navigation system. The average lesion diameter was 13.2 ± 7.0 mm (SD) (range 4.8 mm–29.8 mm) and the mean distance to the lesions from the surface along the planned path was 76.8 ± 21.3 mm (SD) (range 43.5 mm–121.4 mm). The mean needle placement accuracy in the liver was 2.0 ± 0.7 mm (SD) for one-pass procedures and 2.8 ± 1.1 mm (SD) for two passes and the average procedure time was 9.9 ± 0.2 (SD) minutes (range 9.55–10.1 minutes) and 11.9 ± 0.3 (SD) minutes (range 11.8–12.4), respectively. In thoracic procedures, the mean needle placement accuracy was 2.7 ± 1.7 mm (SD) and 3.0 ± 1.4 mm (SD) for one and two passes, respectively. The average time of navigated needle placement was 8.8 minutes ± 1.1 (SD) (range 6.6–9.8 minutes) for one-pass procedures and

TABLE 1: Patient demographics.

	Patient demographics ($n = 21$)
Mean age, years	63.8 (17–85)
Gender	
Male, n	6
Female, n	15
Lung biopsy, n	15
Lung cryoablation, n	2
Liver biopsy, n	5

TABLE 2: Interventional procedure details.

	Interventional procedures ($n = 22$)
Mean target diameter (mm)	14.3 ± 6.7 (7.4–32.0)
Mean target distance from skin (mm)	63.1 ± 25.2 (28.7–109.7)

12.8 minutes $\pm$ 1.2 (SD) (range 10.8–13.8 minutes) for the two-pass method. The average 3D anatomic map registration error was 1.79 mm.

3.2. Clinical Application of Navigation System. In the clinical application segment of this study, a total of 21 patients consented to participate in this study. The average patient was 63.8 years of age (17–85); 68.2% of patients were female; see Table 1. Fifteen procedures were lung biopsy; 5 were targeted liver biopsies; and 2 were lung neoplasm ablations.

The average diameter of targets was 14.3 mm $\pm$ 6.7 (7.4–32 mm) SD with a mean distance from skin of 63.1 $\pm$ 25.2 mm SD (range 28.7–109.7) (Table 2). Eighteen-gauge biopsy needles were used for lung biopsy, while 16-gauge needles were used liver biopsy. Both lung ablations were performed with a 13-gauge cryoablation probe. The mean accuracy of the 3D navigation system in this passive study was 4.6 mm $\pm$ 3.1 (SD) (range 0.88–14.29). Sixteen of the 22 procedures (72.7%) had an accuracy less than 5 mm. There was no significant difference in accuracy between body parts or types of the procedures in this trial ($p = 0.0802$) or the distance to target from the skin surface ($p = 0.2859$). Average time of the system setup was 3.1 minutes.

4. Discussion

The results from this study suggest that (1) this 3D navigational system was able to obtain highly accurate needle placement both in phantoms and in patient's procedures; (2) the use of this system is feasible within the existing workflow for interventional procedures.

The needle placement accuracy was evaluated in multiple scenarios. First, in the controlled environment of a phantom study, in this scenario, we were able to document final needle position accuracy of 2.3 $\pm$ 1.2 mm. Since a phantom procedure is an idealized situation, we extended these experiments to use in patients. In these cases, the device was used in a passive

manner. That is the radiologist performed, the procedure as standard of care without the ability to use or see the 3D navigational system. Accuracy of final needle position was determined by comparing where the 3D navigational system indicated the final needle position and where the CT images indicated the final needle position. This was done to avoid any potential adverse events in patients.

The final aspect of the study was to evaluate this 3D navigational system in clinical scenarios. In addition to determining if this system can generate sufficiently high accuracy in needle position the system must be easily integrated into the clinical workflow. In this study, we measured the time of each part of the procedures. The use of this 3D navigational system added an average of 3.1 minutes. From our experience, using this system, we are confident that adding this system into the clinical workflow should be easily done in an imaging suite as prior EMN image fusion studies have suggested [14–18]. Of interest the degree of variance of the final needle tip position observed with the two-pass method was greater than the degree of variance observed with a one-pass method. There was no clear reason for this difference which was not statistically significantly different.

The navigation system in this study differs from others by providing 3D fully quantified anatomies, making the physician aware of the surrounding structures and facilitating a needle path planning and placement with an intuitive approach. Navigation systems like the one used in this study fuse different 3D imaging modalities (CT, MR, and PET), from previously taken reference datasets to create a 3D workspace. When the target is not well visualized under the 3D working data set (usually US or CT) but had been previously seen, both the 3D working and reference data sets can be superimposed and aligned to create a new 3D working data set in which the electromagnetic needle can be tracked in a real-time multiplanar display. This has shown potential utility for target lesions with FDG avidity in biopsy procedures [15].

Additionally, particularly for ablation treatments, where the delineation of the ablation zone and lesion is more difficult to see during intraprocedural imaging, having the pretreatment image fused with an intraprocedural scan may help to more effectively determine treatment margins. This may translate to better accuracy and treatment outcomes for noninvasive image guided therapies such as cryoablation, radiofrequency ablation (RFA), and microwave ablation (MWA) [23].

The results of this study compare favorably to other studies using similar methodologies. For example, Wallach et al. [24] observed a target positioning error of 4.6 $\pm$ 1.2 mm for liver lesions comparing free hand placement to aiming device-navigation. This is similar to the results we found in our phantom studies. This study goes further in that it shows that this system can be translated to clinical use and in both liver and lung procedures with similar (4.6 $\pm$ 3.1 mm) accuracy.

There are several limitations to this study. This was a pilot study with a small number of patients and future randomized controlled trials in which the trajectory planned by the 3D navigation system is utilized will be necessary to give a clear understanding of the utility and benefits of a 3D electromagnetic navigation device with image fusion capabilities. Although respiratory motion was incorporated into the navigational system, the use of these in patients with erratic respiratory cycles has not been tested. Needle bending was not evaluated in this study; however, the needles used in this study are of a gauge where there is less risk of significant needle bending. The use of these needles also adds an additional bias; the potential for more significant and important needle bending could occur with thinner needle gauges.

Tissue deformation was not considered in this study. This is a common issue in solid organs but is obviated in the extreme scenario of an intraprocedural pneumothorax. Most common tissue deformation refers to the change in shape and position of an organ or target lesion after the introduction of a needle. Despite these limitations and potentially confounding factors this study shows that this 3D electromagnetic navigational system is able to attain extremely high accuracy level of needle placement in both phantoms and humans, in the clinical scenario or liver biopsy, lung biopsy, and lung ablation. This study suggests that this system could be used in many clinical scenarios with limited impact of clinical workflow and potentially with improved clinical outcomes. Future studies using this system to actively guide biopsy and ablation procedures are necessary to fully test this system.

Acknowledgments

This study was funded by a grant from EDDA technology.

References

[1] A. Rose-James and S. Tt, "Molecular markers with predictive and prognostic relevance in lung cancer," *Lung Cancer International*, vol. 2012, pp. 1–12, 2012.

[2] K. Zhu, Z. Dai, and J. Zhou, "Biomarkers for hepatocellular carcinoma: progression in early diagnosis, prognosis, and personalized therapy," *Biomarker Research*, vol. 1, no. 1, p. 10, 2013.

[3] W. Moore, R. Talati, P. Bhattacharji, and T. Bilfinger, "Five-year survival after cryoablation of stage I non-small cell lung cancer in medically inoperable patients," *Journal of Vascular and Interventional Radiology*, vol. 26, no. 3, pp. 312–319, 2015.

[4] D. H. Lee, J. M. Lee, J. Y. Lee et al., "Radiofrequency ablation of hepatocellular carcinoma as first-line treatment: Long-term results and prognostic factors in 162 patients with cirrhosis," *Radiology*, vol. 270, no. 3, pp. 900–909, 2014.

[5] D. V. Sahani and S. P. Kalva, "Imaging the liver," *The Oncologist*, vol. 9, no. 4, pp. 385–397, 2004.

[6] R. Chojniak, R. K. Isberner, L. M. Viana, L. S. Yu, A. A. Aita, and F. A. Soares, "Computed tomography guided needle biopsy:

Experience from 1,300 procedures," *São Paulo Medical Journal*, vol. 124, no. 1, pp. 10–14, 2006.

[7] L. S. Yu, D. Deheinzelin, R. N. Younes, and R. Chojniak, "Computed tomography-guided cutting needle biopsy of pulmonary lesions," *Revista do Hospital das Clínicas*, vol. 57, no. 1, pp. 15–18, 2002.

[8] S. Steil, S. Zerwas, G. Moos et al., "CT-guided percutaneous core needle biopsy in oncology outpatients: Sensitivity, specificity, complications," *Onkologie*, vol. 32, no. 5, pp. 254–258, 2009.

[9] J. M. Lorenz, "Updates in percutaneous lung biopsy: new indications, techniques and controversies," *Seminars in Interventional Radiology*, vol. 29, no. 4, pp. 319–324, 2012.

[10] J. Hur, H.-J. Lee, J. E. Nam et al., "Diagnostic accuracy of CT fluoroscopy-guided needle aspiration biopsy of ground-glass opacity pulmonary lesions," *American Journal of Roentgenology*, vol. 192, no. 3, pp. 629–634, 2009.

[11] J. W. Choi, C. M. Park, J. M. Goo et al., "C-arm cone-beam CT-guided percutaneous transthoracic needle biopsy of small (≤ 20 mm) lung nodules: Diagnostic accuracy and complications in 161 patients," *American Journal of Roentgenology*, vol. 199, no. 3, pp. W322–W330, 2012.

[12] A. Hakime, F. Deschamps, E. G. M. De Carvalho, A. Barah, A. Auperin, and T. De Baere, "Electromagnetic-tracked biopsy under ultrasound guidance: Preliminary results," *CardioVascular and Interventional Radiology*, vol. 35, no. 4, pp. 898–905, 2012.

[13] P. Lei, F. Moeslein, B. J. Wood, and R. Shekhar, "Real-time tracking of liver motion and deformation using a flexible needle," *International Journal for Computer Assisted Radiology and Surgery*, vol. 6, no. 3, pp. 435–446, 2011.

[14] L. Appelbaum, J. Sosna, Y. Nissenbaum, A. Benshtein, and S. N. Goldberg, "Electromagnetic navigation system for CT-guided biopsy of small lesions," *American Journal of Roentgenology*, vol. 196, no. 5, pp. 1194–1200, 2011.

[15] A. M. Venkatesan, S. Kadoury, N. Abi-Jaoudeh et al., "Real-time FDG PET guidance during biopsies and radiofrequency ablation using multimodality fusion with electromagnetic navigation," *Radiology*, vol. 260, no. 3, pp. 848–856, 2011.

[16] J. Krücker, S. Xu, A. Venkatesan et al., "Clinical utility of real-time fusion guidance for biopsy and ablation," *Journal of Vascular and Interventional Radiology*, vol. 22, no. 4, pp. 515–524, 2011.

[17] L. Appelbaum, L. Solbiati, J. Sosna, Y. Nissenbaum, N. Greenbaum, and S. N. Goldberg, "Evaluation of an electromagnetic image-fusion navigation system for biopsy of small lesions: assessment of accuracy in an in vivo swine model," *Academic Radiology*, vol. 20, no. 2, pp. 209–217, 2013.

[18] B. J. Wood, H. Zhang, A. Durrani et al., "Navigation with electromagnetic tracking for interventional radiology procedures: A feasibility study," *Journal of Vascular and Interventional Radiology*, vol. 16, no. 4, pp. 493–505, 2005.

[19] V. A. Moyer, "Screening for lung cancer: U.S. preventive services task force recommendation statement," *Annals of Internal Medicine*, vol. 160, no. 5, pp. 330–338, 2014.

[20] D. J. Brenner, "Should we be concerned about the rapid increase in CT usage?" *Reviews on Environmental Health*, vol. 25, no. 1, pp. 63–68, 2010.

[21] M. K. Gould, T. Tang, I.-L. A. Liu et al., "Recent trends in the identification of incidental pulmonary nodules," *American Journal of Respiratory and Critical Care Medicine*, vol. 192, no. 10, pp. 1208–1214, 2015.

[22] Y.-B. He, L. Bai, Y. Jiang et al., "Application of a three-dimensional reconstruction technique in liver autotransplantation for end-stage hepatic alveolar echinococcosis," *Journal of Gastrointestinal Surgery*, vol. 19, no. 8, pp. 1457–1465, 2015.

[23] B. J. Wood, J. K. Locklin, A. Viswanathan et al., "Technologies for guidance of radiofrequency ablation in the multimodality interventional suite of the future," *Journal of Vascular and Interventional Radiology*, vol. 18, no. 1, pp. 9–24, 2007.

[24] D. Wallach, G. Toporek, S. Weber, R. Bale, and G. Widmann, "Comparison of freehand-navigated and aiming device-navigated targeting of liver lesions," *The International Journal of Medical Robotics and Computer Assisted Surgery*, vol. 10, no. 1, pp. 35–43, 2014.

20

Construction of an Anthropomorphic Phantom for Use in Evaluating Pediatric Airway Digital Tomosynthesis Protocols

Nima Kasraie ⓘ, Amie Robinson, and Sherwin Chan

Department of Radiology, Children's Mercy Hospital, 2401 Gillham Rd., Kansas City, MO 64108, USA

Correspondence should be addressed to Nima Kasraie; nkasraie@cmh.edu

Academic Editor: Henrique M. Lederman

Interpretation of radiolucent foreign bodies (FBs) is a common task charged to pediatric radiologists. The use of a motion compensated technique to decrease breathing motion on images would greatly decrease overall exposure to ionizing radiation and increase access to treatment yielding a great impact on clinical care. This study reports on the methodology and materials used to construct an in-house anthropomorphic phantom for investigating image quality in digital tomosynthesis protocols for volumetric imaging of the pediatric airway. Availability and cost of possible substitute materials were considered and simplifying assumptions were made. Two different modular phantoms were assembled in coronal slab layers using materials designed to approximate a one- and three-year-old thorax at diagnostic photon energies for use with digital tomosynthesis protocols such as those offered on GE's VolumeRAD application. Exposures were made using both phantoms with inserted food particles inside an oscillating airway. The goal of the phantom is to help evaluate (1) whether the currently used protocol is sufficient to image the airway despite breathing motion and (2) whether it is not, to find the optimal protocol by testing various commercially available protocols using this phantom. The affordable construction of the pediatric sized phantom aimed at optimizing GE's VolumeRAD protocol for airway foreign body imaging is demonstrated in this study which can be used to test VolumeRAD's ability to image the airways with and without a low-density foreign body within the airways.

1. Introduction

Accidental impaction of objects in pediatric respiratory tract, known as airway foreign bodies (AFBs), is a common and potentially life-threatening occurrence. Of the 110,000 foreign body ingestions in patients of all ages reported in the United States in 2011, over 85% of these occurred in the pediatric population [1], and this continues to remain the most common cause of mortality owing to unintentional injury in children aged under 1 year [2].

Aspiration of a foreign body can be difficult to diagnose especially in infants and small children as most aspirated objects are radiolucent and are not seen on routine chest X-rays [3]. Thus, conventional radiographs used in the diagnosis have low specificity for radiolucent foreign bodies [3–7]. On the other hand, digital tomosynthesis (DT) volumetric imaging has multiple clinical applications for adults, including airway imaging [8–10]. However, corresponding pediatric applications have yet to be developed, as pediatric

imaging presents a unique set of challenges for DT volumetric acquisition, the largest of these being the challenge of patient cooperation during the exam. In particular, midexposure patient motion remains a resilient obstacle facing tomosynthesis imaging of the thoracic region. This is mainly due to the long time spans (greater than ten seconds) typically used by thoracic protocol exposures to complete their imaging sweep. This motion can be classified into respiratory and patient body motions (e.g., child wiggling and unrest). In pediatric imaging, radiologists are able to compensate for the latter using various immobilization devices for younger aged children as well as child life specialists encouraging patient cooperation. Nonetheless, the majority of pediatric patients will not be able to exercise full control over their breathing during exams, especially if they are acutely symptomatic (e.g., shortness of breath, coughing, or choking).

Quantifying respiratory patient motion may be very useful in assessing which pediatric clinical applications would be appropriate targets for tomosynthesis imaging. In this study, we aim to investigate the proposal to evaluate the amount of respiratory motion in the pediatric airway. Computational modeling studies have shown that DT may add substantial sensitivity and specificity for the detection of low-density aspirated foreign bodies; thus, we believe that airway tomosynthesis would be a highly useful tool for pediatric radiologists. Our preliminary investigation has shown that adding simulated VolumeRAD images to simulated radiographs increased sensitivity from 15% to 67% and increased specificity from 94% to 100% [11].

Interpretation of radiolucent foreign bodies (FBs) is a common task charged to pediatric radiologists. The use of a motion compensated technique to decrease breathing motion on images would greatly decrease exposure to ionizing radiation and increase access to treatment yielding a great impact on clinical care. One of the main disadvantages of tomosynthesis is the long acquisition time which makes it very susceptible to motion degradation of image quality. By improving image quality, we could improve diagnostic performance and tomosynthesis could replace CT as a confirmatory test in some cases. If tomosynthesis is used to replace chest CT for any clinical indication [12], then the dose saving could be considerable since the effective dose from CT for an adult patient is in the range of 4.0–18.0 mSv [13]. Our research group is interested in testing the hypothesis that patient breathing motion will not degrade VolumeRAD image quality enough to significantly affect the ability of radiologists to diagnose a low-density foreign body in the airway. The primary aim of this paper is to describe the construction of a phantom that mimics the breathing motion of infants and small children who are prone to ingesting objects in their airways. The phantom is to be used to test different VolumeRAD protocols to determine which one is optimally suited to minimize breathing artifacts and create the images that are best fit for diagnosis of pediatric AFBs. This report focuses on the design, construction, and feasibility testing of this phantom for the aforementioned purpose.

2. Methods and Materials

First, the tissue-equivalent substitutes used were developed with three design benchmarks in mind: approximating the physical properties of human tissue such as density, attenuation coefficients, and physical dimensions. In regard to the latter design element, the phantom was designed to mimic the thorax habitus of a one- and a three-year-old patient. The selected age is based on the fact that this age group in our practice is known to exhibit a higher occurrence of aspirating a foreign body, and published reports show that 80% of all AFB cases occur below the three-year-old age group [14].

Second is compartmentalizing the phantom into modular segments to enable switching out various elements such as airways of different sizes or to improve or add components if need be, without the need to change the entire phantom set for each modification.

The third design element focused on particular geometry of the tomosynthesis acquisition. Unlike the conventional oval-shaped chest dosimetry or computed tomography (CT) phantoms, the cranial-caudal (CC) direction of the

sweep movement during the sequence of projections in VolumeRAD eases restrictions on having to consider an oval-shaped architecture in the transverse axial plane for this phantom prototype. Thus, the vertical single-plane movement of the sweep allows the use of a simplified Cartesian model design for the shape of the phantom. To accommodate the above stated goals, we employed the materials described in the following sections in constructing the phantom.

The developed lung and tissue-equivalent materials were evaluated by measuring the attenuation properties, namely, the Hounsfield Unit (HU) values for each component, using a Siemens Somatom Flash 64-slice CT scanner operated at a tube voltage of 120 kVp and employing a mA modulated exposure control. The mean HU was determined from three selected regions of interest (ROI) at different axial (z) positions in the phantom, using areas of approximately 100 mm^2.

Density measurements of each sample were taken utilizing Archimedes' principle. A cured sample of each material was weighed on an APX-60 model scale with 0.1 mg precision (Denver Instrument, Bohemia, NY) to find the dry mass of each sample. The samples were then submerged in a beaker of deionized water to estimate the volume of the samples.

The most common site for AFBs is the right lower bronchus or its bronchus intermedius [15]. The positioning of the lodged food particles in our phantom involved the right and left bronchi with equal frequency and was based on pediatric data cited by Rothmann and Boeckman [16]. We used dry food particles, namely, peanuts (the most common food type), accounting for 35%–55% of all aspirated foreign bodies, as well as seeds, popcorn, and other food particles [16].

2.1. Phantom Construction and Imaging Methodology. The design of the phantom consists of three slabs stacked together: a posterior slab, a midsection slab, and an anterior slab. The construction is modular: any slab can be removed or swapped so as to change the configuration (AP length or components) of the phantom if desired.

Two phantom prototypes were made, one with a larger AP dimension and slightly different anterior lung design. The respective thickness (or AP length) of each slab of the first phantom is 80 mm for the anterior section, 22 mm for the middle slab, and 58 mm for the posterior part combining to a sum of 160 mm, roughly corresponding to the chest of an average three-year-old, while the respective thickness (or AP length) of each slab of the second phantom is 52 mm for the anterior section, 22 mm for the middle slab, and 58 mm for the posterior part combining to a sum of 132 mm, roughly corresponding to the chest of an average one-year-old child. The only differences between the two phantom prototypes essentially were the anterior slab AP length and middle slab airway size.

The overall AP thicknesses we used were based on the measurements made by Kleinman et al. where we tried to select an AP thickness above the 50th but below the 95th percentile of AP thorax values for one- and three-year-olds, respectively [17]. The linear equation of the 50th percentile of their data (see (1)) can roughly be used to scale this thickness

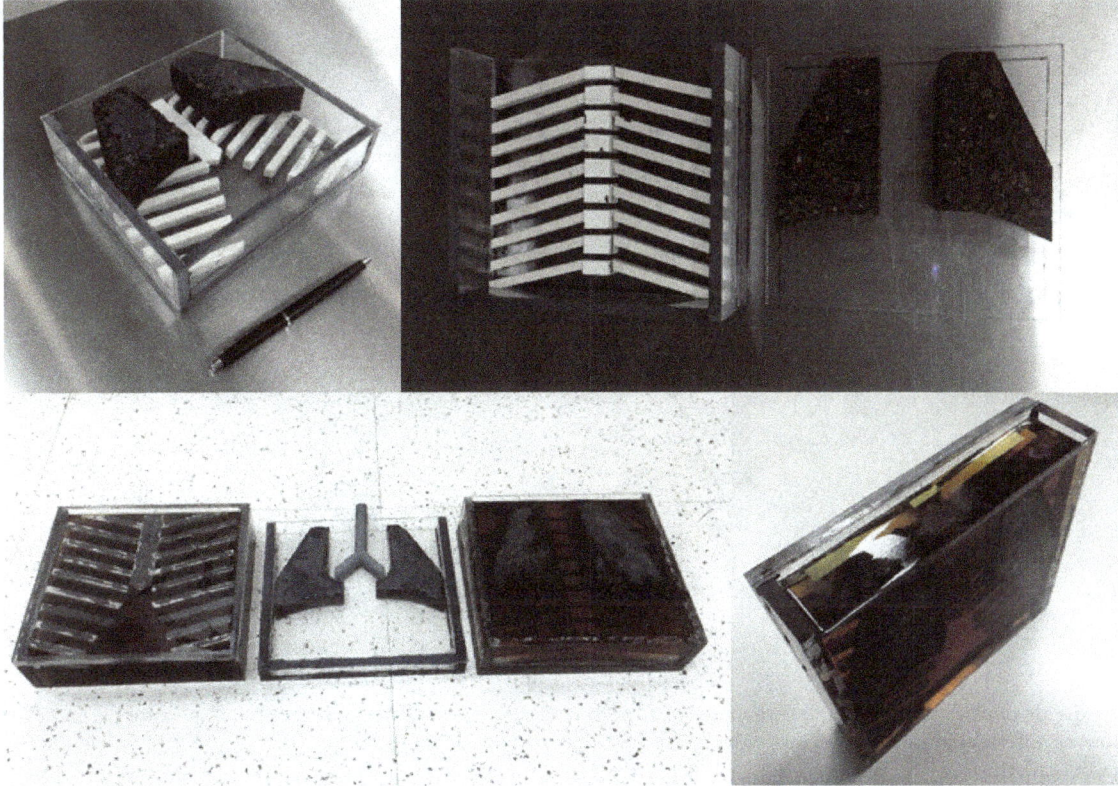

FIGURE 1: Components of the phantom assembly. Clockwise from top left: the anterior frame with LE and BE inserts. The posterior frame with the BE insert and the LE insert not attached yet. The anterior slab view from the side with the SE poured in. All 3 slabs side by side for comparison with the SE poured in A and P frames.

to other thorax sizes (including adult) if need be. Here, y is the AP dimensions in centimeters and x is age in years:

$$y = 0.60x + 11.7. \tag{1}$$

The middle slab is filled with water to enable movement of the airways, which is why we decided to use VolumeRAD's vertical or wall-stand acquisition protocol. The other two sections are constructed as box-shaped frames with bone-tissue-equivalent (BE) inserts glued to the anterior rim of the interior of the container at anatomical spacing and then poured and filled with the soft-tissue equivalent (SE) epoxy resin.

The frame or container itself is made of cast acrylic (Regal Plastics, Kansas City) with dimensions of 20 cm in the transverse and 18 cm in the CC (or vertical) direction for all three slabs (Figure 1) in both phantom types.

All exposures of the phantom were acquired with a GE Discovery XR 650 unit using the "Chest VolumeRAD" protocol. The tomosynthesis angle was 30 degrees and the acquisition time was 11.4 seconds.

2.2. Soft-Tissue Equivalent (SE) Substitute. Adipose tissue was not specifically modeled in the construction of this anthropomorphic phantom. The distribution of subcutaneous as well as intra-abdominal adipose tissue was determined to be too complicated to directly model with a specific tissue-equivalent material. Thus, the SE substitute was developed to be a homogeneous soft-tissue analog that represents skeletal muscle as well as organs, connective tissue, and adipose tissue.

A polyurethane-based SE substitute was used to match the X-ray attenuation and density of human soft tissue within the diagnostic (80–120 kVp) energy range. Polyurethane-based material has been used for constructing lung phantoms in the past [18]. Hence, the SE substitute was designed to have a density similar to that of human soft tissue (1.04 g/cm^3) and with published [19, 20] X-ray mass attenuation coefficients of soft-tissue compositions in mind.

The commercially available, two-part rubber compound PMC 121/30 Wet (Smooth-On Inc., Easton, PA) was used as the template for soft-tissue equivalent inserts. The durable, readily available, polyurethane-based compound was relatively easy to work with at room temperature; however, a hood or sufficient ventilation is required to ensure respiratory protection of the user and nearby occupants. Part A of the compound was a TDI prepolymer composed of diisononyl phthalate and toluene diisocyanate. Part B was composed of diisononyl phthalate, diethyltoluenediamine, and phenylmercury neodecanoate. The two parts were thoroughly mixed in 1 : 1 volume (or mass) ratios in a disposable graduated cylinder, as per instructions by the manufacturer.

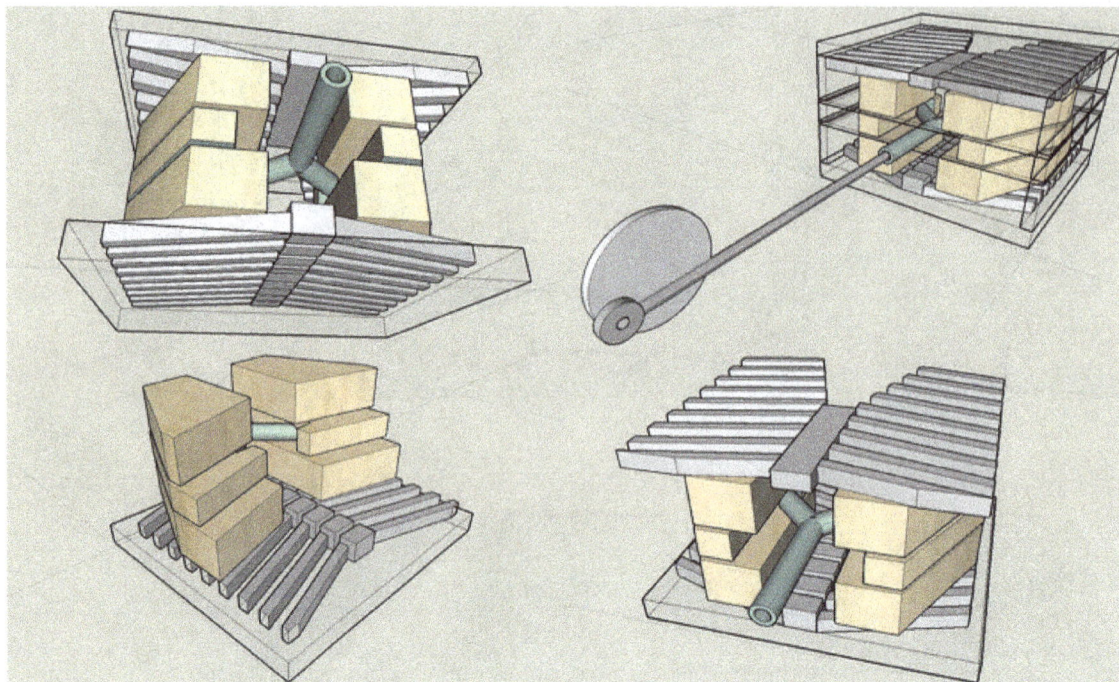

FIGURE 2: Rendering of phantom design and components. 3D perspective view of renderings of the second phantom, using FORMZ CAD software, showing different parts of the phantom without the SE. Notice the gradual stepped contour of the inferior part of the 6-plated lung in the lower left rendering.

We ended up requiring nearly 2000 ml of the mixed compound, per phantom set. The pouring had to be planned ahead of time and the phantom frame constructed beforehand, because once mixed, the composite liquid exhibits high viscosity (1800 CPS, per technical specs) which makes handling rather difficult and has a pot life of less than 30 minutes, with the viscosity gradually increasing by the minute. The pouring has to be slow to avoid trapping air bubbles in the phantom. This is a very crucial factor to ensure a homogenous mix. The poured mixture was given 24 hours of curing time, and four to eight hours of postcuring heating inside an oven to allow the resin to settle in and permanently solidify. Our oven (Mac Medical, Millstadt, IL) was set at 130 F overnight. Our design required no release agent as our phantom frame served as the casting mold to the mixture. The manufacturer's technical overview sheet claims a specific gravity of $1.04 \, g/cm^3$ for this material.

2.3. Lung-Tissue Equivalent (LE) Substitute.

The LE substitute used was designed by combining commercially available dark cork tiles measuring $30.4 \times 30.4 \times 1.0$ cm (ArtMinds, Michaels, Irving, TX) and cutting them into coronal plates in four different quadrants (anterior left, anterior right, posterior left, and posterior right) and gluing them together using a two-part epoxy mix adhesive (Quiksteel Blue Magic, Cleburne, TX) into stacks of 3.0 and 6.0 cm anterior, 3.0 and 4.0 cm posterior, and 1.5 cm midsection thicknesses. The superior lobes were cut to measure 3.0 cm in the transverse direction and widened as we move toward the inferior lobes. When cutting, each of the six plates had a slightly different contour in the bottom (inferior) section, so that when the

stacks are aligned, the overall shape of the lung changed stepwise going from anterior to posterior, in line with the sloped shape of the costodiaphragmatic recess area of the lungs (seen in Figure 2). The right lung was also intentionally slightly elevated compared to the left one, representing normal anatomical configuration. The cork material was selected by trial and error among other candidates due to its amorphous texture, light density, attenuation properties, and ease of handling and reproducibility. While the density of lung tissue can vary widely depending on the level of inspiration, patients undergoing diagnostic procedures are typically asked to hold their breath during the exposure. Therefore, a value of $0.33 \, g/cm^3$ was chosen for the LE substitute, representing the density of a fully inspired lung [19].

2.4. Bone-Tissue-Equivalent (BE) Substitute.

The BE substitute used was a Gammex 450-210 cortical bone-tissue-equivalent material (Gammex Inc., Middleton, WI) used for dosimetry studies. A $20 \times 20 \times 1.0$ cm plate of this material was cut using a precision water jet technique (Kastle Grinding, Lee's Summit, MO) and the input computer-aided design (CAD) spacing dimensions seen in Figure 3. The absorption and scattering properties of this material "are within one percent of living tissue" and provide adequate simulations for electron and photon applications between 0.01 and 100 MeV, according to the manufacturer [21]. The dimensions of the cut pieces were as follows: rib thickness, 0.7 cm; rib spacing, 1 cm; sternum, 0.6 cm AP × 2 cm transverse × 9 cm in CC direction; spine, 2 cm transverse × 2 cm AP, spanning the full length of phantom in the CC direction. These dimensions (see

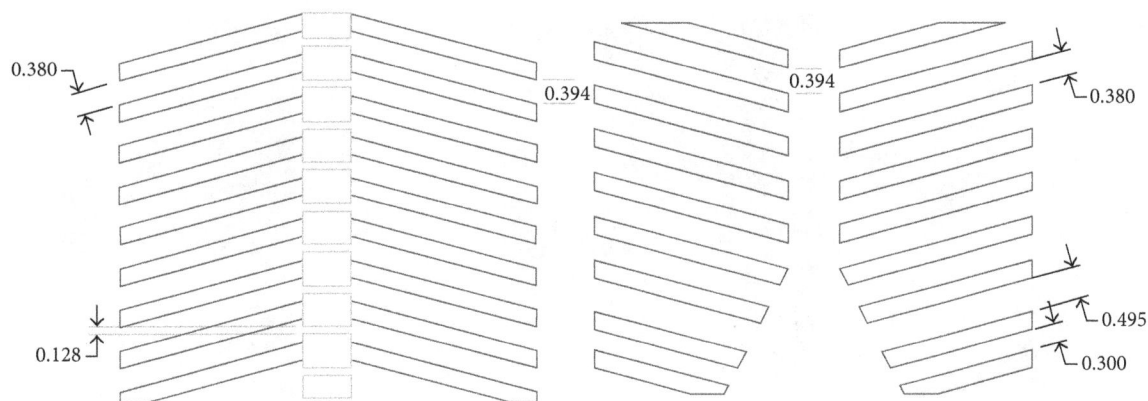

FIGURE 3: Spacing of BE components in inches. Dimensions of the anterior and posterior rib cage used in the second version of the phantom.

Figure 3) were based on a normal CT from a three-year-old patient at our institution.

2.5. The Airway Equivalent (AE) Substitute. The main components of an airway (i.e., trachea, carina, left mainstem bronchus, and right mainstem bronchus) were all made using onsite 3D printers using Platinum Series ABS Filaments (Airwolf 3D Printers, Costa Mesa, CA) which are composed of acrylonitrile-butadiene-styrene copolymer. This material has specific gravity (density) of 1.03–1.10 g/cm^3 and is insoluble in water. Using two Airwolf HDX model units 150526-002 and 150617-0001 (Airwolf 3D Printers, Costa Mesa, CA), we printed 20 airways in two different sizes, as shown in Figure 4: ten airways for a one-year-old and ten larger airway sizes corresponding to a three-year-old. The 3D dataset used to print the models was derived from two normal chest CTs of a one- and a three-year-old who were scanned at our institution. The inner diameter of the printed trachea of the one-year-old was 6 mm and the outer was 10 mm, while the lumen (inner) diameter of the printed trachea in the three-year-old was 6 mm and the outer diameter was 13 mm (Figure 4). The tubes are continuously hollow and airtight when sealed at the ends. The top of the tubes is attached to a shaft that connects to the rotor that oscillates the airway to breathing frequencies of 30 cycles/min (for 1 yr old) and 20 cycles/min (for 3 yr old) [22, 23]. Twenty copies were printed so as to test different types and locations of foreign bodies inserted into the lumen before being sealed and inserted into the phantom. In order for the airway tube to be able to freely move with the breathing frequency, it was necessary to carve out a groove in the medial part of the LE in the middle slab of the phantom, as seen in the lower right image in Figure 4. The remaining space in the middle slab was filled with water to mimic the soft tissues of the mediastinum that surround the airway.

2.6. Simulated Motion. We used a rotating motor with an adjustable frequency and attached the 3D-printed airway to the motor using a rigid rod. As the motor would rotate at a desired frequency based on the estimated heart rates of pediatric patients, the rotational motion would translate into vertical motion of the printed airway. This vertical motion

TABLE 1: Measured (average/standard deviation) attenuation values in HU of key phantom components vs. an actual patient with same ROI (100 mm^2).

	SE	BE	LE	AE (wall)	Acrylic
phantom	9.8/11.0	1111.1/130.9	−664.6/84.8	−122.9/7.3	121.2/9.5
actual	45.6/7.9	346.9/73.5	−652.8/78.9	62/80	NA

TABLE 2: Measured Half Value Layer (HVL) thicknesses of the phantom (in mm) at 60, 80, 100, and 120 kVp energy for the X-ray unit used.

	60	80	100	120
Plain beam (mm Al)	2.4	3.2	3.9	4.7
Phantom (mm)	3.4	4.2	4.8	5.5

simulated the vertical motion of the airway in the chest caused by diaphragm movement.

3. Results and Discussion

To date, two pediatric thorax phantoms, one mimicking a one-year-old's chest and one mimicking a three-year-old's chest, have been constructed using the methods and materials described in the previous section. The major difference between these versions is that the first model was thicker in the AP dimension than the second with different airway sizes. Table 1 shows the average of the measured CT numbers (in HU) of the phantom versus a sample three-year-old patient for the four key components. Table 2 shows the half value layer (HVL) thicknesses (in mm) evaluating the beam itself and the phantom at 60, 80, 100, and 120 kVp using a chest technique with 2 mAs. Table 3 displays the measured density of each component compared to some values in the referenced literature [24, 25].

Figure 5 shows a montage of select frames from the reconstructed images for phantom one, while Figure 6 shows one of those corresponding frames from the second phantom with a food particle lodged in one of the bronchi.

A series of 80 simulated images were interpreted for the presence of a radiolucent AFB by a designated pediatric

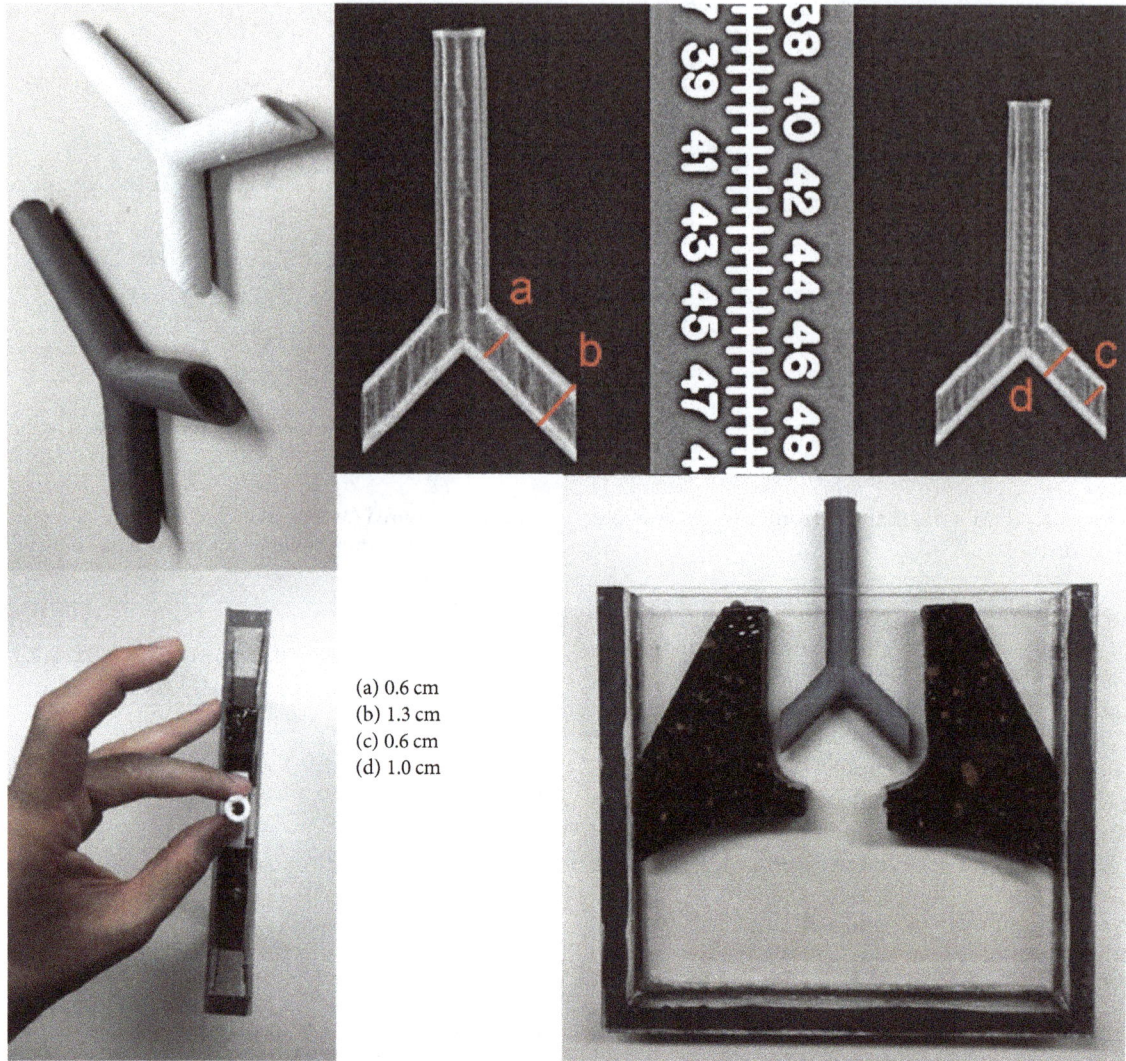

(a) 0.6 cm
(b) 1.3 cm
(c) 0.6 cm
(d) 1.0 cm

FIGURE 4: View of the AE components and how they fit within the middle slab of the phantom. Clockwise from top left: multiple copies of two sizes were printed. The linear dimensions are given for the X-ray image with a centimeter scale appearing for comparison. The angle at the carina between the right and the left mainstem bronchi is 90 degrees. The tubes are continuously hollow and sealed airtight before being inserted and imaged as part of the phantom. A side view showing how the airway fits in the middle slab. A 1 mm gap between the LE component and the container (lower left image) allows for water to uniformly fill any space not occupied by the LE or AE substitutes. An AP view.

TABLE 3: Measured average density values of key phantom components vs. actual reported values from literature (g/cm^3).

	SE	BE	LE	AE (wall)	Acrylic
phantom	0.97	1.89	0.38	0.89	1.23
actual	1.04	1.85	0.33	1.1	

radiologist. 40 simulated images were chest X-rays only and 40 images were DTS images. Twenty images in each group were static and 20 were motion-simulated to represent breathing. Seventeen (ten in motion group and seven in static group) were scored as uninterpretable by the reader and were excluded from our final analysis. Scoring was based on a 5-point probability Likert scale: (1) not probable, (2) somewhat improbable, (3) neutral, (4) somewhat probable, or (5) very probable for right bronchus, mainstem bronchus, and left bronchus. Images were viewed on our institutional PACS system and compared to ground truth.

After removal of the seventeen images, we compared the two groups to the ground truth. Overall, in comparison to the ground truth, the reader correctly identified the presence or absence of a foreign body in 44% ($n = 28/63$) of the images. In comparison to the ground truth and static versus motion images, the static images were correctly identified in 48% ($n = 16/33$) of the cases and in 40% ($n = 12/30$) of the motion group.

Winslow et al. enumerate several advantages of using a polyurethane-based material for constructing a dosimetry phantom [25]. The same reasoning applies to the phantom

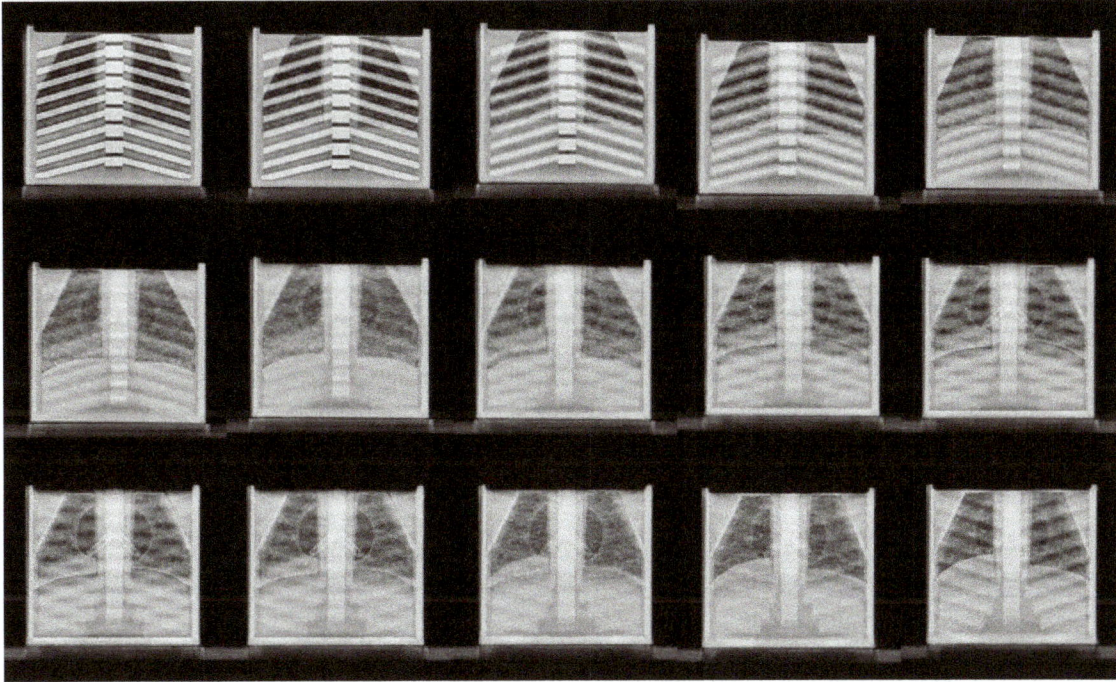

FIGURE 5: A montage of 12 reconstructed frames of the VolumeRAD acquisition for the first phantom. Notice how the airway bronchi are clearly visible in frames 10 through 12 (left to right, top to bottom).

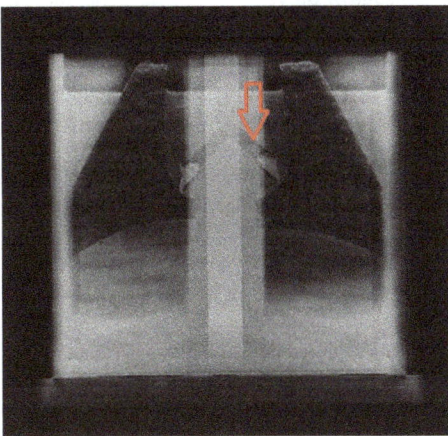

FIGURE 6: Visualization of a food particle in the airway. A reconstructed frame of the VolumeRAD acquisition for the second phantom with a low-density dry food particle lodged in the right airway bronchus (red arrow).

design in this study whose purpose is diagnostic in nature. However, there is room for improvements to be made in the material design and selection. For example, the only material available to us for the 3D printer was the commercial spool of acrylonitrile-butadiene-styrene copolymer threads. A better material can be substituted, which would improve the density and attenuation coefficient values to closer physiological values as those depicted in Tables 1 and 2. Similarly, among the limitations of the phantom also was the not too large but finite difference in CT numbers between the phantom (9.8 HU) and anatomical range (45.6 HU) for the SE material. This

problem can theoretically however be mitigated by adding traces of impurities to the SE mixture before curing. For example, by adding small quantities of hydroxyapatite (number 289396) in powder form (Sigma-Aldrich, St. Louis, MO) to the polyurethane PMC 121/30 liquid form mixture, it is possible to elevate the attenuation of the SE material to higher values, provided that the compound is thoroughly mixed while parts A and B of the mixture are being poured into the phantom template. Likewise, low-density esters or fatty liquids can also be added to the curing mixture to lower the CT numbers closer to desired values. This CT number matching problem was particularly pronounced with the BE (measured 1111.1 HU versus actual 346.9 HU) material. The latter however also can be addressed by noting that a different model of the Gammex tissue-equivalent slab, namely, "inner bone" Model 456 instead of cortical bone (Model 450), which has a much lower attenuation for the area of interest in the study, can be used to construct the BE substitute inserts. An improvement in the DT image quality would be expected using a lesser attenuating bone material.

If a horizontal (instead of vertical) orientation of the setup is desired, a solid tissue-equivalent material can be used in place of water for the midsection slab (e.g., Gammex 452 Muscle or a tissue mimicking gel). The entire phantom can then also be used for hypothetical horizontal sweeps. We however only performed the imaging in vertical mode to be clinically relevant.

Finally, in our practice, we currently use a 2-view plus bilateral decubitus radiographic exam for pediatric foreign body airway imaging. However, standard radiographs with or without special views (decubitus or expiratory) suffer from low diagnostic accuracy [6]. We did not perform any dosimetry measurements in the present study and instead only focused on the visualization aspect of the AFB imaging. However, comparative dosimetry studies have been performed on DT acquisitions [26, 27]. For example, Bath et al. reported the effective dose to a standard-sized patient from a VolumeRAD chest tomosynthesis examination to be close to 2% of an average chest CT and only two to three times the effective dose from the conventional (standard only) two-view chest radiography examination [28].

The purpose of this project was to construct a phantom for use in observer studies to measure the change in diagnostic accuracy for detecting low-density AFB due to breathing motion using a DT radiographic technique. This is the first and only phantom of its kind the authors of this paper are aware of specifically designed for a pediatric target.

4. Conclusions

This study reports a methodology developed to construct anthropomorphic phantoms for use in radiographic tomosynthesis studies. While the value of this methodology has already been proven with the construction of two pediatric phantoms, it should be noted that the same methodology could be applied to the construction of phantoms of other sizes and ages. In particular, our group plans to develop and use these phantoms for dynamic studies in order to accurately model the moving airways. Furthermore, such phantoms may aid optimization studies regarding kVp, number of projections, total angular range, and geometric acquisition parameters that affect DT image quality and dosimetry [27].

While anthropomorphic phantoms have many potential applications, this particular phantom series was created to evaluate tomosynthesis techniques in radiographic units for the purpose of visualizing low-density foreign body particles in pediatric airways. In our small study, we used this phantom that showed that diagnostic accuracy was better in static images compared to images with simulated breathing motion. This result contradicted our main hypothesis that breathing motion would not affect diagnostic accuracy of digital tomosynthesis. More studies are needed to confirm these results and this phantom would be an ideal tool with which to do those studies. It is anticipated that other institutions could create similar customized phantoms for clinical use by following the methodology in this paper and using the described tissue-equivalent materials for a total material cost of less than US$ 1,000.

Acknowledgments

The authors would like to thank Erin Opfer, Rodney Suydam, Kevin Buck, and Stephen Torre of Children's Mercy Hospital as well as Chris Dawson of Kastle Grinding for assisting in preparing components of the phantom.

References

[1] W. Denney, N. Ahmad, B. Dillard, and M. J. Nowicki, "Children will eat the strangest things: a 10-year retrospective analysis of foreign body and caustic ingestions from a single academic center," *Pediatric Emergency Care*, vol. 28, no. 8, pp. 731–734, 2012.

[2] B. S. Pugmire, R. Lim, and L. L. Avery, "Review of ingested and aspirated foreign bodies in children and their clinical significance for radiologists," *RadioGraphics*, vol. 35, no. 5, pp. 1528–1538, 2015.

[3] A. K. Ayed, A. M. Jafar, and A. Owayed, "Foreign body aspiration in children: Diagnosis and treatment," *Pediatric Surgery International*, vol. 19, no. 6, pp. 485–488, 2003.

[4] D. Assefa, N. Amin, G. Stringel, and A. J. Dozor, "Use of decubitus radiographs in the diagnosis of foreign body aspiration in young children," *Pediatric Emergency Care*, vol. 23, no. 3, pp. 154–157, 2007.

[5] A. Boufersaoui, L. Smati, K. N. Benhalla et al., "Foreign body aspiration in children: Experience from 2624 patients," *International Journal of Pediatric Otorhinolaryngology*, vol. 77, no. 10, pp. 1683–1688, 2013.

[6] J. C. Brown, T. Chapman, E. J. Klein et al., "The utility of adding expiratory or decubitus chest radiographs to the radiographic evaluation of suspected pediatric airway foreign bodies," *Annals of Emergency Medicine*, vol. 61, no. 1, pp. 19–26, 2013.

[7] V. E. Mortellaro, C. Iqbal, R. Fu, H. Curtis, F. B. Fike, and S. D. St. Peter, "Predictors of radiolucent foreign body aspiration," *Journal of Pediatric Surgery*, vol. 48, no. 9, pp. 1867–1870, 2013.

[8] S.-J. Park, J. Y. Choo, K. Y. Lee et al., "Usefulness of digital tomosynthesis for the detection of airway obstruction: A case report of bronchial carcinosarcoma," *Cancer Research and Treatment*, vol. 47, no. 3, pp. 544–548, 2015.

[9] J. T. Dobbins III, H. P. McAdams, J.-W. Song et al., "Digital tomosynthesis of the chest for lung nodule detection: Interim sensitivity results from an ongoing NIH-sponsored trial," *Medical Physics*, vol. 35, no. 6, pp. 2554–2557, 2008.

[10] J. Y. Choo, K. Y. Lee, A. Yu et al., "A comparison of digital tomosynthesis and chest radiography in evaluating airway lesions using computed tomography as a reference," *European Radiology*, vol. 26, no. 9, pp. 3147–3154, 2016.

[11] S. Chan, D. Hippe, and G. Kicska, "Pediatric aspirated foreign body: adding digital tomosynthesis improves sensitivity compared to conventional radiographs," *Pediatric Radiology*, vol. 45, pp. 107-108, 2015.

[12] A. A. Johnsson, J. Vikgren, A. Svalkvist et al., "Overview of two years of clinical experience of chest tomosynthesis at Sahlgrenska university hospital," *Radiation Protection Dosimetry*, vol. 139, no. 1-3, Article ID ncq059, pp. 124–129, 2010.

[13] F. A. Mettler Jr., W. Huda, T. T. Yoshizumi, and M. Mahesh, "Effective doses in radiology and diagnostic nuclear medicine: a catalog," *Radiology*, vol. 248, no. 1, pp. 254–263, 2008.

[14] A. M. Salih, M. Alfaki, and D. M. Alam-Elhuda, "Airway foreign bodies: a critical reviewfor a common pediatric emergency," *World Journal of Emergency Medicine*, vol. 7, no. 1, pp. 5–12, 2016.

[15] A. H. Limper and U. B. S. Prakash, "Tracheobronchial foreign bodies in adults," *Annals of Internal Medicine*, vol. 112, no. 8, pp. 604–609, 1990.

[16] B. F. Rothmann and C. R. Boeckman, "Foreign bodies in the larynx and tracheobronchial tree in children: A review of 225 cases," *Annals of Otology, Rhinology & Laryngology*, vol. 89, no. 5, pp. 434–436, 1980.

[17] P. L. Kleinman, K. J. Strauss, D. Zurakowski, K. S. Buckley, and G. A. Taylor, "Patient size measured on CT images as a function of age at a tertiary care children's hospital," *American Journal of Roentgenology*, vol. 194, no. 6, pp. 1611–1619, 2010.

[18] R. J. Traub, P. C. Olsen, and J. C. McDonald, "The radiological properties of a novel lung tissue substitute," *Radiation Protection Dosimetry*, vol. 121, no. 2, pp. 202–207, 2006.

[19] ICRU, Tissue substitutes in radiation dosimetry and measurement. Report 44. In. ICRU report. Bethesda, Md., U.S.A.: International Commission on Radiation Units and Measurements, 1989.

[20] D. R. White, E. M. Widdowson, H. Q. Woodard, and J. W. T. Dickerson, "The composition of body tissues. (II) Fetus to young adult," *British Journal of Radiology*, vol. 64, no. 758, pp. 149–159, 1991.

[21] Gammex. Tissue Equivalent Materials: GAMMEX 450, 452, 453, 454, 455, 456, 481, 482 Data Sheet, https://www.peo-radiation-technology.com/wp-content/uploads/2015/10/gam_15_tissue-equivalent-materials_datasheet_peo.pdf.

[22] E. A. Hooker, D. F. Danzl, M. Brueggmeyer, and E. Harper, "Respiratory rates in pediatric emergency patients," *The Journal of Emergency Medicine*, vol. 10, no. 4, pp. 407–410, 1992.

[23] F. Rusconi, M. Castagneto, L. Gagliardi et al., "Reference values for respiratory rate in the first 3 years of life," *Pediatrics*, vol. 94, no. 3, pp. 350–355, 1994.

[24] J. P. Bilezikian, L. G. Raisz, and G. A. Rodan, *Principles of Bone Biology*, Academic Press, San Diego, CA, USA, 2nd edition, 2002.

[25] J. F. Winslow, D. E. Hyer, R. F. Fisher, C. J. Tien, and D. E. Hintenlang, "Construction of anthropomorphic phantoms for use in dosimetry studies," *Journal of Applied Clinical Medical Physics*, vol. 10, no. 3, pp. 195–204, 2009.

[26] Y. Zhang, X. Li, W. P. Segars, and E. Samei, "Comparison of patient specific dose metrics between chest radiography, tomosynthesis, and CT for adult patients of wide ranging body habitus.," *Medical Physics*, vol. 41, no. 2, p. 023901, 2014.

[27] I. Reiser and S. Glick, *Tomosynthesis Imaging*, CRC Press, Boca Raton, Fla, USA, 2014.

[28] M. Bath, A. Svalkvist, A. Wrangel, H. Rismyhr-Olsson, and A. Cederblad, "Effective dose to patients from chest examinations with tomosynthesis," *Radiation Protection Dosimetry*, vol. 139, no. 1-3, Article ID ncq092, pp. 153–158, 2010.

21

A Current Review of the Meniscus Imaging: Proposition of a Useful Tool for Its Radiologic Analysis

Nicolas Lefevre,[1,2] **Jean Francois Naouri,**[1] **Serge Herman,**[1,2] **Antoine Gerometta,**[1,2] **Shahnaz Klouche,**[1,2] **and Yoann Bohu**[1,2]

[1]*Clinique du Sport Paris V, 75005 Paris, France*
[2]*Institut de l'Appareil Locomoteur Nollet, 75017 Paris, France*

Correspondence should be addressed to Nicolas Lefevre; docteurlefevre@sfr.fr

Academic Editor: Ali Guermazi

The main objective of this review was to present a synthesis of the current literature in order to provide a useful tool to clinician in radiologic analysis of the meniscus. All anatomical descriptions were clearly illustrated by MRI, arthroscopy, and/or drawings. The value of standard radiography is extremely limited for the assessment of meniscal injuries but may be indicated to obtain a differential diagnosis such as osteoarthritis. Ultrasound is rarely used as a diagnostic tool for meniscal pathologies and its accuracy is operator-dependent. CT arthrography with multiplanar reconstructions can detect meniscus tears that are not visible on MRI. This technique is also useful in case of MRI contraindications, in postoperative assessment of meniscal sutures and the condition of cartilage covering the articular surfaces. MRI is the most accurate and less invasive method for diagnosing meniscal lesions. MRI allows confirming and characterizing the meniscal lesion, the type, the extension, its association with a cyst, the meniscal extrusion, and assessing cartilage and subchondral bone. New 3D-MRI in three dimensions with isotropic resolution allows the creation of multiplanar reformatted images to obtain from an acquisition in one sectional plane reconstructions in other spatial planes. 3D MRI should further improve the diagnosis of meniscal tears.

1. Introduction

Arthroscopic knee surgery is the gold standard in the diagnosis and treatment of intra-articular knee lesions. Preoperative imaging is still necessary before any surgery. Indeed, the diagnostic arthroscopy alone has no place in the evaluation of meniscal lesions of the knee. Clinicians (sports doctor, surgeon, or rheumatologist) therefore need to have a precise radiological analysis of meniscal lesions and associated injuries in order to best adapt their treatment. In the literature, many diagnostic radiological examinations were described for the evaluation of meniscal lesions but the magnetic resonance imaging (MRI) is the most accurate and least invasive for the diagnosis of meniscal tears. This technique has revolutionized the imaging of the knee and has become the "gold standard" imaging of the meniscus. Studies have shown excellent results regarding the sensitivity and specificity of MRI in the diagnosis of meniscal tears. They are used to classify the different meniscal lesions, particularly in

the early detection of grade I and grade II lesions to reduce the rate of unnecessary diagnostic knee arthroscopy. This paper describes the various complementary tests used today in the diagnosis of meniscal tears with a precise description of all lesions. All anatomical descriptions were clearly illustrated by MRI, arthroscopy, and/or drawings.

2. Standard Radiography

The value of standard radiography is extremely limited for the assessment of meniscal injuries because the meniscus is not normally visualized with this type of examination. Standard radiography is therefore not useful in the investigation and diagnosis of meniscal injuries. Nevertheless, conventional X-ray of the knee may be indicated to confirm or obtain a differential diagnosis such as osteoarthritis, which often develops in association with meniscal degeneration. AP and lateral X-rays should be performed in the unipodal stance, as well as a standing flexion view (Schuss view) to evaluate and compare the height of the joint space of the weight-bearing area compared to the contralateral side. Thus, a radiographic examination is recommended in case of suspected meniscal injury in patients over the age of 50 because of the risk of associated osteoarthritis. Joint space narrowing of more than 50% or even complete narrowing can create doubt about a potential clinically symptomatic meniscal injury. Radiography can also exclude unsuspected lesions such as osteochondritis or loose bodies. Finally, in the presence of a discoid meniscus, X-rays can identify the relative widening of the involved joint compartment, usually the lateral compartment. Radiography can be used to assess the quality of the bone stock, the width of the tibiofemoral joint spaces, and the thickening of the medial or lateral tibial plateau.

3. Ultrasound

Ultrasound of the knee is a highly valuable diagnostic tool for tendon (patellar tendon, quadricipital tendon, and pes anserinus) and peripheral ligament injuries (medial and lateral collateral ligaments) [1]. Visualization of joint effusion (hydrarthrosis or hemarthrosis) and cysts (which do or do not communicate with the joint) is also good on ultrasound. On the other hand, ultrasound is rarely used as a diagnostic tool for meniscal pathologies. De Flaviis et al. [2] reported a sensitivity of 82% with dynamic ultrasound for the detection of meniscal degeneration based on criteria including meniscal irregularities, cystic lesions, or calcifications. Ultrasound cannot accurately examine the deep structures of the knee and its accuracy depends on the radiologist's experience (operator-dependent). The reliability of ultrasound for the diagnosis of meniscal lesions varies considerably in the literature and existing results suggest that it is not satisfactory [1, 3–5]. It is therefore not a routine test for meniscal imaging. Only meniscal cysts are easily diagnosed and may be punctured and aspirated by ultrasound guidance. Rutten et al. [5] reported a sensitivity of 97%, a specificity of 86%, and accuracy of 94% in the study of meniscal cysts.

4. Arthrography and CT Arthrography

The reliability of arthrography of the knee for the diagnosis of meniscal lesions is well established (tears, bucket-handle tears, and meniscocapsular separation) with reliability between 83 and 94% [6, 7]. Arthrography was the reference technique in the 1970s and 1980s and was given up after 2000 to be replaced by MRI, which has the advantage of being noninvasive and without ionizing radiation. Nevertheless, today, arthrography can be associated with CT to perform CT arthrography, which provides complementary information to MRI. Indeed, thanks to continuous rotation scanning, spiral acquisitions provide high quality 2D multiplanar reconstructions with thin 0.5 mm slices. Coronal, sagittal, and even axial reconstructions can detect tears that are not visible on MRI, as well as meniscocapsular separations based on contrast enhancement between the meniscal wall and the peripheral capsule. This technique also provides a detailed analysis of tibiofemoral and patellofemoral joints with precise mapping of lesions. CT arthrography is not common in Anglo-Saxon countries but is still a gold standard technique for assessment of cartilage in meniscal lesions in Europe [8, 9]. This test has a sensitivity and specificity between 86% and 100% for the evaluation of meniscal lesions. CT arthrography of the knee is a safe technique that provides an accurate diagnosis of meniscal and cartilage injuries in patients who cannot undergo MRI (claustrophobia, pacemaker) or in the postoperative assessment of meniscal sutures and the condition of cartilage covering the articular surfaces [10].

5. Magnetic Resonance Imaging

Magnetic resonance imaging (MRI) is the most accurate and less invasive method for diagnosing meniscal lesions. It is more precise than a clinical examination and has influenced clinical practice and the treatment of patients by eliminating unnecessary diagnostic arthroscopies [11–13]. MRI has revolutionized imaging of the knee and become the "gold standard" for meniscal imaging. Its advantages are the analysis of meniscal lesions on all spatial planes, an excellent resolution using different sequences and high quality assessment of soft tissues. Its multiparametric characteristics allow visualization of specific injuries or structures depending on the sequences chosen. MRI allows characterization of meniscal lesions according to type, extension, association with a cyst, and meniscal extrusion as well as the evaluation of cartilage and subchondral bone. Thus, this technique provides a precise analysis of stability and the risk of propagation of the tear. It also determines whether the meniscal tear can be preoperatively repaired [13–16].

Overall, MRI has the following advantages:

(i) It does not expose the patient to ionizing radiation. Routine MRI does not require intravenous contrast agent administration, which may be associated with adverse events. No manipulation of joints is required. MRI is painless and can be performed in 20 minutes.

(ii) Unlike CT arthrography, MRI does not require intra-articular administration of iodinated contrast agents. MRI has replaced arthrography and CT arthrography, except for patients who are too large to enter the MRI unit, or in patients with contraindications (intracranial aneurysm clips, metallic foreign bodies in the eye, or pacemakers and recent stents). MRI is also very useful for the diagnosis of residual meniscal lesions following meniscal surgery.

The disadvantages and contraindications are the following:

(i) MRI is limited in claustrophobic patients, obese patients (over 170 kg), or patients with pace-makers. With the use of open MRI machines and extremity MRI units, the number of patients who cannot undergo MRI due to claustrophobia or obesity has

(a)

(b)

(c)

(d)

(e)

(f)

(g)

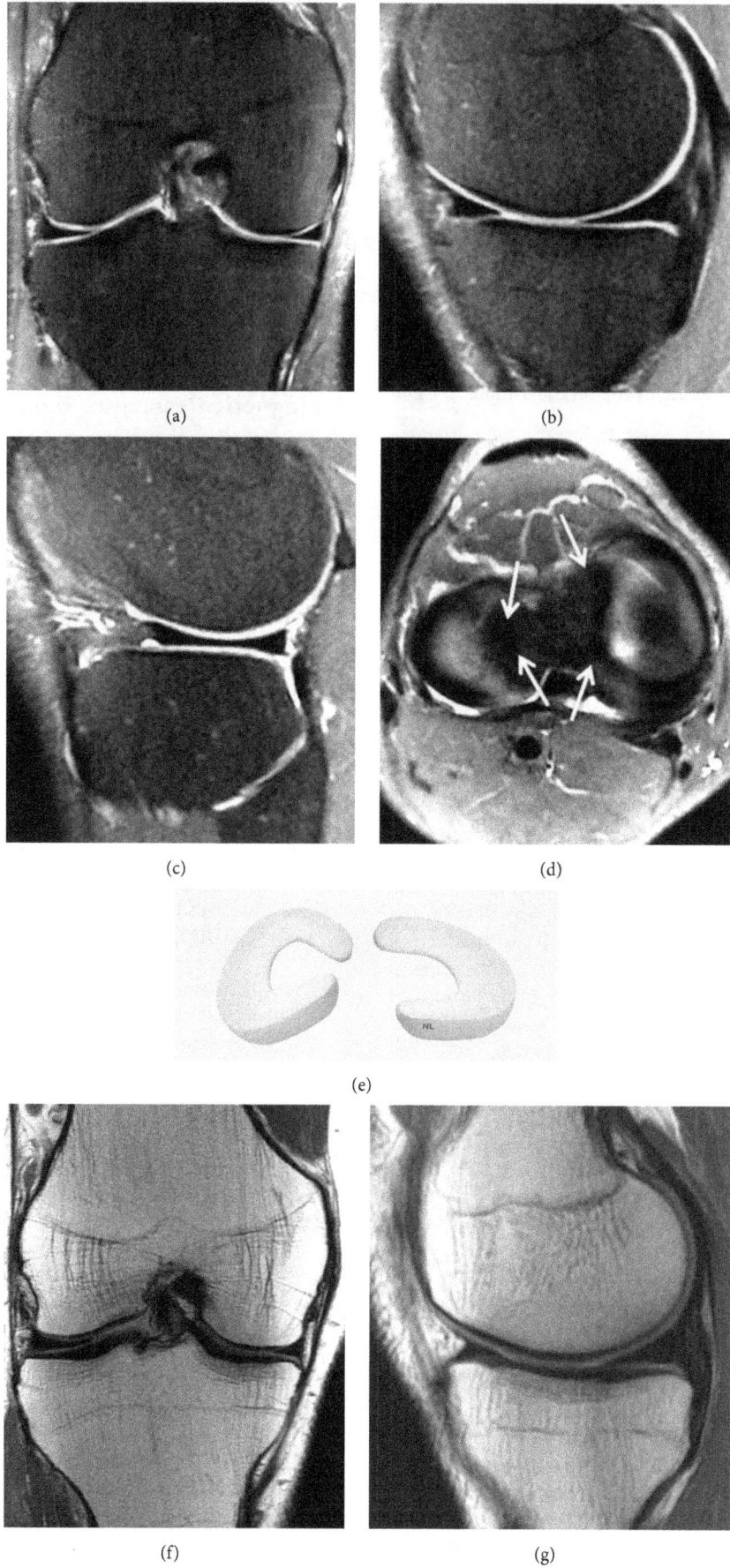

FIGURE 1: Continued.

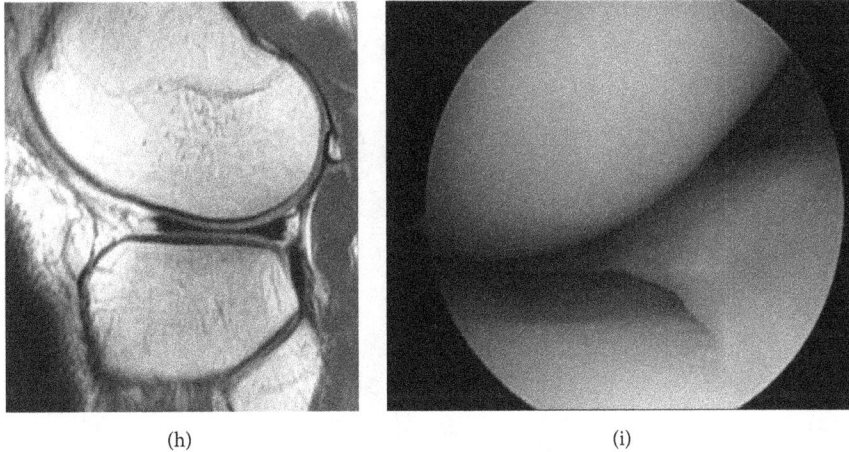

(h)　　　　　　　　　　　　　　　　　(i)

FIGURE 1: Normal meniscus on (a) Coronal T2 FSE Fat Sat MRI; (b) Sagittal T2 FSE Fat Sat MRI (the posterior horn is typically larger than the anterior horn medially); (c) Sagittal T2 FSE Fat Sat MRI (the horns of the lateral meniscus are equal in size and look like opposing triangles); (d) Axial T2 FSE Fat Sat MRI (the shapes of medial and lateral menisci differ, in attachment site (arrow). The medial meniscus is larger and has a more open C-shape configuration, with anterior and posterior tibial attachment sites separated by a greater distance compared to the lateral meniscus which has a more O-shape configuration); (e) three-dimensional diagram of the medial and lateral menisci; (f) coronal proton density weighted sequences; (g) sagittal proton density weighted sequences of the medial meniscus; (h) sagittal proton density weighted sequences of the lateral meniscus; (i) arthroscopic view of meniscus.

decreased. In patients with permanent contraindications to MRI, CT arthrography can be considered the alternative option.

(ii) It is also limited by the presence of artifacts created by nearby orthopedic hardware. Resolution is hampered around the fixation by artifacts that depend upon the implant used. However, the use of nonferromagnetic metals such as titanium minimizes the artifacts in the postoperative knee [17]. Artifacts that hamper MRI results are considerably reduced if bioabsorbable screws are used. Moreover, artifacts associated with bioabsorbable screws tend to decrease over time. STIR sequences should replace fat-sat T2 sequence in the MRI protocol when imaging patients with orthopedic hardware.

5.1. MRI Technique. MRI machines with low, middle, and high field strengths (1, 1.5, or 3 T) can all provide accurate diagnostic images of meniscal lesions. For low-field strength MRI, the number of signals averaged must be increased to obtain a good quality meniscal image. However, this adjustment increases the imaging time and thus increases the risk of movement by the patient. Even the slightest amount of movement can degrade the images, which can compromise the ability to diagnose meniscal lesions [18–20].

Diagnostic sensitivity for medial meniscal lesions is between 86% and 96% with a specificity of 84% to 94%. The diagnostic sensitivity for the lateral meniscus is between 68% and 86%, with a specificity between 92 and 98% [16, 21–30]. The differences in sensitivity and specificity could be due to the sequences used, intraobserver variations or the size of the study population. Sensitivity for the detection of meniscal tears is usually higher for the medial meniscus, whatever the technique used [31]. Mackenzie et al. [32] reported

that the overall sensitivity of MRI for meniscal lesions was 88% with a specificity of 94%. However, diagnostic errors are still possible on MRI. Using conventional coronal and sagittal spin-echo MR imaging, De Smet et al. [23] could not identify 6% of the meniscal tears, even in retrospect compared to arthroscopic findings. False-positive diagnoses due to healed tears or tears missed at arthroscopy occurred in 1.5% of menisci evaluated with MR imaging. Despite the large experience of radiologists, interpretation errors occurred in 21% menisci, due to misinterpretation of normal anatomic structures [23, 33, 34].

The most frequently used MRI is 1.5 tesla machine which provides high quality diagnostic images. There are very few results in the literature comparing musculoskeletal MRI with a 1.5 T and a 3.0 T machine. Faster image acquisition with the 3.0 T should result in more detailed images and improve the diagnostic accuracy [35, 36]. However, several studies [37–39] have shown that knee MRI with a 3.0 tesla machine is as sensitive and specific as with a 1.5 tesla machine. Moreover, 3T imaging has certain disadvantages including increased sensitivity to metallic artifacts.

5.2. Protocols and Imaging Views. The knee is generally extended in slight external rotation to facilitate imaging of the anterior cruciate ligament (ACL). High spatial resolution is necessary to show meniscal tears. This typically requires a field of view of 14 cm × 16 cm. For this review, we use 0.4 mm × 0.4 mm resolution for proton-density-weighted images and 0.5 mm × 0.5 mm resolution for fat sat T2-weighted images. An extremity coil optimizes the signal-to-noise ratio [13, 20, 40, 41].

Images should be obtained on all three planes: sagittal, coronal, and axial. Sagittal images are obtained with the knee in slight external rotation to visualize the anterior

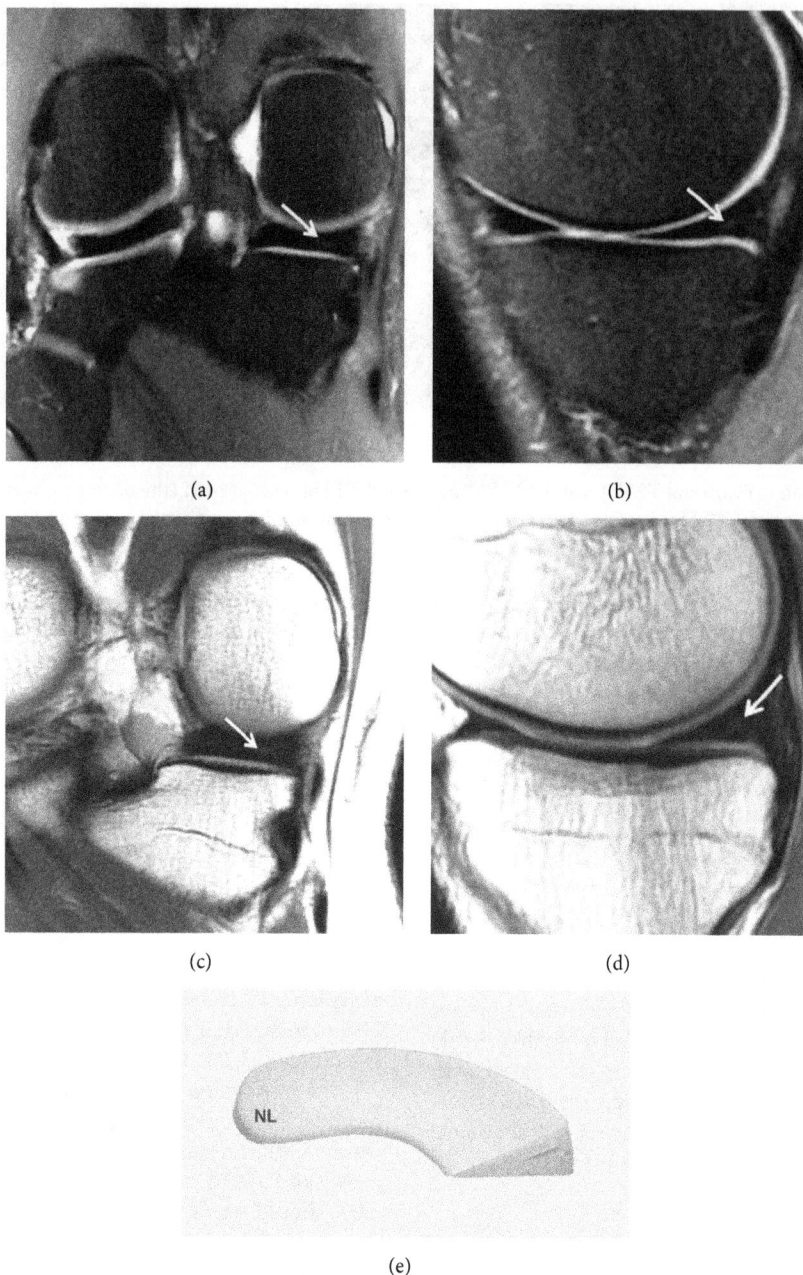

(a)

(b)

(c)

(d)

(e)

FIGURE 2: Grade 1 meniscal lesion (arrow) (a) Coronal T2 FSE Fat Sat MRI; (b) Sagittal T2 FSE Fat Sat MRI; (c) Coronal proton density weighted sequences; (d) sagittal proton density weighted sequences; (e) three-dimensional diagram.

cruciate ligament (indeed, meniscal and ligament lesions are frequently associated). Several factors should be taken into account to optimize the imaging protocols. Although imaging on all three planes is useful, all sequences should not be performed on all planes. Usually T1-weighted sequences are performed on the sagittal plane while T2-weighted sequences are performed on all three spatial planes (sagittal, coronal, and axial) [40].

Sequences defining anatomical structures should be distinguished from those characterizing meniscal pathologies.

Imaging of meniscal structures and contours is better with proton-density T2-weighted sequences:

(i) The so-called anatomical sequences: they are mainly T1-weighted proton density sequences. An MRI of the knee will nearly systematically include a sagittal T1-weighted image to evaluate the cruciate ligaments, the morphology of the menisci, the osteochondral structures, the extensor apparatus (patella, patellar tendon, and quadriceps), and the articular cavity.

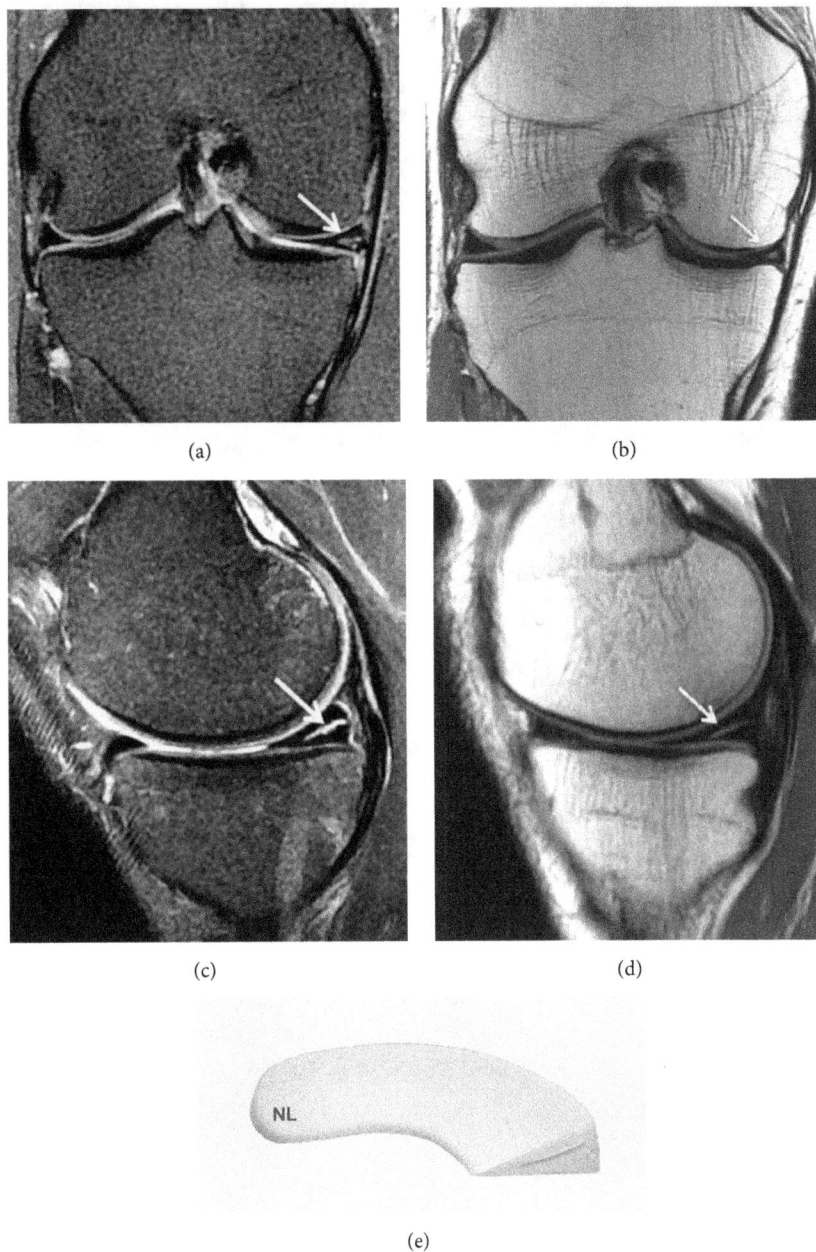

FIGURE 3: Grade 2 meniscal lesion on (a) Coronal T2 FSE Fat Sat MRI (arrow); (b) Coronal proton density weighted sequences (arrow); (c) Sagittal T2 FSE Fat Sat MRI (arrow); (d) sagittal proton density weighted sequences (arrow); (e) three-dimensional diagram.

(ii) Sequences to identify pathologies: these sequences use fat suppression, either STIR or T-2 weighted fast spin-echo with specific fat suppression (T2 and T2 FSE Fat-Sat). This is the reference sequence for the analysis of intra-articular lesions: joint effusion, edematous infiltration, ligament or tendon tears, bone contusions, subchondral bone edemas, muscle lesions, and especially meniscal lesions.

There are other more specific sequences:

(i) T1-weighted Fat-Sat Gadolinium sequence (T1-weighted sequence with fat suppression and intravenous gadolinium administration). This sequence has the advantage of providing anatomical images while still being sensitive to all inflammatory and/or vascularized structures.

(ii) T2-weighted sequence (gradient echo T2-weighted), this sequence is rarely used in other joints (shoulder and ankle) but is sometimes used in the knee. Its main value, besides good sensitivity for the diagnosis of meniscal tears [42], is mainly identifying signs of chronic bleeding in the form of hemosiderin deposition from villonodular synovitis.

The most reliable MRI sequences of the meniscus are proton density-weighted (FSE) sequences and T2-weighted and fast

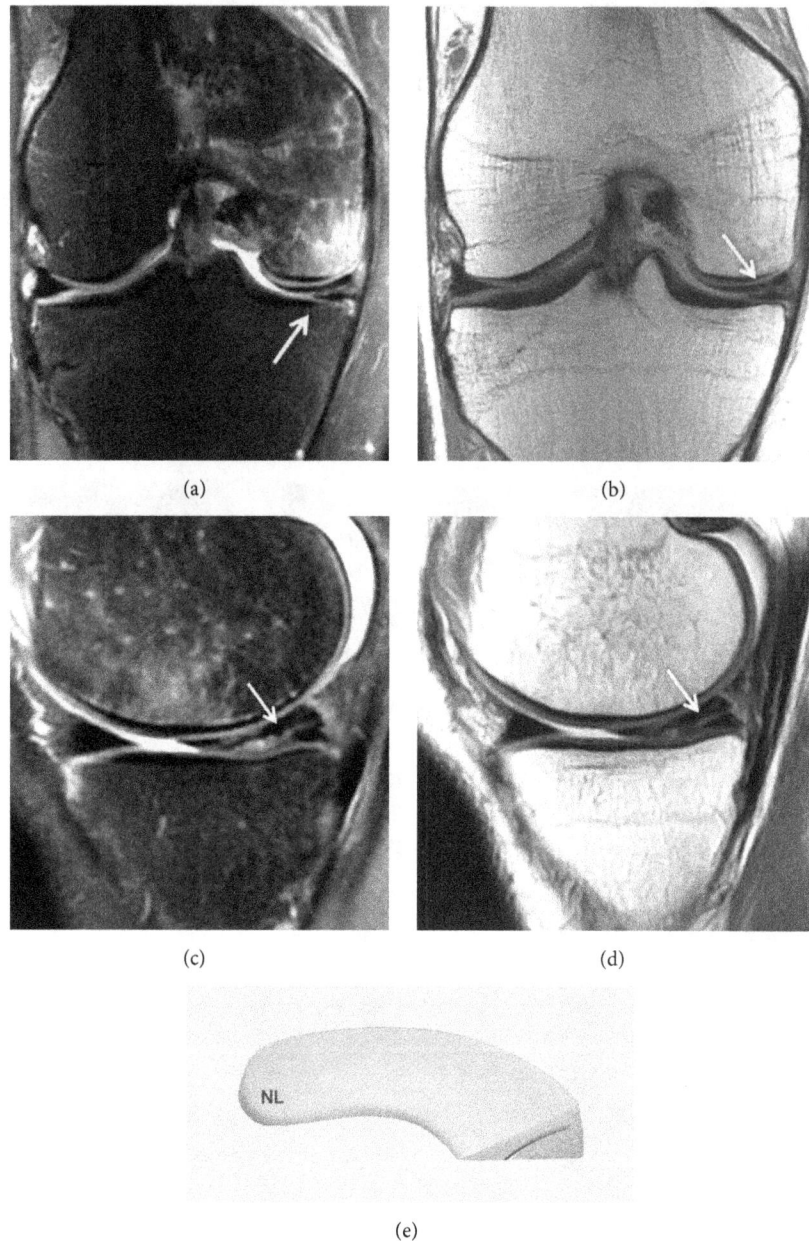

(a)

(b)

(c)

(d)

(e)

FIGURE 4: Grade 3 meniscal lesion on (a) Coronal T2 FSE Fat Sat MRI (arrow); (b) Coronal proton density weighted sequences (arrow); (c) Sagittal T2 FSE Fat Sat MRI (arrow); (d) sagittal proton density weighted sequences (arrow); (e) three-dimensional diagram.

spin-echo T2-weighted sequences [43, 44] but also Rhô FSE Fat Sat sequences. T1-weighted sequences are less sensitive. Fast spin-echo is currently the imaging modality of choice.

5.3. Normal MRI of the Meniscus. A normal meniscus is seen as a triangular shaped low intensity signal on classic T-1 and T-2 weighted sequences or on Fast Spin-Echo (FSE) sequences. The low intensity signal is due to a lack of mobile protons in the fibrocartilage of a normal meniscus (Figure 1).

In children, a grade 2 signal is often visualized in the posterior meniscal horns. This is considered to be normal and corresponds to the vascular system of the meniscus in children. This high intensity signal disappears in adulthood.

5.3.1. Meniscal Stability. Anterior or posterior meniscofemoral ligaments (ligament of Humphrey and Wrisberg ligament) are present and visible on 33% of MRI images. Visualization of the ligament of Humphrey is better on sagittal images. It is sometimes observed on coronal images. The Wrisberg ligament is easier to see on posterior coronal images [5, 45]. The lateral meniscus is stabilized by the coronary ligament, the meniscofemoral ligament, the arcuate ligament, and the meniscotibial ligament [46]. Both menisci are also stabilized by the transverse ligament. If any of these supporting ligaments or the meniscus itself degenerates or is torn, the meniscus may become unstable. The meniscocapsular ligaments including the meniscofemoral and meniscotibial

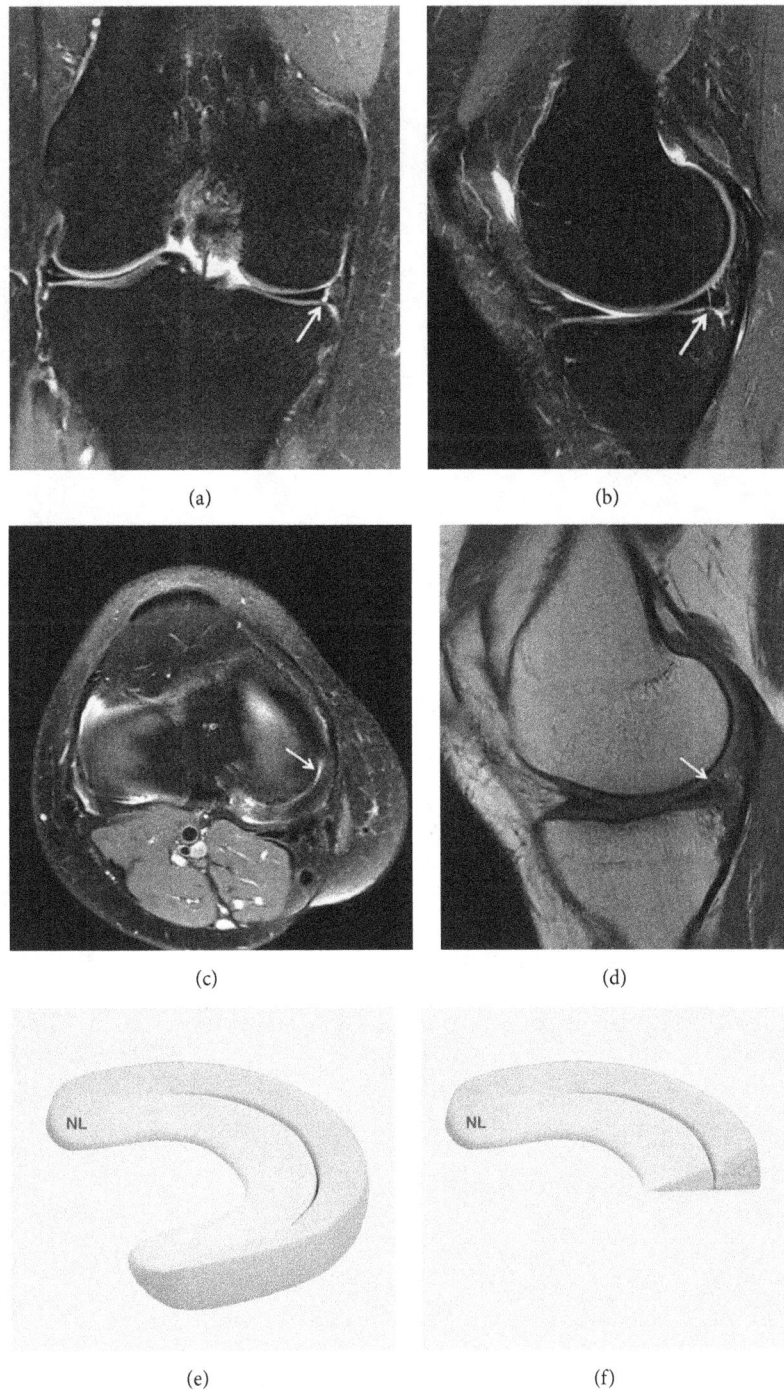

(a)

(b)

(c)

(d)

(e)

(f)

FIGURE 5: A vertical tear in the meniscal tissue communicating with the superior and inferior meniscal articular surfaces completely divides the meniscus into two parts. (a) Coronal T2 FSE Fat Sat MRI (arrow), (b) Sagittal T2 FSE Fat Sat MRI (arrow), (c) Axial T2 FSE Fat Sat MRI (arrow), and (d) sagittal T1-weighted sequence MRI. (e) Three-dimensional diagram shows a vertical and longitudinal tear of the meniscus. (f) Three-dimensional diagram shows a vertical tear.

ligaments attach the menisci to the posterior femur and posterior tibial plateau, respectively [47].

5.4. *Classification System of Meniscal Lesions.* The features of meniscal degeneration are well codified on MRI. The use of Stoller and Crues 3-stage classification [45, 46] has been shown to be reliable, sensitivity: 87 to 97%, specificity: 89 to 98%, reliability: 88 to 95% [46, 48]. Only stage 3 degeneration (linear high intensity signal communicating with the joint) should be considered pathological. This MRI classification was developed in correlation with a histological model. The degenerative areas show a high intensity signal that varies

(a)

(b)

(c)

(d)

(e)

(f)

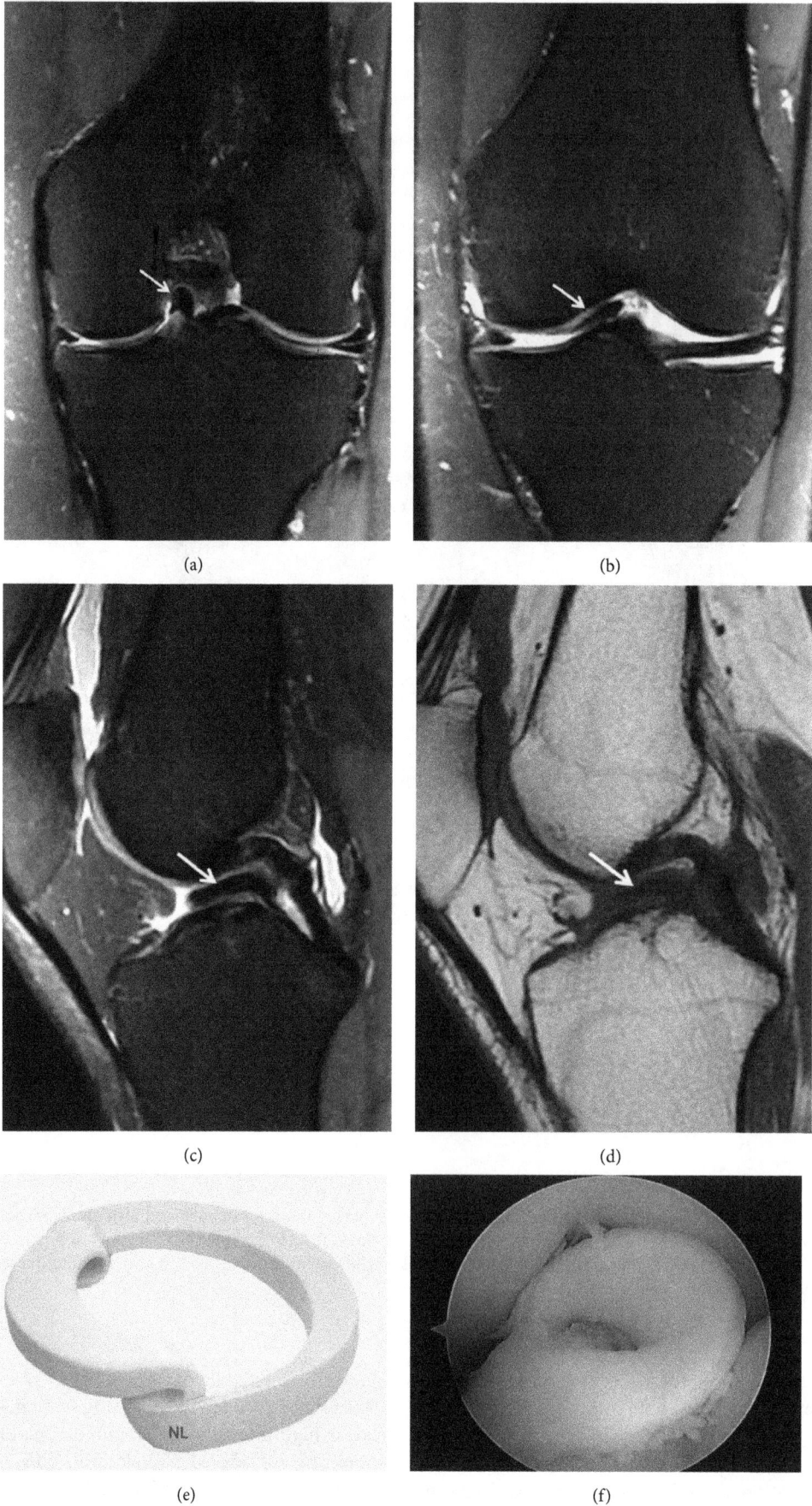

Figure 6: Continued.

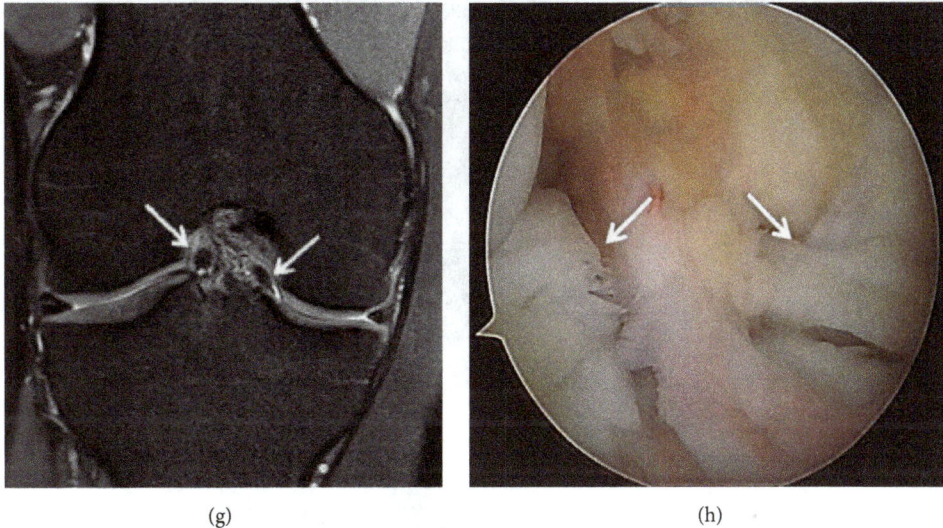

(g) (h)

FIGURE 6: Displaced bucket-handle tear of the medial meniscus. (a) Coronal T2 FSE Fat Sat MRI shows a displaced bucket-handle fragment of the medial meniscus into the intercondylar notch of the knee (arrow). The remnant of the body of the meniscus is small; (b) Coronal T2 FSE Fat Sat MRI shows a displaced bucket-handle fragment of the anterior medial meniscus (arrow); (c) Sagittal T2 FSE Fat Sat MRI shows the "double PCL sign," with a displaced fragment of a bucket-handle tear into the intercondylar notch of the knee; (d) Sagittal T1-weighted sequence MRI (arrow); (e) three-dimensional diagram shows a displaced bucket-handle tear of the medial meniscus; (f) arthroscopic view of a bucket-handle tear; (g) Coronal T2 FSE Fat Sat MRI shows a double displaced bucket-handle fragment of the medial and lateral meniscus into the intercondylar notch of the knee (arrow); (h) arthroscopic view of a double bucket-handle tear (arrow).

depending on the location and severity of the meniscal lesion. This classification does not include peripheral capsular meniscal separations, which are not considered to be articular [45].

5.4.1. Grade 1 Lesion.
A grade 1 lesion is a focal or diffuse nonarticular area (Figure 2).

This finding is correlated with early meniscal degeneration. The terms myxoid degeneration or hyaline degeneration are both used to describe these lesions.

5.4.2. Grade 2 Lesion.
A grade 2 lesion is a horizontal linear image in the body of the mensicus with a high intensity signal that extends to the inferior surface of the meniscus without involving it (Figure 3).

This abnormal signal is more extensive than in grade 1 degeneration but there is no cleavage or tear. Grade 2 degeneration is a progression of grade 1 degeneration. Patients are usually asymptomatic.

There are three types of grade 2 signals [45]:

Type 2A is a linear signal without contact with an articular surface.

Type 2B is an abnormal signal in contact with one of the articular surfaces on a single image.

Type 2C is a very extensive signal without contact with an articular surface [46, 49].

5.4.3. Grade 3 Tears.
Grade 3 corresponds to an abnormal signal in the meniscus that extends over a large part of

the meniscus and communicates with at least one articular surface of the meniscus (Figure 4).

Nevertheless, approximately 5% of grade 3 lesions are intrameniscal with no real meniscal cleavage. They cannot be diagnosed on routine arthroscopy if surface extension is not identified preoperatively [50].

Besides this classification, there are two pathological criteria for meniscal tears. These two MRI criteria were established for the diagnosis of meniscal tears. If no prior surgery has been performed on the meniscus, the diagnostic accuracy of these criteria is more than 90% [13].

5.4.4. Criteria 1.
Criteria 1 correspond to an abnormal signal in the meniscus suggesting a tear that is found on at least two consecutive images. This corresponds to the "two-slice-touch rule" a concept with a positive predictive value of 94% for tears of the medial meniscus and 96% for the lateral meniscus. The positive predictive value was 55% and 36% for medial and lateral meniscal tears, respectively, when they are seen on a single image [4, 13, 51].

The abnormal signal intensity should be in contact with an articular surface, the superior or inferior or the tip (free end) of the meniscus. If the contact with the articular surface appears in two or more consecutive images, the diagnostic accuracy for a meniscal tear increases [13, 50].

5.4.5. Criteria 2.
Criteria 2 involve the morphology of the meniscus. A comprehensive understanding of the normal anatomy of the meniscus on MRI is necessary. Meniscal lesions are analyzed on the sagittal and coronal planes. Visualization of a meniscal tear on these two planes reduces

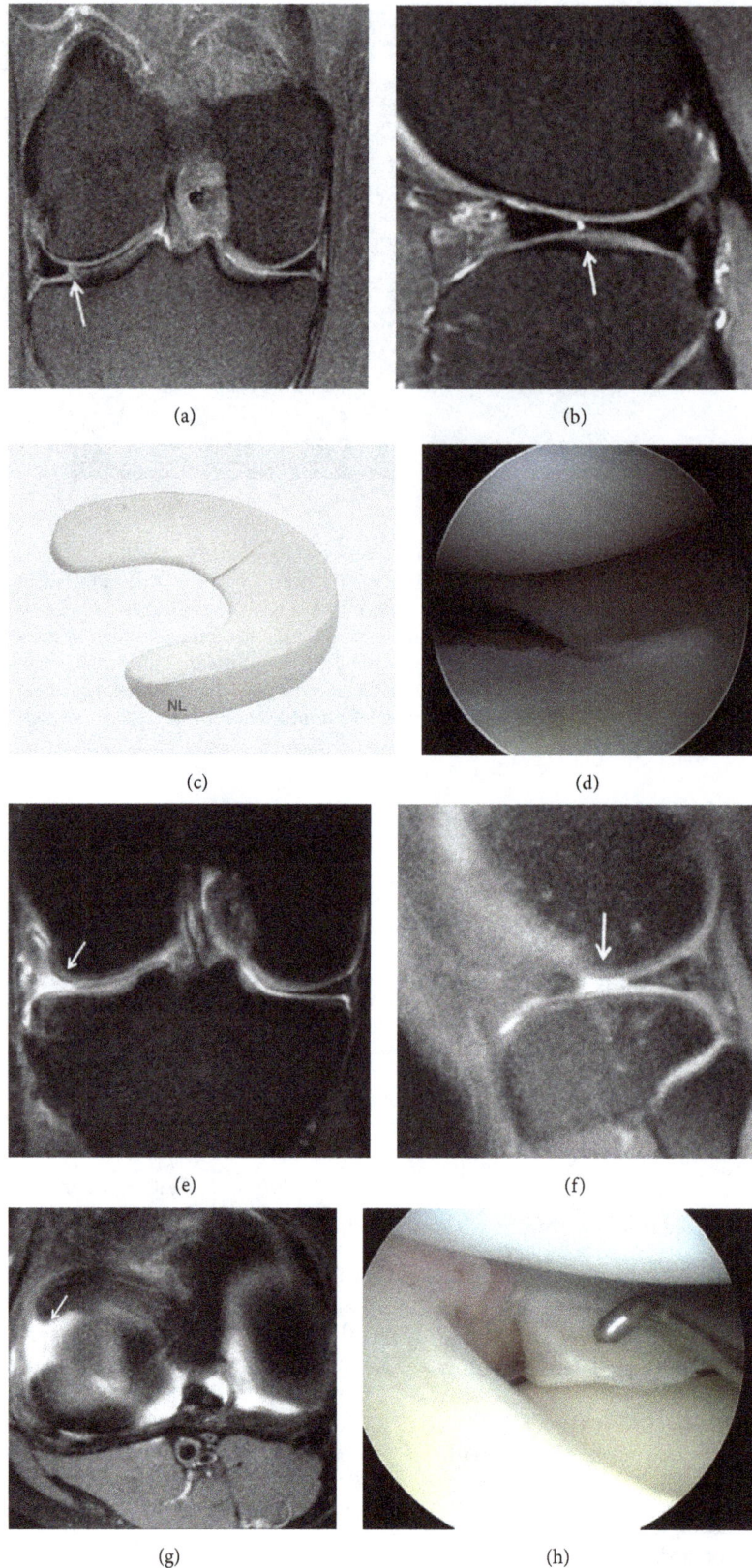

FIGURE 7: Radial tear involving the peripheral aspect of the meniscus. (a) Coronal T2 FSE Fat Sat MRI shows the vertical hyperintense signal (arrow) extends to both articular surfaces of the posterior horn of the medial meniscus; (b) Sagittal T2 FSE Fat Sat MRI shows the cleft sign of a radial tear; (c) three-dimensional diagram showing a radial tear involving the peripheral aspect of the meniscus; (d) arthroscopic view of the radial tear; (e) Coronal T2 FSE Fat Sat MRI: a part of the medial meniscus is not identified on the coronal image due to a large radial tear (arrow); (f) Sagittal T2 FSE Fat Sat MRI shows the large radial tear (arrow); (g) axial reconstruction showing the large radial tear (arrow) extending from the free edge into the posterior horn; (h) arthroscopic view of the large radial tear.

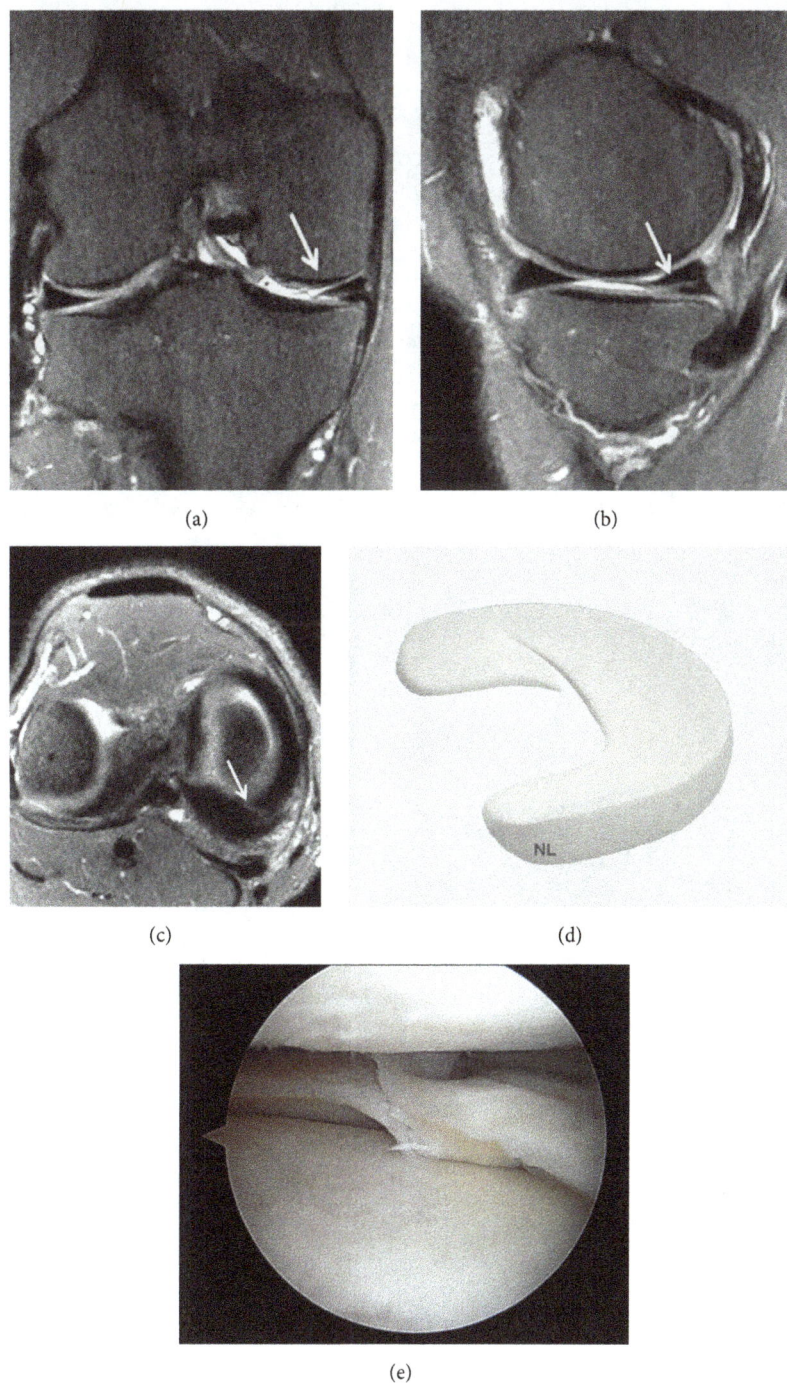

FIGURE 8: Oblique tears are a type of radial tear: (a) Coronal T2 FSE Fat Sat MRI: oblique tear of the body of the medial meniscus (arrow); (b) Coronal T2 FSE Fat Sat MRI: oblique-horizontal tear of the medial meniscus (arrow); (c) Axial T2 FSE Fat Sat MRI reconstruction showing the oblique tear of the posterior part of the medial meniscus (arrow); (d) three-dimensional diagram showing an oblique tear involving the peripheral aspect of the meniscus; (e) arthroscopic view showing a medial meniscus oblique tear.

the rate of false positives. However, several tears at the meniscocapsular junction may only be seen on one of these planes.

5.5. *Description of Lesions: Size, Shapes, and Characteristics.* Multiple images of meniscal tears should be translated into 3D images [13, 15]. Meniscal tears occur on two main planes:

vertical and horizontal. The three basic shapes of meniscal tears are longitudinal, radial, and horizontal. Meniscal tears are either partial or full thickness (through all of the meniscal tissue).

5.5.1. *Vertical Tears.* Vertical tears are perpendicular to the coronal plane of the meniscus and can be subdivided into

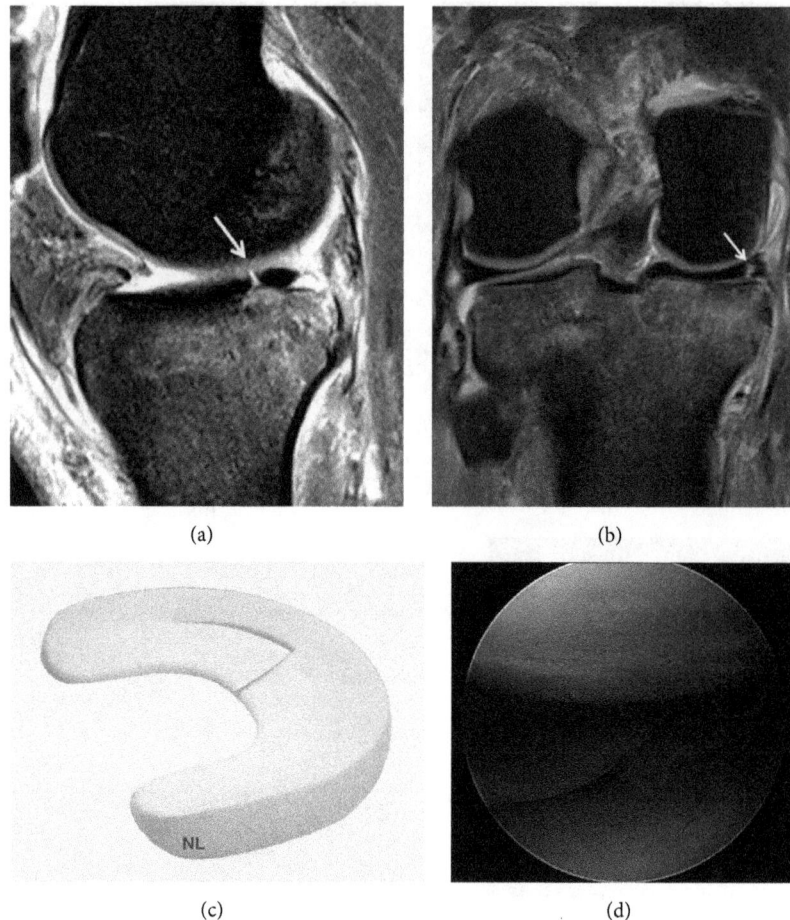

(a)   (b)

(c)   (d)

FIGURE 9: Radial tear extends towards the periphery to longitudinal meniscal tears; (a) Sagittal T2 FSE Fat Sat MRI (arrow); (b) Coronal T2 FSE Fat Sat MRI shows the longitudinal meniscal tears towards the periphery (arrow); (c) three-dimensional diagram showing the radial tear extends towards the periphery to longitudinal meniscal tears towards the periphery; (d) arthroscopic view showing a medial meniscus tear.

peripheral longitudinal or radial tears. They usually occur following a trauma in young patients [52].

A vertical tear in the meniscal tissue communicating with the superior and inferior meniscal articular surfaces completely divides the meniscus into two parts (Figure 5).

These tears can result in the development of bucket-handle tears (Figure 6) [20]. Vertical tears of the posterior horn may not be visible on sagittal images.

5.5.2. Radial (or Transverse) Tears.
Radial tears are vertical tears that extend perpendicular to the main axis of the meniscus. The most frequent location is the middle segment of the meniscus (Figure 7).

This tear begins at the free edge of the meniscus and extends towards the periphery for a distance that varies [20]. A full thickness radial tear extends from the free edge towards the periphery of the meniscus (meniscal wall).

Small tears can be difficult to see on MRI. Radial tears represent a large percentage of the errors made in the interpretation of meniscal pathologies on MRI. The main feature of these tears is that they involve the free edge of the meniscal surface. Thus, if the inner point of the meniscal triangle is absent or blunted on one or more coronal images,

a radial meniscal tear should be suspected. These tears are best seen on sagittal images.

Oblique tears are a type of radial tear (Figure 8).

They begin on the free edge of the meniscus then continue longitudinally (Figure 9), similar to longitudinal meniscal tears, and the tear extends towards the periphery.

These oblique tears are the most frequent meniscal tear [13, 15, 46]. Oblique radial tears of the posterior horn of the lateral meniscus are often associated with ACL tears [53].

5.5.3. Horizontal Tears.
Horizontal tears are also called cleavage or fish-mouth tears (Figure 10).

They divide the meniscus into two superior and inferior parts. They usually begin on the underside of the meniscus [20]. Although horizontal tears may appear to extend deep into the meniscus on MRI, they may only be several millimeters deep on arthroscopy. When the tear extends to the periphery of the meniscus, to the meniscosynovial border, this can form a meniscal cyst. Most of these tears are degenerative and occur in elderly patients with osteoarthritis.

5.5.4. Complex Tears.
Complex tears are a combination of longitudinal, radial, and horizontal tears. Several tears may be

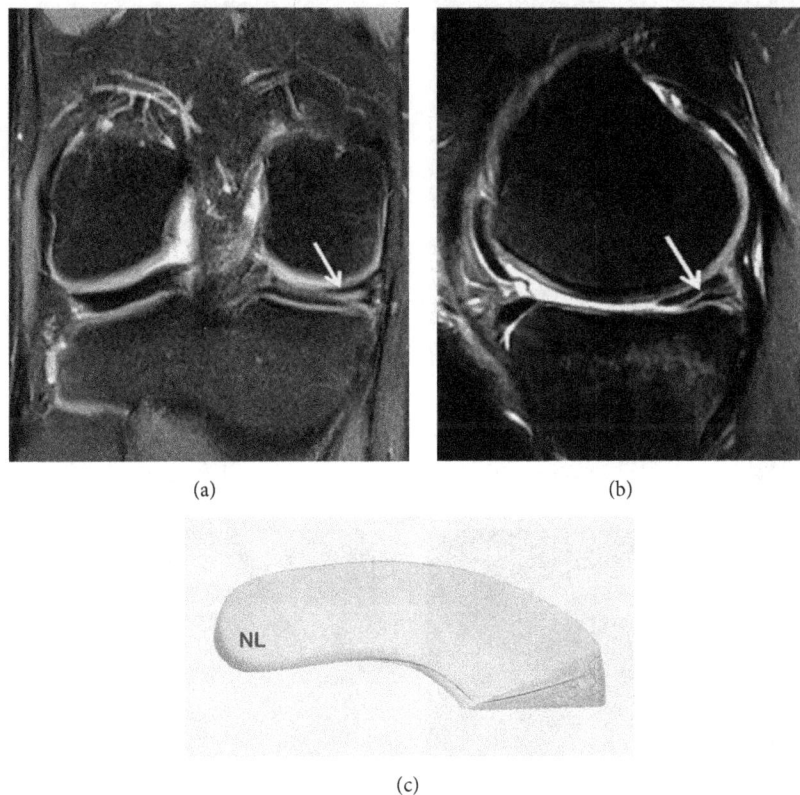

FIGURE 10: Horizontal tears are also called cleavage or fish-mouth tears. (a) Coronal T2 FSE MRI: horizontal tear (arrow) of the body of the medial meniscus; (b) Sagittal T2 FSE MRI (arrow); (c) three-dimensional diagram.

present simultaneously in the meniscus, involving different parts of the same region or several regions. One common complex tear includes a horizontal and radial tear. It is nearly always degenerative [13, 15].

5.5.5. Meniscus Posterior Horn Avulsion.
It is not always easy to diagnose a meniscus avulsion on MRI (Figure 11).

The diagnostic sensitivity of MRI for the detection of root avulsion of the posterior horn is only 66.3%, which is not specific enough to determine the type of tear [54]. However, recent studies have helped improve the sensitivity and specificity of these tears [47, 55–59]. Lee et al. [59] have proposed a diagnostic assessment based on three MRI signs: a "ghost meniscus" on the sagittal plane (100% detection rate), the "vertical linear defect" (truncated aspect) on the coronal plane (100%), and the "radial linear defect" on the axial plane (94%).

5.5.6. Displaced Meniscal Fragments.
Fragments or displaced meniscal loose bodies occur in 9–24% of meniscal tears. All forms of tears can result in displaced fragments [60]. Diagnosis by MRI is based on visualization of the tear with a missing portion of the meniscus and of the displaced meniscal fragment [61].

(i) Bucket-Handle Tear. The bucket-handle tear is caused by a full thickness vertical-longitudinal tear. The fragment (which may or may not be displaced) separated by the meniscal wall, on the axial images, looks like a bucket handle. These tears account for 10% of all meniscal tears [40, 61–63]. The diagnostic accuracy of MRI for bucket-handle tears (Figure 6) is good and the displaced fragment can be clearly visualized in the intercondylar notch on coronal but also on sagittal images when searching for the double posterior cruciate ligament sign (double PCL sign) [50, 62, 64]. These tears can be classified as simple vertical longitudinal tears, displaced or not, torn or not from the middle part of the meniscus (Figure 12) and sometimes with double or triple bucket handles.

These tears are three times more frequent in the medial meniscus than in the lateral meniscus and may be associated with ACL tears.

Pseudohypertrophy of the anterior horn of the lateral meniscus occurs when the anterior horn of the meniscus seems abnormally large. The posterior horn of the lateral meniscus is abnormally weak. This indicates that part of the meniscus has tipped forward into a bucket-handle tear.

(ii) Meniscal Fragments. Meniscal fragments from horizontal meniscal tears can sometimes be displaced in relation to the body of the meniscus, slipping above or below the rest of the meniscal surface (Figure 13).

These fragments generally concern the medial meniscus [60]. Inferomedial displaced fragments under the medial meniscus are rare. When the displaced fragment blocks

(a)

(b)

(c)

(d)

(e)

(f)

(g)

(h)

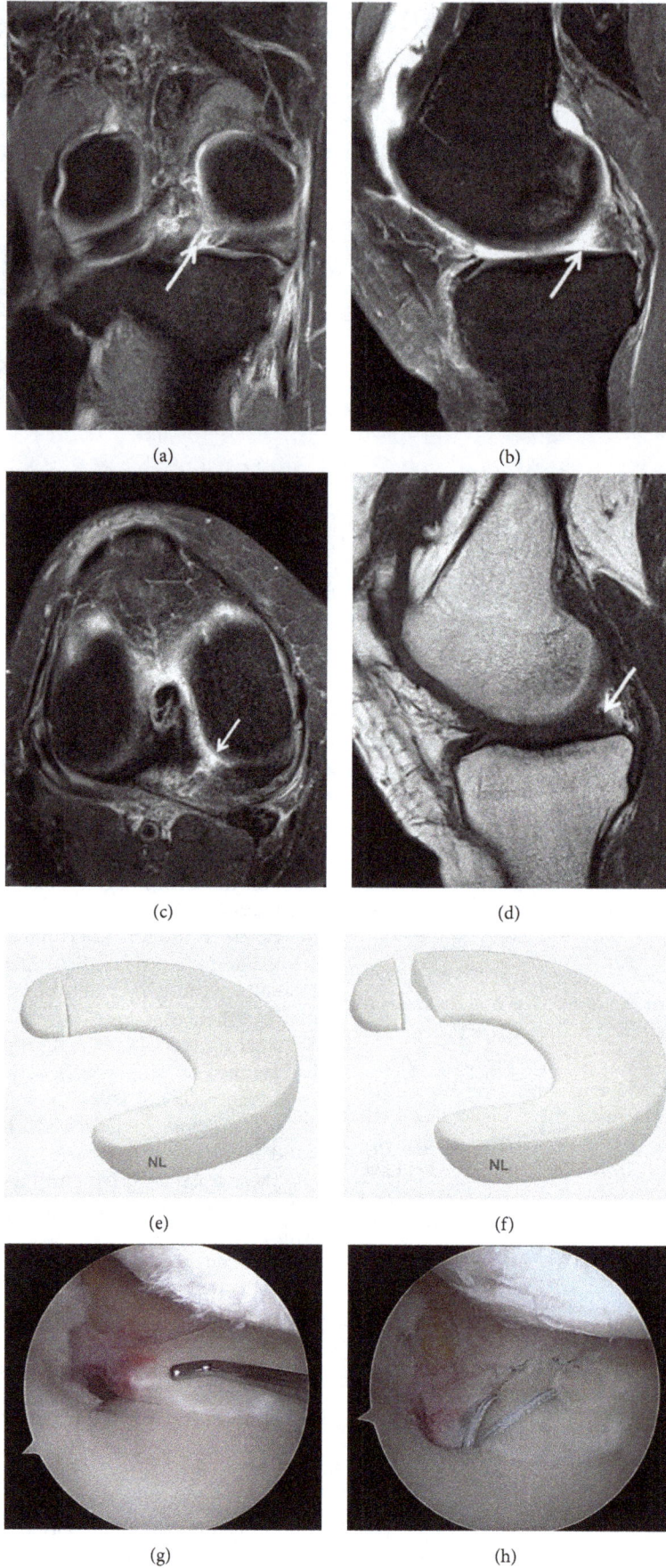

Figure 11: Continued.

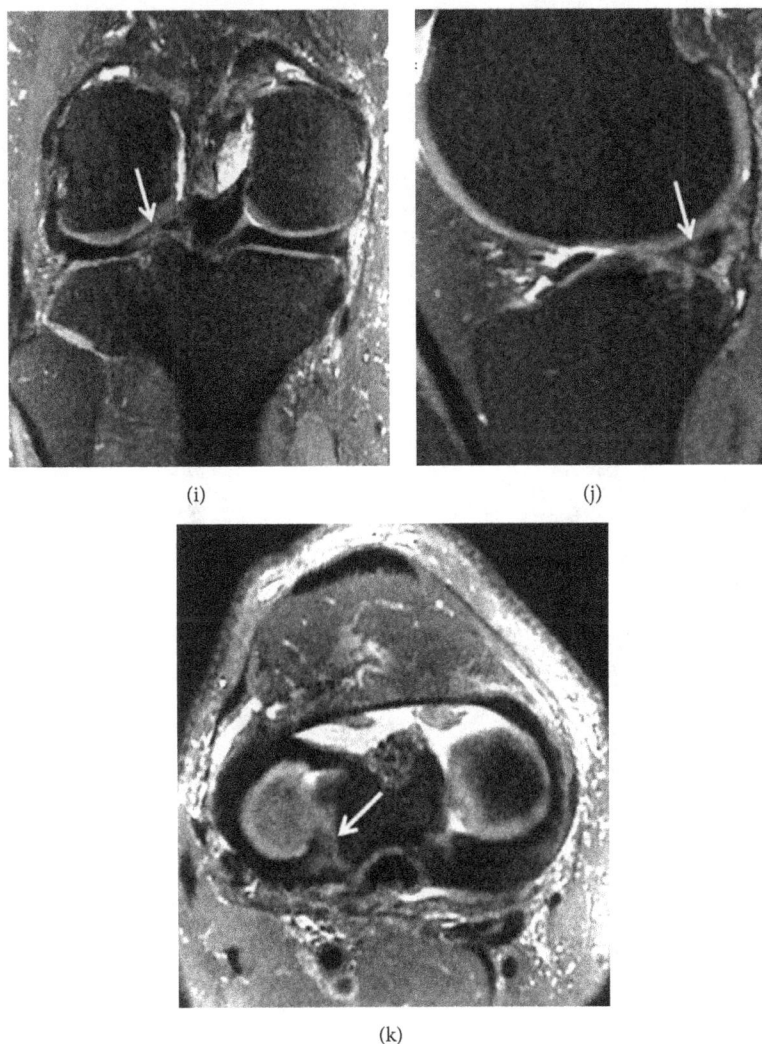

(i)

(j)

(k)

FIGURE 11: Meniscus posterior horn avulsion. (a) T2-weighted fat-saturated images showing a complete posterior root tear of the medial meniscus (arrow); (b) Ghost meniscus sign. The posterior horn of the medial meniscus has been replaced with triangular high signal intensity on the T2-weighted fat-saturated sequence (arrow); (c) axial reconstruction showing the large posterior horn avulsion (arrow) with high signal intensity on the T2-weighted fat-saturated sequence; (d) the posterior horn of the medial meniscus is not identified on the sagittal T1 (arrow); (g) arthroscopic view showing a displaced medial meniscus root tear; (h) arthroscopic view showing a suture of the medial meniscus root tear; (i) identification of root tears of the lateral meniscus can be more difficult on the coronal T2-weighted fat-saturated sequence; (j) ghost meniscus sign is less significant on the sagittal T2-weighted fat-saturated sequence (arrow); (k) axial reconstruction showing the posterior horn avulsion (arrow).

the peripheral edge of the tibial plateau and the deep part of the medial cruciate ligament, it cannot be seen on arthroscopy because the surface of the meniscus appears to be intact. On the other hand, it is more often visible on coronal images (Figure 14).

Superior or inferior displacement of a small meniscal fragment from a vertical tear is less frequent.

5.5.7. Meniscocapsular Separation. Meniscocapsular separation is a tear of the periphery of the meniscus at the meniscosynoval junction. This usually involves the capsular attachment of the posterior horn of the medial meniscus. MRI is much less reliable than arthroscopy for the diagnosis of meniscocapsular separation, positive predictive value: PPV

of 9% for the medial meniscus and 13% for the lateral meniscus [65].

Meniscocapsular separation is frequently associated with knee ligament tears. These entities can heal spontaneously because of the rich vascularization on the periphery of the meniscus, depending on the site of separation in relation to the area of vascularization of the connective tissue.

5.5.8. Meniscal Cyst. Meniscal cysts occur more frequently in the medial compartment [66]. Symptoms of medial parameniscal cysts are more frequent because of their location near the medial collateral ligament. The incidence is between 2% and 8%, and these cysts are usually found in men between 20 and 40 years old. Medial meniscal cysts are usually found

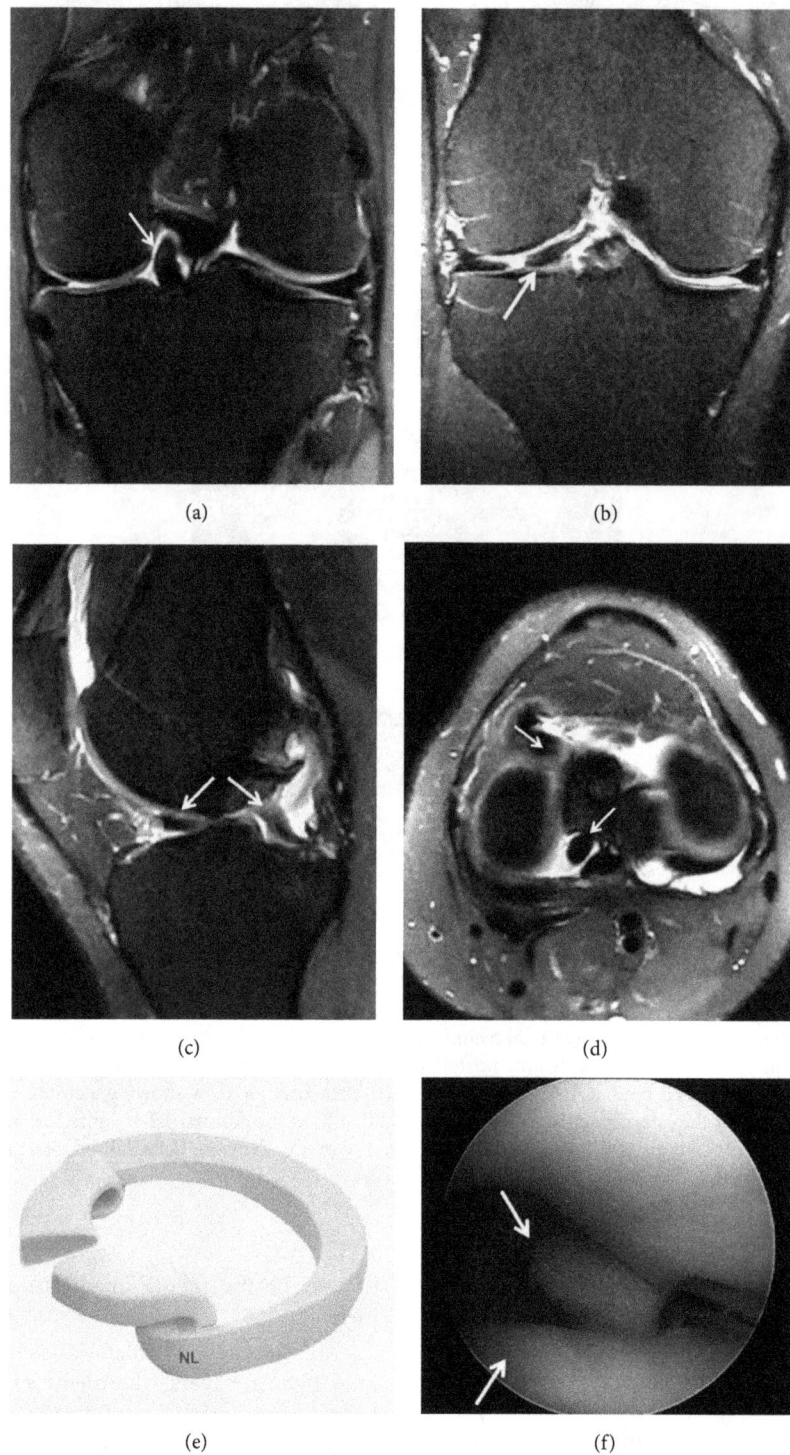

FIGURE 12: Displaced bucket-handle tear of the medial meniscus with tear from the middle part of the meniscus. (a) Coronal T2 FSE Fat Sat MRI: large meniscal fragment (arrow) seen within the intercondylar notch; (b) Coronal T2 FSE Fat Sat MRI: flap tears displaced horizontal under surface tear of the body and anterior horn of the medial meniscus with a flipped fragment (arrow); (c) Sagittal T2 FSE Fat Sat MRI showing a complex tear with a displaced fragment (arrow); (d) Axial T2 FSE Fat Sat MRI reconstruction showing the 2 flap tears of the displaced bucket-handle; (e) three-dimensional diagram; (f) arthroscopic view showing the rupture and the displaced bucket-handle tear.

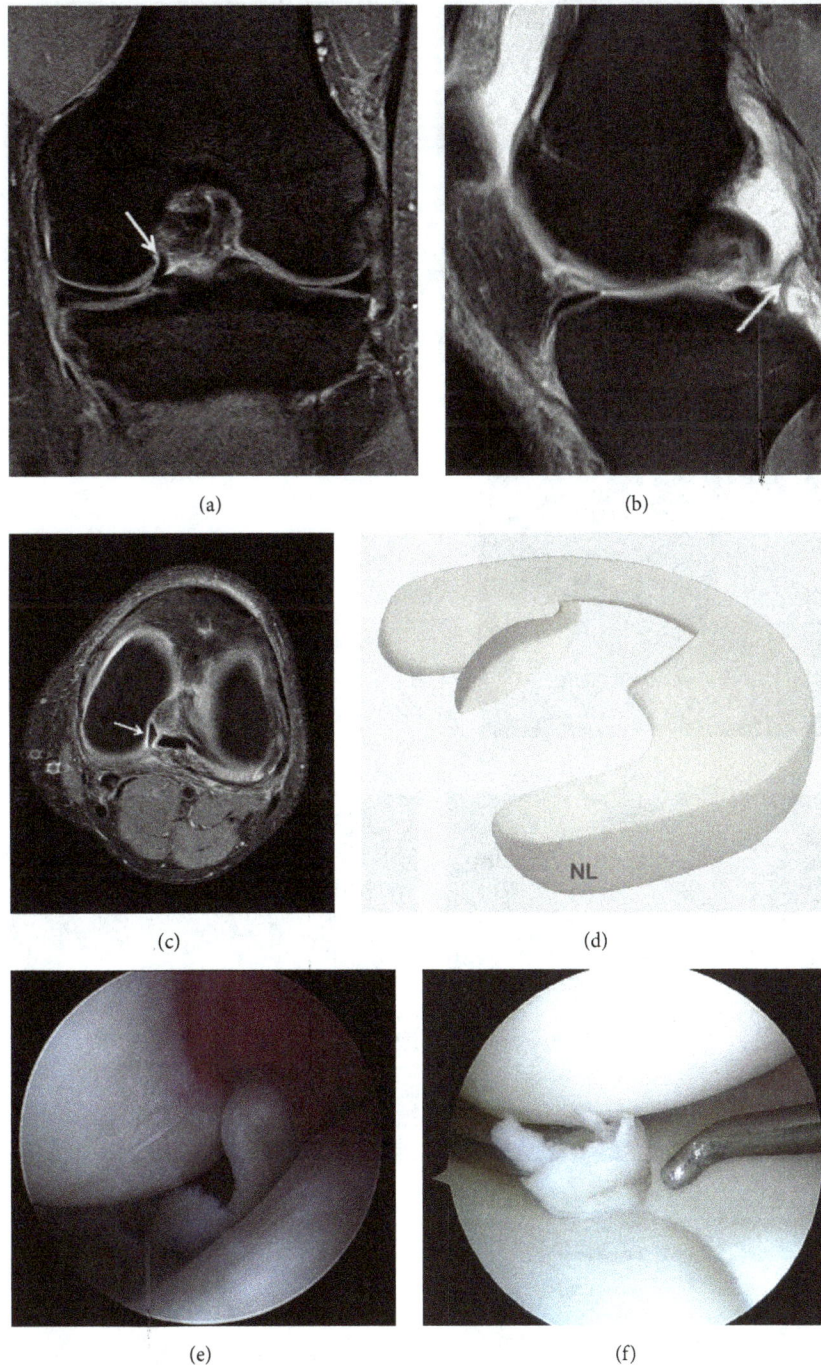

(a)   (b)

(c)   (d)

(e)   (f)

FIGURE 13: Meniscal fragments from horizontal meniscal tears can sometimes be displaced in relation to the body of the meniscus, slipping above or below the rest of the meniscal surface. (a) Coronal T2 FSE Fat Sat MRI showing a displaced fragment of the medial meniscus; (b) a meniscal fragment (arrow) is seen posterior to the PCL in Sagittal T2 FSE Fat Sat MRI; (c) axial reconstruction showing meniscal fragment (arrow) on the T2-weighted fat-saturated sequence; (d) three-dimensional diagram showing the meniscal fragments; (e) arthroscopic views of a displaced tear of the medial meniscus in the intercondylar notch; (f) arthroscopic views of a displaced tear of the medial meniscus in the underlying posteromedial tibial plateau.

at the posterior horn [20], while lateral meniscal cysts are usually located at the anterior meniscal horn (Figure 15).

Tears are usually horizontal and extend to the periphery of the meniscus, allowing synovial fluid to leak from the joint into the parameniscal tissue and form a meniscal cyst.

Sometimes the cyst can be limited to the meniscus. This is called an intrameniscal cyst.

The parameniscal cyst located adjacent to the lateral anterior meniscal horn is less at risk of an underlying meniscal tear than cysts in other meniscal locations [67]. It is

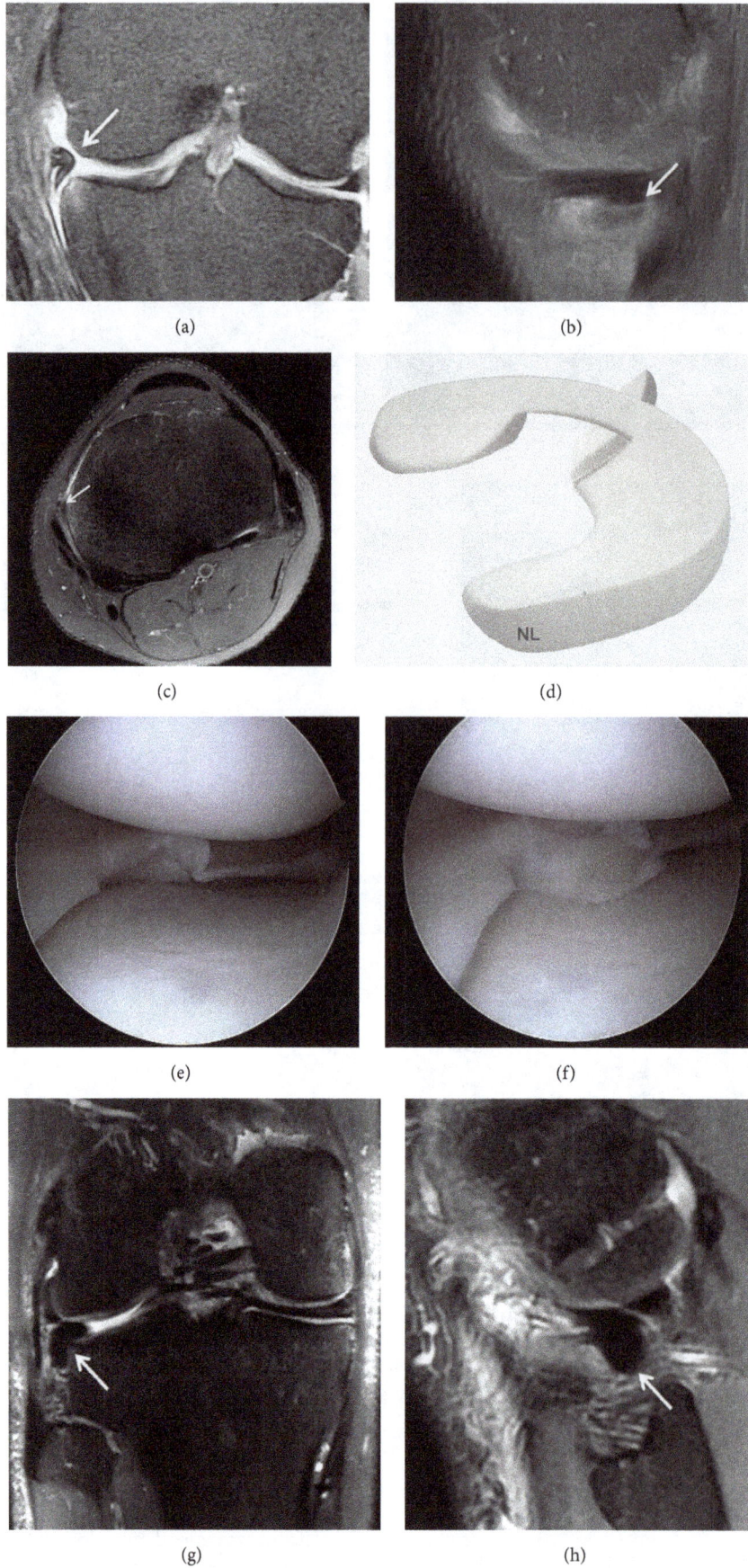

(a)

(b)

(c)

(d)

(e)

(f)

(g)

(h)

FIGURE 14: Continued.

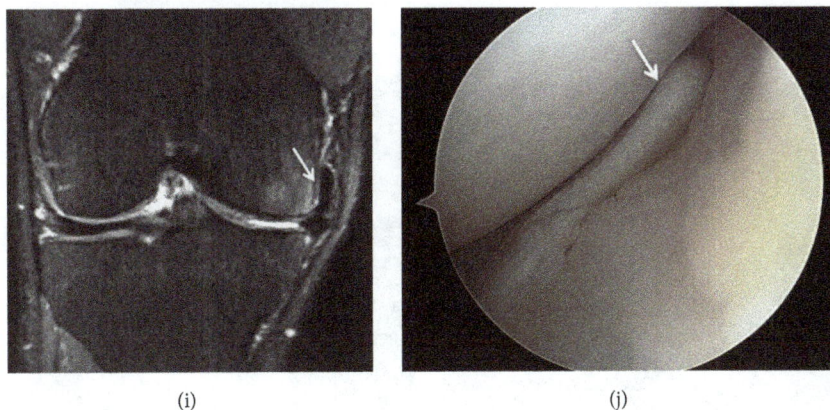

(i)

(j)

FIGURE 14: Meniscal fragments from horizontal meniscal tears displaced under the medial or lateral meniscus. The displaced fragment blocks the peripheral edge of the tibial plateau and the deep part of the MCL or LCL. (a) Coronal T2 FSE Fat Sat MRI showing a displaced horizontal undersurface tear of the body of the medial meniscus with a flipped fragment (arrow) along the undersurface of the native meniscus and extending under MCL; (b) Sagittal T2 FSE Fat Sat MRI showing a displaced fragment of the medial meniscus (arrow); (c) axial reconstruction showing the flipped fragment (arrow) under MCL on the T2-weighted fat-saturated sequence; (d) three-dimensional diagram showing a displaced tear of the medial meniscus; (e) arthroscopic views of a displaced tear of the medial meniscus under the meniscus; (f) arthroscopic view of the medial meniscus tear under the meniscus reduced in intra-articular lesion; (g) Coronal T2 FSE Fat Sat MRI showing a displaced fragment of the lateral meniscus (arrow); (h) Sagittal T2 FSE Fat Sat MRI showing a large fragment of the lateral meniscus under the LCL; (i) complex tear with a displaced fragment (arrow) coursing into the superior recess in Coronal T2 FSE Fat Sat MRI; (j) arthroscopic views of a displaced tear of the medial meniscus into the superior recess.

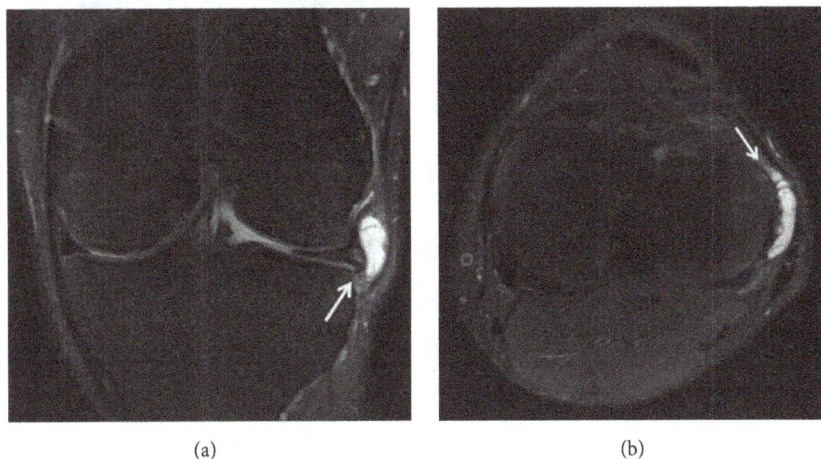

(a)

(b)

FIGURE 15: Lateral meniscal cysts: (a) lateral meniscal cysts are usually located at the anterior meniscal horn (coronal T2 FSE MRI sequences); (b) Axial T2 FSE Fat Sat MRI reconstruction showing the lateral meniscal cysts (arrow).

important to recognize the link between meniscal cysts and tears. If the cyst is treated without treating the tear, the cyst can recur.

5.5.9. Meniscal Extrusion. Meniscal extrusion of the tibiofemoral joint space has been reported in elderly patients with clinically symptomatic osteoarthritis of the knee. In this group, meniscal extrusion preceded the degenerative joint disease [68]. Following meniscal extrusion, direct impaction of the tibial and femoral cartilages increases progression to osteoarthritis.

Tibiofemoral cartilage damage and leg malalignment increase the risk of meniscal extrusion. Poor alignment increases the loads on the meniscal surface that can lead to extrusion. Varus and valgus malalignment are associated with medial and lateral meniscal extrusion, respectively [68].

5.5.10. Postoperative Meniscus and MRI. The diagnosis of a recurrent tear is more complex in patients who have undergone partial meniscectomy or meniscal repair and coronal and sagittal T2-W FSE Fat-Sat sequences are recommended. In sutured menisci, a persistent linear hypersignal

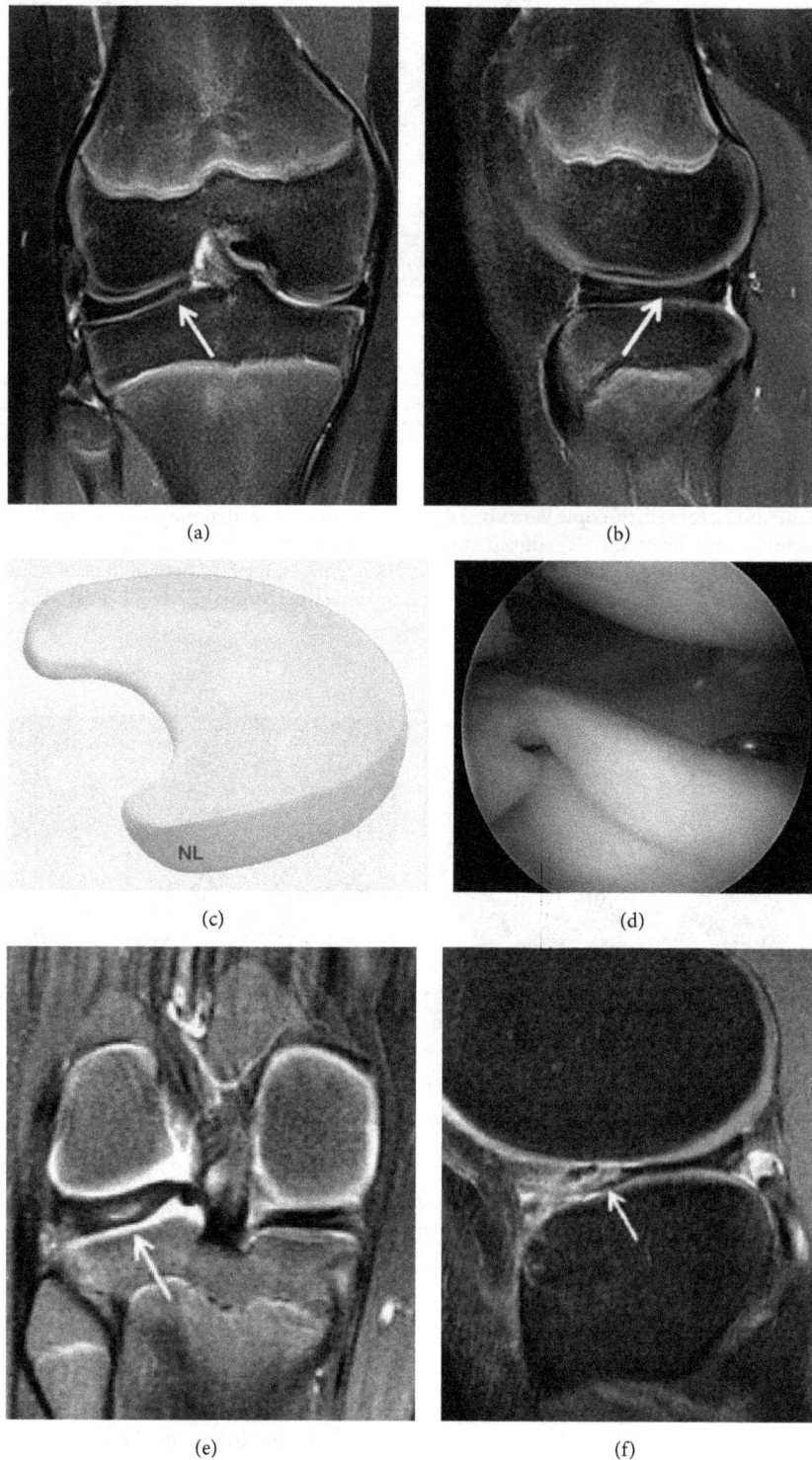

FIGURE 16: Discoid lateral meniscus. (a) Coronal T2 FSE Fat Sat MRI showing meniscal enlargement. The lateral meniscal body (arrow) is enlarged and has a more slab-like configuration compared to the normal-appearing triangular medial meniscal body; (b) Sagittal T2 FSE Fat Sat image of the lateral meniscus demonstrating persistence of the bow tie appearance on the more central slices rather than converting into 2 opposing triangles; (c) three-dimensional diagram showing a discoid lateral meniscus; (d) arthroscopic views of a discoid lateral meniscus; (e) posterior cystic degeneration in a discoid lateral meniscus; (f) anterior cystic degeneration in a discoid lateral meniscus.

in the suture zone makes it difficult to obtain the differential diagnosis between a recurrent tear and a separation that is in the process of healing [69]. If there was more than 25% resection of the meniscal surface or meniscal repair, most authors advise using MR arthrography [12]. Following meniscectomy, the remaining meniscus can present with a heterogeneous signal and irregular borders without being pathological. The diagnostic accuracy of MR-arthrography for recurrent meniscal tears is 88%, while it is 66% with routine MRI. During extensive meniscectomies, MR-arthrography is more accurate than simple MRI. Magee [70] has showed recently that the combined use of MR and MR arthrogram imaging was 98% sensitive and 75% specific in the diagnosis of a meniscal retear.

5.5.11. Discoïd Meniscus. Differentiation between true discoid meniscus and a meniscus that is a little larger than normal can be difficult (Figure 16).

The three types of discoid meniscus are classified as complete, incomplete, and Wrisberg discoid meniscus. The amount of tibial plateau coverage varies between complete and incomplete discoid meniscus. The Wrisberg variant is the least frequent anomaly (it lacks the normal posterior coronary ligament and capsular attachments). This ligament is mobile and can sublux [71].

On sagittal images, a discoid meniscus has a thickened bowtie appearance on three consecutive sagittal images. The anterior horns and the normal meniscus are visible on several MRI images near the intercondylar notch. With a complete discoid meniscus this difference is not seen. The normal meniscus rapidly narrows from the outer periphery to the center. The presence of an equally or nearly equally high meniscus on 2 adjacent 5 mm thick images is a sign of discoid meniscus [45].

Coronal MRI images are more sensitive for the diagnosis of discoid meniscus by showing meniscal enlargement. An asymmetric discoid meniscus can have an enlarged meniscal body on coronal images but have normal posterior and anterior horns on sagittal images, emphasizing the necessity of coronal images. Discoid meniscus is accurately diagnosed on MRI (PPV 92%) [72].

6. 3D Isotropic Turbo Spin-Echo MRI

3D isotropic Turbo Spin-Echo MRI was developed to create multiplanar reformatted images to obtain reconstructions of other spatial planes from a single plane acquisition or even on the axis of a structure defined as a ligament. Besides visualizing 2D and 3D structures, this technique also reduces overall MRI examination time [8, 73–76]. Moreover, small anatomical structures can be visualized with 3D MRI and the partial volume effect can be minimized by thin slices. Finally, the field of study can cover the entire area of interest without interslice gaps [8, 77, 78]. Thus, 3D MRI has received increasing attention for musculoskeletal imaging because most anatomical structures are small and facing in different directions, often oblique, especially the ACL [78, 79]. Until

recently, 3D isotropic images were based on gradient-echo imaging which has certain disadvantages, such as increasing the risk of artifacts and a lack of contrast between normal and diseased tissue [80, 81]. Recently, turbo-spin-echo (TSE) sequences have been shown to provide 3D isotropic images in acceptable acquisition times [82–84]. The knee is one of the most frequent applications of 3D isotropic sequences. TSE is considered to be the best sequence to evaluate the internal structures of the knee because of its high definition of tissue contrast [55, 85]. The diagnostic accuracy of TSE sequences is comparable to routine spin-echo MRI, for cartilage coverage, menisci, ligaments and subchondral bone [86–88]. Recent studies have shown that standardized TSE sequences make it possible to detect more meniscal lesions and in particular the first stages of osteoarthritis [89, 90].

7. Conclusion

MRI is the most accurate and least invasive tool for the diagnosis of meniscal tears. This knee imaging technique is the "gold standard" for the analysis of meniscal lesions. It allows confirming and characterizing the meniscal lesion. The diagnostic arthroscopy alone therefore has no place in the analysis of meniscal lesions of the knee. However, the therapeutic arthroscopy is a feasible treatment of meniscal lesions of the knee. The perfect knowledge of different meniscal lesions described in this paper allows the clinician to adapt treatment, medical or surgical, specifically for each lesion. New 3D MRI in three dimensions with isotropic resolution should help improve the diagnosis of meniscal tears.

Disclosure

Level of evidence is V.

References

[1] M. De Maeseneer, L. Lenchik, M. Starok, R. Pedowitz, D. Trudell, and D. Resnick, "Normal and abnormal medial meniscocapsular structures: MR imaging and sonography in cadavers," *American Journal of Roentgenology*, vol. 171, no. 4, pp. 969–976, 1998.

[2] L. De Flaviis, P. Scaglione, R. Nessi, and W. Albisetti, "Ultrasound in degenerative cystic meniscal disease of the knee," *Skeletal Radiology*, vol. 19, no. 6, pp. 441–445, 1990.

[3] H.-R. Casser, C. Sohn, and A. Kiekenbeck, "Current evaluation of sonography of the meniscus. Results of a comparative study of sonographic and arthroscopic findings," *Archives of Orthopaedic and Trauma Surgery*, vol. 109, no. 3, pp. 150–154, 1990.

[4] H. Gerngross and C. Sohn, "Ultrasound scanning for the diagnosis of meniscal lesions of the knee joint," *Arthroscopy*, vol. 8, no. 1, pp. 105–110, 1992.

[5]   M. J. C. M. Rutten, J. M. P. Collins, A. Van Kampen, and G. J. Jager, "Meniscal cysts: detection with high-resolution sonography," *American Journal of Roentgenology*, vol. 171, no. 2, pp. 491–496, 1998.

[6]   J. M. Dumas and D. J. Edde, "Meniscal abnormalities: prospective correlation of double-contrast arthrography and arthroscopy," *Radiology*, vol. 160, no. 2, pp. 453–456, 1986.

[7]   H. Gillies and D. Seligson, "Precision in the diagnosis of meniscal lesions: a comparison of clinical evaluation, arthrography, and arthroscopy," *The Journal of Bone & Joint Surgery—American Volume*, vol. 61, no. 3, pp. 343–346, 1979.

[8]   C. Gückel, G. Jundt, K. Schnabel, and A. Gächter, "Spin-echo and 3D gradient-echo imaging of the knee joint: a clinical and histopathological comparison," *European Journal of Radiology*, vol. 21, no. 1, pp. 25–33, 1995.

[9]   F. Pelousse and J. Olette, "Arthroscanner of the knee: current indication, examination of the femoro-tibial compartment. Comparative study with classical simple-contrast media arthrography," *Journal Belge de Radiologie*, vol. 76, no. 6, pp. 377–381, 1993.

[10] M. De Filippo, A. Bertellini, F. Pogliacomi et al., "Multidetector computed tomography arthrography of the knee: diagnostic accuracy and indications," *European Journal of Radiology*, vol. 70, no. 2, pp. 342–351, 2009.

[11] B. K. Harrison, B. E. Abell, and T. W. Gibson, "The thessaly test for detection of meniscal tears: validation of a new physical examination technique for primary care medicine," *Clinical Journal of Sport Medicine*, vol. 19, no. 1, pp. 9–12, 2009.

[12] J. C. Nguyen, A. A. De Smet, B. K. Graf, and H. G. Rosas, "MR imaging-based diagnosis and classification of meniscal tears," *Radiographics*, vol. 34, no. 4, pp. 981–999, 2014.

[13] D. A. Rubin and G. A. Paletta Jr., "Current concepts and controversies in meniscal imaging," *Magnetic Resonance Imaging Clinics of North America*, vol. 8, no. 2, pp. 243–270, 2000.

[14] M. J. Matava, K. Eck, W. Totty, R. W. Wright, and R. A. Shively, "Magnetic resonance imaging as a tool to predict meniscal reparability," *The American Journal of Sports Medicine*, vol. 27, no. 4, pp. 436–443, 1999.

[15] D. A. Rubin, J. M. Kettering, J. D. Towers, and C. A. Britton, "MR imaging of knees having isolated and combined ligament injuries," *American Journal of Roentgenology*, vol. 170, no. 5, pp. 1207–1213, 1998.

[16] A. S. D. Spiers, T. Meagher, S. J. Ostlere, D. J. Wilson, and C. A. F. Dodd, "Can MRI of the knee affect arthroscopic practice? A prospective study of 58 patients," *The Journal of Bone & Joint Surgery—British Volume*, vol. 75, no. 1, pp. 49–52, 1993.

[17] J. S. Suh, E. K. Jeong, K. H. Shin et al., "Minimizing artifacts caused by metallic implants at MR imaging: experimental and clinical studies," *American Journal of Roentgenology*, vol. 171, no. 5, pp. 1207–1213, 1998.

[18] A. Cotten, E. Delfaut, X. Demondion et al., "MR imaging of the knee at 0.2 and 1.5 T: correlation with surgery," *American Journal of Roentgenology*, vol. 174, no. 4, pp. 1093–1097, 2000.

[19] N. Subhas, A. Kao, M. Freire, J. M. Polster, N. A. Obuchowski, and C. S. Winalski, "MRI of the knee ligaments and menisci: comparison of isotropic-resolution 3D and conventional 2D fast spin-echo sequences at 3 T," *American Journal of Roentgenology*, vol. 197, no. 2, pp. 442–450, 2011.

[20] D. D. Thornton and D. A. Rubin, "Magnetic resonance imaging of the knee menisci," *Seminars in Roentgenology*, vol. 35, no. 3, pp. 217–230, 2000.

[21] H. N. Chen, Q. R. Dong, and Y. Wang, "Accuracy of low-field MRI on meniscal tears," *Genetics and Molecular Research*, vol. 13, no. 2, pp. 4267–4271, 2014.

[22] A. A. De Smet, D. A. Asinger, and R. L. Johnson, "Abnormal superior popliteomeniscal fascicle and posterior pericapsular edema: indirect MR imaging signs of a lateral meniscal tear," *American Journal of Roentgenology*, vol. 176, no. 1, pp. 63–66, 2001.

[23] A. A. De Smet, M. J. Tuite, M. A. Norris, and J. S. Swan, "MR diagnosis of meniscal tears: analysis of causes of errors," *American Journal of Roentgenology*, vol. 163, no. 6, pp. 1419–1423, 1994.

[24] J. Elvenes, C. P. Jerome, O. Reikerås, and O. Johansen, "Magnetic resonance imaging as a screening procedure to avoid arthroscopy for meniscal tears," *Archives of Orthopaedic and Trauma Surgery*, vol. 120, no. 1-2, pp. 14–16, 2000.

[25] D. A. K. Jaddue, F. H. Tawfiq, and A. S. Sayed-Noor, "The utility of clinical examination in the diagnosis of medial meniscus injury in comparison with arthroscopic findings," *European Journal of Orthopaedic Surgery and Traumatology*, vol. 20, no. 5, pp. 389–392, 2010.

[26] W. W. Justice and S. F. Quinn, "Error patterns in the MR imaging evaluation of menisci of the knee," *Radiology*, vol. 196, no. 3, pp. 617–621, 1995.

[27] R. Nickinson, C. Darrah, and S. Donell, "Accuracy of clinical diagnosis in patients undergoing knee arthroscopy," *International Orthopaedics*, vol. 34, no. 1, pp. 39–44, 2010.

[28] F. Rayan, S. Bhonsle, and D. D. Shukla, "Clinical, MRI, and arthroscopic correlation in meniscal and anterior cruciate ligament injuries," *International Orthopaedics*, vol. 33, no. 1, pp. 129–132, 2009.

[29] M. Ryzewicz, B. Peterson, P. N. Siparsky, and R. L. Bartz, "The diagnosis of meniscus tears: the role of MRI and clinical examination," *Clinical Orthopaedics and Related Research*, vol. 455, pp. 123–133, 2007.

[30] T. G. Sanders and M. D. Miller, "A systematic approach to magnetic resonance imaging interpretation of sports medicine injuries of the knee," *The American Journal of Sports Medicine*, vol. 33, no. 1, pp. 131–148, 2005.

[31] E. H. G. Oei, J. J. Nikken, A. C. M. Verstijnen, A. Z. Ginai, and M. G. M. Hunink, "MR imaging of the menisci and cruciate ligaments: a systematic review," *Radiology*, vol. 226, no. 3, pp. 837–848, 2003.

[32] R. Mackenzie, A. K. Dixon, G. S. Keene, W. Hollingworth, D. J. Lomas, and R. N. Villar, "Magnetic imaging of the knee: assessment of effectiveness," *Clinical Radiology*, vol. 51, pp. 245–250, 1996.

[33] A. T. Watanabe, B. C. Carter, G. P. Teitelbaum, L. L. Seeger, and W. G. Bradley Jr., "Normal variations in MR imaging of the knee: appearance and frequency," *American Journal of Roentgenology*, vol. 153, no. 2, pp. 341–344, 1989.

[34] L. J. Herman and J. Beltran, "Pitfalls in MR imaging of the knee," *Radiology*, vol. 167, no. 3, pp. 775–781, 1988.

[35] D. C. Fithian, M. A. Kelly, and V. C. Mow, "Material properties and structure-function relationships in the menisci," *Clinical Orthopaedics and Related Research*, vol. 252, pp. 19–31, 1990.

[36] L. V. Engelhardt, A. Schmitz, P. H. Pennekamp, H. H. Schild, D. C. Wirtz, and F. Falkenhausen, "Diagnostics of degenerative meniscal tears at 3-Tesla MRI compared to arthroscopy as reference standard," *Archives of Orthopaedic and Trauma Surgery*, vol. 128, no. 5, pp. 451–456, 2008.

[37] T. Magee and D. Williams, "3.0-T MRI of meniscal tears," *American Journal of Roentgenology*, vol. 187, no. 2, pp. 371–375, 2006.

[38] S. Wong, L. Steinbach, J. Zhao, C. Stehling, C. B. Ma, and T. M. Link, "Comparative study of imaging at 3.0 T versus 1.5 T of the knee," *Skeletal Radiology*, vol. 38, no. 8, pp. 761–769, 2009.

[39] P. Van Dyck, F. M. Vanhoenacker, V. Lambrecht et al., "Prospective comparison of 1.5 and 3.0-T MRI for evaluating the knee menisci and ACL," *The Journal of Bone & Joint Surgery—American Volume*, vol. 95, no. 10, pp. 916–924, 2013.

[40] J. A. Carrino and M. E. Schweitzer, "Imaging of sports-related knee injuries," *Radiologic Clinics of North America*, vol. 40, no. 2, pp. 181–202, 2002.

[41] G. E. Antonio, J. F. Griffith, and D. K. W. Yeung, "Small-field-of-view MRI of the knee and ankle," *American Journal of Roentgenology*, vol. 183, no. 1, pp. 24–28, 2004.

[42] S. F. Quinn, T. R. Brown, and J. Szumowski, "Menisci of the knee: radial MR imaging correlated with arthroscopy in 259 patients," *Radiology*, vol. 185, no. 2, pp. 577–580, 1992.

[43] L. P. Cheung, K. C. P. Li, M. D. Hollett, A. G. Bergman, and R. J. Herfkens, "Meniscal tears of the knee: accuracy of detection with fast spin-echo MR imaging and arthroscopic correlation in 293 patients," *Radiology*, vol. 203, no. 2, pp. 508–512, 1997.

[44] E. M. Escobedo, J. C. Hunter, G. C. Zink-Brody, A. J. Wilson, S. D. Harrison, and D. J. Fisher, "Usefulness of turbo spin-echo MR imaging in the evaluation of meniscal tears: comparison with a conventional spin-echo sequence," *American Journal of Roentgenology*, vol. 167, no. 5, pp. 1223–1227, 1996.

[45] D. W. Stoller, C. Martin, J. V. Crues III, L. Kaplan, and J. H. Mink, "Meniscal tears: pathologic correlation with MR imaging," *Radiology*, vol. 163, no. 3, pp. 731–735, 1987.

[46] J. V. Crues and D. W. Stoller, "The menisci," in *MRI of the Knee*, J. H. Mink, M. A. Reicher, J. V. Crues et al., Eds., vol. 2nd, pp. 91–140, Raven, New York, NY, USA, 1993.

[47] R. S. Bikkina, C. A. Tujo, A. B. Schraner, and N. M. Major, "The 'floating' meniscus: MRI in knee trauma and implications for surgery," *American Journal of Roentgenology*, vol. 184, no. 1, pp. 200–204, 2005.

[48] R. Mackenzie, C. R. Palmer, D. J. Lomas, and A. K. Dixon, "Magnetic resonance imaging of the knee: diagnostic performance studies," *Clinical Radiology*, vol. 51, no. 4, pp. 251–257, 1996.

[49] T. R. McCauley, W.-H. Jee, M. T. Galloway, K. Lynch, and P. Jokl, "Grade 2C signal in the meniscus on MR imaging of the knee," *American Journal of Roentgenology*, vol. 179, no. 3, pp. 645–648, 2002.

[50] J. V. Crues III, J. Mink, T. L. Levy, M. Lotysch, and D. W. Stoller, "Meniscal tears of the knee: accuracy of MR imaging," *Radiology*, vol. 164, no. 2, pp. 445–448, 1987.

[51] A. A. De Smet and M. J. Tuite, "Use of the 'two-slice-touch' rule for the MRI diagnosis of meniscal tears," *American Journal of Roentgenology*, vol. 187, no. 4, pp. 911–914, 2006.

[52] T. H. Baxamusa and M. T. Galloway, "Irreducible knee dislocations secondary to interposed menisci," *American Journal of Orthopedics*, vol. 30, no. 2, pp. 141–143, 2001.

[53] B. J. Laundre, M. S. Collins, J. R. Bond, D. L. Dahm, M. J. Stuart, and J. N. Mandrekar, "MRI accuracy for tears of the posterior horn of the lateral meniscus in patients with acute anterior cruciate ligament injury and the clinical relevance of missed tears," *American Journal of Roentgenology*, vol. 193, no. 2, pp. 515–523, 2009.

[54] S.-I. Bin, J.-M. Kim, and S.-J. Shin, "Radial tears of the posterior horn of the medial meniscus," *Arthroscopy*, vol. 20, no. 4, pp. 373–378, 2004.

[55] S.-H. Choi, S. Bae, S. K. Ji, and M. J. Chang, "The MRI findings of meniscal root tear of the medial meniscus: emphasis on coronal, sagittal and axial images," *Knee Surgery, Sports Traumatology, Arthroscopy*, vol. 20, no. 10, pp. 2098–2103, 2012.

[56] C.-J. Choi, Y.-J. Choi, J.-J. Lee, and C.-H. Choi, "Magnetic resonance imaging evidence of meniscal extrusion in medial meniscus posterior root tear," *Arthroscopy*, vol. 26, no. 12, pp. 1602–1606, 2010.

[57] A. A. De Smet, D. G. Blankenbaker, R. Kijowski, B. K. Graf, and K. Shinki, "MR diagnosis of posterior root tears of the lateral meniscus using arthroscopy as the reference standard," *American Journal of Roentgenology*, vol. 192, no. 2, pp. 480–486, 2009.

[58] S. Y. Lee, W.-H. Jee, and J.-M. Kim, "Radial tear of the medial meniscal root: reliability and accuracy of MRI for diagnosis," *American Journal of Roentgenology*, vol. 191, no. 1, pp. 81–85, 2008.

[59] Y. G. Lee, J.-C. Shim, Y. S. Choi, J. G. Kim, G. J. Lee, and H. K. Kim, "Magnetic resonance imaging findings of surgically proven medial meniscus root tear: tear configuration and associated knee abnormalities," *Journal of Computer Assisted Tomography*, vol. 32, no. 3, pp. 452–457, 2008.

[60] L. K. Lecas, C. A. Helms, F. J. Kosarek, and W. E. Garret, "Inferiorly displaced flap tears of the medial meniscus: MR appearance and clinical significance," *American Journal of Roentgenology*, vol. 174, no. 1, pp. 161–164, 2000.

[61] C. A. Helms, "The meniscus: recent advances in MR imaging of the knee," *American Journal of Roentgenology*, vol. 179, no. 5, pp. 1115–1122, 2002.

[62] C. A. Helms, A. Laorr, and W. D. Cannon Jr., "The absent bow tie sign in bucket-handle tears of the menisci in the knee," *American Journal of Roentgenology*, vol. 170, no. 1, pp. 57–61, 1998.

[63] F. Türkmen, İ. H. Korucu, C. Sever, M. Demirayak, G. Goncü, and S. Toker, "Free medial meniscal fragment which mimics the dislocated bucket-handle tear on MRI," *Case Reports in Orthopedics*, vol. 2014, Article ID 647491, 3 pages, 2014.

[64] K. L. Weiss, H. T. Morehouse, and I. M. Levy, "Sagittal MR images of the knee: a low-signal band parallel to the posterior cruciate ligament caused by a displaced bucket-handle tear," *American Journal of Roentgenology*, vol. 156, no. 1, pp. 117–119, 1991.

[65] D. A. Rubin, C. A. Britton, J. D. Towers, and C. D. Harner, "Are MR imaging signs of meniscocapsular separation valid?" *Radiology*, vol. 201, no. 3, pp. 829–836, 1996.

[66] S. E. Campbell, T. G. Sanders, and W. B. Morrison, "MR imaging of meniscal cysts: incidence, location, and clinical significance," *American Journal of Roentgenology*, vol. 177, no. 2, pp. 409–413, 2001.

[67] A. A. De Smet, B. K. Graf, and A. M. del Rio, "Association of parameniscal cysts with underlying meniscal tears as identified on MRI and arthroscopy," *American Journal of Roentgenology*, vol. 196, no. 2, pp. W180–W186, 2011.

[68] W. J. Rennie and D. B. L. Finlay, "Meniscal extrusion in young athletes: associated knee joint abnormalities," *American Journal of Roentgenology*, vol. 186, no. 3, pp. 791–794, 2006.

[69] R. Brostein, P. Kirk, and J. Hurley, "The usefulness of MRI in evaluating menisci after meniscus repair," *Orthopedics*, vol. 15, no. 2, pp. 149–152, 1992.

[70] T. Magee, "Accuracy of 3-Tesla MR and MR arthrography in diagnosis of meniscal retear in the post-operative knee," *Skeletal Radiology*, vol. 43, no. 8, pp. 1057–1064, 2014.

[71] K. Singh, C. A. Helms, M. T. Jacobs, and L. D. Higgins, "MRI appearance of Wrisberg variant of discoid lateral meniscus," *American Journal of Roentgenology*, vol. 187, no. 2, pp. 384–387, 2006.

[72] K. N. Ryu, I. S. Kim, E. J. Kim et al., "MR imaging of tears of discoid lateral menisci," *American Journal of Roentgenology*, vol. 171, no. 4, pp. 963–967, 1998.

[73] S. R. Duc, C. W. A. Pfirrmann, P. P. Koch, M. Zanetti, and J. Hodler, "Internal knee derangement assessed with 3-minute three-dimensional isovoxel true FISP MR sequence: preliminary study," *Radiology*, vol. 246, no. 2, pp. 526–535, 2008.

[74] S. E. Harms, D. P. Flamig, C. F. Fisher, and J. M. Fulmer, "New method for fast MR imaging of the knee," *Radiology*, vol. 173, no. 3, pp. 743–750, 1989.

[75] A. Lu, E. Brodsky, T. M. Grist, and W. F. Block, "Rapid fat-suppressed isotropic steady-state free precession imaging using true 3D multiple-half-echo projection reconstruction," *Magnetic Resonance in Medicine*, vol. 53, no. 3, pp. 692–699, 2005.

[76] S. B. Wieslander, E. D. Rappeport, G. S. Lausten, and H. S. Thomsen, "Multiplanar reconstruction in MR imaging of the knee: comparison with standard sagittal and coronal images," *Acta Radiologica*, vol. 39, no. 2, pp. 116–119, 1998.

[77] R. Kijowski, D. G. Blankenbaker, J. L. Klaers, K. Shinki, A. A. De Smet, and W. F. Block, "Vastly undersampled isotropic projection steady-state free precession imaging of the knee: diagnostic performance compared with conventional MR," *Radiology*, vol. 251, no. 1, pp. 185–194, 2009.

[78] S. L. Solomon, W. G. Totty, and J. K. T. Lee, "MR imaging of the knee: comparison of three-dimensional FISP and two-dimensional spin-echo pulse sequences," *Radiology*, vol. 173, no. 3, pp. 739–742, 1989.

[79] N. Lefevre, J. F. Naouri, Y. Bohu, S. Klouche, and S. Herman, "Partial tears of the anterior cruciate ligament: diagnostic performance of isotropic three-dimensional fast spin echo (3D-FSE-Cube) MRI," *European Journal of Orthopaedic Surgery and Traumatology*, vol. 24, no. 1, pp. 85–91, 2014.

[80] C. W. Heron and P. T. Calvert, "Three-dimensional gradient-echo MR imaging of the knee: comparison with arthroscopy in 100 patients," *Radiology*, vol. 183, no. 3, pp. 839–844, 1992.

[81] H. Yoshioka, K. Stevens, B. A. Hargreaves et al., "Magnetic resonance imaging of articular cartilage of the knee: comparison between fat-suppressed three-dimensional SPGR imaging, fat-suppressed FSE imaging, and fat-suppressed three-dimensional DEFT imaging, and correlation with arthroscopy," *Journal of Magnetic Resonance Imaging*, vol. 20, no. 5, pp. 857–864, 2004.

[82] R. F. Busse, H. Hariharan, A. Vu, and J. H. Brittain, "Fast spin echo sequences with very long echo trains: design of variable refocusing flip angle schedules and generation of clinical T_2 contrast," *Magnetic Resonance in Medicine*, vol. 55, no. 5, pp. 1030–1037, 2006.

[83] G. E. Gold, R. F. Busse, C. Beehler et al., "Isotropic MRI of the knee with 3D fast spin-echo extended echo-train acquisition (XETA): initial experience," *American Journal of Roentgenology*, vol. 188, no. 5, pp. 1287–1293, 2007.

[84] K. J. Stevens, R. F. Busse, E. Han et al., "Ankle: isotropic MR imaging with 3D-FSE-cube-initial experience in healthy volunteers," *Radiology*, vol. 249, no. 3, pp. 1026–1033, 2008.

[85] A. H. Sonin, R. A. Pensy, M. E. Mulligan, and S. Hatem, "Grading articular cartilage of the knee using fast spin-echo proton density-weighted MR imaging without fat suppression," *American Journal of Roentgenology*, vol. 179, no. 5, pp. 1159–1166, 2002.

[86] J. Y. Jung, Y. C. Yoon, S.-H. Choi, J. W. Kwon, J. Yoo, and B.-K. Choe, "Three-dimensional isotropic shoulder MR arthrography: comparison with two-dimensional MR arthrography for the diagnosis of labral lesions at 3.0 T," *Radiology*, vol. 250, no. 2, pp. 498–505, 2009.

[87] R. Kijowski, K. W. Davis, M. A. Woods et al., "Knee joint: comprehensive assessment with 3D isotropic resolution fast spin-echo MR imaging—diagnostic performance compared with that of conventional MR imaging at 3.0 T," *Radiology*, vol. 252, no. 2, pp. 486–495, 2009.

[88] O. Ristow, L. Steinbach, G. Sabo et al., "Isotropic 3D fast spin-echo imaging versus standard 2D imaging at 3.0 T of the knee: image quality and diagnostic performance," *European Radiology*, vol. 19, no. 5, pp. 1263–1272, 2009.

[89] K. Glückert, B. Kladny, A. Blank-Schäl, and G. Hofmann, "MRI of the knee joint with a 3-D gradient echo sequence. Equivalent to diagnostic arthroscopy?" *Archives of Orthopaedic and Trauma Surgery*, vol. 112, no. 1, pp. 5–14, 1992.

[90] T. Ohishi, M. Takahashi, M. Abe, T. Tsuchikawa, M. Mori, and A. Nagano, "The use of axial reconstructed images from three-dimensional MRI datasets for morphological diagnosis of meniscal tears of the knee," *Archives of Orthopaedic and Trauma Surgery*, vol. 125, no. 9, pp. 622–627, 2005.

22

Restrictive Cardiomyopathies: The Importance of Noninvasive Cardiac Imaging Modalities in Diagnosis and Treatment

Aidonis Rammos,[1] **Vasileios Meladinis,**[1] **Georgios Vovas,**[2] **and Dimitrios Patsouras**[1]

[1]*Department of Cardiology, Chatzikosta General Hospital, Ioannina, Greece*
[2]*Department of Cardiology, Agrinio General Hospital, Agrinio, Greece*

Correspondence should be addressed to Aidonis Rammos; aidrammos@yahoo.gr

Academic Editor: Paul Sijens

Restrictive cardiomyopathy (RCM) is the least common among cardiomyopathies. It can be idiopathic, familial, or secondary to systematic disorders. Marked increase in left and/or right ventricular filling pressures causes symptoms and signs of congestive heart failure. Electrocardiographic findings are nonspecific and include atrioventricular conduction and QRS complex abnormalities and supraventricular and ventricular arrhythmias. Echocardiography and cardiac magnetic resonance (CMR) play a major role in diagnosis. Echocardiography reveals normal or hypertrophied ventricles, preserved systolic function, marked biatrial enlargement, and impaired diastolic function, often with restrictive filling pattern. CMR offering a higher spatial resolution than echocardiography can provide detailed information about anatomic structures, perfusion, ventricular function, and tissue characterization. CMR with late gadolinium enhancement (LGE) and novel approaches (myocardial mapping) can direct the diagnosis to specific subtypes of RCM, depending on the pattern of scar formation. When noninvasive studies have failed, endomyocardial biopsy is required. Differentiation between RCM and constrictive pericarditis (CP), nowadays by echocardiography, is important since both present as heart failure with normal-sized ventricles and preserved ejection fraction but CP can be treated by means of anti-inflammatory and surgical treatment, while the treatment options of RCM are dictated by the underlying condition. Prognosis is generally poor despite optimal medical treatment.

1. Introduction

According to a recent position statement of the European Society of Cardiology (ESC) working group on myocardial and pericardial diseases, cardiomyopathy is defined as a myocardial disorder in which there is abnormality in the structure and function of the myocytes, in the absence of coronary artery disease, hypertension, valvular disease, and congenital heart disease that could justify this abnormality. In the past, cardiomyopathies were also separated from systematic disorders that could involve the myocardium. ESC classification proposes a shift from diagnosing by exclusion criteria and focusing on the morphology and function of the heart [1].

Restrictive cardiomyopathy (RCM) is the least common of cardiomyopathies. It is characterized by impaired diastolic function with restrictive filling and reduced diastolic volume of either or both ventricles, preserved systolic function, and invariably normal or mildly increased wall thickness [2]. Due to increased myocardial stiffness, a small increase in volume leads to a precipitous rise of pressure within the ventricle with an accentuated filling in early diastole, which ceases abruptly at the end of the rapid filling phase showing the characteristic "dip-and-plateau" pattern [3] during cardiac catheterization.

There are many classification criteria for the causes of RCM. According to the ESC Working group in myocardial and pericardial disease RCM can be idiopathic, familial (autosomal dominant, autosomal recessive or X-linked inheritance), or secondary to systematic disorders [1] (Table 1). For the purposes of this review, we will refer to the most common of them.

TABLE 1: Causes of restrictive cardiomyopathy.

(1) Amyloidosis (AL, ATTR, SSA)

(2) Sarcoidosis

(3) Hemochromatosis

(4) Eosinophilic myocardial disease

(5) Idiopathic RCM

(6) Progressive systemic sclerosis (scleroderma)

(7) Postradiation therapy (Hodgkin's lymphoma, breast cancer etc)

(8) Anderson Fabry disease

(9) Danon's disease

(10) Friedreich's ataxia

(11) Diabetic cardiomyopathy (restrictive phenotype)

(12) Drug induced (anthracycline toxicity, methysergide, ergotamine, mercurial agents, etc.)

(13) Mucopolysaccharidoses (Hurler's cardiomyopathy)

(14) Myocardial oxalosis

(15) Wegener's granulomatosis

(16) Metastatic malignancies

2. Clinical Presentation and Physical Examination

Patients commonly present with dyspnea, fatigue and limited exercise capacity, palpitations, and syncope, while angina may also occur. Others may present with thromboembolic complications. Physical examination may reveal signs of congestive heart failure (distended jugular veins occasionally with Kussmaul sign, peripheral bilateral edema, respiratory rales, hepatomegaly, ascites, and S_3 and S_4 gallops). The ECG may reveal sinus rhythm with signs of left or biatrial enlargement or atrial fibrillation. There may be nonspecific ST and T wave abnormalities. QRS voltage may be low in the precordial leads and conductive disturbances may also occur, particularly in infiltrative diseases. Specific ECG findings may occur depending on the underlying cause and aid in the diagnostic work-up.

3. Diagnosis

3.1. Laboratory Tests. A complete evaluation should be performed as restrictive cardiomyopathy may originate from systematic disorders or can in turn affect other organs as heart failure develops. Hematocrit (HCT), serum electrolytes, blood urea nitrogen (BUN), creatinine, 24 hr urine total protein, and liver function should be assessed. Arterial blood gas (ABG) should also be obtained to monitor hypoxia. Serum brain natriuretic peptide (BNP) or N-terminal pro-b-type natriuretic peptide (NT-proBNP) and troponin T are indicative of the heart failure and in many cases predictors of survival [5–7]. Specific disorders will require more sophisticated exams (angiotensin converting enzyme (ACE) in sarcoidosis [8], complete blood count (CBC) with peripheral smear helping to establish eosinophilia [9] in hypereosinophilic syndromes, serum iron concentrations, total iron-binding capacity and ferritin levels in hemocromatosis, immunoglobulin free light κ, λ chain testing, and serum and urine immunofixation in amyloidosis, etc.).

3.2. Echocardiography. Echocardiography is the first imaging modality for the assessment of patients with dyspnea and/or heart failure. In patients with RCM, it usually discloses nonspecific findings such as normal (not dilated) ventricles with normal or increased wall thickness (Figures 1(a) and 1(b)) although it can occasionally give specific clues to the diagnosis. Transmitral spectral Doppler often shows restrictive filling pattern (accentuated early diastolic velocity with low or absent late filling velocity with E/A ratio > 2, E wave deceleration time < 150 ms, and short isovolumic relaxation time < 60 ms, Figure 1(c)) although this is commonly a sign of advanced myocardial involvement. There is marked left or biatrial dilatation usually as a consequence of chronically elevated filling pressures (Figures 1(a) and 1(b)). Although classically systolic function as expressed by means of ejection fraction (EF) is normal or near normal, novel techniques like tissue Doppler and speckle tracking echocardiography (STE) reveal the presence of latent systolic myocardial impairment which may be specific to the disease state. Tissue Doppler of the mitral annulus shows reduced systolic waves (s wave), blunted early diastolic waves, and preserved or blunted late diastolic waves, depending on the degree of atrial involvement in the myopathic process [10, 11] (Figures 1(d) and 1(e)).

One of the main utilities of echocardiography is the differential diagnosis between constrictive pericarditis (CP) and RCM. Both present as heart failure with normal-sized ventricles and preserved EF, dilated atria, and Doppler findings of increased filling pressure (often restrictive filling pattern). Differential diagnosis is important since CP can be treated by means of anti-inflammatory drugs or surgery while the treatment options of RCM are dictated by the underlying condition. For the main differences between those disease states, the reader can refer to Table 2 and recent research findings [12, 13].

3.3. Cardiac Magnetic Resonance. Echocardiography is unable to establish the definite diagnosis of specific RCM subtypes due to its inherent poor tissue characterization and limited assessment of the ventricular apex and the right ventricle. Cardiac Magnetic Resonance (CMR) with a higher spatial resolution and late gadolinium enhancement (LGE) can provide detailed information about anatomic structures, perfusion, ventricular function, and tissue characterization [14]. Late gadolinium enhancement (LGE) depending on the pattern of scar formation can direct the diagnosis to specific subtypes of RCM. Finally it can accurately measure pericardial thickness [15, 16] and visualize pericardial inflammation [17], aiding in the diagnosis of CP.

3.4. Cardiac CT. As of this writing, Cardiac CT has no specific role in the work-up of patients with RCM. It can accurately exclude the presence of coronary obstructive artery disease in patients with angina symptom. Its main role is

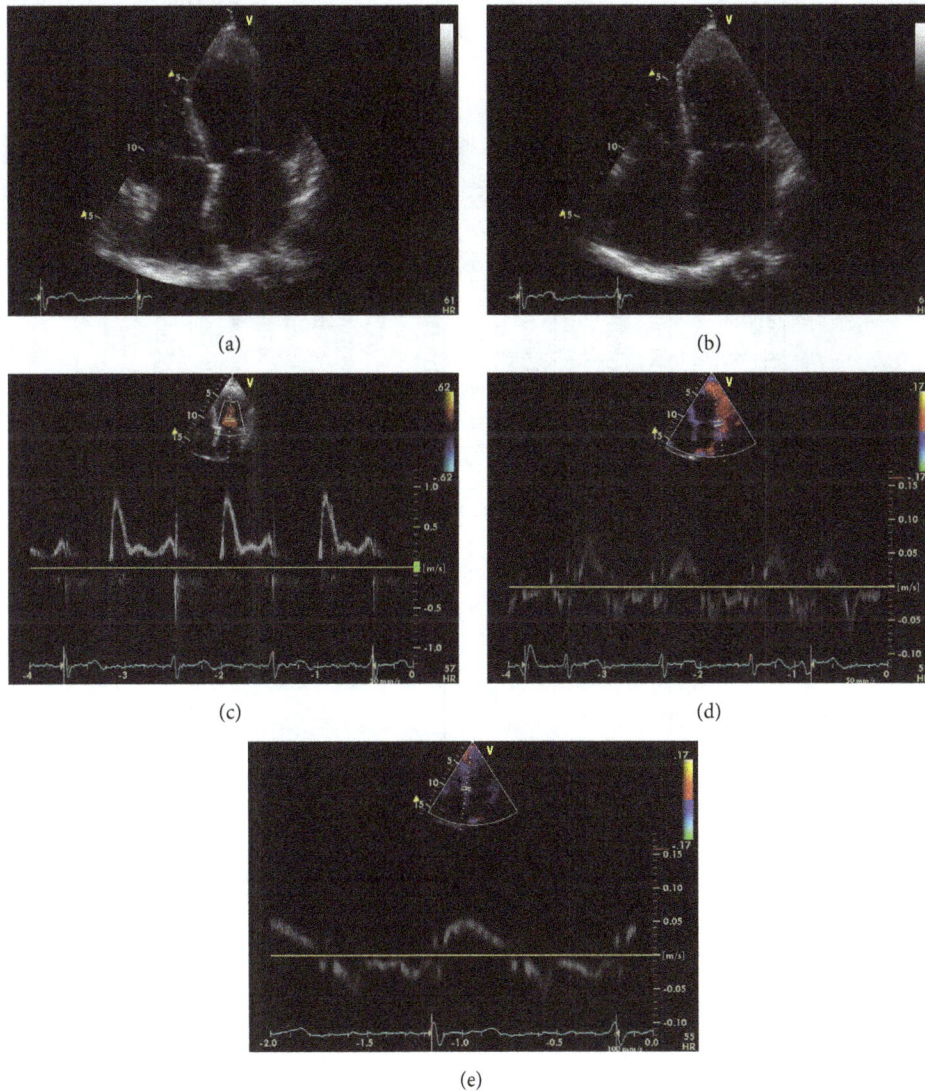

FIGURE 1: Echocardiographic images from a patient with restrictive cardiomyopathy. Two-dimensional 4-chamber view in diastole (a) and systole (b), showing normal left ventricular volume, wall thickness, and systolic function (EF 62%). There is marked biatrial enlargement. Pulse wave Doppler from the left ventricular inflow (c) showing restrictive filling pattern with an E wave velocity of 1 m/sec, an A wave velocity of 0.4 m/sec, and an E wave deceleration time of 145 msec. Spectral tissue Doppler from the lateral (d) and septal (e) mitral annulus. There is marked reduction in systolic annular velocities indicative of latent systolic dysfunction. E/e' (e' measured as the average between the two annular e' velocities) is 16, indicative of increased left ventricular filling pressure. Note the marked reduction in lateral a' velocity (<4 cm/sec) indicative of left atrial systolic dysfunction.

in the differential diagnosis between RCM and CP where it can give invaluable information about the thickness and composition of the pericardium [18].

3.5. *Invasive Catheterization.* In contemporary practice, invasive catheterization and coronary angiography are rarely needed for the establishment of diagnosis. In cases where chest pain is the predominant symptom, it can reveal the presence or absence of obstructive coronary artery disease. Left and right heart catheterization can be used when findings of noninvasive tests, including the differential diagnosis between CP and RCM, are nonconclusive [19].

3.6. *Cardiac Biopsy.* Histological examination can be valuable in setting a definite diagnosis when noninvasive studies have failed, although there are periprocedural risks of endomyocardial biopsy (EMB) [20]. Moreover, in diseases where there is focal involvement of the myocardium (e.g., sarcoidosis), biopsy may miss the area of lesion, giving false negative findings.

4. Prognosis

Prognosis varies among the specific types of RCM but is generally poor with progressive deterioration, particularly in children, despite optimal medical treatment.

TABLE 2: Differential diagnosis between restrictive cardiomyopathy and constrictive pericarditis.

Clinical and investigation features	Restrictive cardiomyopathy	Constrictive pericarditis
History	Systemic disease (e.g., sarcoidosis, hemochromatosis).	Prior history of pericarditis or conditions affecting the pericardium.
Physical examination	± Kussmaul sign, S_3 and S_4 gallop, murmurs of mitral and tricuspid regurgitation	Pericardial knock
Chest X-ray	Atrial dilatation	Pericardial calcification
ECG	Low QRS voltages (mainly amyloidosis), conduction disturbances, nonspecific ST abnormalities	Nonspecific ST and T abnormalities, low QRS voltage (<50%)
2D echocardiography	± Wall and valvular thickening, sparkling myocardium	± Pericardial thickening, respiratory ventricular septal shift.
Doppler echocardiography	Decreased variation in mitral and/or tricuspid inflow E velocity, increased hepatic vein inspiratory diastolic flow reversal, presence of mitral and tricuspid regurgitation	Increased variation in mitral and/or tricuspid inflow E velocity, hepatic vein expiratory diastolic reversal ratio $\geq$ 0.79 medial e'/lateral $e' \geq$ 0.91 (Annulus Reversus) [4]
Catheterization hemodynamics	LVEDP − RVEDP $\geq$ 5 mmHg RVSP $\geq$ 55 mmHg RVEDP/RVSP $\leq$ 0.33	LVEDP − RVEDP < 5 mmHg RVSP < 55 mmHg RVEDP/RVSP > 0.33 Inspiratory decrease in RAP < 5 mmHg Systolic area index > 1.1 (Ref CP in the modern era) Left ventricular height of rapid filling-wave > 7 mmHg
CT	Normal pericardium	Thickened/calcified pericardium
MRI	Measurement of iron overload, various types of LGE (late gadolinium enhancement)	Thickened pericardium
Biopsy	May reveal underlying cause.	Normal myocardium

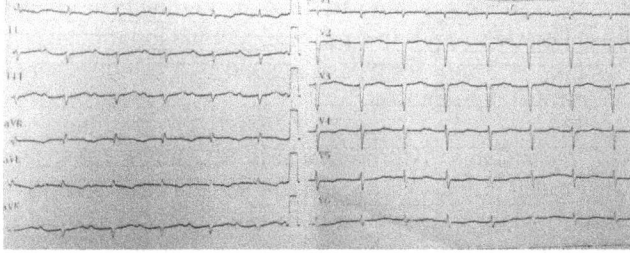

FIGURE 2: ECG from a patient with cardiac amyloidosis. There are low voltage QRS complexes with left axis deviation and marked 1st-degree atrioventricular block.

5. Specific Types of Restrictive Cardiomyopathy

5.1. Cardiac Amyloidosis. This is the most common cause of RCM. It can be either systemic or localized to the heart muscle. It is characterized by deposition of amyloid fibrils in the extracellular space. These fibrils are culprit proteins misfold into β-pleated sheets antiparallel to one another, resistant to proteolysis, and they cause oxidative stress, disruption of the myocardium, and myocardial damage [21, 22]. There are many proteins that can form amyloid but not all of them affect the heart. The main difference among them is the origin of the protein formation, the percentage of heart involvement, and the rate of progress. Amyloid stains pink with hematoxylin and eosin and demonstrates apple-green birefringence when viewed under polarized light.

The deposition begins in the subendocardium and extends within the myocardium between the muscle fibres. Rarely, the pericardium may be the primary site of amyloid deposition without any endomyocardial involvement [23]. Increased wall thickness is therefore the result of interstitial deposition and not of hypertrophied myocardial cells, in contrast to hypertensive heart disease or hypertrophic cardiomyopathy (HCM). Small intramyocardial vessels may also be infiltrated leading to anginal symptoms while epicardial arteries are angiographically normal.

The conductive system is also affected causing several degrees of atrioventricular (AV) block. Other characteristic ECG abnormalities are low voltage QRS complexes which, in combination with the finding of increased wall thickness in echocardiography, can differentiate this disease from HCM. These findings are more commonly seen in light chain amyloid (AL) [24] than in familial transthyretin-related amyloidosis (ATTR) [25] subtype. Other ECG findings include a pseudoinfarct pattern (poor R wave progression in precordial leads), intraventricular conduction delay, and atrial arrhythmias while ventricular arrhythmias are rare [26–30] (Figure 2).

Echocardiographic amyloidosis may present with biventricular hypertrophy, although up to 1/3 of cases may have normal wall thickness. The constellation of low voltage QRS complexes with hypertrophy, often with a restrictive filling pattern, is a classic feature but it indicates advanced disease. Left ventricular EF is commonly preserved in the early stages

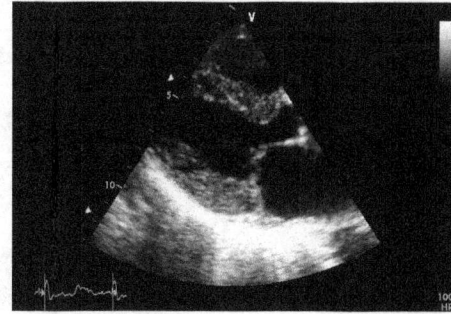

(a)

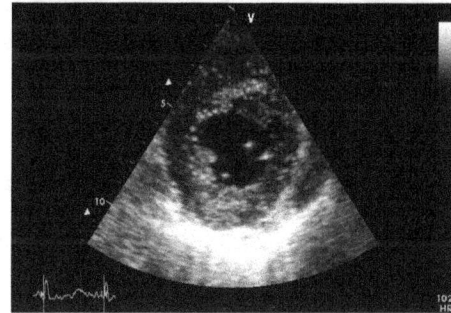

(b)

FIGURE 3: Parasternal long (a) and short axis (b) view from the patient whose ECG appears in Figure 2. There is marked LV hypertrophy. Also note the granular, speckled myocardial appearance.

of the disease process as it is primary calculated from the contraction of the heart along its short axis, while the subendocardial myocytes that are prone to damage are longitudinally oriented and therefore the longitudinal contraction will be impaired [31]. The endocardium may also be infiltrated and there may be thrombi. A granular, speckled appearance of the ventricular myocardium, (Figure 3) while nonspecific (also seen in glycogen storage disease, HCM, Anderson-Fabry disease, hypertensive heart disease, and end-stage renal disease) [32], combined with clinical suspicion and other laboratory findings, is suggestive of cardiac amyloidosis.

Atrioventricular valves, if infiltrated, may be thickened with mild to moderate regurgitation. Mild or moderate pericardial effusion may be present. Thickening of the interatrial septum without sparing of the area of the fossa ovalis is characteristic of the disease but apparent only in late stages [33].

Speckle tracking echocardiography, with the ability of measuring novel indices of deformation, has expanded its role in the diagnosis. It has been found that in cardiac amyloidosis systolic longitudinal strain (LSsys) is impaired in the mid and basal intraventricular septum compared to the apex (Figure 4). In a recent study, septal apical to basal LSsys ratio > 2.1 combined with deceleration time of early filling < 200 msec differentiated amyloidosis from other forms of LV hypertrophy with a sensitivity of 88%, specificity of 85%, positive predictive value of 67%, and negative predictive value of 96% [34] (Figure 4).

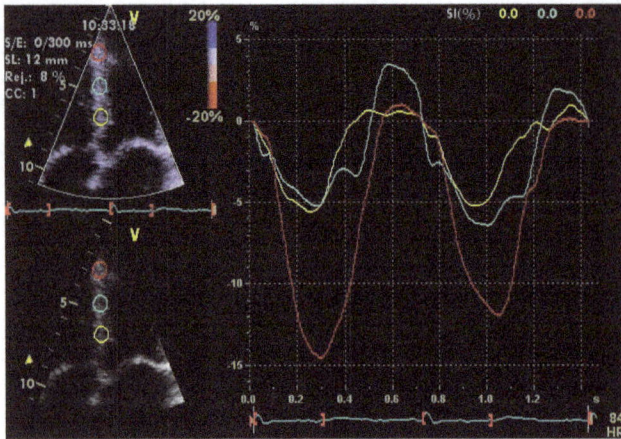

FIGURE 4: Strain curves from the interventricular septum of the same patient appearing in Figures 2 and 3. In this example, strain curves were constructed with the Doppler Myocardial Imaging technique. There is reduced peak systolic strain of the basal (yellow curve) and mid (green curve) septal segments, compared to the apical segment (red curve) with an apex to base ratio > 2.1.

CMR will show diffuse LGE throughout both ventricles, particularly the subendocardium with a characteristic zebra-stripe appearance of the subendocardial enhancement of the LV and RV endocardium, sparing the mid-wall of the interventricular septum [35]. Sometimes there is a patchy transmural pattern [36–38]. There is a faster contrast washout from myocardium and blood pool than normal. Enhancement of the atrial wall has also been reported [39] (Figure 5). The technique of T1 mapping may reveal cardiac involvement at an earlier stage compared to overt LGE images [40] and may also prove useful in patients with end-stage renal dysfunction where the administration of gadolinium based contrast is contraindicated due to the risk of nephrogenic systemic sclerosis. Recent studies have shown high sensitivity of the technique in the diagnosis of AL [41] and its ability to differentiate between AL and ATTR [42]. Moreover the combination of T1 mapping with LGE may have prognostic implications [43].

Radionuclide imaging using single-photon emission computed tomography (SPECT), or positron emission tomography (PET), has been recently introduced in the diagnostic work-up. An intense myocardial uptake of imaging agents Tc-99m pyrophosphate (PYP, available in the USA) or Tc-99m 3,3-diphosphono-1,2-propanodicarboxylic acid (DPD, available in Europe) identifies patients with ATTR and can differentiate them from those with AL [44, 45]. A recent study has shown that Tc-99m DPD uptake is an independent predictor of adverse events [46].

Histological confirmation is mandatory for the diagnosis. Renal, myocardial, or liver biopsy is invasive, expensive with high periprocedural risks [47, 48]. Preferably biopsy can be obtained by the iliac crest bone marrow [49] combined with subcutaneous abdominal fat aspiration [50] which will identify amyloidosis in 85% of cases [51]. If negative, biopsy directly from an involved organ should be obtained. A negative myocardial biopsy in suspected cases practically excludes cardiac amyloidosis, since myocardial involvement is usually widespread. In a positive examination though it is crucial to determine the type of amyloid as this in turn defines treatment and prognosis.

5.1.1. Light Chain (AL) Amyloidosis. AL amyloidosis (formerly called primary) is the commonest and most aggressive form. Amyloid is derived from monoclonal light chains (or chain fragments) secondary to a plasma cell disorder (produced at the bone marrow). The most common plasma cell disorder is multiple myeloma; however only a minority of these patients will develop amyloidosis and vice versa. Cardiac deposition occurs in almost every case of biopsy or autopsy while clinical involvement is found in about half of the cases and has a major prognostic implication [30] with a median survival as low as 4 months [52].

The clinical presentation is that described generally for RCM above. Extracardiac organs infiltrated are the kidneys, skin, liver, peripheral, and autonomic nervous system and symptoms may rise, respectively.

Treatment must combine the underlying plasma dyscrasia and the subsequent heart failure, though patients with amyloidosis respond minimally to conventional heart failure treatment. There is no evidence of beneficial effect of beta blockers, except in atrial fibrillation for relative rate control; angiotensin converting enzyme (ACE) inhibitors and angiotensin receptor blockers (ARBs) are difficultly tolerated because of hypotension which is almost always present (in grounds of low cardiac output and autonomic neuropathy). Calcium channel blockers are contraindicated as they may produce a negative inotropic effect. Cautious titration to diuretics is the most effective treatment. Digoxin should only be used for rate control in atrial fibrillation with extreme caution since the risk of toxicity is high due to possible binding of the drug to amyloid fibrils. Melphalan plus dexamethasone supported with autologous stem-cell transplantation [31, 51] is considered a standard treatment which can increase the median survival. Novel agents such as thalidomide, lenalidomide, and bortezomib are also promising but most of the trials are still ongoing. Recently the results of a phase 1 trial involving the use of a drug called (R)-1-[6-[(R)-2-carboxy-pyrrolidin-1-yl]-6-oxo-hexanoyl]pyrrolidine-2-carboxylic acid (CPHPC) have been reported. The drug succeeded in triggering clearance of amyloid deposits in patients with systemic amyloidosis. Future trials will test its effectiveness in cardiac amyloidosis [53]. The ideal treatment would be a heart transplantation (though most of the patients are unsuitable by precise criteria suggested) with autologous stem-cell transplantation since the underlying systemic disorder still exists.

5.1.2. Familial (ATTR) Amyloidosis. ATTR amyloidosis originates from a number of DNA mutations (autosomal dominant inheritance, more than 100 mutations) of the transthyretin (TTR) protein which is synthesized in the liver. The cardiac deposits vary depending on the mutation and the phenotype may be from exclusive neuropathy to cardiomyopathy or combination of the two [54]. Carpal tunnel syndrome may be an early indicator. Comparatively to

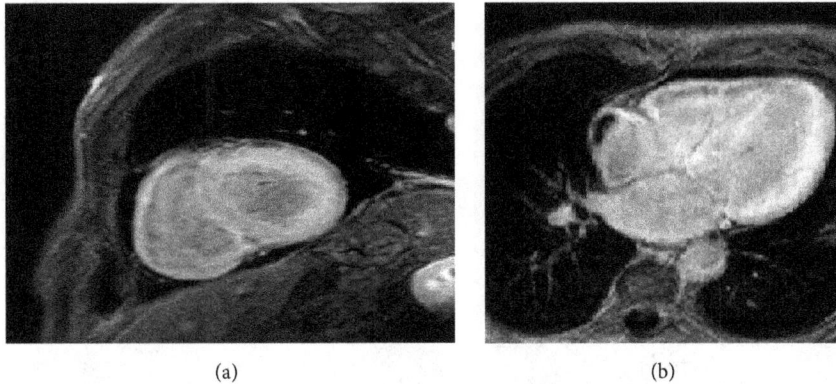

(a)   (b)

FIGURE 5: CMR short axis (a) and four-chamber view (b). LGE images showing diffuse, nonhomogenous myocardial enhancement involving both ventricles and atria. The pattern of enhancement is consistent with cardiac amyloidosis. Note the presence of a right atrial thrombus. Images courtesy of Professor Dr. Jan Bogaert, University Hospital Leuven.

AL amyloidosis ATTR has a more favorable prognosis of 3–5 years as it has a slower clinical course. Heart failure symptoms are treated with beta blockers and ACE inhibitors which are better tolerated than in AL amyloidosis. Liver transplantation is effective in reversing clinical disease in patients with TTR Val30Met mutation but it can accelerate progression of heart disease in the rest. Similar to AL amyloidosis the ideal treatment would be heart transplantation (neuropathy is a major contraindication) along with liver transplantation preferably at an early stage.

5.1.3. Senile Systemic Amyloidosis (SSA). SSA amyloidosis, formerly called wild type amyloidosis, is an exclusive cardiac disease with carpal tunnel syndrome being the only extracardiac manifestation. SSA has a more indolent course than AL with a median survival of 4–6 years after diagnosis [55] and is seen almost always in elderly males. Treatment is currently palliative, with diuretics being the cornerstone of therapy and as the clinical expression is mild, ACE inhibitors or ARBs, beta blockers, or nitrates are generally well tolerated. If atrial fibrillation occurs oral anticoagulants are indicated. Amiodarone is preferred over other antiarrhythmic agents to maintain sinus rhythm. If permanent pacemaker is needed because of high degree AV block, biventricular pacing should be considered as right ventricular pacing may worsen an already affected cardiac output.

Less common forms of amyloidosis are the AA (formerly called secondary) which is a result of chronic inflammatory conditions affecting mostly the liver and kidneys with less than 2% of the cases involving the heart and the isolated atrial amyloid where atrial natriuretic peptide (ANP) is synthesized by atrial myocytes and can be deposited as amyloid and is nowadays considered part of the ATTR or SSA subtypes.

5.2. Sarcoidosis. Sarcoidosis is a systematic noncaseating granulomatous disorder affecting several tissues. Most commonly the respiratory system is affected and patients typically present with hilar lymphadenopathy on chest X-ray. Skin, gastrointestinal, ocular, and nervous system involvement follows in frequency. Cardiac sarcoidosis (CS) is clinically present in about 5% of patients, although an autopsy study showed a prevalence of cardiac involvement in approximately 25% of cases [56] which portends worse prognosis [57].

Sarcoid granulomas consist of macrophages and epithelioid histiocytes and lymphocytes [58]. There are three histological stages: edema, granulomatous infiltration, and fibrosis but the latest is the most severe, and its presence is an independent predictor of mortality [59]. Cardiac granulomas are usually found in the basal septum, AV node, bundle of His, the ventricular free walls, and papillary muscles [60].

Blood test abnormalities are nonspecific but may reveal raised levels of ACE because it is produced by noncaseating granulomas. ECG findings include conduction abnormalities, ventricular arrhythmias (including ventricular tachycardia), and atypical infarction patterns.

There is a wide spectrum of echocardiographic abnormalities that vary from wall thickening due to edema and infiltration, to wall thinning due to fibrosis. Ventricular chambers may be normal or dilated with regional wall motion abnormalities or globally impaired systolic function. Scar retraction may lead to aneurysm formation, particularly after corticosteroid treatment. Compared to idiopathic dilated and ischemic cardiomyopathy, in CS, normokinetic segments may alternate with affected ones [58] and typically do not show a coronary distribution [61].

CMR may display all three stages of edema, inflammation, and scar formation [62]. LGE is patchy and typically found in the myocardium and epicardium of the basal and lateral LV walls [63] (Figure 6), though subendocardial or transmural hyperenhancement has also been observed, resembling an ischemic pattern [35]. The presence, extent, and location of LGE are predictive for the development of ventricular arrhythmias or death and patient response to corticosteroid treatment [59, 64, 65].

Radionuclide imaging with ^{18}fluorodeoxyglucose- (FDG-) PET has also been used in the diagnostic work-up [66]. Perfusion imaging is provided with the tracer rubidium and metabolic activity is assessed according to the degree of ^{18}FDG uptake. Decreased myocardial perfusion with enhanced ^{18}FDG uptake is consistent with inflammation, while decreased perfusion with reduced ^{18}FDG uptake is consistent with scarring. As PET identifies active

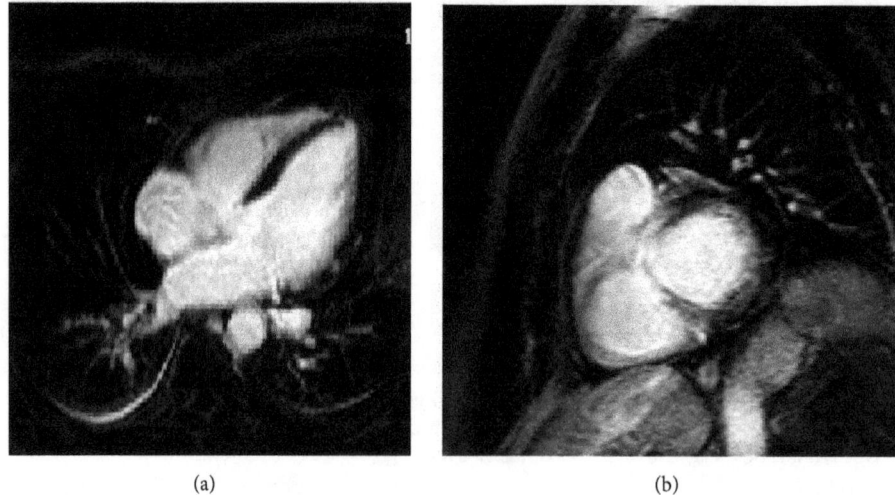

(a)

(b)

FIGURE 6: LGE images of a patient with pulmonary sarcoidosis with cardiac involvement. Four-chamber view (a) showing mid-wall focal enhancement in the lateral wall of the left ventricle and in the apex. Note also the enhancement of the mediastinal lymph nodes. Short axis view (b) demonstrating enhancement of the LVOT and possibly of the RVOT. Images courtesy of Professor Dr. Jan Bogaert, University Hospital Leuven.

inflammation earlier than CMR [67], hybrid techniques, combining PET and CMR scanners enables simultaneous acquisition of structural and functional data, therefore increasing the diagnostic accuracy [68].

The first international guidelines for the diagnosis of CS [69] incorporated the two modalities, PET and CMR in the diagnostic algorithm. When clinical presentation along with imaging findings set the suspicion, biopsy from an affected extracardiac tissue should be obtained to make the diagnosis probable, with the exception of Lofgren's syndrome (bilateral hilar lymphadenopathy, arthritis, and erythema nodosum with an incidence of 30% of cases) where biopsy is not needed [60].

Definite diagnosis is posed only by EMB but it is not preferred because of its potential risks and low sensitivity (20–30%) [20] due to the patchy distribution of granulomas. PET or CMR directed cardiac biopsy has an increased sensitivity, but still a negative EMB cannot definitely exclude CS.

Treatment of CS incorporates the guidelines directed medical therapy (GDMT) of heart failure with the addition of corticosteroids to reduce the inflammatory process (except asymptomatic hilar adenopathy where no therapy is required). FDG-PET is suggested in the treatment algorithm for the follow-up [69], defining whether satisfactory response to steroids is achieved or a second-line agent (i.e., methotrexate) should be added. If sustained VT or VF occurs, particularly in grounds of myocardial scarring, implantable cardiac defibrillator (ICD) is indicated.

5.3. Hemochromatosis. Hemochromatosis is a group of disorders which leads to excessive accumulation of iron within the cells of liver, pancreas, heart, and several endocrine glands leading to cirrhosis, diabetes, heart failure, skin pigmentation, and so forth. It may be hereditary or secondary. In the former, properly called hemochromatosis [70], transferrin

iron-binding capacity (TIBC) falls short of plasma iron content while erythropoiesis is normal. Secondary, properly called hemosiderosis, is due to increased catabolism of erythrocytes and occurs in patients undergoing frequent blood transfusions (e.g., in thalassemia major). Cardiac involvement develops later in comparison to other organs and defines prognosis. In the early stages, ECG is normal while with advanced disease low voltage QRS complexes with nonspecific ST-T segment abnormalities and supraventricular arrhythmias. Echocardiographic features may be those of dilated or less often RCM and are not specific [71]. Liver biopsy is the gold standard to establish diagnosis in hemochromatosis. Serum ferritin concentration which has been traditionally used for establishing diagnosis is a rough estimation of total body iron load.

Recently CMR with the use of T2 star (T2*) technique has been used to quantify myocardial iron overload [72]. T2* values smaller than 20 msec are predictive of adverse cardiac events [73]. It can also accurately predict the development of heart failure and arrhythmias in patients undergoing repeated transfusions [67]. Some authors advocate its use for the assessment of excess cardiac iron from the early age of 5 years in patients with thalassemia major and suboptimal chelation therapy [74]. Consequently it is regarded the gold standard for follow-up of iron chelation therapy and therapeutic guidance [75, 76].

Treatment by limitation of transfusions, phlebotomy, and chelation can reverse cardiomyopathy in hemosiderosis but liver and/or heart transplantation may be needed in advanced disease and in patients with hemochromatosis [77].

5.4. Eosinophilic Endomyocardial Disease. Eosinophilic infiltration of the heart may be caused by a heterogeneous group of disorders, referred to as hypereosinophilic syndromes (HES) and is an uncommon cause of restrictive cardiomyopathy. HES are either primary, first described by

TABLE 3: Causes of eosinophilia.

Infectious (helminths, HIV, tuberculosis)	Allergic reactions
Inflammatory (Churg-Strauss, Crohn's, Wegener, rheumatoid arthritis)	Drug hypersensitivity (NSAIDS, sulfonamides, antimicrobial)
Malignancies (Hodgkin lymphoma, Non-Hodgkin lymphoma, acute leukemia)	Idiopathic hypereosinophilic syndrome

Löffler [78], or secondary (Table 3). Eosinophilia is defined as an eosinophilic count greater than 500 eos/mm^3, while the heart is most commonly affected with a count greater than 5000 eos/mm^3 [79]. Independent of the underlying causative factor, eosinophilic degranulation causes endocardial damage (Löffler endocarditis) [80]. Primary HES is defined as an eosinophilic count greater than 1500 eos/mm^3 for more than 6 months in the absence of a secondary cause without other organ involvement [81, 82].

Cardiac infiltration consists of three stages: (a) acute necrotic stage, (b) thrombotic stage, and (c) fibroting stage. The first stage is characterized by inflammation where eosinophilic degranulation releases toxic proteins that induce endocardial necrosis and apoptosis. Rarely, acute necrotizing myocarditis may ensue with high early mortality without appropriate treatment. If left untreated, the first stage evolves into the thrombotic stage due to continuous eosinophilic activation. It consists of thrombus formation over the affected endocardium. Typically there is thrombotic obliteration of left and/or right ventricular apex which may extend to the ventricular outflow tracts, the basal ventricular segments, or even the atria. Thromboembolic complications dominate the clinical picture at this stage. The final stage is due to scarring and irreversible fibrosis of the endocardium (endomyocardial fibrosis, EMF [1]) which may affect the subvalvular apparatus of both atrioventricular valves. Patients at this stage present with advanced heart failure and prognosis is poor.

ECG findings are nonspecific and include sinus tachycardia with conduction disturbances or nonspecific ST-T segment abnormalities. At the first stage, echocardiography may reveal increased LV wall thickness due to interstitial edema, impaired systolic function with abnormal wall kinetics, although most often ventricular systolic function remains preserved. CMR with LGE may additionally reveal endomyocardial involvement, often with patchy distribution [83]. At the second stage, echocardiography shows the presence and location of thrombi while CMR may be more sensitive for thrombus detection [84] and localization. At the third stage, Doppler echocardiography may show echo-dense regions suggestive of myocardial scarring with restrictive filling pattern. CMR, again, is more sensitive and specific for the detection and localization of fibrosis.

The goals of initial therapy are twofold: first to decrease the eosinophil count and attenuate the inflammatory process and second to treat the underlying cause (if any). Corticosteroids are the mainstay of treatment combined with disease specific interventions, for example, antihelminthic therapy for parasitic infections. Anticoagulation should be initiated at the second stage to prevent thromboembolic complications. Once severe EMF has developed, surgical resection with extended endocardial dissection is the treatment of choice but with poor long-term prognosis. Atrioventricular valve replacement should be undertaken at the time of operation if the valves are affected.

5.5. Anderson-Fabry Disease. Anderson-Fabry disease is a rare X-linked recessive lysosomal storage disorder, caused by mutations of the GLA gene that encodes α-galactosidase A which breaks down neutral glycosphingolipids [85]. This results in intracellular accumulation of glycosphingolipids causing cardiac, renal, and cerebrovascular disease. Males are more commonly affected and diagnosed early in childhood (boys at an average age of 5-6 years and girls approximately 3-4 years older) [86–88] while cardiac involvement occurs in adulthood with a median survival of 50 years. Chronic neuropathic pain, typically affecting hands and feet, can be the first symptom. Children can present with poor growth and difficulties following school activities. Main symptoms are gastrointestinal like postprandial diarrhea and abdominal pain, angiokeratomas, lymphedema, and hypohydrosis. Microalbuminuria, proteinuria, and renal failure present late in the disease process and are a major source of morbidity and mortality [89]. Transient ischemic attacks are also likely to occur. Cardiac disease is caused by accumulation of globotriaosylceramide in all cellular components of the heart. The classic phenotype is that of HCM and less often of the restrictive one. ECG may reveal LV hypertrophy, with preexcitation [90] or prolonged [91] PR interval. Arrhythmias may occur since childhood and include bradycardia, supraventricular tachycardia, atrial fibrillation, or atrial flutter. Echocardiographic concentric LV hypertrophy is the most frequent finding with asymmetric septal hypertrophy developing in approximately 5% of patients [92] (Figures 7(a), 7(b), and 7(c)). RV hypertrophy is a common finding (Figure 7(d)). Systolic anterior motion (SAM) of the anterior mitral valve leaflet, with obstruction of the LV outflow tract, may also occur. Systolic function is preserved and diastolic function is impaired but restrictive physiology is rare [93]. CMR reveals a LGE pattern of the basal inferolateral LV segment and typically spares the subendocardium [35]. Diagnosis in males can be set by measuring α-galactosidase A activity or by GLA gene sequencing, while female carriers have a normal enzyme activity and gene sequencing is needed [86].

Treatment includes GDMT of heart failure (with careful beta blocker use) and enzyme replacement therapy which is effective in myocardial remodeling and improves peak systolic strain and strain rate [94] but its use is limited in advanced cases [95]. Patients should receive genetic counseling. Offsprings of affected families may be screened by means of α-galactosidase A activity or by GLA gene sequencing for

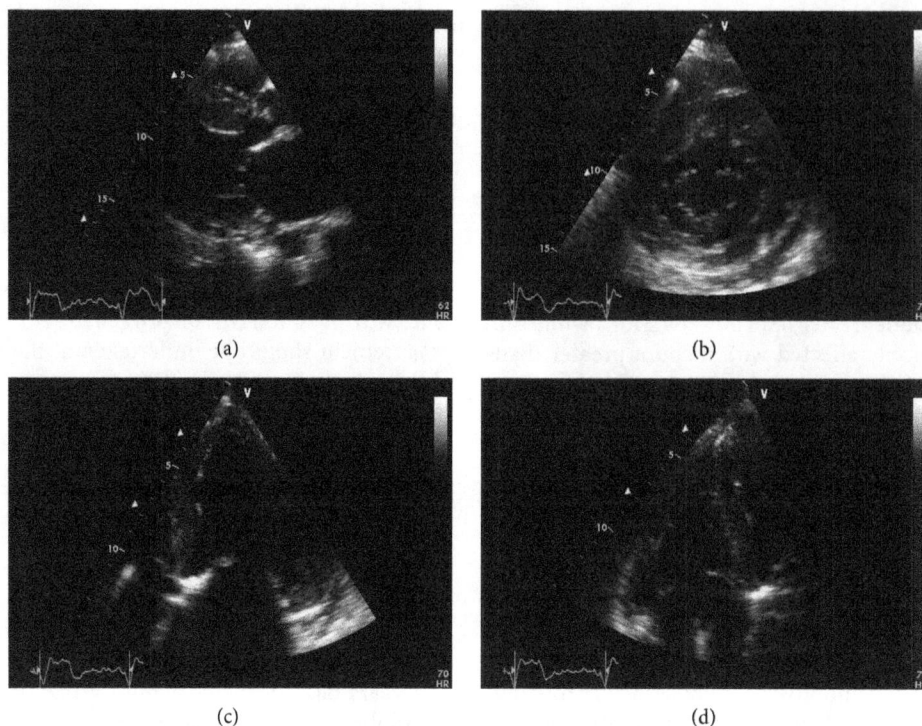

FIGURE 7: Echocardiographic images from a patient with advanced Anderson-Fabry disease and end-stage renal failure. Parasternal long axis (a), short axis (b), and apical four-chamber view (c). There is left ventricular hypertrophy, more pronounced at the interventricular septum. There is also thickening of the right ventricular free wall apparent at the modified apical four-chamber view (d).

males and gene sequencing for females. This can aid in early diagnosis with early implementation of enzyme replacement therapy before overt end-organ damage occurs.

5.6. Diabetic Cardiomyopathy.
Diabetic cardiomyopathy (DMCMP) was firstly described as a dilated phenotype with reduced ejection fraction (HFrEF). Recent studies [96, 97] showed a restrictive phenotype as well with preserved systolic function (HFpEF). These distinct patterns have common pathophysiologic mechanisms (autoimmunity, coronary microvascular rarefaction, hyperglycaemia, lipotoxicity, etc.) [98] which seem to be of variable relevance. This distinction is of therapeutic importance as the standard heart failure treatment is of uncertain value for the restrictive DMCMP. Diagnosis of DMCMP with restrictive phenotype (HFpEF) requires exclusion of CAD, valvular, congenital, or hypertensive heart disease, as well as exclusion of infiltrative cardiomyopathies which may require endomyocardial biopsy.

5.7. Idiopathic Restrictive Cardiomyopathy.
This is the primary restrictive cardiomyopathy, more commonly affecting women, where hemodynamic abnormalities occur without any specific histological changes and in the absence of ischemic, valvular, and congenital heart disease or hypertension. Patients usually present with overt heart failure. Echocardiographic findings are nonspecific as well, with marked dilation of the atria and normal-sized ventricles with preserved systolic function. Doppler demonstrates elevated LV filling pressures [99] more often with restrictive filling pattern.

5.8. Progressive Systemic Sclerosis (Scleroderma).
Systemic sclerosis is an autoimmune disorder that practically affects almost any organ system. Myocardial fibrosis results in heart failure symptoms, while fibrosis of the conduction system may lead to ventricular arrhythmias and sudden cardiac death. Physical examination depends on the organs involved with cardiac manifestations mainly caused by right heart failure (peripheral bilateral edema and raised jugular venous pressure). Echocardiographic findings are consistent with restrictive physiology.

5.9. Postradiotherapy Cardiomyopathy.
Radiotherapy used against thoracic malignancies (Hodgkin's lymphoma, breast cancer, etc.) may provoke several cardiovascular disorders such as coronary artery disease, myocardial fibrosis, valvular heart disease, pericardial disease, and ECG conduction abnormalities. Diffuse interstitial fibrosis after relatively low doses of radiation [100] ultimately leads to decrease in tissue elasticity and distensibility [101] which causes restrictive cardiomyopathy.

5.10. Danon Disease.
Danon disease is an X-linked disorder, due to primary deficiency of lysosome-associated membrane protein 2 (LAMP2). Symptoms occur in adolescence and include heart failure, mental retardation, and skeletal myopathy. Most patients die of heart failure in the third

decade of life [102]. Laboratory tests reveal creatine kinase (CK) elevation two to three times the normal value in males, liver enzyme (aspartate transaminase (AST), alanine aminotransferase (ALT), and lactate dehydrogenase (LDH)) and serum aldolase elevation in at least one-half of patients. As in Anderson-Fabry disease ECG may reveal normal or increased QRS voltage often with extreme hypertrophy (Sokolov score ≥ 50) [103] and/or preexcitation. Other ECG abnormalities include nonspecific intraventricular conduction delay, variable degrees of atrioventricular block, sinus bradycardia, reentrant atrial, and ventricular tachycardia.

Echocardiography reveals severe hypertrophy of both ventricles, resembling HCM but the electrophysiological abnormalities, particularly ventricular preexcitation, may give a clue for differentiating the two conditions [104]. In Danon disease, CMR may show subendocardial LGE [105]. Definite diagnosis is set by biopsy of skeletal muscle. There is no specific treatment.

5.11. Friedreich Ataxia. It is an autosomal recessive disorder caused by repeated Guanine-Adenine-Adenine triplets in the frataxin gene on chromosome 9 [106]. Manifestations include neuromuscular impairment of the respiratory muscles with frequent respiratory infections and heart failure. Echocardiography reveals increased wall thickness of the intraventricular septum or posterior wall with preserved systolic function [107].

6. Conclusions

Restrictive cardiomyopathies are a group of diseases with various genetic or acquired etiologies. They are characterized by marked increase in ventricular filling pressures which cause symptoms and signs of congestive heart failure. Electrocardiogram, echocardiography, CMR with LGE, or novel radionuclide imaging can direct the diagnosis to specific subtypes of RCM which is important as treatment and prognosis differ significantly, but endomyocardial biopsy is the definite means of establishing the diagnosis. Genetic counseling and familial screening are necessary in hereditary forms.

Acknowledgments

Dr. Georgios Vovas has been supported by a grant from the Hellenic Cardiological Society.

References

[1] P. Elliott, B. Andersson, E. Arbustini et al., "Classification of the cardiomyopathies: a position statement from the european society of cardiology working group on myocardial and pericardial diseases," *European Heart Journal*, vol. 29, no. 2, pp. 270–276, 2008.

[2] N. M. Ammash, J. B. Seward, K. R. Bailey, W. D. Edwards, and A. J. Tajik, "Clinical profile and outcome of idiopathic restrictive cardiomyopathy," *Circulation*, vol. 101, no. 21, pp. 2490–2496, 2000.

[3] S. T. Higano, E. Azrak, N. K. Tahirkheli, and M. J. Kern, "Hemodynamic rounds series II: Hemodynamics of constrictive physiology: Influence of respiratory dynamics on ventricular pressures," *Catheterization and Cardiovascular Interventions*, vol. 46, no. 4, pp. 473–486, 1999.

[4] T. D. Welch, L. H. Ling, R. E. Espinosa et al., "Echocardiographic diagnosis of constrictive pericarditis Mayo Clinic criteria," *Circulation: Cardiovascular Imaging*, vol. 7, no. 3, pp. 526–534, 2014.

[5] F. S. Leya, D. Arab, D. Joyal et al., "The efficacy of brain natriuretic peptide levels in differentiating constrictive pericarditis from restrictive cardiomyopathy," *Journal of the American College of Cardiology*, vol. 45, no. 11, pp. 1900–1902, 2005.

[6] J. A. de Lemos, D. K. McGuire, and M. H. Drazner, "B-type natriuretic peptide in cardiovascular disease," *The Lancet*, vol. 362, no. 9380, pp. 316–322, 2003.

[7] A. Dispenzieri, M. A. Gertz, R. A. Kyle et al., "Serum cardiac troponins and N-terminal pro-brain natriuretic peptide: a staging system for primary systemic amyloidosis," *Journal of Clinical Oncology*, vol. 22, no. 18, pp. 3751–3757, 2004.

[8] G. M. Ainslie and S. R. Benatar, "Serum angiotensin converting enzyme in sarcoidosis: Sensitivity and specificity in diagnosis: correlations with disease activity, duration, extrathoracic involvement, radiographic type and therapy," *QJM: An International Journal of Medicine*, vol. 55, no. 3-4, pp. 253–270, 1985.

[9] M. E. Rothenberg, "Eosinophilia," *The New England Journal of Medicine*, vol. 338, no. 22, pp. 1592–1600, 1998.

[10] S. Liu, C. Ma, W. Ren et al., "Regional left atrial function differentiation in patients with constrictive pericarditis and restrictive cardiomyopathy: a study using speckle tracking echocardiography," *The International Journal of Cardiovascular Imaging*, vol. 31, no. 8, pp. 1529–1536, 2015.

[11] C. Pislaru, T. P. Abraham, and M. Belohlavek, "Strain and strain rate echocardiography," *Current Opinion in Cardiology*, vol. 17, no. 5, pp. 443–454, 2002.

[12] D. R. Talreja, R. A. Nishimura, J. K. Oh, and D. R. Holmes, "Constrictive pericarditis in the modern era: novel criteria for diagnosis in the cardiac catheterization laboratory," *Journal of the American College of Cardiology*, vol. 51, no. 3, pp. 315–319, 2008.

[13] W. A. Jaber, P. Sorajja, B. A. Borlaug, and R. A. Nishimura, "Differentiation of tricuspid regurgitation from constrictive pericarditis: Novel criteria for diagnosis in the cardiac catheterisation laboratory," *Heart*, vol. 95, no. 17, pp. 1449–1454, 2009.

[14] G. Quarta, D. M. Sado, and J. C. Moon, "Cardiomyopathies: Focus on cardiovascular magnetic resonance," *British Journal of Radiology*, vol. 84, no. 3, pp. S296–S305, 2011.

[15] J. Bogaert, S. Dymarkowski, and A. M. Taylor, *Clinical Cardiac MRI*, Springer, Berlin, Germany, 1st edition, 2005.

[16] A. J. Misselt, S. R. Harris, J. Glockner, D. Feng, I. S. Syed, and P. A. Araoz, "MR Imaging of the Pericardium," *Magnetic Resonance Imaging Clinics of North America*, vol. 16, no. 2, pp. 185–199, 2008.

[17] A. M. Taylor, S. Dymarkowski, E. K. Verbeken, and J. Bogaert, "Detection of pericardial inflammation with late-enhancement cardiac magnetic resonance imaging: Initial results," *European Radiology*, vol. 16, no. 3, pp. 569–574, 2006.

[18] J. Bogaert and M. Francone, "Pericardial disease: Value of CT and MR imaging," *Radiology*, vol. 267, no. 2, pp. 340–356, 2013.

[19] P. Sorajja, "Invasive hemodynamics of constrictive pericarditis, restrictive cardiomyopathy, and cardiac tamponade," *Cardiology Clinics*, vol. 29, no. 2, pp. 191–199, 2011.

[20] L. T. Cooper, K. L. Baughman, A. M. Feldman et al., "The role of endomyocardial biopsy in the management of cardiovascular disease: a scientific statement from the American Heart Association, the American College of Cardiology, and the European Society of Cardiology. Endorsed by the Heart Failure Society of America and the Heart Failure Association of the European Society of Cardiology," *Journal of the American College of Cardiology*, vol. 50, no. 19, pp. 1914–1931, 2007.

[21] G. Merlini and V. Bellotti, "Molecular mechanisms of amyloidosis," *The New England Journal of Medicine*, vol. 349, no. 6, pp. 583–596, 2003.

[22] K. B. Shah, Y. Inoue, and M. R. Mehra, "Amyloidosis and the heart: a comprehensive review," *JAMA Internal Medicine*, vol. 166, no. 17, pp. 1805–1813, 2006.

[23] V. Singh, J. E. Fishman, and C. E. Alfonso, "Primary systemic amyloidosis presenting as constrictive pericarditis," *Cardiology*, vol. 118, no. 4, pp. 251–255, 2011.

[24] B. Murtagh, S. C. Hammill, M. A. Gertz, R. A. Kyle, A. J. Tajik, and M. Grogan, "Electrocardiographic findings in primary systemic amyloidosis and biopsy-proven cardiac involvement," *American Journal of Cardiology*, vol. 95, no. 4, pp. 535–537, 2005.

[25] P. T. Sattianayagam, A. F. Hahn, C. J. Whelan et al., "Cardiac phenotype and clinical outcome of familial amyloid polyneuropathy associated with transthyretin alanine 60 variant," *European Heart Journal*, vol. 33, no. 9, pp. 1120–1127, 2012.

[26] G. Y. Lee, K. Kim, J.-O. Choi et al., "Cardiac amyloidosis without increased left ventricular wall thickness," *Mayo Clinic Proceedings*, vol. 89, no. 6, pp. 781–789, 2014.

[27] M. Namdar, J. Steffel, S. Jetzer et al., "Value of electrocardiogram in the differentiation of hypertensive heart disease, hypertrophic cardiomyopathy, aortic stenosis, amyloidosis, and fabry disease," *American Journal of Cardiology*, vol. 109, no. 4, pp. 587–593, 2012.

[28] S. Perlini, F. Salinaro, F. Cappelli et al., "Prognostic value of fragmented QRS in cardiac AL amyloidosis," *International Journal of Cardiology*, vol. 167, no. 5, pp. 2156–2161, 2013.

[29] S.-O. Granstam, S. Rosengren, O. Vedin et al., "Evaluation of patients with cardiac amyloidosis using echocardiography, ECG and right heart catheterization," *Amyloid*, vol. 20, no. 1, pp. 27–33, 2013.

[30] A. K. L. Reyners, B. P. C. Hazenberg, W. D. Reitsma, and A. J. Smit, "Heart rate variability as a predictor of mortality in patients with AA and AL amyloidosis," *European Heart Journal*, vol. 23, no. 2, pp. 157–161, 2002.

[31] R. H. Falk and S. W. Dubrey, "Amyloid Heart Disease," *Progress in Cardiovascular Diseases*, vol. 52, no. 4, pp. 347–361, 2010.

[32] W. A. Aljaroudi, M. Y. Desai, W. H. W. Tang, D. Phelan, M. D. Cerqueira, and W. A. Jaber, "Role of imaging in the diagnosis and management of patients with cardiac amyloidosis: State of the art review and focus on emerging nuclear techniques," *Journal of Nuclear Cardiology*, vol. 21, no. 2, pp. 271–283, 2014.

[33] J. K. Oh, J. B. Seward, and A. J. Talik, *The Echo Manual*, 3rd edition, 2007.

[34] D. Liu, K. Hu, M. Niemann et al., "Effect of combined systolic and diastolic functional parameter assessment for differentiation of cardiac amyloidosis from other causes of concentric left ventricular hypertrophy," *Circulation: Cardiovascular Imaging*, vol. 6, no. 6, pp. 1066–1072, 2013.

[35] T. D. Karamitsos, J. M. Francis, S. Myerson, J. B. Selvanayagam, and S. Neubauer, "The Role of Cardiovascular Magnetic Resonance Imaging in Heart Failure," *Journal of the American College of Cardiology*, vol. 54, no. 15, pp. 1407–1424, 2009.

[36] J. B. Selvanayagam, P. N. Hawkins, B. Paul, S. G. Myerson, and S. Neubauer, "Evaluation and Management of the Cardiac Amyloidosis," *Journal of the American College of Cardiology*, vol. 50, no. 22, pp. 2101–2110, 2007.

[37] A. M. Maceira, J. Joshi, S. K. Prasad et al., "Cardiovascular magnetic resonance in cardiac amyloidosis," *Circulation*, vol. 111, no. 2, pp. 186–193, 2005.

[38] A. S. H. Cheng, A. P. Banning, A. R. J. Mitchell, S. Neubauer, and J. B. Selvanayagam, "Cardiac changes in systemic amyloidosis: Visualisation by magnetic resonance imaging," *International Journal of Cardiology*, vol. 113, no. 1, pp. E21–E23, 2006.

[39] J. C. Lyne, J. Petryka, and D. J. Pennell, "Atrial enhancement by cardiovascular magnetic resonance in cardiac amyloidosis," *European Heart Journal*, vol. 29, no. 2, p. 212, 2008.

[40] A. M. Maceira, S. K. Prasad, P. N. Hawkins, M. Roughton, and D. J. Pennell, "Cardiovascular magnetic resonance and prognosis in cardiac amyloidosis," *Journal of Cardiovascular Magnetic Resonance*, vol. 10, no. 1, article no. 54, 2008.

[41] T. D. Karamitsos, S. K. Piechnik, S. M. Banypersad et al., "Noncontrast T1 mapping for the diagnosis of cardiac amyloidosis," *JACC: Cardiovascular Imaging*, vol. 6, no. 4, pp. 488–497, 2013.

[42] J. N. Dungu, O. Valencia, J. H. Pinney et al., "CMR-Based Differentiation of AL and ATTR Cardiac Amyloidosis," *JACC: Cardiovascular Imaging*, vol. 7, no. 2, pp. 133–142, 2014.

[43] M. Fontana, S. M. Banypersad, T. A. Treibel et al., "Native T1 Mapping in Transthyretin Amyloidosis," *JACC: Cardiovascular Imaging*, vol. 7, no. 2, pp. 157–165, 2014.

[44] S. Bokhari, A. Castaño, T. Pozniakoff, S. Deslisle, F. Latif, and M. S. Maurer, "99mTc-pyrophosphate scintigraphy for differentiating light-chain cardiac amyloidosis from the transthyretin-related familial and senile cardiac amyloidoses," *Circulation: Cardiovascular Imaging*, vol. 6, no. 2, pp. 195–201, 2013.

[45] E. Perugini, P. L. Guidalotti, F. Salvi et al., "Noninvasive etiologic diagnosis of cardiac amyloidosis using 99mTc-3,3-diphosphono-1,2-propanodicarboxylic acid scintigraphy," *Journal of the American College of Cardiology*, vol. 46, no. 6, pp. 1076–1084, 2005.

[46] C. Rapezzi, C. C. Quarta, P. L. Guidalotti et al., "Role of 99mTc-DPD scintigraphy in diagnosis and prognosis of hereditary transthyretin-related cardiac amyloidosis," *JACC: Cardiovascular Imaging*, vol. 4, no. 6, pp. 659–670, 2011.

[47] H. Von Hutten, M. Mihatsch, H. Lobeck, B. Rudolph, M. Eriksson, and C. Röcken, "Prevalence and origin of amyloid in kidney biopsies," *The American Journal of Surgical Pathology*, vol. 33, no. 8, pp. 1198–1205, 2009.

[48] B. Kieninger, M. Eriksson, R. Kandolf et al., "Amyloid in endomyocardial biopsies," *Virchows Archiv*, vol. 456, no. 5, pp. 523–532, 2010.

[49] F. Petruzziello, P. Zeppa, L. Catalano et al., "Amyloid in bone marrow smears of patients affected by multiple myeloma," *Annals of Hematology*, vol. 89, no. 5, pp. 469–474, 2010.

[50] I. I. Van Gameren, B. P. C. Hazenberg, J. Bijzet et al., "Amyloid load in fat tissue reflects disease severity and predicts survival in amyloidosis," *Arthritis Care & Research*, vol. 62, no. 3, pp. 296–301, 2010.

[51] M. A. Gertz, "Immunoglobulin light chain amyloidosis: 2014 update on diagnosis, prognosis, and treatment," *American Journal of Hematology*, vol. 89, no. 12, pp. 1133–1140, 2014.

[52] R. A. Kyle and M. A. Gertz, "Primary systemic amyloidosis: clinical and laboratory features in 474 cases," *Seminars in Hematology*, vol. 32, pp. 45–59, 1995.

[53] D. B. Richards, L. M. Cookson, A. C. Berges et al., "Therapeutic clearance of amyloid by antibodies to serum amyloid P component," *The New England Journal of Medicine*, vol. 373, no. 12, pp. 1106–1114, 2015.

[54] C. Rapezzi, C. C. Quarta, L. Obici et al., "Disease profile and differential diagnosis of hereditary transthyretin-related amyloidosis with exclusively cardiac phenotype: An Italian perspective," *European Heart Journal*, vol. 34, no. 7, pp. 520–528, 2013.

[55] F. L. Ruberg, M. S. Maurer, D. P. Judge et al., "Prospective evaluation of the morbidity and mortality of wild-type and V122I mutant transthyretin amyloid cardiomyopathy: The Transthyretin Amyloidosis Cardiac Study (TRACS)," *American Heart Journal*, vol. 164, no. 2, pp. 222–228.e1, 2012.

[56] K. J. Silverman, G. M. Hutchins, and B. H. Bulkley, "Cardiac sarcoid: a clinicopathologic study of 84 unselected patients with systemic sarcoidosis," *Circulation*, vol. 58, no. 6, pp. 1204–1211, 1978.

[57] D. Bejar, P. C. Colombo, F. Latif, and M. Yuzefpolskaya, "Infiltrative cardiomyopathies," *Clinical Medicine Insights: Cardiology*, vol. 9, pp. 29–38, 2015.

[58] S. W. Dubrey and R. H. Falk, "Diagnosis and management of cardiac sarcoidosis," *Progress in Cardiovascular Diseases*, vol. 52, no. 4, pp. 336–346, 2010.

[59] S. Greulich, C. C. Deluigi, S. Gloekler et al., "CMR imaging predicts death and other adverse events in suspected cardiac sarcoidosis," *JACC: Cardiovascular Imaging*, vol. 6, no. 4, pp. 501–511, 2013.

[60] M. C. Iannuzi, B. A. Rybicki, and A. S. Tierstein, "Sarcoidosis," *The New England Journal of Medicine*, vol. 357, pp. 2153–2165, 2007.

[61] Y. Yazaki, M. Isobe, S. Hiramitsu et al., "Comparison of clinical features and prognosis of cardiac sarcoidosis and idiopathic dilated cardiomyopathy," *American Journal of Cardiology*, vol. 82, no. 4, pp. 537–540, 1998.

[62] A. Gupta, G. Singh Gulati, S. Seth, and S. Sharma, "Cardiac MRI in restrictive cardiomyopathy," *Clinical Radiology*, vol. 67, no. 2, pp. 95–105, 2012.

[63] J. Smedema, G. Snoep, M. P. G. van Kroonenburgh et al., "Evaluation of the accuracy of gadolinium-enhanced cardiovascular magnetic resonance in the diagnosis of cardiac sarcoidosis," *Journal of the American College of Cardiology*, vol. 45, no. 10, pp. 1683–1690, 2005.

[64] T. Crawford, G. Mueller, S. Sarsam et al., "Magnetic resonance imaging for identifying patients with cardiac sarcoidosis and preserved or mildly reduced left ventricular function at risk of ventricular arrhythmias," *Circulation: Arrhythmia and Electrophysiology*, vol. 7, no. 6, pp. 1109–1115, 2014.

[65] T. Ise, T. Hasegawa, Y. Morita et al., "Extensive late gadolinium enhancement on cardiovascular magnetic resonance predicts adverse outcomes and lack of improvement in LV function after steroid therapy in cardiac sarcoidosis," *Heart*, vol. 100, no. 15, pp. 1165–1172, 2014.

[66] K. A. Britton, W. G. Stevenson, B. D. Levy, J. T. Katz, and J. Loscalzo, "The beat goes on," *The New England Journal of Medicine*, vol. 362, no. 18, pp. 1662–1726, 2010.

[67] F. Erthal, D. Juneau, S. P. Lim et al., "Imaging of cardiac sarcoidosis," *The Quarterly Journal of Nuclear Medicine and Molecular Imaging*, vol. 60, no. 3, pp. 252–263, 2016.

[68] J. A. White, M. Rajchl, J. Butler, R. T. Thompson, F. S. Prato, and G. Wisenberg, "Active cardiac sarcoidosis first clinical experience of simultaneous positron emission tomography-magnetic resonance imaging for the diagnosis of cardiac disease," *Circulation*, vol. 127, no. 22, pp. e639–e641, 2013.

[69] D. H. Birnie, P. B. Nery, A. C. Ha, and R. S. B. Beanlands, "Cardiac Sarcoidosis," *Journal of the American College of Cardiology*, vol. 68, no. 4, pp. 411–421, 2016.

[70] A. Pietrangelo, "Hereditary hemochromatosis—a new look at an old disease," *The New England Journal of Medicine*, vol. 350, no. 23, pp. 2383–2430, 2004.

[71] D. T. Kremastinos, D. Farmakis, A. Aessopos et al., "β-thalassemia cardiomyopathy: History, present considerations, and future perspectives," *Circulation: Heart Failure*, vol. 3, no. 3, pp. 451–458, 2010.

[72] L. J. Anderson, S. Holden, B. Davis et al., "Cardiovascular T2-star (T2*) magnetic resonance for the early diagnosis of myocardial iron overload," *European Heart Journal*, vol. 22, no. 23, pp. 2171–2179, 2001.

[73] P. Kirk, M. Roughton, J. B. Porter et al., "Cardiac T2* magnetic resonance for prediction of cardiac complications in Thalassemia Major," *Circulation*, vol. 120, no. 20, pp. 1961–1968, 2009.

[74] X. Chen, Z. Zhang, J. Zhong et al., "MRI assessment of excess cardiac iron in thalassemia major: When to initiate?" *Journal of Magnetic Resonance Imaging*, vol. 42, no. 3, pp. 737–745, 2016.

[75] M. A. Tanner, R. Galanello, C. Dessi et al., "A randomized, placebo-controlled, double-blind trial of the effect of combined therapy with deferoxamine and deferiprone on myocardial iron in thalassemia major using cardiovascular magnetic resonance," *Circulation*, vol. 115, no. 14, pp. 1876–1884, 2007.

[76] M. A. Tanner, R. Galanello, C. Dessi et al., "Combined chelation therapy in thalassemia major for the treatment of severe myocardial siderosis with left ventricular dysfunction," *Journal of Cardiovascular Magnetic Resonance*, vol. 10, article 12, 2008.

[77] M. Nishio, T. Endo, S. Nakao, N. Sato, and T. Koike, "Reversible cardiomyopathy due to secondary hemochromatosis with multitransfusions for severe aplastic anemia after successful nonmyeloablative stem cell transplantation," *International Journal of Cardiology*, vol. 127, no. 3, pp. 400–401, 2008.

[78] W. L. Löffler, "Endocarditis parietal fibroplastica with eosinophilia: a strange diseas," *Schweizerische Medizinische Wochenschrift*, vol. 66, pp. 817–820, 1936 (German).

[79] M. J. Chusid, "Eosinophilia in childhood," *Immunology and Allergy Clinics of North America*, vol. 19, no. 2, pp. 327–346, 1999.

[80] P. E. Séguéla, X. Iriart, P. Acar, M. Montaudon, R. Roudaut, and J. B. Thambo, "Eosinophilic cardiac disease: molecular, clinical and imaging aspects," *Archives of Cardiovascular Diseases*, vol. 108, no. 4, pp. 258–268, 2015.

[81] M. J. Chusid, D. C. Dale, B. C. West, and S. M. Wolff, "The hypereosinophilic syndrome: analysis of fourteen cases with review of the literature," *Medicine*, vol. 54, no. 1, pp. 1–27, 1975.

[82] S. K. Feske, M. Goldberg, D. M. Dudzinski, R. G. Gonzalez, and A. E. Kovach, "Case 29-2015—A 38-year-old pregnant woman with headache and visual symptoms," *The New England Journal of Medicine*, vol. 373, no. 12, pp. 1154–1164, 2015.

[83] W. Chun, T. M. Grist, T. J. Kamp, T. F. Warner, and T. F. Christian, "Images in cardiovascular medicine. Infiltrative eosinophilic myocarditis diagnosed and localized by cardiac magnetic resonance imaging," *Circulation*, vol. 110, no. 3, p. e19, 2004.

[84] N. R. Mollet, S. Dymarkowski, W. Volders et al., "Visualization of ventricular thrombi with contrast-enhanced magnetic resonance imaging in patients with ischemic heart disease," *Circulation*, vol. 106, no. 23, pp. 2873–2876, 2002.

[85] C. O'Mahony and P. Elliott, "Anderson-Fabry disease and the heart," *Progress in Cardiovascular Diseases*, vol. 52, no. 4, pp. 326–335, 2010.

[86] U. Ramaswami, C. Whybra, R. Parini et al., "Clinical manifestations of Fabry disease in children: Data from the Fabry Outcome Survey," *Acta Paediatrica*, vol. 95, no. 1, pp. 86–92, 2006.

[87] K. D. MacDermot, A. Holmes, and A. H. Miners, "Anderson-Fabry disease: clinical manifestations and impact of disease in a cohort of 98 hemizygous males," *Journal of Medical Genetics*, vol. 38, no. 11, pp. 750–760, 2001.

[88] K. D. MacDermot, A. Holmes, and A. H. Miners, "Anderson-Fabry disease: clinical manifestations and impact of disease in a cohort of 60 obligate carrier females," *Journal of Medical Genetics*, vol. 38, no. 11, pp. 769–775, 2001.

[89] Y. A. Zarate and R. J. Hopkin, "Fabry's disease," *The Lancet*, vol. 372, no. 9647, pp. 1427–1435, 2008.

[90] A. Linhart and P. M. Elliott, "The heart in Anderson-Fabry disease and other lysosomal storage disorders," *Heart*, vol. 93, no. 4, pp. 528–535, 2007.

[91] W. T. Pochis, J. T. Litzow, B. G. King, and D. Kenny, "Electrophysiologic findings in Fabry's disease with a short PR interval," *American Journal of Cardiology*, vol. 74, no. 2, pp. 203-204, 1994.

[92] M. E. Goldman, R. Cantor, M. F. Schwartz, M. Baker, and R. J. Desnick, "Echocardiographic abnormalities and disease severity in Fabry's disease," *Journal of the American College of Cardiology*, vol. 7, no. 5, pp. 1157–1161, 1986.

[93] A. Linhart, J.-C. Lubanda, T. Palecek et al., "Cardiac manifestations in Fabry disease," *Journal of Inherited Metabolic Disease*, vol. 24, no. 2, pp. 75–83, 2001.

[94] F. Weidemann, F. Breunig, M. Beer et al., "Improvement of cardiac function during enzyme replacement therapy in patients with fabry disease: A prospective strain rate imaging study," *Circulation*, vol. 108, no. 11, pp. 1299–1301, 2003.

[95] F. Weidemann, M. Niemann, F. Breunig et al., "Long-term effects of enzyme replacement therapy on fabry cardiomyopathy. Evidence for a better outcome with early treatment," *Circulation*, vol. 119, no. 4, pp. 524–529, 2009.

[96] T. H. Marwick, "Diabetic cardiomyopathy," in *Cardiology*, M. H. Crawford, J. P. DiMarco, and W. J. Paulus, Eds., pp. 1107–1109, Mosby-Elsevier, Philadelphia, Pa, USA, 3rd edition, 2010.

[97] J. M. Forbes and M. E. Cooper, "Mechanisms of diabetic complications," *Physiological Reviews*, vol. 93, no. 1, pp. 137–188, 2013.

[98] P. M. Seferović and W. J. Paulus, "Clinical diabetic cardiomyopathy: a two-faced disease with restrictive and dilated phenotypes," *European Heart Journal*, vol. 36, no. 27, pp. 1718–1727, 2015.

[99] P. Nihoyannopoulos and D. Dawson, "Restrictive cardiomyopathies," *European Heart Journal - Cardiovascular Imaging*, vol. 10, no. 8, pp. iii23–iii33, 2009.

[100] C. Jaworski, J. A. Mariani, G. Wheeler, and D. M. Kaye, "Cardiac complications of thoracic irradiation," *Journal of the American College of Cardiology*, vol. 61, no. 23, pp. 2319–2328, 2013.

[101] N. K. Taunk, B. G. Haffty, J. B. Kostis, and S. Goyal, "Radiation-induced heart disease: pathologic abnormalities and putative mechanisms," *Frontiers in Oncology*, vol. 5, article 39, 2015.

[102] P. Charron, E. Villard, P. Sébillon et al., "Dano's disease as a cause of hypertrophic cardiomyopathy: A systematic survey," *Heart*, vol. 90, no. 8, pp. 842–846, 2004.

[103] P. M. Elliott, A. Anastasakis, M. A. Borger et al., "2014 ESC Guidelines on diagnosis and management of hypertrophic cardiomyopathy: the Task Force for the Diagnosis and Management of Hypertrophic Cardiomyopathy of the European Society of Cardiology (ESC)," *European Heart Journal*, vol. 35, no. 39, pp. 2733–2779, 2014.

[104] M. Arad, B. J. Maron, J. M. Gorham et al., "Glycogen storage diseases presenting as hypertrophic cardiomyopathy," *The New England Journal of Medicine*, vol. 352, no. 4, pp. 362–372, 2005.

[105] D. Piotrowska-Kownacka, L. Kownacki, M. Kuch et al., "Cardiovascular magnetic resonance findings in a case of Danon disease," *Journal of Cardiovascular Magnetic Resonance*, vol. 11, no. 1, article no. 12, 2009.

[106] A. Dürr, M. Cossee, Y. Agid et al., "Clinical and genetic abnormalities in patients with Friedreich's ataxia," *The New England Journal of Medicine*, vol. 335, no. 16, pp. 1169–1175, 1996.

[107] E. T. Alboliras, C. Shub, M. R. Gomez et al., "Spectrum of cardiac involvement in Friedreich's ataxia: Clinical, electrocardiographic and echocardiographic observations," *American Journal of Cardiology*, vol. 58, no. 6, pp. 518–524, 1986.

23

Diffusion-Weighted Imaging with Color-Coded Images: Towards a Reduction in Reading Time While Keeping a Similar Accuracy

Felipe Campos Kitamura, Srhael de Medeiros Alves, Luis Antônio Tobaru Tibana, and Nitamar Abdala

Departamento de Diagnóstico por Imagem da Escola Paulista de Medicina da UNIFESP, Rua Napoleão de Barros, 800 Vila Clementino, 04024-002 São Paulo, SP, Brazil

Correspondence should be addressed to Felipe Campos Kitamura; kitamura.felipe@gmail.com

Academic Editor: Sotirios Bisdas

The aim of this study was to develop a diagnostic tool capable of providing diffusion and apparent diffusion coefficient (ADC) map information in a single color-coded image and to assess the performance of color-coded images compared with their corresponding diffusion and ADC map. The institutional review board approved this retrospective study, which sequentially enrolled 36 head MRI scans. Diffusion-weighted images (DWI) and ADC maps were compared to their corresponding color-coded images. Four raters had their interobserver agreement measured for both conventional (DWI) and color-coded images. Differences between conventional and color-coded images were also estimated for each of the 4 raters. Cohen's kappa and percent agreement were used. Also, paired-samples t-test was used to compare reading time for rater 1. Conventional and color-coded images had substantial or almost perfect agreement for all raters. Mean reading time of rater 1 was 47.4 seconds for DWI and 27.9 seconds for color-coded images ($P = .00007$). These findings are important because they support the role of color-coded images as being equivalent to that of the conventional DWI in terms of diagnostic capability. Reduction in reading time (which makes the reading easier) is also demonstrated for one rater in this study.

1. Introduction

Nowadays there are many types of diffusion magnetic resonance imaging techniques, ranging from the most common—mapping apparent diffusion coefficient (ADC)—to the most advanced, such as diffusion spectrum imaging and tractography [1].

Diffusion-weighted imaging was first created for brain imaging application, but its use in other anatomical sites has gained wide acceptance due to its undeniable diagnostic contribution [2]. It is well known that signal intensities from corresponding voxels in high "b"-value image and its ADC map may predict tissue diffusion properties [3].

The most common use of these sequences is to analyze diffusion images with high "b"-values and compare them with its corresponding ADC map, side by side. As a general rule, high signal intensities in diffusion (high "b"-value) with low signal in ADC map are related to restricted diffusion, while low signal intensities in diffusion (high "b"-value) with high signal in ADC map are related to facilitated diffusion. Blackout effect is characterized when low signal intensities are seen at the same voxel both in diffusion-weighted images and at the ADC map; on the other hand, T2 shine-through effect happens when high signal is present at the same voxel in diffusion-weighted images and at the ADC map.

Therefore, it is known that a thorough voxelwise analysis of signal intensities in both images, side by side, is necessary to define tissue diffusion properties and aid radiologists in clinical practice. Even though comparing two images side by side does not take too long in the daily clinical practice, the diffusion sequences reading time could be reduced by combining the information of diffusion-weighted images and

ADC map in a single image. Another advantage of combining both information items in a single image is related to the difficulty in analyzing the exact corresponding voxels when reading diffusion-weighted images and ADC map side by side. This is a major problem particularly when examining heterogeneous lesions. Reading a single image can make this task simpler.

The purposes of this study were (I) to develop a diagnostic tool capable of providing diffusion and ADC map information in a single color-coded image and (II) to assess the performance of color-coded images compared to their corresponding diffusion and ADC map.

2. Materials and Methods

2.1. Patients. The study was conducted in a tertiary teaching hospital with 712 beds. The institutional review board approved this retrospective study and waived the need for informed consent. Patients met the inclusion criteria if they were more than 18 years old and had been scanned with 1.5T MRI scanner. Patients were excluded if they lacked diffusion-weighted images with ADC maps or if these images had been made nondiagnostic by artifacts. The hospital's database was used to identify the list of patients who underwent head MRI between August 2015 and September 2015, sequentially enrolled, until sample size was reached.

2.2. Head MRI. All patients were imaged with the institution's protocol for head MRI, which included a diffusion-weighted sequence acquired in the axial plane, with three "b"-values (0, 500, and 1000). Two ADC maps were calculated: one of them was based on $b0$, $b500$, and $b1000$ while the other was based only on $b500$ and $b1000$. The MR scanner used was MAGNETOM Sonata 1.5T (Siemens Healthcare, Erlangen, Germany) with 8-channel head coil; matrix size of 128×128 pixels; FOV: 230×230 mm; slice thickness of 5.0 mm; and gradient strength of 40 mT/m.

2.3. Color-Coded Images. An algorithm was implemented in MATLAB® (MathWorks®, Natick, Massachusetts) to analyze the signal intensities from both diffusion-weighted images and ADC map of a given head MRI scan in order to generate a novel image that assigns a default color for each of the four main possibilities (restriction, facilitation, T2 shine-through, and blackout).

Diffusion sequences and corresponding ADC map were loaded into two three-dimensional matrices with the same size ($128 \times 128 \times 20$), one containing $b1000$ diffusion images (from now on referred to as diffusion) and the other containing the ADC map. Signal intensities of diffusion images were normalized for each axial slice and corrected through plane to account for signal inhomogeneities. In-plane signal inhomogeneities were not sufficiently intense in our images to cause artifacts in the color maps. A more robust correction may be needed to apply this technique to other scanners with different coil sensitivity profiles.

Initially, half-maximum values from normalized diffusion and ADC map in each slice were used as the "zero-effect"

TABLE 1: Voxel classification depending on its ADC and on its normalized $b1000$ signal intensity.

ADC (10^{-5} mm^2/s)	Normalized $b1000$ signal	Effect
≥ 120	≥ 0.6	T2 shine-through
	< 0.6	Facilitated diffusion
< 120	≥ 0.64	Restricted diffusion
	< 0.64	Blackout

point, meaning that there is no restriction, facilitation, T2 shine-through, or blackout.

The following colors were chosen for each situation:

(i) Blue: restricted diffusion.

(ii) Yellow: facilitated diffusion.

(iii) White: blackout.

(iv) Green: T2 shine-through.

These colors were chosen because they yielded good contrast, although any combination of colors could be used.

The Red, Green, and Blue (RGB) color system was used to represent color data, ranging from 0 to 1. In each slice, each voxel is first classified regarding its ADC value Then it is classified regarding its normalized $b1000$ signal intensity. Cut-offs were optimized empirically and became different than the initially mentioned "half-maximum values." See Table 1 for details.

After classification, a color is attributed to each voxel depending on the value of normalized $b1000$ (nDiff) and the normalized ADC (nADC). The formulas were empirically designed taking into account a simple idea:

(i) For restricted diffusion, as the ADC decreases below 120×10^{-5} mm^2/s, the color of the voxel changes from black to blue. This produces a horizontal color gradient in the upper left corner of the color map in Figure 1. The formulas for restricted diffusion are

$$\text{Red} = 0,$$

$$\text{Green} = \frac{(1 - 4\text{nADC})}{2}, \quad (1)$$

$$\text{Blue} = (1 - 4\text{nADC}).$$

(ii) For facilitated diffusion, as the ADC increases above 120×10^{-5} mm^2/s, the color of the voxel changes from dark yellow to light yellow. This produces a horizontal color gradient in the lower right corner of the color map in Figure 1. The formulas for facilitated diffusion are

$$\text{Red} = 1.5\text{nADC},$$

$$\text{Green} = \text{nADC}, \quad (2)$$

$$\text{Blue} = 0.$$

FIGURE 1: Resulting color map for a range of normalized $b1000$ signal intensities and ADC values. Normalized $b1000$ signal intensities range from 0 (lower part) to 1 (upper part). ADC values range from 0 (left) to 300×10^{-5} mm^2/s (right).

(iii) For the T2 shine-through, both ADC and normalized $b1000$ were weighted to generate a color that changes from dark green to light green as the ADC and/or the $b1000$ signal increases. This produces a lower left to upper right diagonal color gradient in the upper right corner of the color map in Figure 1. The formulas for T2 shine-through are

$$Red = 0.5 \, (2nDiff + nADC - 1.2),$$

$$Green = 2.5 \, (2nDiff + nADC - 1.2), \qquad (3)$$

$$Blue = 0.$$

(iv) For the blackout, both ADC and normalized $b1000$ were weighted to generate a color that changes from dark gray to white as the ADC and/or the $b1000$ signal decreases. This produces a lower left to upper right diagonal color gradient in the lower left corner of the color map in Figure 1. The formulas for blackout are

$$Red = 1 - nDiff - nADC,$$

$$Green = 1 - nDiff - nADC, \qquad (4)$$

$$Blue = 1 - nDiff - nADC.$$

The resulting matrix is multidimensional, accounting for 20 slices, 128 × 128 pixels, and 3 colors each (3 × 20 × 128 × 128).

A DICOM file was created for each resulting matrix, to facilitate reading of the resulting images by the radiologists.

Data manipulation, such as windowing the original data, or setting a different "zero-effect" point was necessary prior to the above mentioned algorithm, in order to accomplish better image contrast. Until now, this windowing process is done in a semiautomatic way.

2.4. Measurement of Interrater Agreement and Differences between Conventional and Color-Coded Images.

Conventional and color-coded images were reviewed individually by 2 pairs of raters blinded to clinical data (pair A: raters 1 and 2: radiologists attending a neuroradiology fellowship; pair B: raters 3 and 4: first-year radiology residents). Interrater agreement was evaluated between each combination of raters (total of 6 combinations). Differences between conventional and color-coded images were assessed for each of the 4 raters. To avoid a learning effect, rating was done with conventional images first and a week later with the color-coded images. Scans were categorized into normal or abnormal, regarding the existence of an unexpected effect in a given location. Effect type (restriction, facilitation, blackout, and T2 effect) and location were also assessed to look for false-positive agreements.

2.5. Statistical Analysis.

Cohen's kappa (κ) value and overall percent agreement (OPA) were used to quantify interrater agreement for both conventional and color-coded images. Also, positive percent agreement (PPA) and negative percent agreement (NPA) were used to compare the differences between conventional and color-coded images for all raters [4]. Bonferroni correction was applied to address the multiple comparisons problem. A two-tailed P value less than .05 was considered to be indicating a significant difference (before correction for multiple comparisons). After correcting for multiple comparisons, the cut-off became $P < .0083$. Sample size was estimated to guarantee 90% statistical power [5]. Rater 1 had his reading time computed and compared with paired-samples t-test.

3. Results and Discussion

3.1. Patients.

Fifty-one patients who underwent head MRI between August 2015 and September 2015 were sequentially enrolled. After applying inclusion and exclusion criteria, there were 36 eligible scans, which was the sample size necessary to guarantee 90% statistical power.

3.2. Color-Coded Images.

The algorithm generates a new color-coded image in which, by convention, restriction is shown in blue, facilitation is shown in yellow, T2 shine-through is shown in green, and blackout effect is shown in white.

Examples are given in Figures 2, 3, and 4, demonstrating $b1000$ diffusion image, ADC map, and the resulting color-coded image. In general, ADC maps calculated with $b500$ and $b1000$ (without $b0$) were no different than their respective ADC maps calculated with $b0$, $b500$, and $b1000$, particularly in strokes and in normal scans. This was also true for the corresponding color-coded images. Tumors showed slightly lower ADC values when calculated only with $b500$ and $b1000$, as depicted in Figure 2.

As expected, any factor that deteriorates the diffusion images will also affect the color-coded images. Several factors may contribute to the generation of artifacts in DWI: limitations from the gradient system hardware (gradient amplitude,

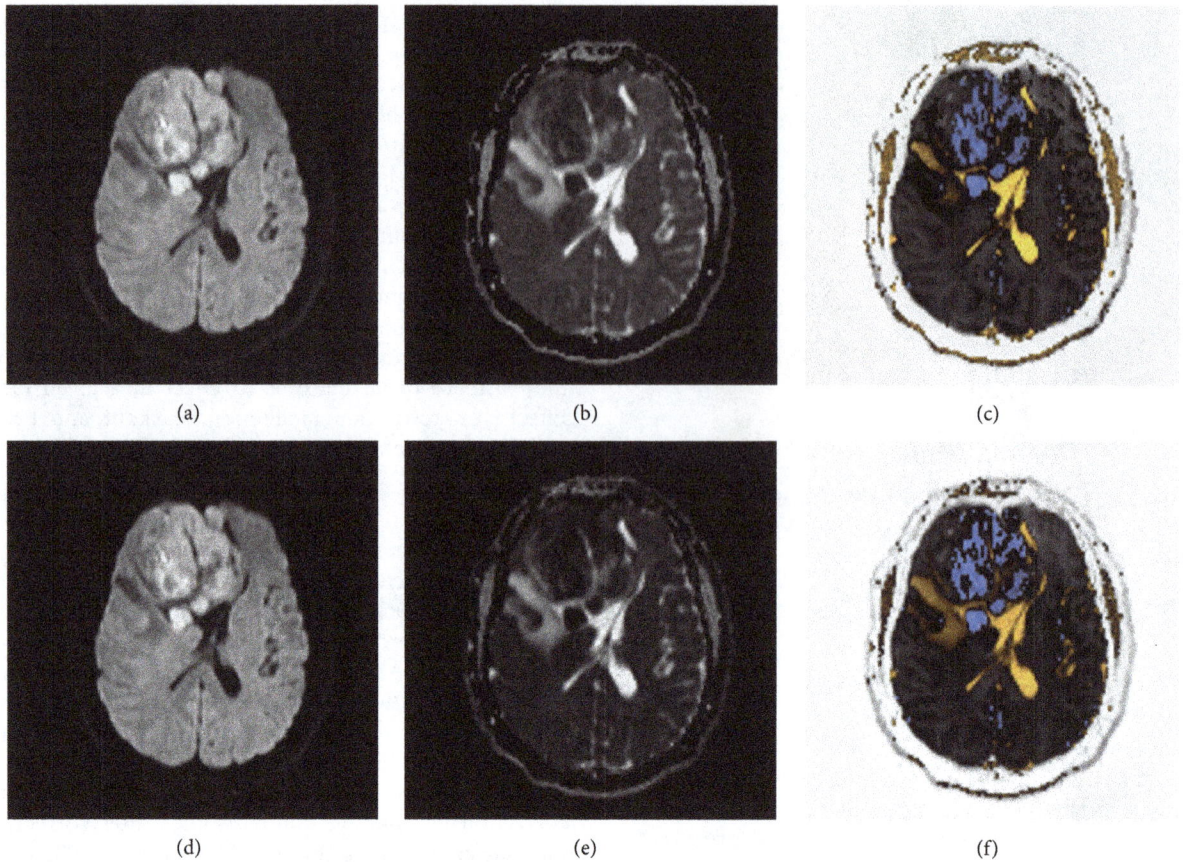

FIGURE 2: From (a) to (c): (a) high "b"-value diffusion (b1000). (b) Corresponding ADC map, calculated with b0, b500, and b1000. (c) Postprocessed image. Note that, for the window chosen, the tumor shows areas with different degrees of restricted diffusion (blue). Also, tumor heterogeneity can be better depicted, since corresponding voxels are matched exactly. Liquor appears as bright yellow. Vasogenic oedema near the tumor appears as dark yellow. From (d) to (f): (d) high "b"-value diffusion (b1000). (e) Corresponding ADC map, calculated with b500 and b1000, without b0. (f) Postprocessed image. All images were shown in the same window.

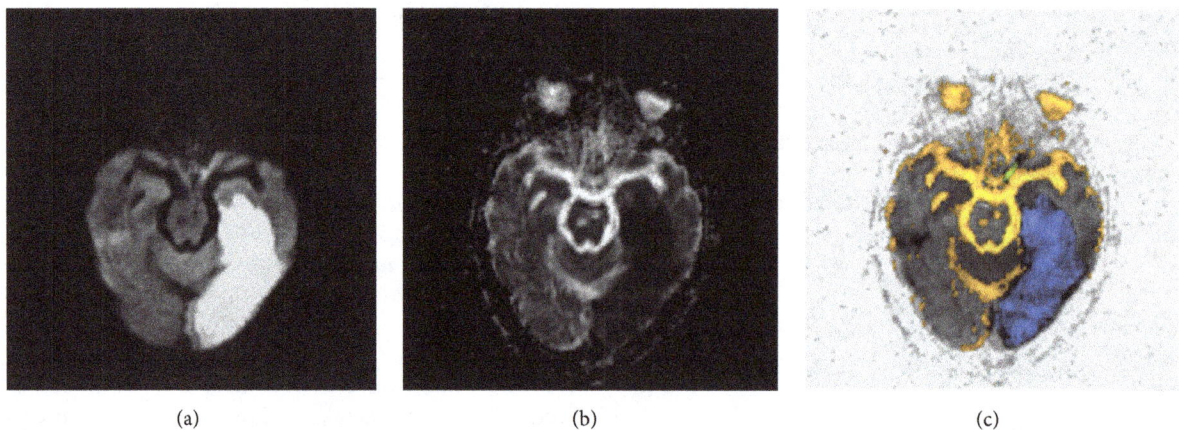

FIGURE 3: (a) High "b"-value diffusion (b1000). (b) Corresponding ADC map. (c) Postprocessed image. This is an acute left posterior cerebral artery stroke (blue). Note chronic lacunar infarcts in the pons (yellow).

slew rate, nonlinearity, and instability) may cause image distortion and widely distributed ghost artifacts; Eddy currents from diffusion sensitizing gradients may cause geometric distortion (contraction, dilation, shift, and shear); Eddy currents from echo-planar imaging (EPI) may cause "N/2" ghost; the low bandwidth of echo-planar imaging (EPI) in the phase-encoding direction may cause significant displacement of fat in this direction, due to chemical-shift; also, the low bandwidth of EPI in the phase-encoding direction causes severe shape distortion in this direction, because, even in

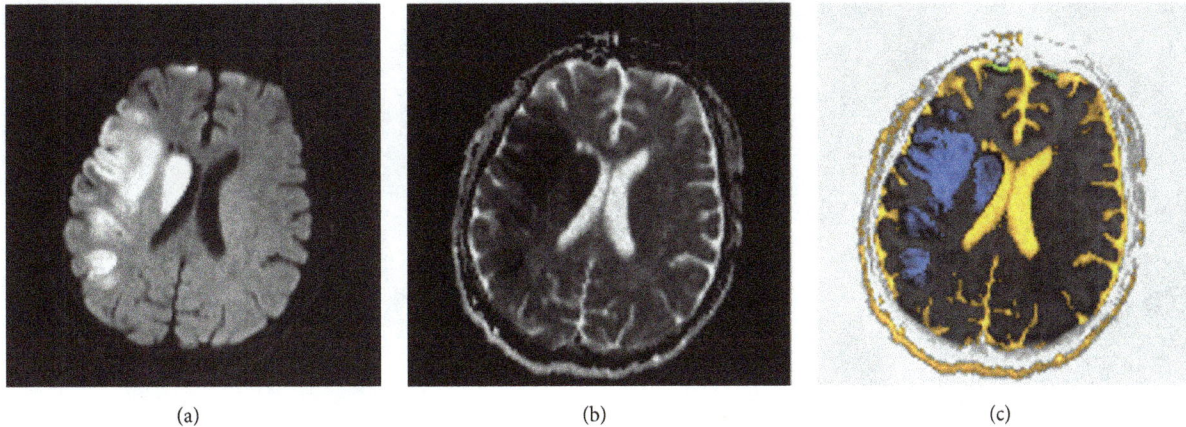

FIGURE 4: (a) High "*b*"-value diffusion (*b*1000). (b) Corresponding ADC map. (c) Postprocessed image. This is an acute right middle cerebral artery stroke (blue).

a well-shimmed magnet, the human head will magnetize unevenly, specially in tissue interfaces with very different magnetic susceptibilities, like bone and air [6].

Considerable progress has been made in the last 30 years to develop high-performance gradient coils available today, capable of providing linear and stable gradients of the utmost intensity (at least 40 mT/m). Adding preemphasis to the gradient shape and using "self-shielded" gradient coils helped to manage Eddy current and its artifacts. The fat misregistration due to chemical-shift can be eliminated in a straightforward manner by applying a fat-saturation pulse prior to imaging. Besides, using lower B_0 field strength (1.5T instead of 3T) can aid in reducing field inhomogeneities. All these techniques were applied to our images. However, spatial misregistering in the phase-encoding direction due to local field inhomogeneities is still difficult to overcome [6]. An example of this last artifact is shown in Figure 5.

3.3. Differences between Conventional and Color-Coded Images

Pair A. For rater 1, conventional and color-coded images had almost perfect agreement (OPA = 91.7%; PPA = 100.0; NPA = 78.6; κ = .818; and P = .000001). For rater 2, conventional and color-coded images had substantial agreement (OPA = 86.1%; PPA = 82.6%; NPA = 92.3%; κ = .713; and P = .000014).

Pair B. For rater 3, conventional and color-coded images had substantial agreement (OPA = 86.1%; PPA = 89.3%; NPA = 75.0%; κ = .615; and P = .000213). For rater 4, conventional and color-coded images had almost perfect agreement (OPA = 91.7%; PPA = 100.0%; NPA = 83.3%; κ = .833; and P < .000001).

After reviewing the 16 cases in which the raters disagreed, a fifth rater considered the color-coded images to be the right ones in 8 of these cases.

There is substantial or almost perfect agreement between the reading of conventional and color-coded images for all

raters. The agreement index (κ) does not seem to correlate with the rater's experience, since the greatest and the lowest κ were found in the least experienced pair of raters (B). These findings are important because they support color-coded images as being equivalent to conventional DWI in terms of diagnostic capability. Reduction in reading time is also demonstrated for one rater in this study, which supports the idea of reading color-coded images being a simpler task when compared to the reading of conventional DWI images.

3.4. Interrater Agreement. In pair A (raters 1 and 2), interrater agreement (κ) was statistically significant with conventional images (OPA = 75.0%; κ = .467; and P = .005) and with color-coded images (OPA = 80.6%; κ = .594; and P = .000198).

In pair B (raters 3 and 4), interrater agreement (κ) was not significant with conventional images (OPA = 66.6%; κ = .333; and P = .016) but significant with color-coded images (OPA = 83.3%; κ = .636; and P = .000042).

For raters 1 and 3, interrater agreement (κ) was significant with conventional images (OPA = 77.7%; κ = .493; and P = .001) and with color-coded images (OPA = 94.4%; κ = .862; and P < .000001).

For raters 1 and 4, inter-rater agreement (κ) was significant with conventional images (OPA = 83.3%; κ = .667; P = .000041) and with color-coded images (OPA = 88.9%; κ = .762; P = .000002).

For raters 2 and 3, interrater agreement (κ) was not significant with conventional images (OPA = 75.0%; κ = .409; and P = .009) but significant with color-coded images (OPA = 75.0%; κ = .471; and P = .002).

For raters 2 and 4, interrater agreement (κ) was significant with conventional images (OPA = 75.0%; κ = .500; and P = .002) and with color-coded images (OPA = 86.1%; κ = .717; and P = .000016).

Interrater agreement is significant for all the 6 pairs of raters when analyzing color-coded images, but not when analyzing conventional images, as seen between rater 3 and raters 2 and 4. Also, interrater agreement index (κ) was higher for color-coded images than for conventional DWI for all the

(a)   (b)   (c)

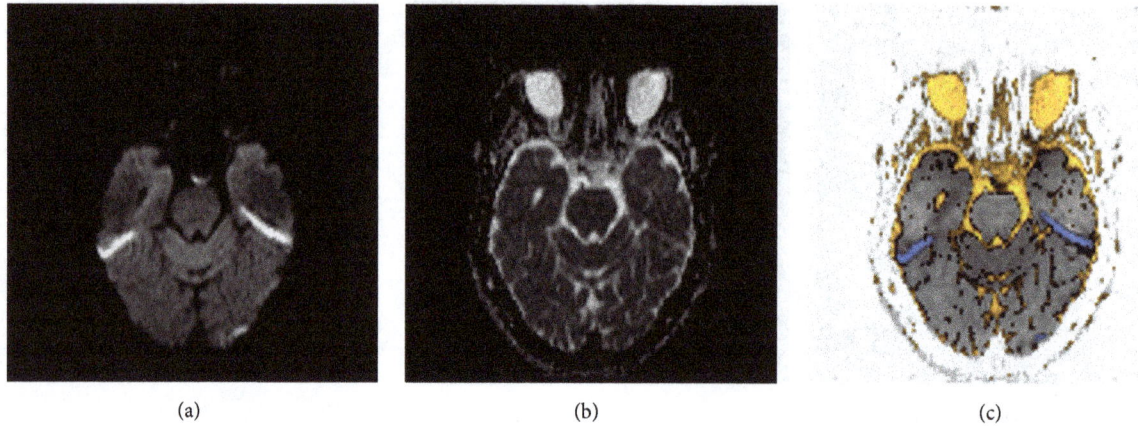

FIGURE 5: (a) High "b"-value diffusion (b1000). (b) Corresponding ADC map. (c) Postprocessed image. This is an example of spatial misregistering due to susceptibility artifacts induced by the temporal bones.

6 pairs of raters. These findings support the hypothesis that color-coded images would be more reproducible than conventional DWI, especially for less experienced radiologists.

Mean reading time of rater 1 was 47.4 seconds for conventional DWI and 27.9 seconds for color-coded images ($P = .00007$).

Another important aspect of this work is the potential to avoid misinterpretation, either by inattention or by those who are not used to reading conventional DWI, as was observed with the 8 cases in which color-coded images were deemed as correct.

Previous authors have demonstrated that using color-coded images increased interrater agreement of FLAIR images and the correlation between time from stroke onset and FLAIR signal. It also yielded higher specificity and positive predictive value for the identification of patients with ischemic stroke within 4.5 h of symptoms onset [7], thus, providing evidence that color-coding images may improve the accuracy of radiologists in reading magnetic resonance scans.

However, the authors in that study applied a different approach for the color-coding FLAIR images method: they applied a color map to a single sequence, which only adds subjective effects in the reading process. The information contained in that color-coded image is essentially the same as that of the conventional one. Our method is different because it combines two source images (high "b"-value DWI and ADC map) to assemble a new one, providing an image with higher information content.

Our study had some limitations. First, one of the raters had already seen three cases among our sample, making it more susceptible to remember clinical and/or image details of the cases, which would make it easier to detect abnormalities in that study. Second, all scans were acquired with only one MRI scanner, which limits extrapolation to scanners from other companies. Third, reading time was assessed only for one observer, limiting conclusions about time reduction.

Our paper, while important, demonstrates the need for additional, multiple reader and, ideally, "perfect-referenced" study.

4. Conclusion

Interpretation of color-coded images seems to be equivalent to or even better than the interpretation of conventional DWI/ADC in terms of reading time and reproducibility.

Competing Interests

The authors declare that there is no conflict of interests regarding the publication of this paper.

Acknowledgments

The authors thank the raters of this study: Dr. Anna Carolina Mendonça de Andrade, Dr. Igor Rodrigues Ramos, and Dr. Stenio Burlin.

References

[1] P. Hagmann, L. Jonasson, P. Maeder, J.-P. Thiran, J. V. Wedeen, and R. Meuli, "Understanding diffusion MR imaging techniques: from scalar diffusion-weighted imaging to diffusion tensor imaging and beyond," *RadioGraphics*, vol. 26, pp. S205–S223, 2006.

[2] P. D. Schellinger, R. N. Bryan, L. R. Caplan et al., "Evidence-based guideline: the role of diffusion and perfusion MRI for the diagnosis of acute ischemic stroke: report of the therapeutics and technology assessment subcommittee of the American Academy of Neurology," *Neurology*, vol. 75, no. 2, pp. 177–185, 2010.

[3] E. O. Stejskal and J. E. Tanner, "Spin diffusion measurements: spin echoes in the presence of a time–dependent field gradient," *The Journal of Chemical Physics*, vol. 42, no. 1, pp. 288–292, 1965.

[4] K. Meier, *Statistical Guidance on Reporting Results from Studies Evaluating Diagnostic Tests*, Guid Ind FDA Staff, 2007, http://www.fda.gov/downloads/medicaldevices/deviceregulationandguidance/guidancedocuments/ucm071287.pdf&sa=U&ved=0ahUKEwilx-TymbbLAhUWBI4KHcClAsYQFggLMAA&usg=AFQjCNG5rSipAzYItThLtlqbvLBfu1oSBg.

[5] H. Hong, Y. Choi, S. Hahn, S. K. Park, and B.-J. Park, "Nomogram for sample size calculation on a straightforward basis for

the kappa statistic," *Annals of Epidemiology*, vol. 24, no. 9, pp. 673–680, 2014.

[6] D. Le Bihan, C. Poupon, A. Amadon, and F. Lethimonnier, "Artifacts and pitfalls in diffusion MRI," *Journal of Magnetic Resonance Imaging*, vol. 24, no. 3, pp. 478–488, 2006.

[7] B. J. Kim, Y.-H. Kim, Y.-J. Kim et al., "Color-coded fluid-attenuated inversion recovery images improve inter-rater reliability of fluid-attenuated inversion recovery signal changes within acute diffusion-weighted image lesions," *Stroke*, vol. 45, no. 9, pp. 2801–2804, 2014.

24

Determination of Epiphyseal Union Age in the Knee and Hand Joints Bones among the Saudi Population in Taif City

Majed O. Aljuaid ⓘ and Osama R. El-Ghamry

Medical College, Taif University, Taif 21974, Saudi Arabia

Correspondence should be addressed to Majed O. Aljuaid; majedoaljuaid@hotmail.com

Academic Editor: Paul Sijens

Introduction. The use of radiographic data for determination of age, according to the epiphyseal union stage, is a widely accepted method and considered scientifically approved. The aim of the present work is to estimate the age of epiphyseal union of hand and knee joints bones among Saudi population in Taif City. *Subjects and Method.* A retrospective cross-sectional study was conducted in the Armed Forces Hospitals (4 hospitals) in Taif City. The five-stage method was used for the union assessment. *Results.* A total of 473 patients' X-ray images were involved. Approximately three-quarters of the knee and hand images were males' images (77.25% and 75.41%, resp.). The means of age of stage 3 (age of recent union) in the knee joint were 23.63 ± 3.12 and 21.19 ± 3.41 in males and females, respectively, and 19.84 ± 3.47 and 17.19 ± 1.61 in hand joints for males and females, respectively. There were significant differences between males and females in the means of age for stages 1, 3, and 4 at the knee joint plates and for stages 0, 2, and 3 in the hand joint plates (P values were <0.05). However, by comparing the mean of age for each stage with the previous stage mean in males and females, there was a significant difference between stages 0–4 (P values ≤ 0.0001, ≤ 0.001, <0.0001, and <0.001, resp.) and stages 2 and 3 (P value $= 0.012$) in knee joint images for males and females, respectively. In addition, there were significant differences between stages 2–4 in hand joints for males and females (P values ≤ 0.0001, <0.0001, <0.0001, and <0.0001, resp.) and stages 0 and 1 for males only (P value $= 0.002$). *Conclusion and Recommendation.* This study suggests that the union of epiphyses of knees and hands in Taif City occurs later than other places. More studies must be done with female samples.

1. Introduction

Determination of human chronological age was extensively investigated by biological anthropologists, archeologists, and anatomists from many perspectives, one of which was the epiphyseal union and its relationship to chronological age [1–3]. This approach used the archeological (autopsied) skeletal collection [2, 4, 5], although radiographic data was used instead, as it is easier to obtain a greater number of images in each phase (of early ages) of the study's population; the epiphyseal union stages are confined to this era of human life [1, 6]. The use of radiographic data for determination of age according to epiphyseal union stage is considered to be scientifically approved [7–9]. The study group on forensic age diagnostics recommended a physical examination, X-ray of the left hand, and a dental examination to determine the age of young people (before epiphyseal union) [10, 11].

The age at each stage of an epiphyseal union is a parameter known to be multifactorial [3, 4, 7, 12–17], which will consequently affect the process of the union at the epiphyses. The differences in geographical distribution, socioeconomic status, climate, metabolism, nutrition, and genetics (race) comprise some of these factors. Also, ethnicity is one of the main reasons for this kind of study with a neglected population in this field [3, 4, 7, 12–17]. The application for this project in a clinical situation, a forensic investigation, and medicolegal aspects has a number of dimensions. In the forensic investigation, we are determining chronological age accurately in cases of young, unknown corpses. Clinically, medical consultation in cases of incorrect dating of birth or absent date of birth in young refugees is necessary [6, 8, 18–20]. On the other hand, it also determines chronological age for judicial responsibility of young people who commit a crime, but do not have an identity. Establishment of accurate linkage between biological and chronological age is used in practical situations mentioned above. The epiphyses are the growth plates for the long bones. The aim of this study was to determine the age of the epiphyseal union in the knee and hand joints of the Saudi population with X-ray images, including males and females. Thus, the primary outcome of this study will identify the ages of different epiphyseal union stages in males and females. The secondary outcome will be the difference between male and female samples of different epiphyseal union stages. This study will concentrate on two areas of the body: the knee and hand. Selecting these areas include a high number of images, largely due to trauma, as young people are more prone to engage in dangerous activities. In this study, the revised method for assessment of the union of the epiphysis was used [1, 17]. This method was first outlined by McKern et al. in 1957, who divided the epiphyseal union into five stages: nonunion, beginning of union, active union, recent union, and complete union [1, 17]. McKern et al. worked on osseous specimens of the knee joint, first applied via knee radiographic image assessment by O'Connor and colleagues [1]. This method was also applied on hand joint radiographic image assessments by Bhise et al. [17].

2. Methods

The current study is retrospective and cross-sectional, including all patients who have X-ray images over the last 6 years (between the end of July 2010 and July 2016) in the Armed Forces Hospitals (4 hospitals) in Taif City; this fulfilled inclusion criteria and was kept separate from exclusion criteria. Inclusion criteria included images of Saudi patients, between 4 and 30 for females and 6 and 32 for males, who lived in Taif since birth; they must also verify their date of birth and have X-rays with available reports and radiographic images at the Armed Forces Hospitals. Exclusion criteria were fracture of the epiphysis, congenital anomaly of the bones, and/or bone disease. Data was collected from patients' electronic health records onto an Excel sheet with a hospital computer, thereby maintaining any nominative information: patients were identified by a serial study code and initials. These were linked to patients' names and medical record numbers (MRNs) on a separate identification log sheet, kept in a locked location. After verification, data were transferred to the statistical database with SPSS (Statistical Package for the Social Sciences) program v. 20. The X-ray reports for these patients were examined to separate them from exclusion criteria. Patient files were examined in both the presence of exclusion criteria and in the presence of a defective report, or else the case was excluded. Those patients were statistically investigated. The IRB (Institutional Review Board) for both hospitals and the University Ethical Committees approved the waiver of the informed consent, as this was a retrospective study.

2.1. The Method of Assessment of the Epiphyseal Union. In the assessment of radiographic images of the knee and hand joints, the revised method for epiphyseal union assessment was used [1, 17]. The bones of the knee joint that had been included were the lower part of the femur and the upper part

of the tibia and fibula. The bones of the hand joints that had been included were the metacarpals and phalanges without the distal ulna, radius, or carpals. If there were different stages in the same radiographic image, we considered the last one. This approach was used to obtain the age of union for the joint bones as a whole without segregation.

In stage 0, a radiolucent area was observed between the epiphysis and the diaphysis (Figure 1). In stage 1, there is a continuous radiolucent gap between the epiphysis and diaphysis, which is separable at the extremes (Figure 1). In stage 2, a radio-opaque thick line was observed between the epiphysis and diaphysis (Figure 2). In stage 3, a continuous radiopaque thin line was observed, called the union scar (Figure 2). In stage 4, the union scar disappeared and both the epiphysis and diaphysis appeared fused as one bone (Figure 2). Similarly, stages 0–4 on hand plates were assessed in the same manner (Figures 3 and 4). Moreover, X-rays showed more advanced results in the active union stage compared to the macroscopic results; this showed less advanced results in the complete union stage [2].

After deleting the patient data on the images, hand and the knee joints were assessed. Training for this method was done by our mentor (Professor Osama Elghamri).

2.2. Statistical Analysis. All continuous variables were expressed as mean ± SD. Categorical variables were compared with the X^2 test and t-test for comparing means of continuous variables. A P value must be less than 0.05 to be considered significant, except for the correlation coefficient (spearman's rho) and linear regression in which the P value must be less than 0.01 to be considered significant. Linear regression was used to detect the best fitting line between the stages of epiphyseal union and the exact age of cases. This method will analyze the predictability of the relationship between the two variables (age and stage). Also, linear regression was used to calculate the regression equation to predict the age of a case with the stage number of involved cases.

3. Results

A total of 473 patients' X-ray images ($N = 473$) was involved in this retrospective cross-sectional study. Approximately half of this sample involved knee joint images ($n1 = 233$) while the other half was hand images ($n2 = 240$). Approximately three-quarters of the knee images and hand images were male images (77.25% and 75.41%, resp.). The number of the knee and hand images for each age stage interval of the epiphyseal union in each gender is shown in Tables 1 and 2. Patients' ages ranged from 4 to 32 years, with a different means of age in each stage, as shown in Table 3. The epiphyseal union in the knee joint was first recorded (stage 1: beginning of union) at age 13 in the female group and at age 15 in the male group (Figure 5). However, the means of the age in stage 1 were 16.77±1.24 and 14.51±0.87 in males and females, respectively. On the other hand, the hand joints had started the epiphyseal union at age 12 in the male group. Nevertheless, at age 12 in the female group, there was an active union case, indicating that the beginning of the union of hand joints in the female group was younger than the male group (Figure 6). Recent

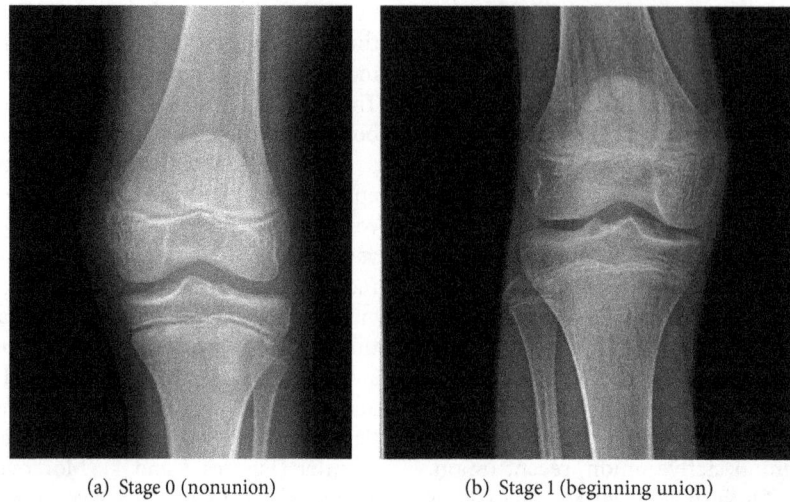

(a) Stage 0 (nonunion)

(b) Stage 1 (beginning union)

FIGURE 1: Radiographic images of knee joint showing stage 0 labeled as (a) and stage 1 labeled as (b).

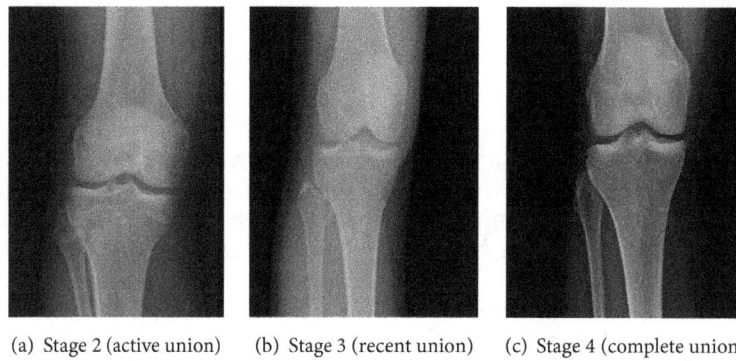

(a) Stage 2 (active union) (b) Stage 3 (recent union) (c) Stage 4 (complete union)

FIGURE 2: Radiographic images of knee joint showing stage 2 labeled as (a) and stage 3 labeled as (b) and stage 4 labeled as (c).

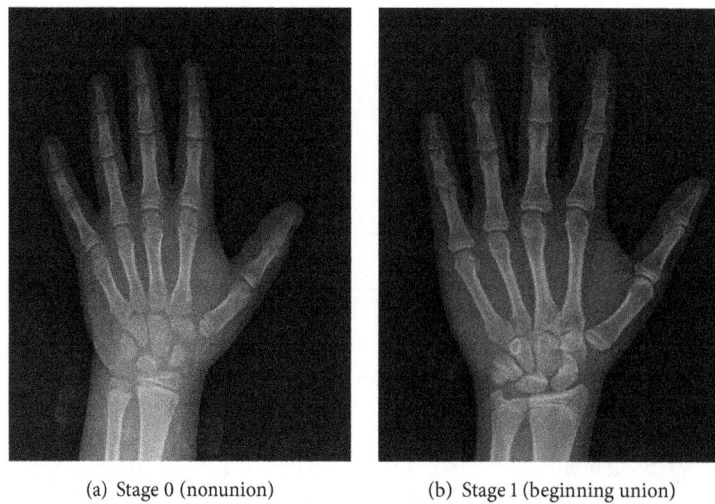

(a) Stage 0 (nonunion)

(b) Stage 1 (beginning union)

FIGURE 3: Radiographic images of hand joints showing stage 0 labeled as (a) and stage 1 labeled as (b).

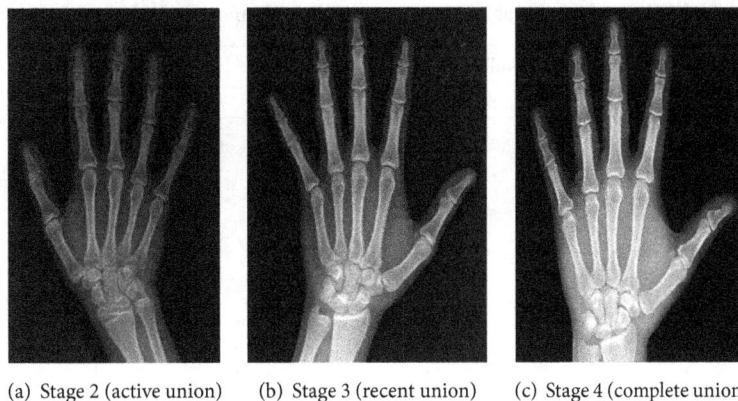

(a) Stage 2 (active union)   (b) Stage 3 (recent union)   (c) Stage 4 (complete union)

FIGURE 4: Radiographic images of hand joints showing stage 2 labeled as (a) and stage 3 labeled as (b) and stage 4 labeled as (c).

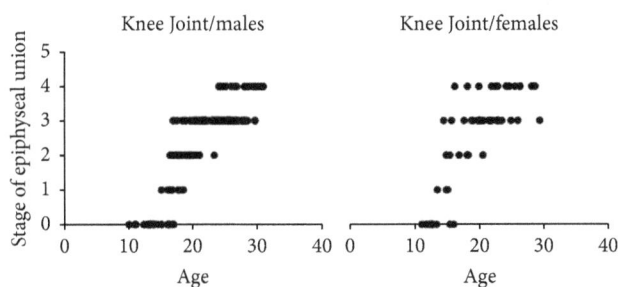

FIGURE 5: The graphical presentation of our sample range of age in the different epiphyseal union stages in knee joint.

completion of epiphyseal union (stage 3) at the knee joint was noted at age 14 in the female group and at age 16 in the male group (Figure 5). United epiphyses of the hand joints were observed at the age of 16 years in the male group and 15 years in the female group (Figure 6). Stage 3 means of age in the knee joint included 23.63 ± 3.12 and 21.19 ± 3.41 in males and females, respectively; in hand joints, it was 19.84 ± 3.47 and 17.19 ± 1.61 in males and females, respectively. Correlation coefficients (spearman's rho) were 0.851 and 0.887 for knee and hand joints, respectively, in males (P value ≤ 0.0001) and 0.752 and 0.901 in females (P value ≤ 0.0001), and the best fit line for the correlation between age and the epiphyseal union of knee and hand joints is depicted in Figures 7 and 8, respectively. There were significant differences between males and females in the means of age for stages 1, 3, and 4 at knee joint plates and for stages 0, 2, and 3 at hand joint plates (P values shown in Table 3). However, by comparing the means of age for each stage with the previous stage means in males and females, there was a significant difference between stages 0 and 4 (P values ≤ 0.0001, 0.001, <0.0001, and <0.0001, resp.) in a male group of knee joint images. Significant differences between the means of age stages 2 and 3 in the female group of knee joint images were observed (P value = 0.012). In addition, there were significant differences between stages 2 and 4 in hand joints for males and females (P values ≤ 0.0001, <0.0001, <0.000, and <0.0001, resp.). Similarly, male group images of the hand joints showed significant differences between stages 0 and 1 (P value = 0.002). Otherwise, there

was no significant difference found by comparing means of age of each stage with the previous one. A regression formula was calculated, as shown in Table 4.

4. Discussion

In the literature, there were many studies conducted on different parts of the body using various methods and modalities. Also, there were a few studies that used the radiological approach compared to that used for bone remains [1, 3, 6–20]. These studies were done on different populations in race, ethnicity, or residency, which had an influential but comparative effect on the epiphyseal union and on the results [8, 12]. The variation in the ages of epiphyseal union stages between different ethnic groups was the main purpose for previous studies, which ended up demonstrating that there is indeed variation between different ethnic groups [3, 4, 7, 12–17]. The socioeconomic status was one of the factors that influenced the epiphyseal union process [21]. The same author suggested that previous factors do not actually affect this process [21].

However, by reviewing previous study results regarding age of union, we found a wide range [14–23] for knee joint plate unions [11–18] and for hand joint plate unions [1, 9, 15–18, 20–23]. Some previous studies are summarized in Table 5. This variation mandates a wider range of ages in the samples selection process. We will conduct a 7-year margin for the lowest and oldest ages to accurately determine the initiation of union at the completion of the recent union stage. During analysis of results, we extended the latter margin by 2 years (with a year by year approach) to determine the end of stage 3. As a result of this change, the range of sample ages was 4–32 years. This range was used according to the available data in different groups and different areas.

Determination of the union age for each epiphyseal plate was done in previous studies, revealing that the knee and hand joint plates showed the same union stage [1, 17]. Other studies showed that different plates were in different stages; based on this study, there is variation of union age for different plates [1, 7, 8]. This study dealt with plates in hand and knee joints as a whole, without segregation. The relationships between the chronological age of the patient at the time of radiological examination and the stages in males and females

TABLE 1: Numbers of images at each stage of epiphyseal union of the knee joint bones.

Age interval	n	Staging of knee epiphyses (males)					n	Staging of knee epiphyses (females)				
		0	1	2	3	4		0	1	2	3	4
4–4.99	-	-	-	-	-	-	-	-	-	-	-	-
5–5.99	-	-	-	-	-	-	-	-	-	-	-	-
6–6.99	-	-	-	-	-	-	-	-	-	-	-	-
7–7.99	-	-	-	-	-	-	-	-	-	-	-	-
8–8.99	-	-	-	-	-	-	-	-	-	-	-	-
9–9.99	-	-	-	-	-	-	-	-	-	-	-	-
10–10.99	2	2	-	-	-	-	-	-	-	-	-	-
11–11.99	1	1	-	-	-	-	2	2	-	-	-	-
12–12.99	7	7	-	-	-	-	4	4	-	-	-	-
13–13.99	8	8	-	-	-	-	2	1	1	-	-	-
14–14.99	4	4	-	-	-	-	3	-	1	1	1	-
15–15.99	3	2	1	-	-	-	4	1	1	1	1	-
16–16.99	12	5	4	2	1	-	3	1	-	1	-	1
17–17.99	11	1	1	7	2	-	1	-	-	-	1	-
18–18.99	12	-	2	5	5	-	5	-	-	2	1	2
19–19.99	11	-	-	9	2	-	4	-	-	-	3	1
20–20.99	14	-	-	3	11	-	4	-	-	1	3	-
21–21.99	15	-	-	1	14	-	4	-	-	-	3	1
22–22.99	4	-	-	-	4	-	4	-	-	-	2	2
23–23.99	10	-	-	1	9	-	2	-	-	-	2	-
24–24.99	13	-	-	-	10	3	3	-	-	-	1	2
25–25.99	12	-	-	-	11	1	2	-	-	-	1	1
26–26.99	14	-	-	-	11	3	2	-	-	-	-	2
27–27.99	6	-	-	-	6	-	-	-	-	-	-	-
28–28.99	13	-	-	-	7	6	3	-	-	-	-	3
29–29.99	4	-	-	-	2	2	1	-	-	-	1	-
30–30.99	3	-	-	-	-	3	-	-	-	-	-	-
31–31.99	1	-	-	-	-	1	-	-	-	-	-	-
Sum	180	30	8	28	95	19	53	9	3	6	20	15

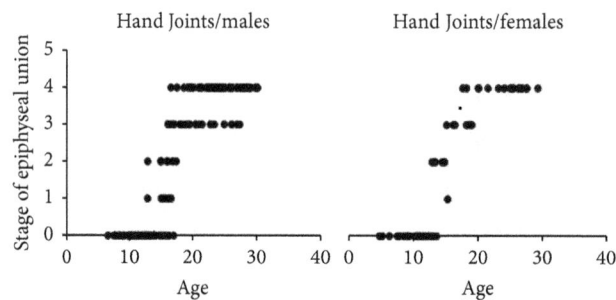

FIGURE 6: The graphical presentation of our sample range of age in the different epiphyseal union stages in hand joints.

were used to determine the most accurate method of union age. This study showed a stronger correlation in the hand joint bones for males and females, compared to knee joint bones. However, a stronger relationship indicates a more accurate method to determine union age; bilateral asymmetry could not be examined in this study due to scarcity of radiographic images depicting both limbs. The right and left discrepancy in the epiphyseal union was not observed in a previous study using the same staging method. However, this could not be examined in the present study.

There were different methods used in previous studies to determine union age. One of these methods considered the

TABLE 2: Numbers of images at each stage of epiphyseal union of the hand joints bones.

Age interval	n	Staging of hand epiphyses (males)					n	Staging of hand epiphyses (females)				
		0	1	2	3	4		0	1	2	3	4
4–4.99	-	-	-	-	-	-	1	1	-	-	-	-
5–5.99	-	-	-	-	-	-	1	1	-	-	-	-
6–6.99	1	1	-	-	-	-	-	-	-	-	-	-
7–7.99	3	3	-	-	-	-	2	2	-	-	-	-
8–8.99	5	5	-	-	-	-	2	2	-	-	-	-
9–9.99	4	4	-	-	-	-	3	3	-	-	-	-
10–10.99	12	12	-	-	-	-	10	10	-	-	-	-
11–11.99	6	6	-	-	-	-	5	5	-	-	-	-
12–12.99	14	12	1	1	-	-	7	6	-	1	-	-
13–13.99	13	13	-	-	-	-	3	1	-	2	-	-
14–14.99	8	5	1	2	-	-	2	-	-	2	-	-
15–15.99	6	3	2	1	-	-	2	-	1	-	1	-
16–16.99	12	2	2	2	6	-	2	-	-	-	2	-
17–17.99	7	2	-	1	2	2	1	-	-	-	-	1
18–18.99	5	-	-	-	4	1	4	-	-	-	3	1
19–19.99	7	-	-	-	4	3	1	-	-	-	-	1
20–20.99	3	-	-	-	2	1	1	-	-	-	-	1
21–21.99	9	-	-	-	2	7	1	-	-	-	-	1
22–22.99	8	-	-	-	1	7	-	-	-	-	-	-
23–23.99	8	-	-	-	-	8	2	-	-	-	-	2
24–24.99	9	-	-	-	-	9	1	-	-	-	-	1
25–25.99	10	-	-	-	1	9	2	-	-	-	-	2
26–26.99	6	-	-	-	1	5	3	-	-	-	-	3
27–27.99	8	-	-	-	2	6	2	-	-	-	-	2
28–28.99	10	-	-	-	-	10	-	-	-	-	-	-
29–29.99	5	-	-	-	-	5	1	-	-	-	-	1
30–30.99	2	-	-	-	-	2	-	-	-	-	-	-
31–31.99	-	-	-	-	-	-	-	-	-	-	-	-
Sum	181	68	6	7	25	75	59	31	1	5	6	16

TABLE 3: Mean, standard deviation (SD), range of age (years), and significance of difference between males' and females' ages at each stage of epiphyseal union of the knee joint and hand joints bones.

Site	Stage	Males					Females					Sig.
		n	Min	Max	Mean	SD	n	Min	Max	Mean	SD	
Knee	0	30	10.04	17.01	13.7542	1.72372	9	11.09	16.04	13.0457	1.67232	0.240
	1	8	15.08	18.54	16.7736*	1.24244	3	13.51	15.13	14.5105	.87442	0.012**
	2	28	16.42	23.38	18.8349*	1.49106	6	14.87	20.55	17.3662	2.07975	0.062
	3	95	16.89	29.65	23.6318*	3.12421	20	14.51	29.38	21.1886*	3.40694	0.003**
	4	19	24.13	31.02	27.8489*	2.26147	15	16.23	28.67	23.4716	3.96549	0.001**
Hand	0	68	6.65	17.01	12.0113	2.35966	31	4.67	13.50	10.3398	2.09470	<0.001**
	1	6	12.78	16.61	15.2434*	1.35211	1	-	-	-	-	0.969
	2	7	12.81	17.43	15.6543	1.63450	5	12.77	14.72	13.6455	.83013	0.031**
	3	25	14.85	27.42	19.8365*	3.47392	6	15.01	18.96	17.1913*	1.61258	0.038**
	4	75	16.53	30.18	24.6715*	3.22954	16	17.50	29.21	23.9502*	3.56247	0.395

* indicates that the mean of the marked stage is significantly (P value < 0.05) different from the mean of the previous stage; ** indicate that the male group mean of the marked stage is significantly (P value < 0.05) different from the mean of the female group of the same stage.

TABLE 4: Regression formulae for male and female groups in knee and hand joints.

Epiphyseal union	Regression formula in males	Sig.	Regression formula in females	Sig.
Knee joint	13.203 + 3.463* the least stage	**<0.001***	12.726 + 2.715* the least stage	**<0.001***
Hand joints	11.792 + 3.128* the least stage	**<0.001***	10.042 + 3.202* the least stage	**<0.001***

* indicates that the P value was <0.05.

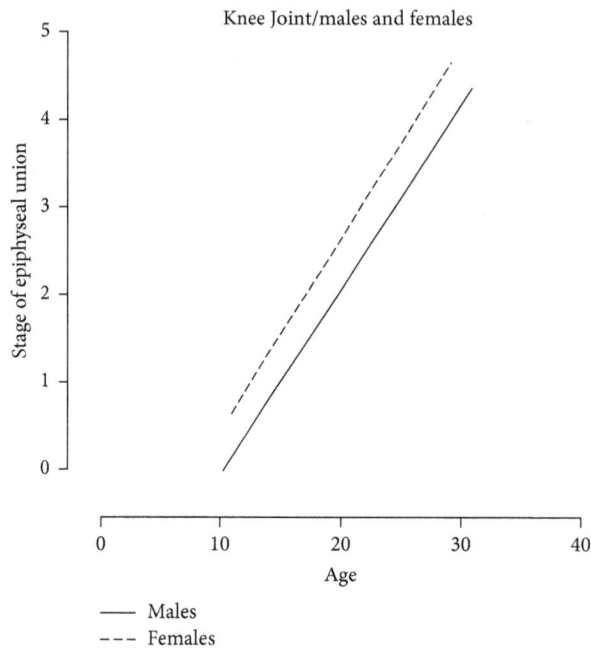

FIGURE 7: The graphical presentation of correlation best fit line between the age and stages of epiphyseal union in knee joint.

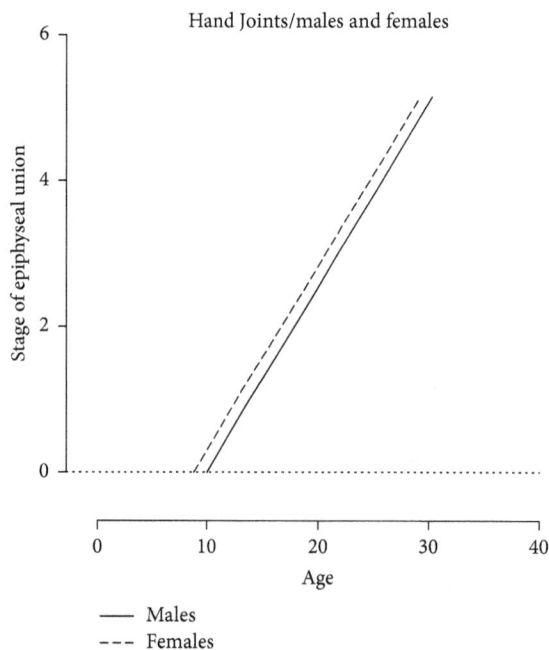

FIGURE 8: The graphical presentation of correlation best fit line between the age and stages of epiphyseal union in hand joints.

TABLE 5: Some of the previous studies that were done at the knee and hand regions.

Author	Year	Population	Number of sample	Number of stages	Knee joint	Hand joints
Washburn [22]*	1958	US	450	5	Males: 22-23	----------
Garn et al. [21]	1961	US	107	3	----------	Males: 15.9–16.4 Females: 13.6–14.6
Schaefer and Black [23]*	2005	Bosnian	114	5	Males: 17–20	----------
O'Connor et al. [1]	2008	Irish	234	5	Males: 17–18.9 Females: 17–17.9	----------
Bhise et al. [17]	2011	Indian	299	5	----------	Males: 16–18 Females: 15–17

* indicates the use of bone remains instead of imaging studies; the studies were chronologically ordered.

age at which more than 50% of the group was completely fused [24]. However, other methods used 85% and 100% as cut-off points [25, 26]. These studies examined different staging methods from those used in this study. Thus, stages 3 and 4 were considered to be united plates (stage 3 in the old classification). Accordingly, applying any approach of the previously mentioned studies must include both stages as one pool. The first method was used in this study to minimize falsified results that could create unequal distribution of images and absence of them at certain ranges. The ages of union were 24 and 21 for knee joints (males and females, resp.), while hand joints were united at 23 and 21 for males and females, respectively. Our findings fell in the range of the previous studies, using the same staging method [1, 17]. In this study, the nonunion of epiphyses was observed at 17 and 16 in knee joints for males and females, respectively, although it was 17 and 13 in hand joints for males and females. These findings are not surprising, compared to documented cases in previous studies, as they revealed older cases with nonunion as well [1].

Age means of males and females in each stage of knee and hand joint bones were statistically examined and regression formulae were calculated to predict age based on images that could be used in many fields (previously mentioned). The insignificant differences were seen between males and females in stages 0 and 2 in the knee joint and stage 2 and 4 in hand joints. These findings could be justified by the discrepancy between the two groups, regarding sample sizes in those stages in this retrospective study, which is limited to available images. However, the gender difference found in the other stages was expected and it confirmed what was revealed in other studies [1]. The males display delayed epiphyseal union compared to females in knee and hand joints. The means of differences between them were 2.25 and 1.5 in hand and knee joint bones [1]. These findings were linear to what other studies had found: 1.5 in the knee joint in one study and 2 in same joint in another. In addition, the means of age in each stage was significantly different from the means of the previous stages in males and females, except in stages 0 and 1 and stages 1 and 2 in hand and knee joints among females. Also, stages 3 and 4 in the knee joint among females and stages 1 and 2 in the hand joint among males were insignificantly different. These findings are justified by the discrepancy of sample numbers at compared stages (Table 3). The

same condition was discussed in a previous study, using the same staging method and reviewing the study's sample numbers at each stage: it was the same statistical issue [1].

In the process of determination of sample age, we faced some difficulties that could be seen from three perspectives. First was the absence in the previous study of the same environments or even nearby areas, such as gulf countries. Second, the presence of extensive data was widely disparate regarding the age of union. Third, previous studies' methods and sample types (osseous versus radiological) were widely varied.

5. Conclusion and Recommendations

This study suggests that the union of epiphyses of knee and hand in the Saudi population in Taif City occurs later than in other locations. The application of this project in estimating age could be used by many fields, being the ultimate goal the authors have in our own society. It is expected to come across some difficulties in the first time, which will be resolved with more investigations. Future projects in other cities and environments in the same country are being recommended to find a valid formula. We also suggest a greater number of studies with more female samples.

Disclosure

This work preliminary results were presented in the 6th International Academic and Research Conference that was held at the University of Manchester, United Kingdom (2016), as an oral presentation.

Acknowledgments

The authors would like to thank the staff of radiology departments in the Armed Forces Hospitals of Taif city for their cooperation and assistance. Also, they acknowledge

Adbulmajed G. Alharbi and Abdulrhman D. Alsofyani's assistance during this work.

References

[1] J. E. O'Connor, C. Bogue, L. D. Spence, and J. Last, "A method to establish the relationship between chronological age and stage of union from radiographic assessment of epiphyseal fusion at the knee: An Irish population study," *Journal of Anatomy*, vol. 212, no. 2, pp. 198–209, 2008.

[2] H. F. V. Cardoso and R. S. S. Severino, "The chronology of epiphyseal union in the hand and foot from dry bone observations," *International Journal of Osteoarchaeology*, vol. 20, no. 6, pp. 737–746, 2010.

[3] K. S. Nemade, N. Y. Kamdi, and M. P. Parchand, "Ages of epiphyseal union around wrist joint - A radiological study," *Journal of the Anatomical Society of India*, vol. 59, no. 2, pp. 205–210, 2010.

[4] H. F. V. Cardoso, "Age estimation of adolescent and young adult male and female skeletons II, epiphyseal union at the upper limb and scapular girdle in a modern Portuguese skeletal sample," *American Journal of Physical Anthropology*, vol. 137, no. 1, pp. 97–105, 2008.

[5] M. C. Schaefer, "A summary of epiphyseal union timings in Bosnian males," *International Journal of Osteoarchaeology*, vol. 18, no. 5, pp. 536–545, 2008.

[6] U. Baumann, R. Schulz, W. Reisinger, A. Heinecke, A. Schmeling, and S. Schmidt, "Reference study on the time frame for ossification of the distal radius and ulnar epiphyses on the hand radiograph," *Forensic Science International*, vol. 191, no. 1-3, pp. 15–18, 2009.

[7] S. Patond, B. Tirpude, P. Murkey, P. Wankhade, N. Nagrale, and V. Surwade, "Age determination from epiphyseal union of bones at ankle joint in girls of central india," *Journal of Forensic Medicine, Science and Law*, vol. 21, no. 2, 2012.

[8] S. S. Bhise, B. G. Chikhalkar, S. D. Nanandkar, G. S. Chavan, and A. P. Rayamane, "Age determination from of ossification center fusion around knee joint in Mumbai region: A radiological study," *Journal of Indian Academy of Forensic Medicine*, vol. 37, no. 1, pp. 19–23, 2015.

[9] P. Memchoubi, "Age determination of manipuri girls from the radiological study of epiphyseal union around the elbow, knee, wrist joints and pelvis," *Journal of Indian Academy of Forensic Medicine*, vol. 28, no. 2, pp. 63-64, 2006.

[10] J. A. Krämer, S. Schmidt, K.-U. Jürgens, M. Lentschig, A. Schmeling, and V. Vieth, "Forensic age estimation in living individuals using 3.0T MRI of the distal femur," *International Journal of Legal Medicine*, vol. 128, no. 3, pp. 509–514, 2014.

[11] P. Saint-Martin, C. Rérolle, F. Dedouit et al., "Age estimation by magnetic resonance imaging of the distal tibial epiphysis and the calcaneum," *International Journal of Legal Medicine*, vol. 127, no. 5, pp. 1023–1030, 2013.

[12] K. K. Banerjee and B. B. L. Agarwal, "Estimation of age from epiphyseal union at the wrist and ankle joints in the capital city of India," *Forensic Science International*, vol. 98, no. 1-2, pp. 31–39, 1998.

[13] P. Bokariya, D. Chowdhary, B. Tirpude, B. Sonatakke, V. Wankhede, and A. Tarnekar, "Age determination in girls of jodhpur region by epiphyseal union of bones at ankle joint," *Journal of the Indian Academy of Forensic Medicine*, vol. 32, no. 1, pp. 42–44, 2007.

[14] J. E. O'Connor, J. Coyle, L. D. Spence, and J. Last, "Epiphyseal maturity indicators at the knee and their relationship to chronological age: Results of an Irish population study," *Clinical Anatomy*, vol. 26, no. 6, pp. 755–767, 2013.

[15] B. Tirpude, S. Patond, P. Murkey, and N. Nagrale, "A radiological study of age estimation from epiphyseal fusion of distal end of femur in the central India population," *Journal of Indian Academy of Forensic Medicine*, vol. 37, no. 1, pp. 8–11, 2015.

[16] P. Bokariya, D. S. Chowdhary, B. H. Tirpude, R. Kothari, J. E. Waghmare, and A. Tarnekar, "A review of the chronology of epiphyseal union in the bones at knee and ankle joint," *Journal of Indian Academy of Forensic Medicine*, vol. 33, no. 3, pp. 258–260, 2011.

[17] S. S. Bhise, B. G. Chikhalkar, S. D. Nanandkar, and G. S. Chavan, "Age determination from radiological study of epiphysial appearance and union around wrist joint and hand," *Journal of Indian Academy of Forensic Medicine*, vol. 33, no. 4, pp. 292–295, 2011.

[18] R. Prasad, P. K. Deb, D. Chetri, R. Maitra, and S. Kavita, "Study of epiphyseal union around the wrist joint & extended hand in males of himalayan area," *Journal of Indian Academy of Forensic Medicine*, vol. 35, no. 2, pp. 113–115, 2013.

[19] C. M. Davies, L. Hackman, and S. Black, "The utility of the proximal epiphysis of the fifth metatarsal in age estimation," *Journal of Forensic Sciences*, vol. 58, no. 2, pp. 436–442, 2013.

[20] A. Kausar and P. Varghese, "Estimation of age by epiphyseal union of knee joint by radiological examination in bijapur district," *International Journal of Biomedical and Advance Research*, vol. 3, no. 2, 2012.

[21] S. M. Garn, C. G. Rohmann, and B. Apfelbaum, "Complete epiphyseal union of the hand," *American Journal of Physical Anthropology*, vol. 19, no. 4, pp. 365–372, 1961.

[22] S. L. Washburn, "Skeletal Age Changes in Young American Males, Analyzed from the Standpoint of Age Identification. Thomas W. McKern and T. D. Stewart. Technical Report EP-45, Environmental Protection Research Division, Quartermaster Research and Development Center, U.S. Army, Natick, 1957. viii + 179 pp., 87 figs., 52 tables," *American Antiquity*, vol. 24, no. 2, pp. 198-199, 1958.

[23] M. C. Schaefer and S. M. Black, "Comparison of ages of epiphyseal union in North American and Bosnian skeletal material," *Journal of Forensic Sciences*, vol. 50, no. 4, pp. 777–784, 2005.

[24] F. E. Johnston, "Sequence of epiphyseal union in a prehistoric Kentucky population from Indian Knoll," *Human biology; an International Record of Research*, vol. 33, no. 1, pp. 66–81, 1961.

[25] J. S. Saksena and S. K. Vyas, "Epiphyseal union at the wrist, knee and iliac crest in residents of Madhya Pradesh.," *Journal of the Indian Medical Association*, vol. 53, no. 2, pp. 67-68, 1969.

[26] S. M. Das Gupta, V. Prasad, and S. Singh, "A roentgenologic study of epiphyseal union around elbow, wrist and knee joints and the pelvis in boys and girls of Uttar Pradesh (a pilot study)," *Journal of the Indian Medical Association*, vol. 62, no. 1, pp. 10–12, 1974.

Permissions

All chapters in this book were first published in RRP, by Hindawi Publishing Corporation; hereby published with permission under the Creative Commons Attribution License or equivalent. Every chapter published in this book has been scrutinized by our experts. Their significance has been extensively debated. The topics covered herein carry significant findings which will fuel the growth of the discipline. They may even be implemented as practical applications or may be referred to as a beginning point for another development.

The contributors of this book come from diverse backgrounds, making this book a truly international effort. This book will bring forth new frontiers with its revolutionizing research information and detailed analysis of the nascent developments around the world.

We would like to thank all the contributing authors for lending their expertise to make the book truly unique. They have played a crucial role in the development of this book. Without their invaluable contributions this book wouldn't have been possible. They have made vital efforts to compile up to date information on the varied aspects of this subject to make this book a valuable addition to the collection of many professionals and students.

This book was conceptualized with the vision of imparting up-to-date information and advanced data in this field. To ensure the same, a matchless editorial board was set up. Every individual on the board went through rigorous rounds of assessment to prove their worth. After which they invested a large part of their time researching and compiling the most relevant data for our readers.

The editorial board has been involved in producing this book since its inception. They have spent rigorous hours researching and exploring the diverse topics which have resulted in the successful publishing of this book. They have passed on their knowledge of decades through this book. To expedite this challenging task, the publisher supported the team at every step. A small team of assistant editors was also appointed to further simplify the editing procedure and attain best results for the readers.

Apart from the editorial board, the designing team has also invested a significant amount of their time in understanding the subject and creating the most relevant covers. They scrutinized every image to scout for the most suitable representation of the subject and create an appropriate cover for the book.

The publishing team has been an ardent support to the editorial, designing and production team. Their endless efforts to recruit the best for this project, has resulted in the accomplishment of this book. They are a veteran in the field of academics and their pool of knowledge is as vast as their experience in printing. Their expertise and guidance has proved useful at every step. Their uncompromising quality standards have made this book an exceptional effort. Their encouragement from time to time has been an inspiration for everyone.

The publisher and the editorial board hope that this book will prove to be a valuable piece of knowledge for researchers, students, practitioners and scholars across the globe.

List of Contributors

Sachin Gupta and Pamela C. Roehm
Department of Otolaryngology, New York University School of Medicine, New York, NY 10016, USA

Francine Mends, Mari Hagiwara and Girish Fatterpekar
Department of Radiology, New York University School of Medicine, New York, NY 10016, USA

Osama Raslan, James Matthew Debnam, Leena Ketonen, Ashok J. Kumar and Dawid Schellingerhout
Department of Radiology, Section of Neuroradiology, MD Anderson Cancer Center, The University of Texas, 1400 Pressler Street, Unit 1482, Houston, TX 77030, USA

JihongWang
Deparament of Imaging Physics, MD Anderson Cancer Center, The University of Texas, 1400 Pressler Street, Unit 1482, Houston, TX 77030, USA

Monica Neagu and Carolina Constantin
Immunology Department, Immunobiology Laboratory, "Victor Babes" National Institute of Pathology, 99-101 Splaiul Independentei, sector 5, Bucharest 050096, Romania

Diana Martin, Nicusor Iacob and Daniel Ighigeanu
National Institute for Laser, Plasma and Radiation Physics, 409 Atomistilor Street, Magurele 077125, Romania

Lucian Albulescu
Department of Infectious Diseases and Immunology, Virology Division, Faculty of Veterinary Medicine, Utrecht University, Yalelaan 1, 3584 CL Utrecht, The Netherlands

Arnav R. Mistry and Daniel Uzbelger Feldman
Department of Endodontology, Temple University Kornberg School of Dentistry, 3223 North Broad Street, Philadelphia, PA 19140, USA

Jie Yang
Oral and Maxillofacial Radiology Department, Temple University Kornberg School of Dentistry, 3223 North Broad Street, Philadelphia, PA 19140, USA

Eric Ryterski
E3Medical, Inc., 941 Garfield Avenue, Louisville, CO 80027, USA

Shikha Goyal and Tejinder Kataria
Division of Radiation Oncology, Medanta Cancer Institute, Medanta-The Medicity, Gurgaon, Haryana 122001, India

Priyanka Naranje, Mahesh Prakash and Niranjan Khandelwal
Department of Radiodiagnosis, Postgraduate Institute of Medical Education and Research (PGIMER), Chandigarh 160012, India

Aman Sharma
Department of Internal Medicine, Postgraduate Institute of Medical Education and Research (PGIMER), Chandigarh 160012, India

Sunil Dogra
Department of Dermatology, Venereology and Leprology, Postgraduate Institute of Medical Education and Research (PGIMER), Chandigarh 160012, India

Paolo F. Felisaz, Francesco Balducci, Giulia Maugeri and Fabrizio Calliada
Radiology Department, University of Pavia, 27100 Pavia, Italy

Eric Y. Chang
Radiology Service, VA San Diego Healthcare System, San Diego, CA 92161, USA

Irene Carne
Medical Physics Department, IRCCS Salvatore Maugeri Foundation, Scientific Institute of Pavia, 27100 Pavia, Italy

Stefano Montagna and Maurizia Baldi
Radiology Department, IRCCS Salvatore Maugeri Foundation, Scientific Institute of Pavia, 27100 Pavia, Italy

Anna Pichiecchio and Stefano Bastianello
Neuroradiology Department, C. Mondino National Neurological Institute, 27100 Pavia, Italy

Fabrizio Calliada
Institute of Radiology, IRCCS Policlinico S. Matteo Foundation, 27100 Pavia, Italy

Stefano Bastianello
Department of Brain and Behavioral Sciences, University of Pavia, 27100 Pavia, Italy

Venkata V. Chebrolu
Department of Biomedical Engineering, University of Wisconsin-Madison, Madison, WI 53706, USA

Venkata V. Chebrolu, Daniel Saenz, Dinesh Tewatia and Bhudatt R. Paliwal
Department of Human Oncology, University of Wisconsin-Madison, Madison, WI 53792, USA

Venkata V. Chebrolu
Wisconsin Institute of Medical Research, 1111 Highland Avenue, Madison, WI 53705, USA

Daniel Saenz
Department of Medical Physics, University of Wisconsin-Madison, Madison, WI 53792, USA

William A. Sethares
Department of Electrical and Computer Engineering, University of Wisconsin-Madison, Madison, WI 53706, USA

George Cannon
Department of Radiation Oncology, Intermountain Healthcare, Salt Lake City, UT 84107, USA

João Palas, António P. Matos and Miguel Ramalho
Department of Radiology, Hospital Garcia de Orta, Avenida Torrado da Silva, Almada, 2801-951 Setúbal, Portugal

Vasco Mascarenhas
Department of Radiology, Hospital da Luz, Avenida Lusíada 100, 1500-650 Lisbon, Portugal

Vasco Herédia
Department of Radiology, Hospital Espírito Santo, Largo do Senhor da Pobreza, 7000-811 Évora, Portugal

Thomas Westermaier, Stefan Koehler, Thomas Linsenmann, Michael Kiderlen, Paul Pakos and Ralf-Ingo Ernestus
Department of Neurosurgery, University Hospital Wuerzburg, Josef-Schneider-Strasse 11, 97080 Wuerzburg, Germany

Gernot Rott and Frieder Boecker
Department of Radiology, Bethesda Hospital Duisburg, Heerstraße 219, 47053 Duisburg, Germany

Letícia da Silva Lacerda, Úrsula David Alves, José Fernando Cardona Zanier, Dequitier Carvalho Machado and Gustavo Bittencourt Camilo
Department of Radiology, State University of Rio de Janeiro, 20551-030 Rio de Janeiro, RJ, Brazil

Dequitier Carvalho Machado, Gustavo Bittencourt Camilo and Agnaldo José Lopes
Postgraduate Programme in Medical Sciences, State University of Rio de Janeiro, 20550-170 Rio de Janeiro, RJ, Brazil

Lin Yang, Xiao Ming Zhang, Yong Jun Ren, Nan Dong Miao, Xiao Hua Huang and Guo Li Dong
Sichuan Key Laboratory of Medical Imaging, Department of Radiology, Affiliated Hospital of North Sichuan Medical College, Nanchong, Sichuan 637000, China

Marek Tagowski, Hendryk Vieweg, Christian Wissgott and Reimer Andresen
Institute of Diagnostic and Interventional Radiology and Neuroradiology, Westkuestenklinikum Heide, Academic Teaching Hospital of the Universities of Kiel, Luebeck and Hamburg, Esmarchstraße 50, 25746 Heide, Germany

Aditi Agarwal, Mahesh Prakash, Pankaj Gupta and Niranjan Khandelwal
Department of Radiodiagnosis and Imaging, Postgraduate Institute of Medical Education and Research (PGIMER), Chandigarh 160012, India

Satyaswarup Tripathy
Department of Plastic Surgery, Postgraduate Institute of Medical Education and Research (PGIMER), Chandigarh 160012, India

Nandita Kakkar
Department of Histopathology, Postgraduate Institute of Medical Education and Research (PGIMER), Chandigarh 160012, India

Radhika Srinivasan
Department of Cytopathology, Postgraduate Institute of Medical Education and Research (PGIMER), Chandigarh 160012, India

Sunny Goel, Avraham Miller and Chirag Agarwal
Department of Medicine, Maimonides Medical Center, Brooklyn, NY 11219, USA

Elina Zakin
Department of Neurology, Icahn School of Medicine at Mount Sinai, New York, NY 10029, USA

Umesh Gidwani
Department of Cardiology, Icahn School of Medicine at Mount Sinai, New York, NY 10029, USA

Abhishek Sharma
Division of Cardiovascular Medicine, State University of New York Downstate Medical Centre, Brooklyn, NY 11203, USA

Guy Kulbak, Jacob Shani and On Chen
Department of Cardiology, Maimonides Medical Center, Brooklyn, NY 11219, USA

P. F. Felisaz, G. Maugeri, V. Busi, R. Vitale and F. Balducci
Radiology Department, University of Pavia, Pavia, Italy

S. Gitto
Postgraduation School in Radiodiagnostics, Universit`a degli Studi di Milano, Milan, Italy

P. Leporati and L. Chiovato
Unit of Internal Medicine and Endocrinology, IRCCS Salvatore Maugeri Foundation, Scientific Institute of Pavia, Pavia, Italy

A. Pichiecchio and S. Bastianello
Neuroradiology Department, C. Mondino National Neurological Institute, Pavia, Italy

M. Baldi
Radiology Department, IRCCS Salvatore Maugeri Foundation, Scientific Institute of Pavia, Pavia, Italy

F. Calliada
Institute of Radiology, IRCCS Fondazione Policlinico San Matteo, Pavia, Italy

S. Bastianello
Department of Brain and Behavioral Sciences, University of Pavia, Pavia, Italy

Shuchi Bhatt, Nipun Rajpal and Vineeta Rathi
Department of Radiodiagnosis, University College of Medical Sciences and GTB Hospital, Dilshad Garden, Delhi 110095, India

Rajneesh Avasthi
Department of Medicine, University College of Medical Sciences and GTB Hospital, Dilshad Garden, Delhi 110095, India

Priya Bhattacharji and William Moore
Department of Radiology, State University of New York at Stony Brook University Hospital, HSC Level IV, Room 120, Stony Brook, NY 11794, USA
Department of Radiology, New York University Medical Center, 650 First Avenue, Third Floor, Room 355, New York, NY 10016, USA

Nima Kasraie, Amie Robinson and Sherwin Chan
Department of Radiology, Children's Mercy Hospital, 2401 Gillham Rd., Kansas City, MO 64108, USA

Nicolas Lefevre, Serge Herman, Antoine Gerometta, Shahnaz Klouche and Yoann Bohu
Clinique du Sport Paris V, 75005 Paris, France

Nicolas Lefevre, Serge Herman, Antoine Gerometta, Shahnaz Klouche and Yoann Bohu
Institut de l'Appareil Locomoteur Nollet, 75017 Paris, France

Aidonis Rammos, Vasileios Meladinis and Dimitrios Patsouras
Department of Cardiology, Chatzikosta General Hospital, Ioannina, Greece

Georgios Vovas
Department of Cardiology, Agrinio General Hospital, Agrinio, Greece

Felipe Campos Kitamura, Srhael de Medeiros Alves, Luis Antônio Tobaru Tibana and Nitamar Abdala
Departamento de Diagnóstico por Imagem da Escola Paulista de Medicina da UNIFESP, RuaNapoleão de Barros, 800 Vila Clementino, 04024-002 São Paulo, SP, Brazil

Majed O. Aljuaid and Osama R. El-Ghamry
Medical College, Taif University, Taif 21974, Saudi Arabia

Index